Infections of Leisure

THIRD EDITION

Infections of Leisure

THIRD EDITION

edited by

David Schlossberg

Temple University School of Medicine and
Jefferson Medical College of Thomas Jefferson University
Philadelphia, Pennsylvania

ASM
PRESS WASHINGTON, D.C.

Address editorial correspondence to ASM Press, 1752 N St. NW,
Washington, DC 20036-2904, USA

Send orders to ASM Press, P.O. Box 605, Herndon, VA 20172, USA
Phone: (800) 546-2416 or (703) 661-1593
Fax: (703) 661-1501
E-mail: books@asmusa.org
Online: www.asmpress.org

Library of Congress Cataloging-in-Publication Data

Infections of leisure / edited by David Schlossberg.—3rd ed.
    p. ; cm.
 Includes bibliographical references and index.
 ISBN 1-55581-299-6 (pbk.)
 1. Communicable diseases—Popular works. 2. Leisure—Health aspects—Popular
works. 3. Zoonoses—Popular works.
 [DNLM: 1. Infection—etiology. 2. Disease Vectors. 3. Leisure Activities. 4. Zoonoses.
WC 195 I438 2004] I. Schlossberg, David.

 RC113.I54 2004
 616.9′0471—dc22

                    2004008585

10 9 8 7 6 5 4 3

This volume is dedicated to Yuan:

She walks in beauty, like the night
Of cloudless climes and starry skies
. . .
And on that cheek, and o'er that brow,
So soft, so calm, yet eloquent,
The smiles that win, the tints that glow,
But tell of days in goodness spent . . .

Byron

CONTENTS

CONTRIBUTORS

Bertha Ayi • Department of Medical Microbiology and Immunology and Department of Internal Medicine, Section of Infectious Diseases, Creighton University Medical Center, Omaha, NE 68131

Buddha Basnyat • Nepal International Clinic, Himalayan Rescue Association, and Patan Hospital, Lal Durbar, GPO Box 3596, Kathmandu, Nepal

Bruno B. Chomel • Department of Population Health and Reproduction, School of Veterinary Medicine, University of California, Davis, Davis, CA 95616

Mark A. Clemence • Department of Internal Medicine, St. Luke's Hospital and Medical Center, Milwaukee, WI 53715

C. Glenn Cobbs • Division of Infectious Diseases, University of Alabama at Birmingham, THT 229, 1530 3rd Ave. S., Birmingham, AL 35294-0006

Thomas A. Cumbo • Division of Infectious Diseases, SUNY Buffalo School of Medicine and Biomedical Sciences, Buffalo VAMC, 3495 Bailey Ave., Buffalo, NY 14215

Burke A. Cunha • Infectious Disease Division, Winthrop-University Hospital, Mineola, NY 11501, and State University of New York School of Medicine, Stony Brook, NY 11790

David Dworzack • Department of Medical Microbiology and Immunology and Department of Internal Medicine, Section of Infectious Diseases, Creighton University Medical Center, Omaha, NE 68131

Robert Edelman • Center for Vaccine Development, Division of Geographic Medicine, Department of Medicine, and Division of Infectious Diseases and Tropical Pediatrics, Department of Pediatrics, University of Maryland School of Medicine, 685 West Baltimore St., Room 480, Baltimore, MD 21201

James G. Fox • Division of Comparative Medicine, Massachusetts Institute of Technology, 77 Massachusetts Ave., Cambridge, MA 02139

Ellie J. C. Goldstein • R. M. Alden Research Laboratory, Santa Monica, CA 90404, and UCLA School of Medicine, Los Angeles, CA 90024

Craig E. Greene • Department of Small Animal Medicine, College of Veterinary Medicine, University of Georgia, Athens, GA 30602

Jeffrey K. Griffiths • Graduate Programs in Public Health, Department of Community Medicine and Family Health, and Department of Medicine, Tufts University School of Medicine, 136 Harrison Ave., Boston, MA 02111

Richard L. Guerrant • Division of Infectious Diseases, University of Virginia Health Sciences Center, Charlottesville, VA 22908

Richard F. Jacobs • Department of Pediatrics, UAMS College of Medicine, and Pediatric Infectious Diseases, Arkansas Children's Hospital, Little Rock, AR 72202

Diane H. Johnson • Infectious Disease Division, Winthrop-University Hospital, Mineola, NY 11501, and State University of New York School of Medicine, Stony Brook, NY 11790

John W. Krebs • Viral and Rickettsial Zoonoses Branch, Division of Viral and Rickettsial Diseases, Centers for Disease Control and Prevention, 1600 Clifton Rd. NE, G-13, Atlanta, GA 30333

Todd Levin • Section of Infectious Diseases, Temple University Hospital, Philadelphia, PA 19140

Matthew E. Levison • Drexel University College of Medicine, 3300 Henry Ave., Philadelphia, PA 19129

Bennett Lorber • Section of Infectious Diseases, Temple University School of Medicine and Hospital, Philadelphia, PA 19140

Arezou Minooee • University of Vermont College of Medicine, Box 298, 89 Beaumont Ave., Burlington, VT 05405

Mukesh Patel • Division of Infectious Diseases, University of Alabama at Birmingham, THT 229, 1530 3rd Ave. S., Birmingham, AL 35294-0006

Leland S. Rickman (deceased) • Epidemiology Unit, Division of Infectious Diseases, University of California, San Diego, San Diego, CA 92103

Gordon E. Schutze • Departments of Pediatrics and Pathology, UAMS College of Medicine, and Pediatric Infectious Diseases, Arkansas Children's Hospital, Little Rock, AR 72202

Sofia Sherman-Weber • Section of Infectious Diseases, Temple University Hospital, Philadelphia, PA 19140

Martin S. Wolfe • Traveler's Medical Service, 2141 K St. NW, Suite 408, Washington, DC 20037

Jonathan M. Zenilman • Division of Infectious Diseases, Johns Hopkins Bayview Medical Center, Johns Hopkins University, 4940 Eastern Ave., Baltimore, MD 21224

PREFACE

The third edition of *Infections of Leisure* continues to identify and organize the infectious risks associated with our leisure time activities. As a by-product of our prosperity, more time is available to travel, swim, camp, hike, garden, and taste exotic foods. We continue to pamper our (sometimes unusual) pets and to play increasingly challenging sports. However, all these activities expose us to an expanding list of pathogenic microbes, some of which are entirely new and others of which are resistant to current therapy. For this edition, all the chapters from the second edition have been thoroughly updated, and two new ones have been added: "Infections from Body Piercing and Tattoos" and "Infectious Diseases at High Altitude." All the activities described herein carry risks with their attendant pleasures, and, as in the previous editions, the risks are outlined and discussed in a convenient, user-friendly, and accessible format. I hope this edition continues to provide a practical resource for this fascinating and challenging group of infections.

Marianne Anderson provided invaluable secretarial assistance, and I am deeply grateful for the friendship and professionalism of the ASM staff, particularly Jeffrey Holtmeier, Kenneth April, and Jennifer Adelman. Working with them is an honor and a pleasure.

PREFACE TO THE FIRST EDITION

Many of us spend our leisure time hiking, sailing, snorkeling, and camping. We like to sample new foods, pamper our pets, and travel to magical places. All these pursuits enrich our lives but carry attendant risks. This book details the infections that complicate exposure to vacation climates, pets, recreational activities, and exotic cuisine.

There are many infectious disorders that fit this category, and they frequently overlap. Thus, touring a tropical paradise affords one the opportunity to eat poisoned food, swim in contaminated waters, and sustain serious injury from marine life. The great outdoors adds arthropod-borne infection and polluted water to the dangers of zoonoses. Clearly, risks are multiple, and a comprehensive guide is necessary. This book attempts to organize the wealth of information about these interesting and varied infections in a convenient and accessible format.

Infections of Leisure, Third Edition
Edited by David Schlossberg
© 2004 ASM Press, Washington, D.C.

Chapter 1

At the Shore

Mark A. Clemence and Richard L. Guerrant

FISH AND SHELLFISH INTOXICATIONS

Introduction

In the United States, the consumption of seafood in 2001 alone totaled more than 4.2 billion lb, or 14.8 lb per person per year (327). An increase in the consumption of seafood is occurring, with a resultant increase in the number of cases of fish- and shellfish-related food poisonings. Seafood was the third most common source of food-borne disease outbreaks between 1983 and 1992 in the United States (274). In addition, improved reporting of cases due to a greater awareness by the public and health care personnel of the association between seafood consumption and illness has also contributed to this observed increase (205, 206, 385). Food-borne disease from fish and shellfish can be categorized into allergic, infectious, and toxin-mediated etiologies (385). The Centers for Disease Control and Prevention (CDC) and U.S. Department of Health and Human Services reported on all types of food-borne illness in the United States from 1988 to 1992. Bacterial causes were involved in more than 79% of confirmed outbreaks, whereas chemical poisonings from fish and shellfish toxins were responsible for 12.3% of outbreaks of confirmed etiology (91).

Vertebrate fish intoxication can be divided into three groups: (i) that by ichthyosarcotoxic fish, which contain toxin in their viscera, mucus, skin, or musculature; (ii) that by ichthyo-otoxic fish, which contain toxin in their gonads; and (iii) that by ichthyohemotoxic fish, which contain toxin in their blood. At least nine types of ichthyosarcotoxism are known, of which ciguatera, scombroid, and puffer fish poisonings are the most common (205).

The term "shellfish" includes crustaceans, which are mobile animals that have a hard articulated exoskeleton, and mollusks, which have hard shells and are sedentary or have limited locomotion. Crustacean species include lobsters,

Mark A. Clemence • Department of Internal Medicine, St. Luke's Hospital and Medical Center, Milwaukee, WI 53215. *Richard L. Guerrant* • Division of Infectious Diseases, University of Virginia Health Sciences Center, Charlottesville, VA 22908.

Table 1. Fish and shellfish poisoning

Disease	Source	Toxin	Mechanism	Epidemiology	Clinical	Mortality	Treatment
Shellfish poisoning Paralytic shellfish[a]	Alaskan butter clam (*Saxidomus giganteus*), mussels, oysters, scallops, cockles	Saxitoxin (heat stable)	Like tetrodotoxin; blocks Na$^+$ channels	Low temp; >30°N or S; 10 outbreaks with 63 cases from 1971–1977 in New England, Southwest, Alaska	0.5–3 h; paresthesias or dysesthesias of mouth and extremities; 14% with N/V/D[e]	8–9% die (usually within 12–24 h)	Supportive
Neurotoxic shellfish[b]	May be aerosolized in the surf	Brevetoxins (heat and acid stable) A, B, C (polycyclic ethers)	Probably via altering Na conductance	Gulf coasts of Florida and Texas	<3 h; paresthesias; temp reversal; cerebellar and GI[f] symptoms	Rare	Supportive; B$_2$ agonists; cholinergic antagonists; Ca^{2+} channel blockers
Amnesic shellfish (neurovisceral toxic syndrome)	*Nitzschia pungens* diatoms in mussels	Domoic acid (heat stable)	Neuroexcitatory like glutamic acid; causes hippocampal necrosis	Atlantic, Pacific, and Indian Oceans	0.25–38 h ($\bar{x}$ = 5.5 h); N/V, GI bleeding; HA[h]; memory loss	3%	
Diarrheic shellfish	Shellfish with dinoflagellate *Dinophysis fortii* or *D. acuminata*	Okadaic acid	Blocks phosphatase that degrades A/G kinase products	Japan and The Netherlands	5–6 h (range, 0.5–30 h); N/V/D with abdominal cramps		

2

Fish poisoning (ichthyosarcotoxic)

Puffer fish[c]	Puffer fish, shellfish, salamanders, frogs, newts	Tetrodotoxin (heat stable, nonprotein)	Blocks Na channels; axonal transmission	Japan, New Jersey, Long Island	10–45 min (<3 h); paresthesias; weakness; paralysis; hypotension; bradycardia; respiratory paralysis	59% (in first 24 h)	Supportive
Ciguatera[d]	Larger (>5-lb) carnivorous reef fish (barracuda, herring, jacks, grouper, snapper, moray eels, etc.)	Ciguatoxins and maitotoxin (heat-stable tasteless polyether)	Blocks Ca^{2+} regulation of Na^+ channels (opens voltage-dependent Na^+ channels)	<35°N and S; subtropical/tropical (Florida, Hawaii, S. Pacific); most common marine food poisoning in United States	2–30 h ↑ or ↓ BP[g] N/V/D with abdominal pain; temp reversal; teeth "loose"	<12% (rare)	Symptomatic (mannitol; opiates are dangerous)
Scombroid fish	Tuna, mackerel, skipjack, bonito, albacore, bluefish, mahimahi	Histamine (heat stable) from bacterial decarboxylation of histidine	Histamine reaction	Common worldwide, especially coastal United States	Minutes–hours ($\bar{x}$ = 30 min); flush; HA, dizziness, burning	Rare	Antihistamine (intravenous cimetidine)

[a]Primary causes are red tides and dinoflagellates such as *Protogonyaulax catenella* and *P. tamarensis.*
[b]Primary causes are red tides and unarmored dinoflagellates such as *P. brevis.*
[c]Tetraodontiae; also known as fugu.
[d]The primary cause is the dinoflagellate *Gambierdiscus toxicus.*
[e]N/V/D, nausea, vomiting, diarrhea.
[f]GI, gastrointestinal.
[g]BP, blood pressure.
[h]HA, headache.

shrimp, crabs, scampi, and crawfish. Mollusks can be divided into the bivalves, which have two shells joined by a hinge, and the gastropods, which have a whorled snaillike shell. The bivalves include oysters, mussels, clams, and scallops. Gastropods of commercial importance include whelks and periwinkles. With the exception of scallops, which reside in deeper waters, all mollusks grow in and are harvested from nearshore coastal waters (465). Ingestion of shellfish containing toxins produced by dinoflagellates may induce dramatic and sometimes fatal illness (Table 1).

Dinoflagellates and Red Tides

Dinoflagellates, or plankton, are unicellular plantlike organisms with a worldwide distribution which serve as an important element of the food chain in marine animals. During blooms, these organisms may achieve concentrations high enough to impart a reddish or yellow discoloration to the sea due to the local production of neurotoxins and pigmented proteins, hence the name "red tide" (391). There are 15 species of toxic dinoflagellates known to inhabit the waters surrounding the United States, of which 4 are related to human poisoning and 6 are associated with the formation of red tides (385).

The association of red tides with human illness has been known since ancient times, the earliest description being from the Bible (Exodus 7:20–21): "And all the water that was in the Nile was turned to blood. And the fish that were in the Nile died, and the Nile became foul, so that the Egyptians could not drink water from the Nile." North American Indians were aware of red tides and their association with poisoning due to mussel ingestion (68). In 1798, Vancouver provided what may be the first description of poisoning due to shellfish ingestion among sailors exploring passages off the mainland coast of what is now British Columbia, Canada; several men became ill after eating roasted mussels, and one of them died within 5 h (449). Walker, in 1884, described several people who became ill after eating oysters in Florida, possibly related to a red tide (456).

Red tides can be caused by nontoxigenic dinoflagellates, and shellfish may become poisonous even in the absence of a red tide (205). Vectors of shellfish poisoning are mainly filter feeders that ingest large quantities of these dinoflagellates, many of which are toxigenic. The continuous filtration can result in the accumulation of large quantities of toxin within the digestive glands of the shellfish or, in the case of the Alaskan butter clam, the siphon (177).

Paralytic Fish Poisoning

Paralytic shellfish poisoning results from the ingestion of marine mollusks containing potent neurotoxins, the best known being saxitoxin, named after the Alaskan butter clam, *Saxidomus giganteus*. Several other toxins are known, each of which shares the ability to invoke a variety of biological effects, including occasionally severe and sometimes fatal impairment in sensory, cerebellar, and motor function.

During the period from 1973 to 1987, state health departments reported 19 outbreaks of paralytic shellfish poisoning (mean, eight persons) to the CDC's Food-borne Disease Outbreak Surveillance System (81), which accounted for 1.1% of all outbreaks of food-borne disease in the United States from 1972 to 1977 and 1.0% from 1978 to 1982 (391). The implicated mollusks included mussels, oysters, clams, scallops, and cockles. Puffer fish were the cause of 13 cases of paralytic shellfish poisoning in Florida in 2002 (94). Worldwide, it was estimated that more than 1,600 cases occurred in 1974 alone, with more than 300 deaths (A. Prakash, *Proc. 1st Int. Conf. Toxic Dinoflagellate Blooms*, p. 5, 1975). In 1990, two outbreaks occurred in the United States: one involved six people who ingested mussels harvested off the Nantucket coast in Massachusetts, and another involved four people, with one fatality, in Alaska (7, 81). The incidence of paralytic shellfish poisoning in Old Harbor and Kodiak, Alaska, has been estimated at 15 and 1.5 cases per 1,000 persons per year, respectively (154). The case fatality ratio is about 8 to 9%, usually secondary to respiratory failure (291). No deaths, however, were reported in 10 outbreaks involving 63 cases reported to the CDC from 1971 to 1977 (2). In one analysis of two outbreaks of paralytic shellfish poisoning in Alaska, those residents who knew nothing about paralytic shellfish poisoning reported the same frequency of symptoms as those who knew about the potentially lethal effects of paralytic shellfish poisoning (154).

The effects of paralytic shellfish poisoning are harmful not only to humans but also to fish, birds, and other wildlife that rely on aquatic sources of food. The ecological consequences can be devastating. One of the earliest signs of a toxic bloom is the sudden and unexplained death of large numbers of fish and wildlife in the vicinity of a bloom. The American Indians were aware of these associations and avoided fish and shellfish ingestion during such times (68). These ecological effects may persist for months following the onset of an outbreak and require a year or more for affected shellfish to become safe for human consumption (177). Economic consequences can be equally devastating, as the shellfish industry becomes paralyzed during this period. Widespread reporting by the news media and strict adherence to public safety measures lead to the significant depression of demand for fish and shellfish not only in affected areas but also in unaffected areas. It is estimated that the cost of surveillance and enforcement during outbreaks of paralytic shellfish poisoning in the United States is about $1.2 million per year (177).

The dinoflagellates responsible for paralytic fish poisoning are widely distributed globally; however, actual outbreaks usually occur endemically in specific geographic areas. Such blooms are usually unpredictable and can occur with rapid accumulation of toxic concentrations. Most cases of paralytic shellfish poisoning occur in cold, temperate waters above 30°N and below 30°S (134, 205); however, tropical cases have been reported in Thailand (248), Singapore (426), India (231), Guatemala (375), Malaysia (226), New Guinea (177), the Solomon Islands (133), Mexico (9), and El Salvador (9). Most North American cases occur along the Pacific coast, from central California to Alaska and the Aleutian Islands, and on the East Coast, in the New England coastal area as well as Nova Scotia, New Brunswick, and Quebec, Canada (177). The majority of outbreaks are reported in coastal areas; however, inland cases have occurred, occasionally remote from the seas (391).

Cases tend to occur along the West Coast from May to October and on the East Coast from July to September (177). The Alaskan butter clam can be dangerous year-round (180). The period of toxicity usually lasts for a few days during each outbreak, but toxic levels may persist for many months. Factors favoring toxic blooms include warm water temperatures (usually when water temperatures reach 16°C), periods of high solar radiation, the attainment of optimal concentrations of trace vitamins and minerals, and periods of turbulence, such as during hurricanes, dredging, and the transplantation of shellfish (177, 391). Afflicted shellfish can be found along open coasts, in bays, and in estuarine areas. The most important hydrographic factor is probably a thermocline imposed barrier, i.e., areas where water temperatures are greater than 16°C (177). Occasionally, red tides may be precipitated by the lowering of salinity, such as at sites of river discharge or during periods of heavy rainfall.

Many types of molluscan shellfish may become toxic. The 19 outbreaks reported to the CDC from 1973 to 1987 were due to the ingestion of mussels, clams, oysters, scallops, and cockles. In Alaska, from 1976 through 1989, 55% of the 42 reported outbreaks were due to the ingestion of Alaskan butter clams. Other shellfish implicated in Alaskan outbreaks included mussels, cockles, steamer clams, sea snails, and razor clams (81). In addition to the ingestion of shellfish, cases of paralytic shellfish poisoning have also been linked to the ingestion of mackerel, scads, and several species of crabs (177).

Mollusks become toxic when they ingest toxic dinoflagellates. The toxins accumulate in the digestive glands and can remain there for a long time. This toxic accumulation can occur even in the absence of the buildup of numbers of dinoflagellates sufficient to discolor the water. If placed in dinoflagellate-free seawater, it can take up to 12 days for the shellfish to become nontoxic. In the case of the Alaskan butter clam, the toxins tend to accumulate in the siphon, from which it is eliminated very slowly (177). Scallops, on the other hand, do not accumulate toxins in the adductor muscle, which is the part usually ingested, although toxins may accumulate in the other tissues.

Several species of toxic dinoflagellates have been implicated in outbreaks of paralytic shellfish poisoning. In North America, *Protogonyaulax catenella* is the principal dinoflagellate species responsible for outbreaks along the northwest Pacific coast of the continent, whereas *Protogonyaulax tamarensis* is responsible for most outbreaks along the northern Atlantic coast in addition to some outbreaks on the Pacific coast (177, 385). In the tropics, *Pyrodinium bahamense* is responsible for most outbreaks (133, 226, 231, 375, 426). Each of these species is armored, ranges in size from 25 to 46 μm, and has a tendency to become highly bioluminescent during blooms (385). During the winter months, most toxic dinoflagellates exist as cysts in the sediment beneath the sea. Turbulent conditions can disperse these cysts; when water temperatures reach optimal conditions (16°C), blooming occurs by excystment and the formation of motile cells (177, 391).

There are 21 molecular forms of paralytic shellfish poisoning toxins, of which saxitoxin is the primary toxin responsible for the biological effects of this type of poisoning (362). Other toxins include neotoxin and the gonyautoxins, designated by roman numerals in the order of their discovery (391, 406). These toxins are pharmacologically similar to tetrodotoxin and are estimated to be 50 times more potent than curare and 1,000 times more potent than cyanide (362, 484). Saxitoxin is an alkaloid, nonprotein, low-molecular-weight, water-soluble toxin that is heat stable (426). Cooking does not inactivate it, and it tends to become concentrated in broth (81). It bears some resemblance to guanine and may undergo trimethylation to form a toxic acetylcholine-like compound (406). The toxic effects result from binding of the toxin to either the cell membrane, a cation receptor, or both to inhibit sodium influx, thus blocking the action potential along neuronal axons or skeletal muscle (134, 205, 391, 406, 426). Higher concentrations may have a similar electrophysiological effect on cardiac and smooth muscle (7). Evidence exists that under acidic conditions, as in the stomach or in pickling containers, nontoxic products may become converted to toxins (5, 231). Furthermore, shellfish may be capable of converting nontoxins to potent neurotoxins (5). Children may be more susceptible to the toxic effects (375). The lethal dose of saxitoxin has been estimated to be 0.3 to 1.0 mg; a single mussel may contain 30 to 50 mg (134). The safe level of toxin in shellfish has been defined as 80 μg/100 g of shellfish (75).

The symptoms of paralytic shellfish poisoning usually begin within 30 min after the ingestion of toxic shellfish but can occur up to 3 h later. The incubation period appears to be inversely related to the amount of toxin ingested. Initially there may be paresthesias and dysesthesias of the lips, tongue, and face which subsequently can progress to involve the neck, arms, fingertips, legs, and toes. Gastrointestinal symptoms, usually nausea, vomiting, and diarrhea, were seen in only 14% in one series (40). Many people have described a "feeling of floating" (289). Progression of symptoms is usually dependent on the dose of toxin ingested (391); more severe cases may be accompanied by weakness, ataxia, incoordination, and cranial nerve findings such as bulbar paresis, iridoplegia, dysphonia, and dysphagia (177, 205, 277, 426). Other associated symptoms include headache, salivation, intense thirst, and temporary blindness (177). High toxin intake can result in muscular paralysis and respiratory failure, which is the usual cause of death in fatal cases. The illness can be sufficiently severe to require hospitalization in 30 to 60% of affected patients (203). When it does occur, death usually ensues within 12 h (205, 426). If the patient survives 12 to 18 h, the prognosis for recovery is good (73). Recovery usually occurs within a week without complications (385); however, several patients in one outbreak described persistent headaches, memory loss, and fatigue lasting for several weeks (375).

The diagnosis is based on a history of recent shellfish ingestion in the appropriate clinical setting. Routine laboratory tests are usually nonspecific and not helpful in establishing the diagnosis (134). The myocardial band fraction of creatine kinase may be elevated in the absence of myocardial damage (97). Diagnosis can be confirmed by a standard mouse bioassay method in which toxin concentrations of the suspect shellfish are calculated by determining the dilution of a shellfish homogenate required to kill a 20-g mouse in 5 to 7 min. The value can then be used to calculate an absolute concentration by comparison with a known control (5, 177). Drawbacks include a precision of ±20%, interference from sodium chloride, and the need to keep a constant supply of mice (419). Other techniques have been developed, such as a fluorimetric assay, an immunologic assay, a colorimetric assay, and high-pressure liquid chromatography (419). Efforts to isolate the toxin from gastric contents have been limited (426).

Treatment is largely supportive. Attempts should be made to remove unabsorbed toxin through gastric lavage or the administration of a cathartic or enema (134, 205, 299, 385). Mechanical ventilation may become necessary in the event of respiratory failure. Hemodialysis was used successfully in one patient (24). Atropine should be avoided because saxitoxin and its derivatives may be anticholinergic (385).

Neurotoxic Shellfish Poisoning

Ptychodiscus brevis (formerly *Gymnodinium breve*) is the dinoflagellate responsible for neurotoxic shellfish poisoning. This syndrome is similar to paralytic shellfish poisoning; however, symptoms are usually milder, and paralysis and respiratory failure do not occur (205). This dinoflagellate produces neurotoxins and is responsible for the formation of red tides off the Gulf coasts of Florida and Texas; occasionally, sea currents can carry the organism to Florida's Atlantic coast (183, 205, 323). In 1987, a red tide due to *P. brevis* formed off the coast of North Carolina and was associated with an outbreak of neurotoxic shellfish poisoning involving 48 people (316). The source of this bloom was probably a red tide carried from Florida's southwest coast by Gulf Stream currents (432). Five cases were reported to the CDC from 1970 through 1974 (205).

P. brevis ranges from 20 to 40 μm in length and about 13 μm in width. It has been referred to as a "naked organism" because it lacks the shell of polysaccharide plates which characterizes *Protogonyaulax* species and other dinoflagellates (415). The neurotoxins produced by the dinoflagellate probably do not accumulate in fish but concentrate in filter-feeding shellfish in the vicinity of a bloom. Shellfish are not affected by the toxins; however, humans become affected by ingestion of those shellfish containing high levels of neurotoxin. Shellfish which may become toxic include oysters, clams, coquinas, and other bivalve mollusks (21).

Five or more separate nonprotein toxins or toxin components are produced by *P. brevis*. These are termed "brevetoxins" and include brevetoxins A, B, C, and Gb-4. Brevetoxins A, B, and C are polycyclic ethers which have similar structures and may be convertible among each other (385, 406). The toxins are lipid soluble, acid stable, and base labile; some are heat stable (22). They probably act by altering sodium conductance at or near sodium channels (372). Animal studies have demonstrated various and diverse biological effects, including smooth muscle contraction through postganglionic parasympathetic acetylcholine release in dogs, inhibition of neuromuscular transmission in skeletal muscle, central nervous system stimulation with cardiovascular and respiratory impairment in dogs and cats, and norepinephrine release from nerve endings in rats (15, 22, 47, 253, 386). Brevetoxin B has been used as a model for a red tide pigment toxin (406).

Symptoms of neurotoxic shellfish poisoning usually begin within 3 h after ingestion of contaminated shellfish and include circumoral paresthesias which progress to involve the pharynx, trunk, and extremities (205, 385). Reversal of hot and cold temperature sensation as in ciguatera fish poisoning (406) can occur, as well as cerebellar symptoms such as vertigo, ataxia, and incoordination (21, 205, 385). Gastrointestinal symptoms are common and include nausea, diarrhea, and abdominal and rectal pain. Bradycardia, headache, cramping of the lower extremities, and dilated pupils have been reported (21). Severe cases may be accompanied by convulsions, with subsequent need for respiratory support (385). Paralysis and respiratory failure are not seen. No deaths are known to have been reported (134, 385).

The diagnosis is based on clinical grounds in the appropriate setting. There is no known antidote, and treatment is supportive and symptomatic, including airway management, intravenous fluids, atropine, and pressors if required. Symptoms are self-limiting and usually resolve completely without sequelae in a few days (134, 205, 385). One patient in North Carolina required admission to an intensive care unit for severe symptoms of bilateral carpopedal tremor and myalgia, total body paresthesia, ataxia, and vertigo after the ingestion of 45 oysters. Recovery was complete in approximately 9 h (316).

The lack of an armored shell allows for aerosolization of the dinoflagellate during red tides by turbulent surf. This results in a unique syndrome seen along Florida's beaches characterized by respiratory and conjunctival irritation with the development of a nonproductive cough, shortness of breath, lacrimation, rhinorrhea, and sneezing. Asthmatics may develop a wheeze. The syndrome is reversible upon leaving the beach (134, 205). Beta-2 agonists, cholinergic antagonists, and calcium channel blockers may alleviate some of the respiratory symptoms (385).

Amnesic Shellfish Poisoning

In 1987, a previously unrecognized illness occurred among several hundred people who had ingested mussels harvested from cultivation beds located in three river estuaries on the eastern coast of Prince Edward Island, Canada (349, 431). The affected individuals developed an acute illness characterized by severe nausea, gastrointestinal bleeding, and a severe and protracted neurological disorder which included disorientation, confusion, dizziness, seizures, coma, and persistent memory loss. Many individuals required prolonged hospitalization, and several deaths were reported. This syndrome, also known as neurovisceral toxic syndrome, was subsequently linked to domoic acid, a toxin produced by the diatom *Nitzschia pungens* f. *multiseries*. A nontoxic form of the species, *N. pungens* f. *pungens*, is a coastal diatom common during the warmer months in the estuaries of Prince Edward Island and Galveston, Tex., and is replaced by *N. pungens* f. *multiseries* when fall and winter storms occur (125; G. B. Glavin, R. Bose, and C. Pinsky, Letter, *Arch. Intern. Med.* **150:**2425, 1990).

The implicated organism is widely distributed in the coastal waters of the Atlantic, Pacific, and Indian oceans; however, not all strains have been shown to produce domoic acid. Gulf Coast oysters were recently shown to contain this toxin, indicating a potential for human poisoning in this area (125). Mussels from the Canadian outbreak were shown to have high concentrations of this toxin in their digestive tracts. During the outbreak, a substantial bloom of *N. pungens* was noted by marine biologists patrolling the area (418). A possible reason for this is that freshwater runoff from record-breaking storms that year may have stratified the ocean layers of the estuaries, thereby enhancing the nutrients at just the right time in the diatom's life cycle. Similar blooms have been recorded since the initial outbreak; however, proper surveillance measures enacted for domoic acid after the initial outbreak have effectively protected the public as well as the shellfish industry. Shellfish can clear the toxin from their tissues once exposed to clean seawater free of the toxic diatom (360).

Domoic acid is a heat-stable neuroexcitatory amine similar to glutamic and kainic acids. Its effects are about two to three times more potent than those of kainic acid and 30 to 100 times more potent than those of glutamic acid. Extracts of seaweed containing this toxin have been used in Japan as an ascaricidal agent for many years, although concentrations are significantly less than those causing illness and no adverse effects have been documented (349). In rats, domoic acid stimulates kainic acid receptors in the hippocampus and can produce limbic seizures, memory and gait abnormalities, and degeneration of the hippocampus (349). Autopsy reports of victims of the Canadian outbreak revealed neuronal necrosis and astrocytosis in several areas of the brain, particularly the hippocampus and amygdala (431).

At least 107 individuals were involved in the outbreak. Symptoms began 15 min to 38 h (median, 5.5 h) after the ingestion of mussels (349). In approximate order of appearance, they included nausea and vomiting (76% of the patients), abdominal cramps (50%), gastric bleeding, diarrhea (42%), incapacitating headache (43%), dizziness, confusion, loss of short-term memory (25%), weakness, lethargy, somnolence, coma, and seizures. Eighteen percent were hospitalized; death occurred in three patients (140, 349). The memory loss was anterograde in all but the most severe cases and persisted for at least 2 years in a few individuals. Cognitive functioning remained intact. Cardiovascular instability, presumably due to the early excitatory effects of domoic acid, was also noted. Alternating hemiparesis and ophthalmoplegia were noted in two patients (431). Evidence suggests that elderly individuals may be more susceptible to the neurological effects of domoic acid, possibly due to diminished renal function (349, 477).

Puffer Fish Poisoning

Ingestion of fish in the order Tetraodontoidea, which includes puffer fish (Fig. 1), porcupine fish, and the ocean sunfish, can result in an acute illness referred to as puffer fish poisoning or tetrodotoxication. This syndrome, although rare in the United States, is not all that uncommon in Japan, where 6,386 cases were reported in a 78-year period, with a mortality rate of 59% (405). Also known as fugu-fugu in Japan, puffer fish there is considered a delicacy and is specially prepared by trained individuals who require licenses to serve this popular dish, which can cost up to $400 for one meal in Japan (93). In spite of these precautions, about 50 cases of fugu poisoning occur annually in association with fugu specialty restaurants (180). Although personal importation of fugu into the United States is illegal, the Food and Drug Administration has permitted fugu to be imported and served in Japanese restaurants in the United States by certified fugu chefs on special occasions (93). Captain James Cook, on his second voyage, ate a piece of puffer fish liver and became acutely ill, requiring 4 days to recover (299). Species of fish in this

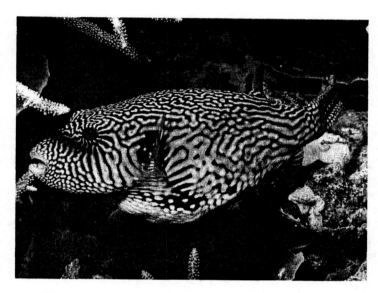

Figure 1. The puffer fish is considered a delicacy in Japan and must be prepared by specially trained chefs to avoid fugu poisoning. The photo is from *Reef: a Safari through the Coral World* (413a) by Jeremy Stafford-Deitsch (Sierra Club Books, San Francisco, Calif., 1991), copyright © Jeremy Stafford-Deitsch, and is reproduced with permission from the author.

family are widespread and are found in warm and temperate waters throughout the world; some species are eaten in New Jersey and Long Island (299). In April 1996, three cases of fugu poisoning occurred in three chefs in San Diego, Calif., who shared prepackaged, ready-to-eat fugu illegally imported from Japan (93).

Tetrodotoxin is a heat-stable nonprotein toxin which is concentrated in the liver, ovaries, and intestine of infected fish. It is not unique to puffer fish and has been isolated from six different classes of animals, including shellfish, salamanders, and a newt found on the campus of Stamford University in Stamford, Conn. (150). Certain frogs and newts in Central and South America harbor this toxin; their skins are used to manufacture poison darts (299).

Tetrodotoxin has its own receptor located at or near the sodium channel of the external nerve axon cell membrane. Binding at this receptor inhibits nerve impulse propagation along preganglionic cholinergic, somatic motor, sensory, and sympathetic nerves in the central, peripheral, and autonomic nervous systems. Direct effects on the brain stem medulla can induce emesis or hyperemesis and respiratory depression. It is not a curare-like agent and does not act directly on the acetylcholine receptor at the motor endplate. Structurally it resembles morphine, which may explain some of its narcotic activity. Primary pharmacological effects include local anesthesia, hypotension, hypothermia, emesis, respiratory depression, and decreased systemic vascular resistance. High levels of toxin can inhibit impulse relay in skeletal or cardiac muscle (405).

Symptoms usually begin within 3 h of ingestion of affected fish (usually 10 to 45 min). Symptoms include lethargy, weakness, paresthesias (including a numbness of the face and extremities), a floating sensation, emesis or hyperemesis, ataxia salivation, and dysphagia (134). The extent of symptomatology varies with the amount of toxin ingested (180). Muscular weakness can progress to total paralysis, including respiratory paralysis. Hypotension, bradycardia, and fixed dilated pupils can occur in severe cases (134). Symptoms usually resolve over a period of days; the prognosis is good if the patient survives 18 to 24 h (49). Death occurs in about 60% within the first 24 h (180).

The diagnosis is based on clinical grounds. Treatment consists of airway support and volume expansion with intravascular fluids such as normal saline, and possibly pressors. Attempts should be made to remove unabsorbed toxins through gastric lavage and emesis (405). Some evidence exists that gastric lavage with 2% sodium bicarbonate is effective if performed within the first hour of intoxication (487). Atropine is useful in the management of bradycardia. The anticholinesterases edrophonium, physostigmine, neostigmine, and galanthamine as well as veratrine-like agents and cysteine may have some benefits, although none of these have proven useful in large-scale studies. Apomorphine currently appears to have the best antiemetic properties (405). Other potential treatment options include hyperbaric oxygen, the narcotic antagonist naloxone, and possibly monoclonal neutralizing antibodies (405, 406).

Ciguatera Food Poisoning

Ciguatera is a distinct clinical syndrome that may follow the ingestion of certain tropical reef fishes which have acquired toxicity through the food chain. The name was give by Don Antonio Parra in Cuba in 1787 from the Spanish *cigua*, which refers to the poisonous turban shellfish of the Turbinidae (175). Sailors with Captain Cook suffered from this malady during his voyages (109). Outbreaks of ciguatera occur in tropical and subtropical regions between 35°N and 35°S latitudes (207). Ciguatera is the most commonly reported food-borne illness of marine origin in the United States; overall, it accounted for 5.8% of all disease-related food-borne outbreaks from 1972 to 1977 and 7.4% of outbreaks from 1978 to 1982 (391). The CDC has reported that 90% of cases in the United States occur in Florida and Hawaii (205). In Miami, Fla., alone, there were 43 outbreaks reported involving 129 cases from 1974 to 1976, which probably represented less than 10% of the actual cases due to the inability of the public and medical profession to recognize the illness; the actual incidence was estimated to be 50 cases/100,000 population/year (261). In 1987, an outbreak occurred in North Carolina involving 10 persons in what is probably the first case of ciguatera associated with consumption of fish harvested from mainland U.S. coastal waters outside Florida (315). In 1995, an outbreak of ciguatera occurred in U.S. soldiers serving in Haiti who had eaten locally caught fish (354). A number of cases have been reported in nontropical areas such as Vermont and Iowa due to the retail of affected fish from Florida (307). In some areas of the world, the disease is so prevalent that only the largest outbreaks are reported. An epidemiological analysis reported on more than 3,000 cases in the South Pacific (25). On one Pacific atoll, a 43% annual incidence was found during a routine survey of households in one such epidemic (391).

Gambierdiscus toxicus is the primary dinoflagellate responsible for the production of a number of closely related but distinct toxins responsible for the complex symptomatology of ciguatera (315). Other dinoflagellates may also be toxigenic, including *Procentrum lima* (470, 485). These dinoflagellates adhere to dead coral, bottom-associated marine algae, and seaweed (391). Herbivorous fishes ingest the dinoflagellates and the toxins are subsequently passed up the food chain to the larger carnivorous reef fishes, which concentrate the toxins in their tissues, resulting in human poisoning when they are consumed. Toxins are ultimately accumulated in viscera, although muscle tissue may also contain lethal amounts. Contamination of reef fishes is more likely to occur during storms or other periods of turbulence (391). Larger fish are more likely to be contaminated (158, 185). Fish are unaffected by the toxins (180). More than 400 species of fish have been implicated in ciguatera, including anchovies, barracuda, filefish, herring, jacks, moray eels, oceanic bonito, parrot fish, porgies, seabass or grouper, red snapper, squirrelfish, surgeonfish, triggerfish, trunkfish, and wrasses (180). In Miami, the high incidence of ciguatera due to the ingestion of barracuda has resulted in the ban of the sale of this fish (386).

The toxins recovered from fish implicated in ciguatera include ciguatoxin(s), maitotoxin, lysophosphatidylcholine (maitotoxin-associated hemolysin), scaritoxin(s), palytoxin, and ciguatoxin-associated ATPase inhibitor (246, 406). The toxins are lipid soluble, colorless, odorless, and heat stable; thus, affected fish lack any unusual taste, odor, or appearance, and cooking does not inactivate the toxins (158). Ciguatoxin is a polyether compound that probably acts by competitive inhibition of calcium regulation of the sodium channel (158, 361). For this reason, calcium gluconate has been advocated in the treatment of ciguatera, although its efficacy has not been proven (391, 406). The toxin appears to act by opening voltage-dependent sodium channels in all cell membranes with initial neural stimulation followed by conduction block primarily in skeletal muscle and neuronal membranes and less so in cardiac muscle. Higher doses can result in phrenic nerve paralysis and respiratory arrest (158). Maitotoxin is cardiotoxic and is also the most potent marine toxin known. Its cardiotoxic effects are due to enhanced calcium influx through the cardiac membrane with a resultant calcium overloaded state. These effects are abolished by verapamil in a rat model (245). In ciguatera, maitotoxin can result in hypotension, whereas ciguatoxin has hypertensive effects; the former may be responsible for ciguatera shock, whereas the latter may play a role in the chronic hypertension seen in chronic ciguatera (406). Immune sensitization to polycyclic ethers occurs in ciguatera by a T-cell-dependent mechanism which results in serotonin release via abnormally released immunoglobulin E (IgE). Subsequently, hypotension can ensue in response to certain medications (e.g., paraldehyde), foods, and factors generated in shock (e.g., thromboxane A2). Morphine may form polycyclic ethers on epoxidation or endoperoxidation of the olefin moiety; this may account for the dramatic hypotension seen in some victims of ciguatera when administered opiates (406).

The symptoms of ciguatera have an ethnic variation which may be due to differences in diet; persons of Philippine or Chinese extraction are more severely affected, Hawaiians are least affected, and other groups are interposed between

(406). Overall, 175 symptoms have been noted (406). The incubation period has been reported to be from 2 to 30 h (25, 261, 315). Gastrointestinal symptoms such as watery diarrhea, nausea and vomiting, and abdominal pain tend to predominate early, followed by neurological symptoms, although great variation exists (315, 385). Virtually all experience gastrointestinal symptoms during the course of their illness which usually resolve in 24 to 48 h (134, 385). Myalgia and weakness, particularly of the lower extremities, may occur at any time. Intense generalized pruritus may occur, and women may even complain of pruritus of the vaginal vault (180). Bradycardia with hypotension occurs in 10 to 15% of cases (406); higher doses of toxin(s) may elicit a biphasic response where the bradycardia with hypotension is followed by tachycardia with hypertension (313). Shock and respiratory failure may occur within minutes. Skin lesions and a distinct erythematous desquamative rash have occasionally been reported (134). Fever, lacrimation, severe muscle spasms, and dysuria may also occur (246, 385).

Initial neurological symptoms usually consist of circumoral and distal paresthesias. Vertigo and ataxia are common and are accompanied by a wide variation of other neurological manifestations, such as cranial nerve palsies, motor paralysis, blurred vision, and coma (385). Pregnant women may complain of bizarre seizure-like fetal activity (134). Temperature reversal is an unusual characteristic commonly seen in ciguatera which usually occurs in 2 to 5 days (406). Hot objects may seem cold, and cold objects can elicit an electric shock-like sensation. Serious thermal injury has been reported due to the individual's failure to recognize extreme heat as being such (391). In the Bahamas, natives may be seen holding beer cans wrapped in towels to keep their fingers from touching the cold metal (180). Teeth may seem painful or loose. Nightmares are quite common, whereas others may complain of auditory hallucinations and zoopsia (134, 470). All food may taste metallic (180).

Symptoms may wax and wane during any 24-h period and give a "pseudodiurnal periodicity" (158). Alcohol may exacerbate or induce the recurrence of symptoms in up to 28% of patients who recover (158). Other conditions that increase blood flow such as increased temperature or physical exertion can also exacerbate symptomatology (261, 315). Whereas gastrointestinal symptoms usually resolve in 24 to 48 h, neurological, musculoskeletal, and cardiovascular symptoms may persist for months to years (134, 158, 385). Furthermore, recurrence of symptoms may intermittently appear for several months after recovery. The total duration of symptoms is usually several days to months, with neurological symptoms and pruritus being the slowest to resolve (391). Sensitization is common, and immunity does not occur (134). Some individuals may never eat fish again, as exposure to even minuscule amounts of ciguatera toxins may reproduce dramatic symptoms (180, 391). Malignancy has developed in a few individuals (406). Death is rare, occurring in up to 12% of reported cases; no deaths occurred in 184 cases reported to the CDC from 1970 to 1974 (205).

The diagnosis is based on clinical grounds. Laboratory abnormalities, if present, are usually due to fluid and electrolyte disturbances secondary to gastrointestinal manifestations. Elevated serum ammonia levels with abnormal prothrombin and partial thromboplastin times may reflect liver toxicity (406). When severe muscle spasms are present, there may be marked elevations of creatinine phosphokinase, serum glutamic oxaloacetic acid, and lactic acid dehydrogenase (246). Reversible T-wave changes on electrocardiograms have been reported (450). The toxins may be detected by a mouse bioassay which is subject to the same limitations as detection of saxitoxin and its derivatives in paralytic shellfish poisoning (see above). Radioimmunoassay, often referred to as a "poke" or "stick" test, and chromatography have also been utilized to detect ciguatera toxins, though they are expensive and subject to other limitations as well (246, 391).

Treatment is primarily symptomatic and supportive. Attempts to remove toxin through emesis or gastric lavage with activated charcoal should be made if vomiting has not occurred. A cathartic may be administered to remove toxin from the lower intestinal tract (134, 205). Intravenous mannitol provided rapid and dramatic relief in 24 patients with ciguatera in one study, with rapid recovery from shock and coma in 2 patients. The effect of mannitol on the course of ciguatera is unknown but may be due to competitive inhibition of the toxin(s) on the sodium channels or the neutralization of toxin(s) (344). Atropine may be used to control symptomatic bradycardia (406). Calcium gluconate and dopamine infusions have been effective in the treatment of hypotension (406). Amitriptyline has been used successfully to alleviate paresthesias (50). Pruritus has responded to antihistamines and avoidance of alcohol, excessive exercise, and high ambient temperatures (391, 406). Myalgia may respond to acetaminophen and indomethacin. Opiates and barbiturates should be avoided, as they may aggravate hypotension (406).

A ciguatera diet has been devised to be used in the treatment of affected patients (406). It is a diet high in protein, carbohydrates, and vitamins which avoids fish, shellfish, seeds, nuts, mayonnaise, and their products. In addition, alcohol, marijuana, solvents, herbicides, insecticides, glues, epoxies, ethers, resins, and cosmetics should be avoided as well. These restrictions should be maintained for at least 3 to 6 months after complete resolution of symptoms, and probably 12 months in the severely affected. Ingestion of fish weighing more than 2.3 kg (5 lb) or fish caught during red tides should be avoided by the general public, as these are more likely to contain ciguatera toxins (269).

Scombroid-Fish Poisoning

Scombroid-fish poisoning is an acute clinical syndrome characterized by symptoms of histamine toxicity resulting from the ingestion of spoiled fish (317). It represents the most common form of ichthyosarcotoxism in the world (23). In the United States, 30 to 153 cases of scombroid-fish poisoning were reported annually to the CDC from 1978 to 1982 in a total of 73 outbreaks; this accounted for 7.2% of all food-borne disease outbreaks (82, 134, 391). Among 697 outbreaks of food-borne disease caused by chemical agents from 1973 through 1987, scombroid-fish poisoning was responsible for 29% of the outbreaks and 27% of the cases (206). One-half of the 18 outbreaks reported to the CDC in 1982 were due to fish served in restaurants and cafeterias (391). In March 1998, 24 people on a Hollywood movie set became ill after eating trays of escolar, a trendy seafood that has caught on with many West Coast crowds (108). The escolar was traced to a Florida supplier who had also sent a shipment to a celebrity ski resort in Utah where several other cases were reported. Tuna burgers were the cause of five outbreaks of scombroid-fish poisoning involving 18 people in North Carolina from July 1998 to February 1999 (32). Most cases in the United States are reported from coastal states and Hawaii, although cases have occurred in the Midwest (134, 391).

The disease is associated with ingestion of fish which belong to the families Scombridae, which includes tuna, mackerel, skipjack, bonito, and albacore, and Scomberesocidae (sauries). Nonscombroid fish, such as mahimahi, bluefish, amberjack, herring, sardines, and anchovies, as well as cheese, have also been implicated (138, 429). Scombroid fish are distributed worldwide throughout temperate and tropical waters and have occasionally been found in polar waters (205).

Histamine has been identified as the toxin responsible for the symptoms of scombroid-fish poisoning (317). The affected fish do not contain high levels of histamine in their flesh at the time of capture; instead, they contain histidine. Histamine is produced during the process of spoilage by the enzymatic decarboxylation of histidine by certain marine bacteria, particularly *Morganella morganii*, *Klebsiella pneumoniae*, *Escherichia coli*, clostridia, *Achromobacter histamineum*, *Plesiomonas shigelloides*, *Enterobacter intermedius*, *Serratia marcesens*, *Serratia plymuthica*, *Serratia fonticola*, and *Hafnia alvei*, which are common surface bacteria on fish (138, 265, 278, 324, 429). This occurs optimally at temperatures between 20 and 30°C (205). Typically, this takes place when previously refrigerated fish is allowed to warm for a period of time before it is prepared. Histamine is heat stable and not destroyed by cooking. It is also stable in freezing temperatures. Oral histamine administered in large doses is rapidly metabolized in the liver and intestinal mucosa, and symptoms, if present, are generally mild. For this reason the presence of an unknown synergistic substance(s) has been proposed to account for the high levels of histamine noted in individuals afflicted with scombroid-fish poisoning (138, 317).

Symptoms generally appear within several minutes to several hours of ingestion (median of 30 min), with a median duration of 4 h (205). Symptoms may persist for 12 to 24 h (134). The fish has been occasionally described as tasting sharp, peppery, or bitter but usually not described as unpleasant (391). Symptoms initially appear as flushing and a hot sensation of the skin, dizziness, headache, a burning sensation in the mouth and throat, shortness of breath in the absence of bronchospasm, itching with or without urticaria, and palpitations. Gastrointestinal symptoms appear as diarrhea, nausea, and, rarely, vomiting. A sunburned-appearing skin rash with sharply demarcated borders may develop, as well as conjunctival injection. More severe symptoms include difficulty swallowing, respiratory distress with bronchospasm, hypotension, tachycardia, and blurred vision (134, 138, 205, 391). People receiving isoniazid and other inhibitors of endogenous histaminase may have more severe symptoms (391). Deaths have occurred but are very rare.

The diagnosis is made on clinical grounds and is usually fairly evident, as the incubation period is relatively short and several people are usually affected at once. Many people are erroneously diagnosed as having a "fish allergy" and are told to abstain from eating fish for the rest of their lives (134). Laboratory data are usually not helpful. Levels of histamine and its metabolite N-methylhistamine are elevated in urine samples at the time of onset of symptoms and may persist for more than

24 h, although urine is not routinely tested (317). Laboratory confirmation of scombroid-fish poisoning is accomplished by measurement of histamine in suspect fish. The concentration may vary from one portion of the fish to another, so several areas must be sampled. The Food and Drug Administration has established the maximum safe level of histamine in tuna to be 450 μmol per 100 g of fresh tuna; fresh tuna contains less than 9 μmol per 100 g (138, 317). In one recent outbreak in Tennessee, marlin was the implicated fish and contained levels of histamine greater than 2,500 μmol per 100 g (317).

Treatment is supportive and symptomatic. If the gastrointestinal symptoms are not severe, gastric lavage or catharsis may be employed to remove unabsorbed histamine (39). Depending on the severity of symptoms, management can best be accomplished by the use of any one or combination of agents such as epinephrine, oxygen, diphenhydramine, hydroxyzine, and corticosteroids (406). Aminophylline may be used for the rare case of severe respiratory distress due to bronchospasm (134). Intravenous cimetidine has been reported to provide rapid and complete resolution of symptoms in severe cases that had not responded to antihistamines (39). Caution must be exercised in the simultaneous use of H1 and H2 blockers to avoid hypotension (406).

Diarrheic Shellfish Poisoning

Diarrheic shellfish poisoning has not been reported in the United States to date but has been implicated in a number of short-lived outbreaks of acute onset of diarrhea following shellfish ingestion in other parts of the world, particularly Japan and The Netherlands. It is caused by the ingestion of okadaic acid and other toxins concentrated in shellfish that feed on the dinoflagellates that produce the toxins. Okadaic acid does not directly stimulate intestinal secretion but instead causes a significant increase in paracellular permeability (442). During the period from 1976 to 1982, more than 1,300 cases were diagnosed in Japan, while sporadic cases occurred in The Netherlands and Chile (472). In 1989, 150 people on the Adriatic coast of Italy were afflicted by this illness after the ingestion of contaminated mussels. This was the first case of diarrheic mussel poisoning observed in the Mediterranean area (G. Bolleta, I. Bacchiochi, G. Durante, and C. Maffei, Letter, *Arch. Intern. Med.* **150:**2425, 1990). Okadaic acid has been detected in Gulf of Mexico shellfish and phytoplankton (125).

Dinophysis fortii is the responsible toxin-producing dinoflagellate in Japan, whereas *Dinophysis acuminata* produces the toxin in outbreaks occurring in The Netherlands (177, 234). Mussels, clams, and scallops are the shellfish implicated in causing human outbreaks (Bolleta et al., letter). Outbreaks are associated with dinoflagellate blooms (234).

Symptoms usually begin about 5 to 6 h after shellfish ingestion, with a range of 30 min to 12 h (234; Bolleta et al., letter). Although usually mild, the severity of the illness is dependent on the amount of toxin ingested (234). The symptoms consist of diarrhea, abdominal cramps, nausea, and vomiting. No fatalities have been reported, and recovery generally occurs within 2 days. Treatment is supportive, as the symptoms are self-limiting (61, 234).

Pfiesteria piscicida

P. piscicida is an estuarine dinoflagellate first described in 1991 (160). This usually nontoxic organism feeds on aquatic organic material but can produce toxins that can kill fish. The toxin can induce formation of open ulcerative lesions, hemorrhaging, and death of fish and shellfish. Beginning in autumn 1996, fish with "punched-out" skin lesions and erratic behavior caused by exposure to toxins produced by *P. piscicida* or *Pfiesteria*-like species were seen in the Pocomoke River and adjacent waterways on the eastern shore of Maryland. In August 1997, similar fish kills were reported (166). That same month, 24 sportsmen, environmental workers, and commercial fishermen who had contact with the water had reported illness (166). Human illness, known as possible estuary-associated syndrome, has been a topic of much debate due to the lack of specific testing and possible implication of unrelated factors (92). Possible estuary-associated syndrome is not an infectious disease, and there have been no cases associated with eating fish or shellfish harvested from waters where *P. piscicida* has been found. Thirty-seven cases had been reported to the CDC prior to 1998, and very few have been reported since then (370). The reason for the drop-off in cases since 1998 is likely due to the paucity of "fish events" due to *P. piscicida* since 1 June 1998 (92).

Symptoms were more likely to occur in those with the highest level of exposure to the contaminated water and included neuropsychiatric symptoms (including new or increased forgetfulness), severe respiratory distress (including asthma), headache, narcosis, severe stomach cramping, nausea with vomiting, and eye irritation, with reddening and blurred vision (108, 160, 166). Neuropsychiatric symptoms tended to last the longest and completely resolve by 6 months, usually by 10 to 12 weeks.

Why *Pfiesteria* suddenly became toxic is unknown; however, the toxicity has been linked to coastal chicken and hog farms in Maryland and North Carolina (108).

THE VIBRIOS

Introduction

Before the 1960s, the focus of vibrios as pathogens of human disease focused primarily on *Vibrio cholerae*, the etiologic agent of cholera. Pacini originally described a vibrio-like organism as the etiologic agent of Asiatic cholera in 1854 (216). The organism was not isolated until 32 years later by Koch, who called the bacillus "Kommabacillus," referring to its curved shape. *V. cholerae* was the only currently recognized vibrio known to cause human disease until 1951, when Fujino described a bacterium resembling *V. cholerae* which was responsible for an epidemic of acute gastroenteritis in Japan involving 272 people, with 20 deaths. He named this organism *Pasteurella parahaemolyticus*, which was subsequently placed in the genus *Vibrio* in 1963. Two distinct biotypes were recognized at that time which were found to be separate species. In 1968, biotype 1 became known as *Vibrio parahaemolyticus*, whereas biotype 2 became known as *Vibrio alginolyticus* (225). Since then, 34 species of vibrio, of which about a dozen are known to be pathogenic to humans (Table 2), have been recognized. Furthermore, several un-named species have been recently identified, so the list is likely to grow (216).

Pathogenic members of the genus *Vibrio* are gram-negative, curved, rod-shaped facultative anaerobes which are capable of both fermentative and respiratory me-tabolism. They are motile organisms which measure 1.5 to 3.0 μm in length and 0.5 to 0.8 μm in width. They contain a single, sheathed polar flagellum in liquid medium and occasionally may display shorter lateral flagella on solid media. They are anaerogenic (with the exception of *Vibrio furnissii* and some strains of *Vibrio damselae*), are oxidase positive (except *Vibrio metschnikovii*), and have the ability to reduce nitrate to nitrite. Most are susceptible to the vibriostatic effects of the compound O/129 (30).

The pathogenic vibrios can be divided into two groups based on their ability to grow in a saline environment (188). Nonhalophilic vibrios can grow in the pres-ence or absence of sodium chloride and include *V. cholerae*, *V. cholerae* non-O1, and *Vibrio mimicus*. Halophilic vibrios, on the other hand, require sodium chloride to support growth and survival and reach very high concentrations in waters of 5 to 8% salinity (216).

Isolated vibrios can occasionally be confused with other bacteria of medical im-portance, such as *Enterobacteriaceae* and *Pseudomonas*, *Aeromonas*, and *Plesiomonas* spp. The *Enterobacteriaceae* are straight rather than curved and are oxidase nega-tive, with peritrichous or circumferential flagella. *Pseudomonas* species, although oxidase positive, have an oxidative rather than fermentative metabolism. Species of *Aeromonas* and *Plesiomonas* do not require sodium chloride for growth and are able to grow in the presence of vibriostatic O/129 (437).

Table 2. Clinical presentations of pathogenic *Vibrio* infections in humans[a]

Pathogen	Symptom			
	Diarrhea (watery/dysentery)	Wound	Otitis	Sepsis
Nonhalophilic				
V. cholerae O1	+	±		
V. cholerae non-O1[b]	+/+	+	+	±
V. mimicus[b]	+/+		+	
Halophilic				
V. parahaemolyticus	+/+	+	±	±
V. hollisae (EF13)[b]	+/±			±
V. fluvialis (EF6)	+/+			
V. furnissii	+			
V. alginolyticus		+	+	
V. vulnificus (L+)[b]	±			++
V. damselae (EF5)		+		
V. metschnikovii (gp16)		+		±

[a]Single cases of *V. cincinnatiensis* and *V. carchariae* infection have been reported with sepsis and shark bite wound in-fections, respectively.
[b]Especially associated with oyster consumption.

Most standard laboratory media used for biochemical testing contain 0.5% sodium chloride and therefore support the growth of both halophilic and non-halophilic vibrios. Isolation is usually accomplished through selective or enrichment media. Alkaline peptone broth is the most suitable general enrichment medium for all pathogenic *Vibrio* species (141). A modified two-step method has been successfully utilized to prevent overgrowth by other bacteria in peptone broth (369). Thiosulfate-citrate-bile salts-sucrose (TCBS) agar is the most widely used selective agar medium for isolation of pathogenic *Vibrio* species; however, several newly described pathogens may fail to grow on this agar medium (186). Furthermore, individual variations of commercially available TCBS agar may affect recovery of the organism (464).

Vibrios are aquatic organisms that can be found in a wide variety of environmental water sources, such as oceans, estuaries, lakes, and ponds. The highest concentrations are generally achieved in the marine waters along the eastern and Gulf coasts, primarily in the summer months; lower concentrations exist along the West Coast. Their numbers fluctuate widely, with marked variation due to such variables as temperature, salinity, sediments, and the presence of certain marine organisms, particularly the copepods and other plankton, in which the vibrios may play a role in salt retention (107).

Water temperature appears to be the single most important variable affecting the growth and survival of the vibrios. Pathogenic vibrios are usually isolated from waters where temperatures exceed 10°C for at least several consecutive weeks (41, 407). They are less frequently found in waters where temperatures exceed 30°C (401, 468). Variation occurs worldwide and among different species; *V. cholerae*, for example, prefers temperatures between 20 and 35°C (216).

Individual *Vibrio* species have different optimal sodium chloride requirements, with a range of 5 to 30%, which accounts for the primary isolation of these organisms from marine and estuarine waters (41, 401, 439, 464). Although *V. cholerae*, *V. cholerae* non-O1, and *V. mimicus* do not require sodium chloride for growth, they achieve higher numbers in its presence. *V. cholerae* has an optimal requirement of 2 to 20% salinity, whereas halophilic vibrios usually achieve optimal concentrations in sodium chloride concentrations of 5 to 8% (216). Pathogenic vibrios may be isolated from freshwater where salinity is less than 5%, probably due to a complex interaction between high water temperatures and increased organic content which may compensate for the detrimental effects of low to absent salinity (298, 392, 407, 408). Evaporation of freshwater and brackish water during summer months may increase the sodium chloride content (369).

As temperatures drop below 10°C, the pathogenic vibrios rapidly disappear from the water, but they can persist throughout the winter in the sediment. This has been shown for *V. parahaemolyticus*, *V. cholerae*, and *V. alginolyticus* and may well hold true for all pathogenic vibrios (227, 228, 464, 468). As water temperatures increase during the spring and summer months, the organisms can reemerge once again to reach high concentrations in water, accounting for as much as 26 to 40% of the total bacterial population in some areas (340).

By associating themselves with higher organisms such as shellfish, plankton, and fish, the vibrios may maintain high numbers and prolong their existence. Adsorption onto the chitinous component of plankton has been shown to significantly prolong the survival of some pathogenic vibrios, and it is possible that this represents a major means of prolonging survival for all pathogenic species (209, 210, 227, 233, 340, 392). Bivalve molluscan shellfish which filter feed on zooplankton may themselves become rapidly contaminated during periods of high bacterial counts. Improper storage of the shellfish may then allow proliferation of the pathogenic bacteria, with resultant outbreaks of food poisoning (121, 139, 232, 389). Crustacean shellfish and fish can also become contaminated during such periods of abundant *Vibrio* growth (34, 209, 345, 392). *Vibrio* species have also been cultured from the teeth, skin, and gum lines of sharks (20, 63).

The spectrum of human disease due to the pathogenic vibrios is mainly dependent on the causative species and ranges from mild self-limiting gastroenteritis and soft tissue infections to severe necrotizing wound infections and fulminant bacteremia primarily in patients with underlying diseases. Illness can result from a variety of means, such as ingestion of contaminated shellfish or exposure of open wounds to contaminated seawater. Raw-oyster eaters, particularly those with liver disease, have been shown be at risk of developing *Vibrio* illness (122). An increase in reports of *Vibrio*-related illness is occurring due to a variety of reasons, including increased awareness by the public and medical profession of *Vibrio* infections, improved biochemical and serologic means for the detection of vibrios, increased recreational exposure to coastal regions, increased foreign travel, increased seafood ingestion, and enhanced survival in immunocompromised individuals (122, 216).

Vibrio species have been isolated from virtually every geographic region within the United States, although most cases occur along coastal areas. Of 713 isolates reported to the CDC from various human anatomical sites, 75% belong to one of three species: *V. cholerae*, *V. parahaemolyticus*, and *Vibrio vulnificus*, with gastrointestinal symptoms predominating (141). Between 1974 and 1978 in a Chesapeake Bay community, 40 *Vibrio* isolates were recovered from 32 patients, with *V. parahaemolyticus*, *V. vulnificus*, and *V. cholerae* non-O1 accounting for 33 of the total isolates. Illnesses were mild and self-limiting, and no mortalities were reported (192). Over a 10-year period in a Gulf Coast community, 23 cases of *Vibrio* infections were reported, with *V. vulnificus*, *V. parahaemolyticus*, and *V. cholerae* non-O1 accounting for all but 2 cases; the 23 cases included gastroenteritis in 3 patients, wound infection in 14 patients, and bacteremia in 12 patients (45). The CDC estimates that 8,028 *Vibrio* infections and 57 *Vibrio*-related deaths occur annually in the United States (292).

V. cholerae

Seven cholera pandemics have been recorded since 1817, six of which began before the 20th century (378). The current (seventh) one began in Sulawesi, Indonesia, in 1961 and then spread to Asia, Africa, the Middle East, Oceania, and parts of Europe while sparing the Western Hemisphere (36, 475). No cases of domestically acquired cholera were reported in the United States after 1911 until 1973, when it was diagnosed in a resident of the Gulf Coast of Texas (460). In 1978, 11 people were involved in an outbreak of cholera following the ingestion of crabs gathered from a Louisiana coastal marsh (36), and in 1981, 16 oil workers were involved in a cholera outbreak on a Texas oil rig after eating rice cooked in water which had been contaminated by canal water containing sewage discharged from the rig (221). These and similar cases account for a total of more than 65 cases of domestically acquired cholera reported to the CDC, most of which have been only isolated incidents (420). Almost all of these cases have been reported in the Gulf of Mexico region; however, there has been at least one such case acquired from the Chesapeake Bay (271). All of the Gulf Coast isolates were of the El Tor biotype, serotype Inaba, which strongly suggests that this organism is endemic along the Gulf Coast of Mexico. *V. cholerae* serogroup O1 has been isolated from U.S. coastal waters of the Gulf of Mexico and Chesapeake Bay throughout the year, including toxin-producing strains (106, 229). Numbers tend to be highest in the warmer summer months, and they are frequently associated with plankton and shellfish. Toxigenic and nontoxigenic strains of *V. cholerae* O1 have been cultured from shellfish harvested from commercial U.S. waters (62, 199, 374, 448). Pollution does not appear to be a necessary factor, as the organism can be found in waters with no evidence of human waste (374). Case-controlled studies of localized outbreaks of *V. cholerae* O1 in the United States have shown that recent ingestion of raw or partially cooked seafood or contact with contaminated water is a significant risk factor (36, 221, 473). Contaminated imported food can be a source of localized outbreaks in the United States. In 1994, a cluster of cases occurred in Indiana and was traced to food imported from El Salvador (86).

In January 1991, toxin-producing strains of *V. cholerae* O1, biotype El Tor, serotype Inaba, appeared in several cities in Peru, which marked the first time in the 20th century that cholera was reported in South America (77, 85). As of January 1992, over 300,000 cases of cholera were reported in 14 countries in North and South America, with almost 4,000 deaths. U.S. citizens accounted for 17 of these cases, 6 associated with travel to South America and 11 associated with the ingestion of crabs imported illegally from Ecuador. Between 1 January and 29 February 1992, 42 cases were identified in the United States among travelers to and from South America; 40 of these cases, including one death, were reported among passengers on the same airline flight from South America to the United States (420).

Over 70 different serotypes of *V. cholerae* exist based on a somatic O antigen (463). These strains are phenotypically indistinguishable and share a common flagellar H antigen. *V. cholerae* serotype O1 is the strain associated with cholera. All others are referred to as noncholera vibrios, *V. cholerae* non-O1, or nonagglutinable vibrios due to their inability to agglutinate in O1 antiserum. Most strains of *V. cholerae* O1 produce an enterotoxin (cholera toxin) which is responsible for the severe fluid losses seen in cholera. Non-O1 *V. cholerae* strains do not produce cholera toxin but may produce toxins capable of eliciting an illness identical to cholera (312, 338, 482). *V. cholerae* can be divided into two biovars, classical and El Tor. Classical strains tend to be more virulent than El Tor strains. El Tor strains were originally detected by their ability to lyse sheep erythrocytes; however, this trait has not been shown to be consistent. They agglutinate chicken erythrocytes, are not sensitive to polymyxin B, and are Voges-Proskauer positive. Classical strains fail to lyse sheep erythrocytes or agglutinate chicken erythrocytes, are Voges-Proskauer negative, and are sensitive to polymyxin B. The biotypes may also be distinguished by phage susceptibility, a tool mainly used for epidemiological purposes. Additionally, both biotypes can be further classified into one of three serotypes: Inaba, Ogawa, and Hikojima (437). The El Tor biotype initially appeared in 1969 in regions in the Ganges Delta where cholera is endemic and quickly became the dominant biotype for most of the world (29). The more severe classical strain reappeared in Bangladesh in 1982 and has become the dominant strain in that region (390). At the time of this writing, all strains in the Western Hemisphere have been of the El Tor biotype. Reasons for the persistence of El Tor strains include its greater ability to survive in the environment and a larger ratio of symptomatic cases to asymptomatic carriers (1:30 to 100 for El Tor and 1:2 to 4 for the classical biotype) (169).

Under adverse environmental conditions, *V. cholerae* O1 can enter a state of dormancy in which the organism remains viable and potentially pathogenic yet fails to grow on conventional culture medium. The presence of the organism under such conditions has clearly been demonstrated by fluorescent and immunologic techniques in the absence of a positive culture. It has been proposed that in this way, *V. cholerae* O1 may persist indefinitely and go undetected in waters such as the Gulf Coast, only to emerge periodically under more favorable conditions to cause disease. This may also explain the periods between epidemics in areas where cholera is endemic. This phenomenon has been referred to as "viable but nonculturable" (463).

In the United States, cases of cholera have usually occurred in the summer or fall months following the ingestion of raw or undercooked shellfish (194). Once in the intestinal tract, the organism may adhere by means of a specialized pilus to the intestinal cell wall, where it may grow and produce enterotoxin (184, 195). Factors diminishing transit time, such as the ingestion of solid foods rather than liquids, may increase the chances of colonization and development of cholera (268). Furthermore, because the organism is less likely to survive in an acidic environment, the use of antacids or previous gastrectomy may increase one's chances of developing disease (396). Adherence of the organism to chitin particles in shellfish may also enhance survival in acidic environments (473). For some reason, persons with blood type O have been noted to be at a higher risk for cholera (409).

Cholera toxin is a heat-labile protein produced by most strains of *V. cholerae* O1. The molecule is composed of five B subunits arranged in a circle around an A1 and an A2 subunit. The B subunits are responsible for binding of the toxin to the receptor ganglioside GM1 on cell membranes. The A1 subunit, bound to the complex by the A2 subunit, stimulates adenylate cyclase activity, causing increased levels of cyclic AMP and hypersecretion of chloride, with the result of massive losses of salt and water (146). Cholera victims may lose over 1 liter of fluid per h and up to 100% of their body weight in 4 to 7 days of diarrhea as a result of the toxin (130, 189). Cholera toxin is not the only factor capable of causing the severe diarrhea in cholera victims; an identical illness has been noted in individuals infected with nontoxigenic variants of *V. cholerae* O1 (309, 314). Factors other than cholera toxin which have been proposed to play a role in producing illness include a heat-stable toxin similar to a toxin produced by *V. parahaemolyticus* (197), lecithinase (285), phospholipase (96), and prostaglandin E (351). *E. coli* may produce a plasmid-mediated toxin that is very similar in structure and mode of action to cholera toxin (146).

The incubation period in cholera varies from 6 h to 5 days. The average is 2 days in areas of endemicity (62). Initial symptoms may include anorexia, abdominal cramping, and mild diarrhea. Vomiting without nausea typically begins within hours of the onset of diarrhea. Fever is usually absent or low-grade. Stools are initially brown and loose, but within hours they become watery and pale gray in appearance and lose all odor except for perhaps a "fishy" smell. Scattered flecks of mucus give the stools a "rice water" appearance. A feeling of relief, rather than tenesmus, accompanies each bowel movement. Peak stool losses occur around 24 h of illness. Shock may occur within 12 h in untreated cases, with death ensuing in 18 h to 5 days. Gallbladder disease has been reported, including one case of acute cholecystitis in Alabama in which *V. cholerae* O1 was isolated from the gallbladder and bile. Serum vibriocidal antibodies were present as well (473). Chronic, asymptomatic gallbladder carriage has also been documented, especially in areas of endemicity where the risk of exposure is great (164, 457). Extraintestinal infections are rare; occasionally nontoxigenic strains may be isolated from wound infections (222, 473).

Cholera is fatal in less than 1% of properly recognized and treated cases, although the mortality rate can be as high as 50% if the disease is left untreated (62, 309, 473). The mainstay of therapy consists of rapid and effective fluid and electrolyte replacement. Oral rehydration is effective for most patients who are able to tolerate this mode of therapy. Currently, oral rehydration salt packets are available, as well as a variety of other premixed rehydration solutions which have been shown to be effective in the treatment of cholera. In the event that vomiting is severe enough or the patient is too obtunded to tolerate enteral hydration, intravenous infusion of lactated Ringer solution has been effective in initial rehydration, with oral therapy being initiated as soon as the patient is able to tolerate it. Normal saline is less effective because it lacks bicarbonate and potassium. The amount of fluids administered should be determined on the basis of dehydration at presentation as well as the rate of ongoing losses (420).

Antibiotics may decrease the duration of illness, the period of *Vibrio* excretion, and the amount of fluids needed for rehydration (309). Ciprofloxacin is the drug of choice in the treatment of cholera (156). It is given as a single dose of 1.0 g. Doxycycline may also be administered as a single dose of 300 mg. Trimethoprim-sulfamethoxazole is recommended for children and pregnant women. It should be noted that fluid rehydration is still considered to be the mainstay of therapy. Antispasmodics, antidiarrheal agents, and corticosteroids are not indicated in the treatment of cholera (420). Although a parenteral vaccine is currently available within the United States, it is not likely to be of benefit because of the low risk of infection in international travelers and the small number of cases acquired to date in the United States (74).

Non-O1 *V. cholerae*

Strains of *V. cholerae* that do not agglutinate in O1 antiserum, or non-O1 *V. cholerae*, are common inhabitants of both sewage-contaminated and sewage-free waters of bays, estuaries, brackish inland lakes, and seafood. Besides being an environmental contaminant, the organism has been isolated from domestic animals, waterfowl, and a variety of wildlife (121). Non-O1 species have even been implicated in enteric infections of horses, lambs, and bison in western Colorado (368). Most disease-associated isolates have been obtained from the coastal waters of Florida, the Gulf of Mexico, and the Chesapeake Bay, although isolates may be found all along the East Coast (384). Fewer isolates are noted along the West Coast, possibly due to colder water temperatures. Infections due to non-O1 strains have also been acquired from freshwater lakes distant from the sea (110, 320). Infections are more common during the warmer-water months of summer and fall.

The first reported case of human disease due to non-O1 strains of *V. cholerae* acquired in the United States occurred in 1972 in Louisiana in an individual who developed profuse and prolonged diarrhea following the ingestion of raw oysters (120). Since then, this organism has been increasingly recognized as a cause of human illness in this country; infection usually manifests as cases of sporadic illness (194). In a Chesapeake Bay hospital over a 15-year period, 40 *Vibrio* isolates were obtained, of which 10 were strains of non-O1 *V. cholerae* (192). Similarly, in a Gulf Coast community over a 10-year period, 4 of 23 *Vibrio* isolates were non-O1 *V. cholerae* (45). Although diarrheal illness is the most common manifestation of disease due to non-O1 *V. cholerae* strains, 10% of the cases are wound infections and an additional 10% are ear infections (309). Septicemia, meningitis, and acalculous cholecystitis have been reported (101, 239, 461). Unlike the strain which causes cholera, non-O1 species are rarely linked to epidemic disease (312). Isolated outbreaks of illness have occurred usually in association with a common contaminated food source. Of three previous outbreaks of diarrheal illness linked to non-O1 *V. cholerae* in Czechoslovakia, the Sudan, and Australia, two were linked to food sources (potatoes and an asparagus salad) and the other was linked to polluted well water (3, 114, 474). In 1992, an epidemic of cholera-like illness occurred in Madras, India, associated with an atypical strain of *V. cholerae* which has subsequently been designated *V. cholerae* O139 (T. Ramamurthy, S. Garg, and R. Sharma, Letter, *Lancet* **341**:703–704, 1993). Infection with the strain has been described as identical to cholera, and imported cases have been described in the United States (88).

More than half the non-O1 *V. cholerae* isolates received by the CDC are from stool samples (309). Gastroenteritis is the most common manifestation of illness in the United States and is almost always due to the ingestion of raw oysters (122, 312, 384, 469). In the United States, the incubation period has generally been less than 48 h; however, it has been as long as 4 days in at least one foreign outbreak (473). The following symptoms were noted in one review of U.S. cases: diarrhea (100%), abdominal cramps (93%), fever (71%), and nausea and vomiting (21%) (312). Another review reported nausea and vomiting occurring more frequently (77 and 69%, respectively) (204). The diarrhea can be severe, with up to 30 watery stools per day, and up to 25% of patients have bloody diarrhea (309). In some cases fluid losses may equal that seen in cholera (38). Illness generally lasts an average of 6.4 days in the cases reported in the United States (range, 2 to 12 days) but has lasted less than 2 days in some overseas outbreaks (3, 114, 312).

Non-O1 strains of *V. cholerae* exert their pathogenic effects through a variety of extracellular toxins and hemolysins. Enterotoxins identical or nearly identical to cholera toxin have been detected (482). Although rare in the United States (312), up to 40% of isolates in India and Bangladesh may produce this toxin (38, 117). In fact, severity of diarrheal illness seems to correlate with production of this toxin (117, 216). The lack of this cholera-like toxin in U.S. isolates indicates that other mechanisms are involved in their pathogenicity. Other factors which may be produced include enterotoxins other than the cholera-like toxin, including an enterotoxin that is also produced by *V. mimicus* and *Vibrio fluvialis* (13, 309, 333, 334); several hemolysins (481), including a hemolysin similar to the Kanagawa hemolysin produced by *V. parahaemolyticus* (T. Honda, M. Arita, T. Takeda, M. Yoh, and T. Miwatani, Letter, *Lancet* ii:163–164, 1985); and a Shiga-like toxin which may be responsible for the occasional bloody diarrhea (337).

Septicemia due to non-O1 strains of *V. cholerae* is a less frequent complication of infection. From 1977 through 1979 there were 70 isolates of *V. cholerae* reported to the CDC, of which 12 were obtained from the blood (384). The case fatality rate for septicemia has been estimated at 61.5% based on previously reported cases in the United States (384). Predisposing factors include alcohol abuse, previous gastric surgery, advanced age, and chronic underlying conditions such as hematologic malignancy, liver disease, immune deficiency, diabetes mellitus, peripheral vascular disease, and achlorhydria (122, 124, 216, 242, 309, 384). The source of the vibrio in many cases is raw-oyster ingestion (122). In addition to septicemia and gastroenteritis, non-O1 *V. cholerae* has been implicated in cases of wound infections (216, 309, 384), otitis media and otitis externa (147, 309, 434), prostatic abscess (384), cholecystitis (350), pneumonia (242), and meningitis (239, 306; E. L. Fearrington, C. H. Rand, A. Mewborn, and J. Wilkerson, Letter, *Ann. Intern. Med.* 81:401, 1974), including one case of neonatal meningitis in an infant who drank milk from a bottle stored near live crabs (380). Extraintestinal infections are usually the result of contact with seawater (309).

Most cases of non-O1 *V. cholerae* infection are relatively mild cases of gastroenteritis which are usually self-limiting in nature; only a minority require hospitalization (3, 312). Treatment should consist of supportive care, with intravenous hydration in severe cases of gastroenteritis (188). Septicemic cases and severe localized infections such as meningitis should be treated with intravenous antibiotics. In cases of gastroenteritis, antibiotics may decrease the severity of illness and shorten its duration (188). Non-O1 *V. cholerae* strains are susceptible in vitro to a wide range of antibiotics, including tetracycline, trimethoprim-sulfamethoxazole, chloramphenicol, and nalidixic acid (311). Susceptibilities to ampicillin and gentamicin are variable (311).

V. parahaemolyticus

V. parahaemolyticus has a worldwide distribution in both tropical and temperate inshore coastal and estuarine waters. Isolates have been obtained from water, sediment, suspended particulates, plankton, fish, and shellfish in a marine environment (309). Although halophilic, the organism can occasionally be isolated from freshwater areas, possibly through association with the chitin of plankton and shellfish or sediments, which may allow it to survive in areas of lower salinity (225). Most cases of illness occur in the summer, when warmer water temperatures favor growth of the organism. During the winter, the organism can be isolated from sediment (463). *V. parahaemolyticus* has been isolated from nearly every coastal state in the United States and is frequently found in Canadian waters as well (225). Outbreaks of diarrheal illness are the most common form of disease caused by this organism, and this usually follows the ingestion of raw or improperly cooked seafood, particularly crabs, shrimp, lobsters, and raw oysters. Most U.S. outbreaks have been caused by gross mishandling of seafood, such as improper refrigeration, insufficient cooking, cross contamination, and recontamination (374). Incubation of the organism in seafood can reduce the generation time to as little as 12 min (149). Previously thought to be a rare strain of *V. parahaemolyticus* and not described in the United States until 1982 (258, 336), a urease-positive strain of *V. parahaemolyticus* representing a new serovar has been established as the predominant cause of *V. parahaemolyticus*-associated gastroenteritis on the West Coast of the United States and Mexico (1, 238).

In Japan, over 70% of food-borne diarrheal illness is caused by *V. parahaemolyticus* (374). First described as a pathogen in the United States in 1971 following the ingestion of improperly cooked crabs in Maryland (304), the organism has been increasingly recognized as a cause of sporadic cases of diarrheal illness, usually in association with food-borne outbreaks (38). During the years 1973 to 1998, 40 outbreaks of *V. parahaemolyticus* were reported to the CDC, with most cases occurring in the warmer months (116). In a Chesapeake Bay hospital over a 15-year period, *V. parahaemolyticus* was the most common vibrio identified and accounted for 16 of 40 isolates obtained from 32 patients (192). During an outbreak of *Vibrio* gastroenteritis among attendees at a scientific congress in New Orleans, La., *V. parahaemolyticus* was found in 35 of the 51 stool specimens yielding a *Vibrio* species (282). In 1997, the largest reported outbreak of *V. parahaemolyticus*-confirmed infections occurred in North America (89). A total of 209 cases were identified, with one fatality. The outbreak was associated with raw oysters harvested from California, Oregon, Washington, and British Columbia. Extraintestinal manifestations may also occur, including sometimes fatal septicemia.

The incubation period has ranged from 4 to 96 h (28). In a review of eight *V. parahaemolyticus* outbreaks in the United States (28), the clinical manifestations included diarrhea (98%), abdominal cramps (82%), nausea (71%), vomiting (52%), headache (42%), fever (27%), and chills (24%). The illness was self-limiting in most cases, with a median duration of 3 days. Fever rarely exceeds 38.9°C. Abdominal pain can be severe (149). The diarrhea is acute in onset and usually watery and mild, although it can, rarely, be severe enough to cause dehydration, hypotension, and acidosis (287, 297). A dysentery-like illness with fecal leukocytes, superficial ulcerations of the colonic mucosa, and blood and mucus in the stool have been described in India and Bangladesh (38, 43, 159). This form of disease has rarely been encountered in the United States (43, 309). The incubation period in dysentery-like disease is shorter (as short as 2.5 h), although the duration of illness approximates that of the more common form of illness (473).

The ability to cause human disease has been associated with a heat-stable enterotoxin capable of lysing erythrocytes on Wagatsuma agar (225). Strains producing this thermostabile direct hemolysin (TDH) are known as "Kanagawa positive," named after the prefecture in Japan where it was first studied (198, 309). The observation that over 95% of clinical isolates and less than 1% of environmental isolates are Kanagawa positive has suggested that TDH is the toxin associated with pathogenicity (225, 309). In several studies involving animal models, purified TDH was able to produce clinical and histopathological effects similar to those seen in disease due to *V. parahaemolyticus* (303, 335, 491). In one report from the Pacific Northwest, only 6 of 13 clinical isolates from patients with diarrhea or wound infections due to *V. parahaemolyticus* were Kanagawa positive (238). The ability of Kanagawa-negative strains lacking TDH to produce diarrheal illness has led to the discovery of other enterotoxins (190, 437). In addition to several hemolysins with unclarified or potential roles in pathogenicity, including a Shiga-like toxin (190, 225), a TDH-related hemolysin has been suggested to be an important virulence factor in TDH-negative clinical isolates (403). The presence of specific intestinal adherence factors may contribute to the pathogenicity of some strains (172).

In rare instances, *V. parahaemolyticus* can result in extraintestinal infections. A history of trauma or insult to the infected anatomical site can be elicited in the majority of cases (216). Wound infections or cellulitis can develop as a primary focus of infection or can result from secondary hematogenous seeding (270). Although less common than stool isolates, wound isolates can constitute a significant number of *V. parahaemolyticus* isolates. Five of sixteen *V. parahaemolyticus* isolates collected over a 15-year period in the Chesapeake Bay region were acquired from wounds (192). Vascular thrombosis and gangrene have been reported (256). In some instances, *V. parahaemolyticus* and another *Vibrio* species may be isolated concurrently (353). Ocular (416, 422) and ear (192, 309) infections can occur, as well as pneumonia (S. L. Yu and O. Uy-Yu, Letter, *Ann. Intern. Med.* **100**:320, 1984) and osteomyelitis (376).

Most cases of *V. parahaemolyticus* gastroenteritis are self-limiting and resolve in a matter of days. Rarely are cases severe enough to require vigorous fluid support. Mortality is unusual, and the mortality rate has been estimated to be 0.04% in Japan (38). From 1981 to 1988, there were four fatalities due to *V. parahaemolyticus* in Florida. All patients were bacteremic and had either cirrhosis or an underlying malignancy (242). In view of the fact that most cases of infection due to *V. parahaemolyticus* manifest as gastroenteritis, methods to avoid such illness include the proper handling of seafood. Heating at 60°C for 15 min kills *V. parahaemolyticus*. In addition, storage at or below 4°C inhibits growth of the organism (447). Persons susceptible to septicemia, such as those with liver disease or any other immunosuppressive condition, should probably avoid raw-seafood ingestion (122, 192).

V. vulnificus

Beginning in 1964, the CDC began receiving extraintestinal isolates that were thought to be variants of *V. parahaemolyticus* but were shown to be different by means of a variety of biochemical tests, including the ability to ferment lactose (38). The species was referred to initially as the "halophilic lactose-positive marine vibrio"; the name *Beneckea vulnifica* was proposed but not widely accepted (366, 437). The virulence of this particular species was first recognized in 1976 by a review of clinical isolates reported to the CDC which revealed that 53% of the isolates were recovered from blood (193). The name *Vibrio vulnificus* was formally recognized in 1979 (142). This organism has been found in seawater, sediments, zooplankton, and shellfish (188). In two separate studies, over 50% of oysters sampled during selected months (425) and 11% of crabs harvested during summer months (119) yielded *V. vulnificus*. Water temperature seems to be an important factor; organisms are rarely isolated from waters with temperatures lower than 17°C (194). Almost all cases of infection have been reported between the months of May and October (374). Cases have been reported along both the Pacific and Atlantic coasts (as far north as Cape Cod), Hawaii, and the Gulf of Mexico and occasionally in such inland areas as New Mexico, Oklahoma, Kentucky, and the Great Salt Lake (4, 6, 35, 45, 192, 330, 414). In a Gulf Coast community over a 10-year period, 12 of 23 *Vibrio* isolates obtained were *V. vulnificus*, of which 9 were wound isolates (45). Similarly, in a Chesapeake Bay hospital over a 15-year period, 10 of 40 *Vibrio* isolates were *V. vulnificus*, of which 7 were obtained from wounds (192). The organism can proliferate in seafood at room temperature but is killed by storage at or near freezing temperatures or by cooking seafood at boiling temperatures (339). *V. vulnificus* has been isolated in oysters that have been refrigerated for 4 days (218).

V. vulnificus is one of the most invasive and rapidly lethal human pathogens ever described. Two major syndromes can result from infection with this organism (220). Primary septicemia typically follows the ingestion of raw oysters by individuals with liver disease. This syndrome can have a rapidly fatal course in up to 60% of cases (423). The other major presentation is that of wound infections, which may occur by either primary inoculation or secondary hematogenous spread in a bacteremic individual. Antibiotics, vigorous debridement, and occasionally amputation are necessary to control the massive necrosis and systemic spread which can occur (235). Unlike other vibrioses, gastroenteritis is not a major hallmark of infection with this species, and although gastrointestinal symptoms may accompany other forms of illness, the relationship is unclear (216, 219). In one epidemiological study of *V. vulnificus* infections in Florida from 1981 to 1987, 7 patients out of a total of 62 (11%) had gastrointestinal symptoms as their only manifestation of disease (244). Stool specimens yielded *V. vulnificus*, and blood cultures were negative. The diarrhea was described as watery, profuse, and accompanied by vomiting and abdominal pain. Six patients (86%) were hospitalized for a median of 6 days. Medications that reduce gastric acidity may be a factor in the development of gastroenteritis (219). Of 62 cases reported in Florida between 1981 and 1987, 38 were primary septicemia (62%), 17 were wound infections (27%), and the remaining 7 were gastrointestinal illness referred to above (11%) (244). Other infections due to *V. vulnificus* include pneumonia (113, 237), endocarditis (443), osteomyelitis (452), ocular infections (126), and meningitis (193). One reported case of endometritis due to *V. vulnificus* occurred in a female who had engaged in sexual intercourse in seawater (438).

The severity of infections due to *V. vulnificus* is dependent on host as well as bacterial factors. The presence of an acidic polysaccharide capsule correlates strongly with virulence (479). This capsule may confer resistance to phagocytosis and bactericidal activity of human serum (251, 308, 488). Strains may shift between encapsulated and unencapsulated forms at a very low frequency by poorly understood mechanisms. Growth of both encapsulated and unencapsulated phenotypes is enhanced significantly by the presence of iron (479). The organism is able to use transferrin-bound iron for growth if the transferrin is 100% iron saturated (normal human serum is 30% saturated). Iron in hemoglobin and hemoglobin-haptoglobin complexes may also be utilized (308). *V. vulnificus* also produces siderophores, which are low-molecular-weight chelators that bind available iron (404). Mouse studies have shown that passage of the organism through the animal may enhance virulence significantly, which suggests that the reintroduction of environmental or food-borne strains into the environment by infected individuals may increase the potential pathogenicity of the strains (236). Various toxins and enzymes may be produced by the organism. They include mucinase, protease, lipase, DNase, chondroitin sulfatase, hyaluronidase, cytolysin, and collagenase (168, 341, 410). The contribution to virulence by each of these factors has not yet been fully determined. Cytolysin-directed antibody has been detected in the sera of individuals with invasive disease, suggesting that this toxin may play a major role in invasive forms of disease (167).

Individuals susceptible to primary septicemia are most commonly those with liver disease, particularly alcoholic cirrhosis. Adults with liver disease who eat raw oysters are 80 times more likely to develop illness with *V. vulnificus* than those without liver disease and are 200 times more likely to die from *V. vulnificus* infections (95). This is due in part to shunting of blood around the liver, thereby bypassing the hepatic reticuloendothelial system and subsequent clearing by hepatic macrophages. Additionally, these individuals may also have deficiencies in leukocyte chemotaxis and complement that can impair host defenses (188). Patients with hepatic disease commonly have high serum iron levels due to liberation of iron stores from damaged hepatocytes (478). In addition, other conditions leading to increased serum iron levels, such as thalassemia major and hemochromatosis, can also contribute to primary septicemia (216). Alcoholics without liver disease are at risk for primary septicemia probably due in part to saturated transferrin levels (56). Other conditions predisposing to primary septicemia include hematopoietic disorders, chronic renal insufficiency, dyspeptic disease or a history of gastric resection, the use of immunosuppressive drugs, and diabetes mellitus (383). Primary septicemia occasionally occurs in previously healthy persons (244).

There is little doubt that the gastrointestinal tract is the portal of entry in primary septicemia. The organism can survive between pH 3.6 and 12.5 when incubated at 37°C for 1 h and grows best between pH 7 and 9 (347). Therefore, the organism is capable of surviving passage through the stomach. Most commonly, this occurs following the ingestion of raw oysters. An epidemiological study in Florida of oyster eaters between 1981 and 1988 estimated the age-standardized annual incidence of any *Vibrio* illness per million as 95.4 for raw-oyster eaters with liver disease, 9.2 for raw-oyster eaters without liver disease, and 2.2 for non-raw-oyster eaters (122). Although these estimates were based on the chances of developing any *Vibrio* illness, the risk was shown to be greatest for *V. vulnificus*. Other types of raw fish or shellfish may cause septicemia, and on previous occasions, illness followed ingestion of deep-fried fish, grilled crab, boiled shrimp, and broiled grouper (135, 244). *V. vulnificus* invades the gastrointestinal mucosa at the level of the proximal small bowel into the systemic circulation to produce sepsis (346, 355). On occasion, the organism may penetrate the intestinal wall into the ascitic fluid of cirrhotics to produce peritonitis (346).

The mean incubation period is 16 h, although it has been as long as 2 weeks in some cases (37, 423). The chief symptoms associated with septicemia include fever (94%), chills (91%), and nausea (58%) (216). Diarrhea occurs in less than half of the patients with primary septicemia (220, 244). Approximately one-third become hypotensive within 12 h of admission to a hospital (191). Signs and symptoms of disseminated intravascular coagulation and septic shock may appear (191). Thrombocytopenia and leukopenia are common, although leukocytosis can appear less frequently (309). Arthritis and arthralgias may develop, and the organism has been cultured from affected joints (37, 220). Other associated clinical characteristics may include the rapid development of anemia, adult respiratory distress syndrome, and heart block (188).

Over 70% of patients with primary septicemia develop skin lesions usually within the first 36 h of illness (309, 414). Lesions are more common on the trunk and extremities and frequently begin as tender erythematous or ecchymotic areas which may progress to bullae or vesicles that develop into necrotic ulcers (430, 437). They may occasionally appear as ecthyma gangrenosum-like lesions, erythema multiforme, cellulitis, and papular or maculopapular eruptions (216, 466). Similar lesions have been reported for individuals who had bacteremia due to *Pseudomonas aeruginosa*, *Aeromonas hydrophila*, and *Yersinia enterocolitica* (414). Gangrene of a limb can develop as a result of major vessel occlusion (430). Histological examination reveals cellulitis with subcutaneous tissue necrosis and septal panniculitis characterized by paucity of an inflammatory infiltrate in the dermis (430). Necrotizing vasculitis and subepidermal bullae can be seen, as well as gram-negative coccobacilli. Gram stain and culture of vesicular or bullous fluid may yield the organisms, which have been described as resembling "seagulls" (135).

Localized wound infections with *V. vulnificus* may occur in otherwise healthy people after an open wound comes in contact with seawater or seafood contaminated with the organism. A typical scenario is the development of a wound infection following injuries sustained while peeling shrimp, cleaning crabs, or shucking oysters (188, 244, 309). Infection may also follow exposure of a preexisting wound to seawater. Approximately one-third to one-half of cases of wound infections due to *V. vulnificus* occur in patients who have underlying illnesses such as alcohol abuse, congestive heart failure, stasis ulcers, arthritis, liver disease, diabetes mellitus, and malignancy (37, 220, 423). Initially, the wound may appear trivial; however, in a matter of hours, it characteristically becomes edematous and erythematous, with development of lymphadenopathy and lymphangitis. Intense pain may develop at the wound site. Patients are frequently ill with fever and chills (37, 423). Anorexia, nausea, and vomiting may occur, although less frequently than in primary septicemia (37, 220). Occasionally, more than one *Vibrio* species may be isolated from the wound (353). Unlike primary septicemia, wound infections usually remain localized; however, bacteremia with secondary development of cutaneous infections can occasionally occur (383). Approximately one-third of individuals with localized wound infections have positive blood cultures (309). Individuals with underlying diseases (rarely healthy persons) may develop progressive cellulitis, myositis, or fasciitis (188). Leukocytosis is usually noted; thrombocytopenia and disseminated intravascular coagulation generally do not occur (383). Severe necrotizing fasciitis can occasionally occur, with gross purulence and easy separation of fascial planes. Findings of fascial necrosis separate this entity from cellulitis (148). The histopathology of wound infections is similar to that which occurs in primary septicemia, although it is generally not as severe. Mortality ranges from 7 to 22% of cases, being higher in those individuals with underlying diseases who are more likely to develop progressive soft tissue involvement and bacteremia (188).

Treatment of *V. vulnificus* infections consists of rapid recognition with prompt institution of antibiotics and supportive measures, along with management of adult respiratory distress syndrome, disseminated intravascular coagulation, and shock if present (188, 309, 346). Surgical debridement of all necrotic tissue is recommended (200). Proximal amputation of infected limbs may be necessary in severe cases of wound infection (188). Tetracycline has been shown to be highly effective against *V. vulnificus* in a mouse model (48). Low efficacy was noted for ampicillin, cefotaxime, and cefazolin. Carbenicillin and gentamicin were not effective. Current antibiotic regimens consist of ceftazidime (2 g intravenously three times a day) and doxycycline (100 mg per os or intravenously twice a day) or doxycycline in combination with ciprofloxacin or an aminoglycoside (156). The data supporting use of fluoroquinolones are limited. Ciprofloxacin has been used effectively in the treatment of one case of infection due to *V. vulnificus;* however, conclusive clinical studies are lacking (10; M. C. Meadors and G. A. Pankey, Letter, *J. Infect.* **20:**88–89, 1990).

V. mimicus

In 1981, a new *Vibrio* species was detected by virtue of DNA and biochemical analysis. Previously thought to be a biochemical variant of *V. cholerae*, the new species differed in its inability to ferment sucrose and its negative Voges-Proskauer reaction. The name *Vibrio mimicus* was proposed because of its similarity to *V. cholerae* (118). The organism is nonhalophilic and has been isolated from both salt water and freshwater (100). A high percentage of strains (49%) are able to grow in 6% sodium chloride (141). Brackish water with an average salinity of 4.0% was found to be suitable for *V. mimicus*. It has been isolated from fish and shellfish (usually oysters), as well as from freshwater prawns (99, 247, 402). Unlike, *V. cholerae*, it probably does not adhere to plankton samples in the environment (100). Over the period from 1977 through 1981, the CDC received 21 clinical isolates of this organism, although the true incidence is unknown (402). Nineteen of the isolates were obtained from stool samples, and the other two were obtained from human ears. Clinical isolates have been obtained from the waters of the Gulf of Mexico, the mid-Atlantic Coast, and the Chesapeake Bay (402). Among 40 *Vibrio* isolates collected over a 15-year period in a Chesapeake Bay hospital, 3 were identified as *V. mimicus;* all were isolated from stool samples (192). The organism has also been implicated along with *V. fluvialis* in a case of terminal ileitis (459).

Gastrointestinal illness is the predominant manifestation of disease, and this typically follows the ingestion of seafood, primarily raw oysters (402). In the largest reported review of illness due to *V. mimicus* in the United States, involving 21 cases, the median incubation period was shown to be 24 h, with a range of 3 to 72 h (402). Symptoms included diarrhea (94%); nausea, vomiting, and abdominal cramps (67%); fever (44%, occasionally up to 38.3°C); and headache (39%). Three of the 17 patients with diarrhea had bloody diarrhea (18%). The median leukocyte count was 13,400, with a median differential of 73% polymorphonuclear cells, 7% bands, 16% lymphocytes, and 4% monocytes. Electrolytes were all within normal limits. Diarrheal illness lasted a median of 6 days. Two cases were ear infections acquired from contact with seawater. Outbreaks of seafood-associated gastroenteritis caused by *V. mimicus* have been described in Japan (100).

Approximately 10% of clinical strains and 16% of all strains produce a heat-labile toxin that appears to be identical to cholera toxin (309). An enterotoxin similar to that described for non-O1 *V. cholerae* and *V. fluvialis* has been described (333).

Antimicrobial testing has shown that *V. mimicus* is susceptible to tetracycline, which may be the drug of choice in severe infections (402). The combination of trimethoprim and sulfamethoxazole, aminoglycosides, chloramphenicol, and ampicillin have been shown to be effective in vitro. Eighty-three percent of environmental isolates in one study were shown to be resistant to ampicillin, with intermediate sensitivity and no resistance to tetracycline in 17% (100).

V. fluvialis

V. fluvialis was first isolated in 1975 from the stool of a patient with diarrhea in Bahrain (151). In 1976 to 1977, it was responsible for an outbreak of diarrheal illness involving over 500 persons in Bangladesh (211). About one-half of the patients were children under 5 years of age. Originally referred to as group F by the British Public Health Laboratories in Maidstone, England, and enteric group EF-6 by the CDC, it was named *Vibrio fluvialis* (from the Latin word for "river") in 1980 on the basis of its original isolation from river and estuarine waters (264, 473). This organism has marked biochemical similarities to *Aeromonas* species and can be distinguished by its ability to grow in 6 to 7% sodium chloride (*Aeromonas* species do not grow) and its inability to grow in the presence of the vibriostatic agent O/129 (*Aeromonas* species do grow) (473). Based on these similarities, it is probable that many clinical isolates previously reported as *Aeromonas* species may have in actuality been

V. fluvialis (400). One-third of organisms labeled as *Aeromonas* in the past by the British Public Health Laboratories were found to actually be *V. fluvialis* on reexamination (264). In the United States, the organism has been isolated from water and sediment in New York Bay (400), shellfish in Louisiana, and water and shellfish in the Pacific Northwest and Hawaii (424). Almost all cases of infection due to *V. fluvialis* in the United States have been gastrointestinal illness. A history of seafood ingestion prior to the onset of illness is reported in most cases (243). In Florida between 1982 and 1988, 12 clinical isolates of *V. fluvialis* were recovered, of which 10 were obtained from stool samples, 1 was obtained from the drainage of a colostomy bag, and 1 was recovered from a wound (243). One isolate was recovered from a stool sample in a Chesapeake Bay hospital in a 15-year period (192). A fatality occurring in the United States due to *V. fluvialis*-related illness has been reported in the case of a Texas man who developed profuse diarrhea with electrolyte imbalance (424). Outbreaks of gastroenteritis linked to a common food source have been reported (433). Occasionally, wound infections can occur in association with injuries sustained near seawater (243, 424). The organism was recovered from purulent bile in one patient in Japan with acute suppurative cholangitis (489).

The median incubation period for gastrointestinal illness has been reported as 39 h (range, 16 to 60 h), with a median duration of illness of 6 days (range, 1 to 60 days) (243). In the Bangladesh outbreak, reported clinical features included diarrhea (100%), vomiting (97%), abdominal pain (75%), moderate to severe dehydration (67%), and fever (35%) (211). Invasive disease probably occurs, as 75% of the patients in that outbreak had fecal leukocytes and blood in the stools. Secondary infection occurs rarely (240).

V. fluvialis is capable of stimulating fluid accumulation in rabbit ileal loops (400). An enterotoxin similar to that described for non-O1 *V. cholerae* and *V. mimicus* has been described (333). Other factors associated with toxicity may also be produced with a variety of effects, including cytolytic activity against mammalian erythrocytes, lethal activity in mice, and nonhemolytic cytotoxicity (225, 276).

Severe cases of gastroenteritis should be treated with intravenous fluid and electrolyte replacement and antibiotics (437). *V. fluvialis* is sensitive to tetracycline, ampicillin, chloramphenicol, gentamicin, and the combination of trimethoprim and sulfamethoxazole (240).

Vibrio hollisae

V. hollisae was known as enteric group EF-13 until 1982, when it was shown to be a separate species by DNA hybridization studies (186). It was named after the researcher at the CDC who first identified it. *V. hollisae* grows inconsistently on TCBS agar and so may not be isolated routinely (310). Isolation may rely on recovery of colonies on blood agar plates (310). There are few ecological studies on *V. hollisae*; however, it has been isolated from deep-sea invertebrates and healthy coastal fish (127, 331). Fifteen clinical isolates were received by the CDC from 1971 to 1981, of which fourteen were stool isolates and one was a blood isolate (310). Cases occurred in states along the Atlantic and Gulf coasts, with three cases in Florida, four in Maryland, and one each in Virginia and Louisiana. In

Florida in the years 1981 to 1988, 34 isolates of *V. hollisae* were identified from clinical cases, of which 28 were obtained from individuals with gastrointestinal illness, 4 were from individuals with septicemia, and 2 were isolated from wounds (122). The risk of infection is most often associated with raw-seafood ingestion, particularly raw oysters, although cases of illness have followed ingestion of fried fish and fish preserved by drying and salting, which suggests that this organism may be resistant to some methods of cooking and preservation (122, 283, 310, 365).

In nine selected cases of gastrointestinal illness reported to the CDC, all patients had diarrhea and abdominal pain, 5 had vomiting, and 5 had fever (310). Diarrhea was bloody in one case. The median white blood cell count was 11,200 per microliter. The median duration of illness was 1 day (range, 4 h to 13 days). Reported cases of septicemia include one fatal case occurring in an individual with hepatic cirrhosis (310) and another case occurring in a 65-year-old man who developed septicemia following consumption of a freshwater catfish who was successfully treated with tobramycin, cefamandole, and tetracycline (283).

Several toxins may be produced, including a hemolysin with potential virulence activity (486) and a heat-sensitive enterotoxin which has been associated with some virulent strains (250). *V. hollisae* possesses gene sequences homologous with those coding for TDH in *V. parahaemolyticus* (332).

V. damselae

V. damselae, previously known as enteric group EF-5, was renamed in 1981 after the damselfish, for which it is an important pathogen (281). This organism is known to cause skin ulcerations and death in fish and has been isolated from seawater (281). Between 1971 and 1981, eight clinical isolates were reported to the CDC of which seven were obtained from wounds (one was a urine isolate) (310). Cases occurred on the Atlantic, Pacific, and Gulf coasts and were reported in Florida, Louisiana, Hawaii, and the Bahamas. Typically, infection is the result of injuries sustained to the foot or leg while swimming or handling fish (103). Infection is usually seasonal and is probably dependent on water temperature and possibly its interaction with certain fish species (103, 310, 394).

Lesions usually began as erythematous and indurated areas which may later exhibit a purulent discharge (310; M. Dryden, M. Legarde, T. Gottlieb, L. Brady, and H. K. Ghosh, Letter, *Med. J. Aust.* **151**:540–541, 1989). Immunocompetent patients may require little more than local wound care; however, severe necrotizing and occasional fatal infections have been described (103, 310). One fatal case involved a diabetic, alcoholic patient who had sustained a small laceration to his hand while cleaning catfish (103). The initial superficial wound evolved into an edematous and necrotizing process with bulla formation. He subsequently died of medical complications, including disseminated intravascular coagulation. Tissue damage may be toxin mediated (10; Dryden et al., letter). *V. damselae* may produce an extracellular hemolytic toxin which has been shown to be lethal in mice (252). Of five *V. damselae* isolates tested, all were sensitive to gentamicin and chloramphenicol, four were sensitive to tetracycline and cephalothin, and none were sensitive to sulfonamides, ampicillin, or penicillin (310).

V. alginolyticus

Originally classified as biotype 2 of *V. parahaemolyticus*, this organism was found to be a separate and distinct species on the basis of several fermentative and biochemical properties. It was renamed *Vibrio alginolyticus* in 1968 (387). This organism was not known to be pathogenic in humans until 1973, when six isolates from tissue specimens collected in 1969 thought to be *V. parahaemolyticus* were found to be in actuality *V. alginolyticus* (38). The ecological niche of this organism is probably similar to that of *V. parahaemolyticus*, and it has been isolated from seawater, fish, shrimp, crabs, oysters, and clams (225). Numbers of this organism in seawater are generally higher than those of *V. parahaemolyticus* and are associated with warm water temperatures (225, 463). This organism fails to grow at temperatures lower than 8°C (38). In the United States, clinical isolates of *V. alginolyticus* have been obtained from waters along the Atlantic, Pacific, and Gulf coasts, as well as in Hawaii and the Chesapeake Bay (38, 45, 192).

Clinically, wound and ear infections represent the majority of cases of illness due to this organism (38, 216). Wound infections almost always follow exposure of open wounds to seawater (437). Frequently, a number of different organisms may be isolated, making the pathogenic role of *V. alginolyticus* uncertain (216). In one study in Western Australia, 56% of infected wounds contaminated with seawater yielded *V. alginolyticus* (359). In a similar study in Hawaii, the organism was isolated from 11% of traumatic marine injuries (352). In Florida between 1981 and 1988, 14 clinical isolates of *V. alginolyticus*, of which 11 were wound isolates, were reported (79%) (122). The incubation period is about 24 h (38, 359). Most wound infections are self-limiting and consist of mild cases of cellulitis with various amounts of a seropurulent exudate; however, more severe cases with bacteremia may be noted for immunocompromised individuals (38, 45, 215, 397). One fatal case of bacteremia involved a 37-year-old woman who was doused in seawater after an explosion on a recreational boat (136). The organism was isolated from burn wounds as well as blood. The organism may produce extracellular protease and collagenase, although the role of these factors in the virulence of this organism has not yet been established (178, 309). Local wound care is probably sufficient for superficial wounds in immunocompetent individuals; however, patients with impaired host defenses or severe or complicated infections should be treated with antibiotics. In vitro, *V. alginolyticus* is susceptible to tetracycline, the combination of trimethoprim and sulfamethoxazole, aminoglycosides, and chloramphenicol (260).

V. alginolyticus has a predisposition towards individuals with ear disorders (463). These infections are generally associated with swimming in seawater. Both otitis media and otitis externa have been reported (38, 397). This organism has rarely been associated with gastrointestinal illness, although cases have been reported (122, 257, 325). Conjunctivitis, pneumonia, osteomyelitis, and a case of an epidural abscess due to *V. alginolyticus* have been reported (225, 266, 342, 397). Peritonitis has been reported for an individual undergoing peritoneal dialysis who had changed his peritoneal dialysis fluid bag on the beach without taking adequate precautions (428).

V. furnissii

V. furnissii was originally classified as biovar II of *V. fluvialis*. This species differs from *V. fluvialis* in its aerogenicity (it produces gas from glucose). In 1983 in was renamed *Vibrio furnissii* in honor of a researcher at the British Public Health Laboratories in Maidstone (55). The organism has been recovered from the marine environment (264). Most clinical isolates have been from Japan and other parts of the Orient (309). Illness related to this species consists of gastroenteritis most likely due to ingestion of raw or undercooked seafood (55). Occasional outbreaks of gastroenteritis have been recorded, including one such episode onboard a flight from Tokyo, Japan, to Seattle, Wash., involving 23 passengers (70, 72). Symptoms included diarrhea (91%), abdominal cramps (79%), nausea (65%), and vomiting (39%). Two patients required hospitalization, and one died. The organism has also been recovered from the feces (along with *V. fluvialis*) of an infant with diarrhea and has also been isolated from stools of asymptomatic individuals (187, 259). *V. furnissii* is capable of producing an enterotoxin similar to that described for *V. fluvialis* and *V. mimicus* (333).

V. metschnikovii

Previously known as enteric group 16, *V. metschnikovii* was first described in 1888 (263). In 1978 it was redefined on the basis of DNA homology studies (263, 437). Freshwater and marine isolates of this organism have been obtained from rivers, estuaries, sewage, cockles, lobsters, oysters, clams, and a bird that died of a cholera-like illness (263). Human disease involving this organism was not recognized until 1978, when it was recovered from the blood of an 82-year-old diabetic female in Chicago, Ill., who presented to a hospital with septicemia due to an inflamed gallbladder (217). She was treated successfully with a cholecystectomy and antibiotic treatment with clindamycin and tobramycin. Although the organism has been isolated from the stools of asymptomatic individuals (437), diarrheal illness has been described in at least one instance (302). An extracellular cytolysin has been characterized, although its role in virulence is uncertain (301).

Vibrio cincinnatiensis

Only one case of human disease involving *V. cincinnatiensis* has been reported to date (42). A 70-year-old man with a history of alcohol abuse developed disorientation and questionable nuchal rigidity upon admission to a hospital. A spinal tap was performed which revealed a gram-negative bacillus; an identical isolate was obtained from his blood. Genetic and biochemical analysis revealed that this was a new *Vibrio* species which was subsequently named *Vibrio cincinnatiensis* (54). The patient was treated successfully with 9 days of moxalactam. There was no history of exposure to salt water or ingestion of seafood.

Vibrio carchariae

First isolated from a brown shark that died in captivity in 1984, *V. carchariae* has been known to be a pathogen to fish (170). This species, whose name comes from the Greek *carcharias*, meaning shark, had not been implicated as a human pathogen until a single report described a wound infection occurring in an 11-year-old girl who was attacked by a shark off the South Carolina coast (348). She suffered extensive trauma to her left calf, requiring plastic surgery. A swab of the leg obtained on the day of the shark bite revealed *V. carchariae*. Minimal drainage occurred from the wound, which subsequently healed well. Antimicrobial testing showed the organism to be susceptible to cephalothin, cefamandole, cefoxitin, gentamicin, and the combination of trimethoprim and sulfamethoxazole. Resistance to ampicillin and carbenicillin was noted; amikacin sensitivity was intermediate.

MYCOBACTERIUM MARINUM

Mycobacterium marinum was first isolated by Aronson in 1926 from saltwater fish that died in a Philadelphia, Pa., aquarium (14). In 1942, Baker and Hagan isolated this mycobacterium from freshwater platyfish in Mexico; they named it *Mycobacterium platypoecilus* (26). Human disease attributed to this organism was not recognized until 1951, when an epidemic of self-limiting skin granulomas occurred in a town in Sweden involving 80 individuals; 75 were children, and lesions were mostly on the elbows (272). All five adult patients were avid swimmers, which suggested that a common swimming pool may have been involved. Tissue specimens from patients and cultures of the swimming pool yielded an atypical mycobacterium which the investigators termed *Mycobacterium balnei* (Latin, meaning "of the bath"). In order to affirm the association between the organism and the clinical findings, the investigators inoculated themselves with the mycobacterium and were able to produce the lesions. In 1959, the previously reported mycobacterial isolates were found to represent the same species (104). *Mycobacterium marinum* became the officially recognized name, as this was the earliest term proposed by Aronson. The first association of this organism with tropical fish tanks was made in 1962 (421). Since then, *M. marinum* has become a well-recognized cutaneous pathogen with a strong association with an aquatic environment and water-related activities. The organism has been called a "leisure-time pathogen," and the disease has been referred to as a "hobby hazard" (144, 181). Manifestations of disease have also been referred to as "fish fancier's finger" and "swimming pool granuloma."

M. marinum belongs to Runyon group I (the photochromogens) of atypical mycobacteria, along with *Mycobacterium kansasii* and *Mycobacterium simiae*. These organisms are capable of producing a yellow carotene pigment when exposed to a strong light. *M. marinum* grows optimally on Löwenstein-Jensen medium, and unlike with other mycobacteria, growth occurs at 28 to 32°C rather than 37°C. This is an important distinction which may be responsible for the fact that most *M. marinum* infections do not invade beyond the superficial cooler regions of the skin (102). Colonies may be visible in as early as 7 days, although they may, rarely, take up to 2 months (8, 104, 255). Growth also occurs on blood agar, though not on MacConkey agar. The organisms are acid-fast and appear as long, slender, occasionally beaded rods; however, they may appear short and compact. Biochemical reactions include a negative response to niacin, neutral red, and arylsulfatase and a positive response to Tween 80 hydrolysis in 10 days (8, 104).

M. marinum is a pathogen of salt- and freshwater fish. It is widely distributed in the environment and may be isolated from contaminated water, the walls of swimming pools or aquariums, and dead or diseased fish (329). Affected fish may be cachectic and frequently show skin changes consisting of pigment changes, loss of scales, blood spots with eventual formation of ulcers, and fin and tail rot (453). Microscopically, miliary tubercles may be found in virtually every organ system. The disease is thought to spread among fish by the ingestion of infective material. In humans, the organism most commonly causes benign superficial cutaneous illness, although destructive tenosynovitis, osteomyelitis, septic arthritis, sclero-keratitis, and, rarely, disseminated systemic illness have been reported (98, 102, 137, 163, 212, 223, 224, 241, 398, 455). The organism is usually acquired through abrasions, lacerations, or punctures sustained in an aquatic environment. Commonly associated activities include swimming, boating, fishing, handling of fish and shellfish, and the keeping of tropical fish tanks. Occasional nonaquatic exposures from an asphalt school yard, school desks, an electrical installation, rose thorns, and even a laboratory have been documented (104, 144, 223, 451). Cases have been reported along the Gulf, Pacific, and Atlantic coasts as far north as Oregon and Long Island (212). Inland cases also occur. An epidemic in Colorado involving 290 individuals was linked to community swimming pools (305).

The incubation period ranges from 2 weeks to 2 months (208). Superficial lesions appear which usually range in number from one to six and appear as chronic, dusky erythematous plaques or verrucous papules or nodules in areas subject to trauma (201). More than 75% of reported cases involved the hand and upper extremity, usually the dominant right hand (208, 212). The lesions can appear as solitary granulomas or verrucous papules 1 to 2.5 cm in diameter which may ulcerate and drain purulent material. Most lesions are asymptomatic and cause only cosmetic inconvenience. Symptoms, if present, are mainly slight tenderness and discharge. Limitation in movement of the affected extremity may be noted. Lymphadenopathy occurs rarely (208). Occasionally, spread in a sporotri-choid fashion may occur. Rarely, disseminated cutaneous spread develops (60, 241). One such case involved a 16-month-old child who developed disseminated lesions after being bathed in a bathtub which her father had previously used to clean his fish tanks (241). The time lag between appearance of the lesion and its correct diagnosis ranges from a few weeks to a few years. Left untreated, 80% of the lesions may resolve completely in an average of 14 months, the longest time noted being 45 years (358, 455). Truncal cutaneous dissemination has been described for an AIDS patient who kept tropical fish as a hobby (371). Histologically, the lesions of *M. marinum* change their appearance according to the age of the infection (60). Early lesions (2 to 3 months' duration) show nonspecific inflammatory infiltrates in the upper corium. Multinucleated giant cells and epithelioid cell granulomas generally appear at 4 to 6 months of infection, and typical tuberculoid structures appear in older lesions. All stages can be observed simultaneously. Staining of tissue specimens reveals the organism in only about 10% of cases. Ten or more slides of thick smears from homogenized tissues are often required for examination after preparation with auramine-rhodamine fluorochrome stain (98).

Deep tissue infections were first widely recognized in 1973 (467). Superficial lesions may invade deeper tissues by attempted self-excision, by intralesional cortisone injections, or by incomplete surgical excision that is not combined with appropriate antibiotics (212). These infections are more destructive and more resistant to treatment than are superficial lesions. Tendon and synovial structures of the wrist and hand are affected in most cases. Diffuse edema at the site of infection is the most common finding (201). A slight fullness may be palpated at the site of the affected tendon sheath. Unlike in pyogenic infections, the dorsum of the hand does not swell and a throbbing pain does not occur. Joint limitation with subsequent development of draining sinus tracts may occur. Up to one-half of the deep infections involving the hand and wrist may be associated with carpal tunnel syndrome (255). Systemic complaints, fever, and lymphadenopathy are usually absent. The erythrocyte sedimentation rate is usually normal, and X-ray findings are nonspecific (201). Factors associated with a poor prognosis include persistent pain, the presence of a draining sinus tract, and previous local injection of corticosteroids (98).

Diagnosis relies primarily on isolation of the organism by staining or culture. A thorough history should be obtained, including such informational items as hobbies and recreational interests. *M. marinum* rarely grows at temperatures utilized for the incubation of most other mycobacteria. If *M. marinum* is suspected, specimens should be incubated at 30°C on Löwenstein-Jensen medium (in addition to 37°C for the isolation of other mycobacteria) (104). Specific mycobacterial skin testing has been utilized, although with inconsistent results (208, 223). The differential diagnosis of *M. marinum* infections includes sporotrichosis, tularemia, nocardia, yaws, syphilis, leishmaniasis, common warts, coccidioidomycosis, blastomycosis, histoplasmosis, tuberculosis cutis verrucosa, sarcoidosis, gout, rheumatoid arthritis, iodine or bromine granuloma, and benign or malignant tumors (201). Although usually self-limiting, superficial infections should probably be treated with antimicrobial agents. Minocycline has long been considered the drug of choice; however, clarithromycin and doxycycline have been equally efficacious (59, 156, 213, 279). Resistance to doxycycline has been described (275). *M. marinum* does not respond to many of the antimycobacterial agents. It is usually susceptible to rifampin, ethambutol, trimethoprim-sulfamethoxazole, and amikacin (129). Ciprofloxacin has shown good in vitro activity against *M. marinum* (105). In vitro susceptibility testing has also shown that gatifloxacin, levofloxacin, and moxifloxacin display activities similar to that of ciprofloxacin (51). Treatment should probably be continued for at least 6 to 12 weeks (129). Patients should be instructed not to "pick at" their lesions to reduce the risk of deeper tissue involvement (212). Deeper tissue involvement usually requires surgical intervention, which may include excision, tenosynovectomy, synovectomy, arthrodesis, or incision and drainage of infected bone or joints (212). Superficial lesions should not be excised or biopsied without the addition of appropriate drug therapy in order to decrease the risk of deeper tissue spread (212).

MARINE TRAUMA

Sharks

Shark attacks have been a popular focus of many books and movies, which often depict these creatures as ruthless savage predators randomly attacking swimmers or divers along beaches or other aquatic recreational areas. Attacks have been recorded in the United States for several hundred years. In the years between 1670 and 2003, there were 833 shark attacks reported in the United States, with 52 fatalities (G. H. Burgess, *International Shark Attack File 2003 Shark Attack Summary* [http://www. flmnh.ufl.edu/fish/sharks/statistics/2003attacksummary.htm]). In 2003 alone, 55 confirmed unprovoked attacks occurred, a number lower than the 63 unprovoked attacks reported in 2002, 68 reported in 2001, and 79 reported in 2000. Of the 350 species of sharks, only 32 have been implicated in the 30 to 100 shark attacks reported annually worldwide (16). In the United States, the most common offenders are the great white (Fig. 2), gray reef, blue, and mako sharks. Most shark attacks occur in temperate waters between 46°N and 47°S latitude. Associated risk factors include murky, warm water (70°F); sewer outlets; late afternoon and early evening hours; recreational areas; deep channels or drop-offs; movement; and bright objects (16). The victim does not see the shark in most cases, although skin abrasions from "bumping" (due to the shark's skin denticles) may precede the bite. In more than 70% of reported attacks, the victim was bitten one or two times (57).

Sharks can range in length from 9 in. to 50 ft (the whale shark). The largest great white shark verified was 19.5 ft long (57). They are extremely well adapted as predators in their environment, with exceptional sensory systems enabling them to detect electrical fields and motion which may compensate for their poor color vision. Specialized telereceptors known as the ampullae of Lorenzini are exquisitely sensitive to vibration and low-frequency sound waves; this sensitivity allows

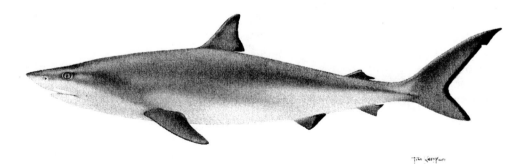

Figure 2. A number of shark species have been implicated in shark attacks in North American waters. Specialized sensory systems compensate for poor color vision by allowing a shark to detect motion as well as electrical fields of its prey. Ripsaw teeth are replaced every few months. Source: U.S. Fish and Wildlife Service. Artist: Timothy Knepp.

these animals to detect struggling creatures (16). Keen olfactory and gustatory chemoreceptors allow them to sense body fluids.

The shark's jaws consist of multirowed crescent-shaped sets of ripsaw teeth which are replaced every few months. The biting force has been estimated at 18 tons per in^2! The jaw opening of some sharks may be large enough to accommodate a horse's head (16).

Sharks usually feed slowly and purposefully; however, they occasionally become frenzied, snapping at anything in sight, usually by an inciting event. Humans are usually mistaken for food (seals). Recent shark attacks in northern California have been focused on surfers who entered migratory habitats of the elephant seal, which the shark feeds on (16). Possible explanations for the precipitation of a shark attack include anomalous behavior by the shark, the violation of courtship patterns, or territorial invasion (27).

Initial management of the shark attack victim consists of basic trauma management: airway, breathing, bleeding control, and management of hemorrhagic blood loss (16, 57). The immediate life threat is hypovolemic shock and occasionally primary pulmonary or cardiac injury. Bleeding is controlled with compression and occasionally ligation of vessels. Wounds should be irrigated and debrided and packed open with primary closure. Tetanus toxoid at 0.5 ml intramuscularly, tetanus immune globulin at 250 to 400 U intramuscularly, and prophylaxis with penicillin, imipenem-cilastatin, an expanded-spectrum cephalosporin, chloramphenicol, or an aminoglycoside have been indicated (16, 17, 57). Wounds are susceptible to contamination by both aerobes and anaerobes, including *Aeromonas*, *Vibrio*, and clostridia (57). Buck and his colleagues cultured the teeth of a great white shark caught off Long Island and isolated the following organisms: *V. alginolyticus*, *V. parahaemolyticus*, *V. fluvialis*, *Pseudomonas putrefaciens*, and *Staphylococcus* species (63). As stated above (see "*Vibrio carchariae*"), *V. carchariae*, a newly recognized human pathogen, was responsible for a wound infection following a shark bite off the South Carolina coast (348).

Measures to be taken to avoid a confrontation with a shark include avoidance of shark-infested waters or waters near sewage outlets or deep channels (especially at night or dusk), never swimming with open wounds or in isolated waters, and storing captured fish away from divers (16, 57). If confronted with a shark, the swimmer should leave the water with slow, purposeful movements, facing the shark and avoiding the urge to flee rapidly. In deeper waters, the diver should seek refuge near a wall or other object offering protection from behind or find a confined area which the shark would have difficulty accessing. The shark may desist upon receiving blows to the snout, gills, or eyes.

Barracudas

Sphyraena barracuda, or the great barracuda, is the only species implicated in human attacks (16, 57). These fish may grow to 10 ft in length and weigh 100 lb. They can be found in tropical and semitropical waters of the Atlantic (Brazil to Florida) and the Pacific (Hawaii). Barracudas involved in attacks are usually solitary, although attacks by schools have occurred. Attacks are swift and ferocious and usually occur out of confusion in turbid waters or when barracudas are attracted by shiny objects. Their teeth are canine-like and sharp. The bite produces V-shaped or straight lacerations, often in rows. Treatment is analogous to that for shark bites.

Moray Eels

Moray eels (Fig. 3) are found in tropical, semitropical, and some temperate waters (16). They are fierce and muscular bottom dwellers that hide in crevices and under rocks and coral. Some species may grow up to 15 ft in length. Divers usually confront these creatures while probing around rocks and coral with their hands. Most smaller species flee when confronted. If provoked or cornered, an eel may inflict a serious laceration with its viselike jaws and fanglike teeth.

Occasionally, an eel does not release its grip. Attempts to disarticulate the jaw or kill the animal may be necessary. An eel's skin is leathery and may not be easily cut. Treatment is similar to that for shark bites (16).

Other Marine Animals

Needlefish are long, streamlined surface fish found in tropical waters that may attain lengths up to 2 m (16). They have a long, sharp snout which has been reported to occasionally impale people as this fish frequently jumps out of the water (273). Injuries have involved the chest, abdomen, neck, and head, with one case of a fatal brain injury (288).

Sea lions, especially mating males or females and their pups, can occasionally be aggressive (19). As these animals are mammals, rabies prophylaxis should be considered after sea lion bites (57).

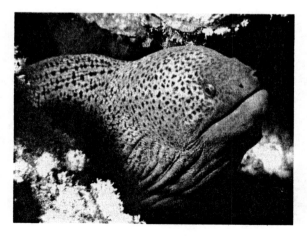

Figure 3. Moray eels usually flee when confronted. Fanglike teeth and viselike jaws allow it to inflict serious damage if confronted. Source: http://www.abc-kid.com/eel/index5.html.

Microbiology of Traumatic Marine Wounds

Most of the pathogenic bacteria in seawater are halophilic, heterotrophic, motile, gram-negative rods (17). The genus *Vibrio* represents one such group. The potential for a wound to become infected is based on several factors, including the size and extent of the wound and the colonization of the waters. Host factors tend to play a role as well, with immunosuppressed individuals more likely to develop systemic spread. One study in Hawaii of acute marine infections revealed an 11% incidence of *V. alginolyticus* wound isolates, with most of the other bacteria comprising flora typical of cutaneous infections (352).

Table 3. Microorganisms associated with marine wound infections and recommended antimicrobial therapies[a]

Microorganism	Therapy	
	First choice	Alternative
Aeromonas hydrophila	TMP-SMX[b]	Gentamicin; tetracycline
Bacteroides fragilis	Metronidazole	Clindamycin
Chromobacterium violaceum	Treatment should be guided by clinical presentation and in vitro susceptibility testing (mezlocillin and aminoglycoside have been used, according to a case report)	
Citrobacter diversus	Imipenem	Ciprofloxacin (or others if susceptible in vitro)
Clostridium perfringens	Penicillin G	Clindamycin; metronidazole
Enterobacter cloacae	Cefotaxime, ceftriaxone, or ceftizoxime + aminoglycoside	Imipenem; aminoglycoside; TMP-SMX; ciprofloxacin
Erysipelothrix rhusiopathiae	Penicillin G or ampicillin	Cephalosporins (e.g., cephalexin)
Escherichia coli	TMP-SMX	Cephalosporin; ampicillin; quinolones; aminoglycoside
Mycobacterium marinum	Minocycline	Rifampin + ethambutol; rifampin + TMP-SMX
Providencia stuartii	Cefotaxime, ceftriaxone, or ceftizoxime + aminoglycoside	Imipenem; aminoglycoside; sulfa-trimethoprim; ciprofloxacin
Pseudomonas aeruginosa	Aminoglycoside + antipseudomonal penicillin	Aminoglycoside + ceftazidime
Salmonella enterica serovar Enteritidis	Ceftriaxone	Ampicillin; ciprofloxacin; TMP-SMX
Staphylococcus aureus		
Methicillin sensitive	Penicillin-resistant synthetic	Vancomycin
Methicillin resistant	Penicillin-vancomycin	TMP-SMX (?)
Streptococcus species	Penicillin G	Erythromycin; clindamycin
Vibrio species (see text)	Tetracycline ± aminoglycoside (if systemic spread is suspected)	TMP-SMX (possibly quinolones if susceptible in vitro)

[a]With rapid emergence of antimicrobial resistance, these empirical recommendations should be confirmed by in vitro susceptibility testing.
[b]TMP-SMX, trimethoprim-sulfamethoxazole.

Minor wound infections may do well without antibiotics; however, individuals with liver disease, immunosuppressed individuals, and those with iron overload states may benefit from oral ciprofloxacin or the combination of trimethoprim and sulfamethoxazole (17). Penicillin, ampicillin, narrow-spectrum cephalosporins, and erythromycin are not acceptable alternatives. Potentially serious or complicated wounds should probably be treated with intravenous antibiotics, including cefoperazone, cefotaxime, ceftazidime, gentamicin, chloramphenicol, and tobramycin. Fulminant infections may be treated with a combination of imipenem and cilastatin. A minor wound infection with a classic erysipeloid reaction (*Erysipelothrix rhusiopathiae*) may be treated with penicillin, erythromycin, or cephalexin (Table 3).

VERTEBRATE ENVENOMATIONS

Stingrays

Eleven species of stingray are found in U.S. waters, of which seven are found in the Atlantic Ocean and four are found in the Pacific Ocean (17). Stingrays are frequently implicated in cases of human envenomation, with at least 2,000 stingray injuries recorded in the United States annually (57). They may be subdivided into four categories, which are (in ascending order of toxicity) the butterfly rays (gymnurid type), the eagle and bat rays (myliobatid type), the stingrays and whiprays (dasyatid type), and the round rays (urolophid type) (17). Stingrays are found in tropical, subtropical, and warm temperate waters in shallow intertidal areas such as bays, lagoons, river mouths, and sandy areas between reefs. These marine animals, which may reach up to 50 to 60 ft^2 in size, are round, diamond-shaped, or kite-shaped objects with wide winglike pectoral fins. They often lie on the surface bottom covered by sand with only their eyes, spiracles, or parts of their elongated, whiplike tail exposed. Stingrays have one to four venomous stingers arranged on the dorsum of the tail. The stingers consist of dentine spines which are tapered and retroserrated so they may enter the skin easily but are extracted with difficulty and worsening of the laceration (17). Each spine is covered by an integumentary sheath which houses a venom gland in the ventrolateral groove along either side. The spine is covered by a layer of venom and mucus. The venom is a highly unstable and very heat-labile protein consisting of at least 10 amino acids with toxic components such as serotonin, 5' nucleotidase, and phosphodiesterase (17, 173). Envenomation usually occurs when an unwary swimmer steps on the stingray while wading in shallow waters. The stingray in turn strikes the individual by lashing its tail upward, forcing its spines into the victim. The lower extremities are involved in most cases, although any part of the body is susceptible.

Initial manifestations consist of intense localized pain and soft tissue edema with bleeding (17, 411). The pain may intensify and spread over a period of 30 to 90 min and then gradually diminish over the next 6 to 48 h. Minor wounds resemble cellulitis; however, more severe wounds may appear dusky and cyanotic, with progression to rapid hemorrhage and necrosis of fat and muscle. Secondary infection is common (57).

The venom affects the cardiovascular system and can cause peripheral vasoconstriction or dilatation and cardiac arrhythmias (411). Respiratory depression (via the medullary centers) and convulsions may also occur. Other symptoms include nausea, vomiting, generalized edema (with truncal wounds), limb paralysis, and hypotension (17).

Initial treatment should consist of irrigation with cool water or saline to produce local vasoconstriction and debridement with exploration to remove any sheath contents left in the wound (17, 57). X rays should be obtained to identify any missed fragments. The wound should be soaked in hot water (113°F) for 30 to 90 min. The benefit of this probably has to do with the thermolabile nature of the protein. Narcotics and infiltration with 1 to 2% lidocaine without epinephrine may provide pain control. Regional-nerve anesthesia with 0.5% bupivacaine may be necessary (17). The wound should be packed open for primary closure or sutured loosely. Antibiotic prophylaxis is recommended. Steroids and antihistamines are without documented efficacy (57).

Scorpion Fish

Scorpion fish can be found in shallow reef waters of the Gulf of Mexico, the Florida Keys, and the coastlines of California and Hawaii (16). Members of this group are responsible for about 300 envenomations annually in the United States (381). Several hundred species are known to exist; they can be divided into three genera based on the structure of the venom glands: *Synanceja* (stonefish), *Scorpaena* (sculpin, scorpion fish, and bullrout), and *Pterois* (zebra fish, lionfish, and butterfly cod) (17, 57). Scorpion fish often hide under rocks, in coral crevices, or buried in the mud, blending in excellently with their surroundings due to their colorful and ornate camouflage. Stonefish are unattractive bottom dwellers which are regarded as the most lethal of these poisonous marine denizens. The potency of their venom is comparable to that of cobra venom. A small number of domestic envenomations occur in tropical fish hobbyists who carelessly handle illegally obtained scorpion fish (441). The venom organs consist of 12 to 13 dorsal, 2 pelvic, and 3 anal spines. The ornate pectoral spines are not venomous. Paired glands exist at the base of the anterolateral spines, and venom flows along grooves in these spines. Approximately 5 to 10 mg of venom may be found in each paired gland (17). When threatened, these fish erect the dorsal spines, flare out the armed gill covers, and protrude the pectoral and anal fins (18). Venom is injected in a manner analogous to a stingray envenomation. The potency of the venom varies according to the species. The pharmacology of scorpion fish venom is poorly understood (446). Wounds inflicted by lionfish are mild compared to those of scorpion fish, with stonefish wounds being the most severe (17).

Intense pain occurs immediately after the injury and radiates up the extremity (17, 57). If untreated, the pain peaks in 60 to 90 min, often lasting 6 to 12 h or perhaps days. Stonefish envenomation may produce pain severe enough to precipitate delusions (18). The wounds initially appear ischemic and cyanotic, with surrounding areas of erythema, edema, and warmth (17). Progressive cellulitis and local induration may follow, occasionally with vesicle formation. Tissue necrosis with sloughing may occur within 48 h. Wounds may take months to heal, with occasional soft tissue fibrous defects or cutaneous granulomata persisting. Secondary infection or deep abscesses may occur. Systemic effects include paresthesias, skin rash, nausea, vomiting, arthralgias, fever, diarrhea, delirium, seizures, abdominal pain, hypertension, arrhythmias, limb paralysis, congestive heart failure, hypotension, and death. In the case of stonefish envenomation, dyspnea and circulatory collapse may occur within 1 h, with death ensuing within 6 h (57).

Initial treatment of scorpion fish injuries is analogous to treatment of stingray injuries, with proper irrigation and debridement to ensure removal of any persistent source of venom (17, 57). Inadequate debridement may predispose to ulceration with tissue extension. Immersion in hot water (113°F) for 30 to 90 min may alleviate the pain possibly secondary to toxin inactivation; longer durations may be needed for persistent pain. Wounds should be packed open for primary closure or sutured loosely to allow drainage. Antibiotic therapy is recommended for deep puncture wounds of the hand or foot because of the high incidence of tissue complications (17). Recommended antibiotics include expanded-spectrum cephalosporins, trimethoprim-sulfamethoxazole, chloramphenicol, tetracycline, aminoglycosides, or imipenem-cilastatin (17). Severe systemic reactions due to *Synanceja* species (and less rarely from other scorpion fish) necessitate the use of intravenous stonefish equine antivenin. It is supplied in 2-ml ampoules; 1 ml is capable of neutralizing 10 mg of dried venom. Antivenins are produced in Australia and India and may be acquired in the United States from the Department of Health and Human Services; Sea World in San Diego; Sea World in Aurora, Ohio; and the Steinhart Aquarium in San Francisco, Calif. Physicians may alternatively locate antivenin by contacting an accredited regional poison center (17).

Sea Snakes

Sea snakes are probably the most abundant reptiles in the world. Fifty-two species are known, and all are venomous (18). At least 7 species have been implicated in fatal envenomations (57). Sea snakes are marine-adapted serpents belonging to the family Hydrophidae and are close relatives of cobras and kraits. They are widely distributed in tropical and subtropical waters along the coasts of the Indian and Pacific Oceans and the Gulf of California. There are no sea snakes in the Atlantic Ocean or Caribbean Sea (18, 57). These reptiles have a flat tail which assists them in propulsion. They can travel with ease in both the forward and reverse directions. Some species may attain lengths of up to 10 ft. These creatures can remain submerged in the water for hours, utilizing an air retention system to control buoyancy. Although usually docile, they may attack when provoked, especially during the mating season (18). Sea snakes have 2 to 4 maxillary fangs, each of which is associated with a pair of venom glands. The fangs of most species are too short to penetrate a diver's wet suit (17). Many envenomations are avoided by the fact that the fangs are easily dislodged. The venom is more potent than terrestrial-snake venom, and its toxicity is derived primarily from potent neurotoxins (446). Neurotoxins may exert their effects through the inhibition of cholinesterase or by blocking presynaptic or postsynaptic impulses. Most sea snake venom contains only postsynaptic neurotoxin, which strongly binds to the acetylcholine receptor at the neuromuscular junction. The venom may contain other toxins, including hyaluronidase, phosphodiesterase, phospholipase A, and proteases (446). Phospholipase A and other myotoxins may cause muscle necrosis with myoglobin release (412). These myotoxic, hemolytic, neurotoxic, and vasoactive components constitute a serious medical emergency if envenomation occurs.

The bites are extremely small and characterized by multiple pinhead, hypodermic-like puncture wounds numbering from 1 to 20 (18). Initially, the pain is only minimal, without any local reaction. Neurological symptoms occur within 2 to 3 h in most cases and always within 8 h of the bite. If no symptoms develop within 8 h, significant envenomation did not occur. Typical signs and symptoms include painful muscle movement, myoglobinuria, euphoria, trismus, malaise, anxiety, ascending paralysis, slurred speech, dysphagia, ptosis, and ophthalmoplegia. Death is rare and is usually due to more severe reactions, including myonecrosis, respiratory insufficiency, bulbar paralysis, and hepatic, cardiac, or renal failure (17, 19).

Diagnosis is based on several factors, such as location (sea snake bites occur only in the water), absence of pain (initial pain is unusual), typical appearance of the fang bites (usually 1 to 4), identification of the snake (it should be caught if possible), and development of characteristic symptoms within 8 h (occasionally as early as 5 min) (16).

Treatment is similar to that for most terrestrial-snake bites (17). Local suction without incision can be performed if done immediately with a plunger device. Incision and drainage are of no value if delayed for several minutes after the bite, and cryotherapy is contraindicated. The affected limb should be immobilized with application of a proximal venous and lymphatic occlusive band or use of the pressure immobilization technique (a cloth pad is pressed directly over the wound by a circumferential elastic wrap at a pressure of ≤70 mm Hg) to minimize systemic toxicity. Antivenin is effective if used within 24 to 36 h and should be used quickly (445). The minimum initial dose of sea snake antivenin is 1 to 3 vials; up to 10 vials may be required. Polyvalent equine antivenin to *Enhydrina schistosa* (the beaked sea snake) and *Notechis scutatus* (the terrestrial tiger snake) neutralizes the bites of most sea snakes. Anaphylaxis and serum sickness may occur, and intradermal sensitivity testing with 0.02 ml of a 1:10 antivenin dilution should be done. *N. scutatus* antivenin is a second-choice alternative (17). Antivenin in the United States may be obtained from the sources listed above for scorpion fish.

Weeverfish

Weeverfish, also referred to as sea cats, sea dragons, adderpike, and stang, are found in the temperate waters of the Atlantic Ocean and Mediterranean Sea and in European coastal waters (19). Weeverfish are among the most venomous fish found in these waters. They are small fish (<50 cm) that can be found buried in the mud or soft bottom with only their head exposed. They produce a venom located in glands associated with dorsal and opercular dentine spines which are capable of piercing a leather boot. Weeverfish are generally docile, yet if provoked, they may become extremely aggressive and strike. Victims are usually professional fishermen or wading swimmers.

The venom is a heat-labile protein substance which also contains 5-hydroxytryptamine, histamine, epinephrine, and norepinephrine (446). An intense burning pain is felt immediately following the sting (19). The pain often spreads throughout the entire limb and generally peaks in intensity within the first hour and usually subsides within 24 h, although it may persist for days. The initial wound is pale and edematous and becomes erythematous, warm, and ecchymotic, with increasing edema. It may take months to heal. Headache, delirium, fever, dyspnea, diaphoresis, nausea, vomiting, seizures, hypotension, and cardiac arrhythmias may occur (16).

Treatment is analogous to that for stingray envenomations. The pain is often poorly controlled even with the liberal use of narcotics (16). An antivenin may be available soon (57). Weeverfish should never be handled when alive; they may survive for hours out of water (19).

Catfish

More than 1,000 species of freshwater and saltwater catfish exist (57). These fish are named for the sensory barbels, resembling cat whiskers, surrounding the mouth. Catfish have long thin venom glands covered by an integumentary sheath located on lateral ridges along the dorsal and pectoral spines (321). Catfish may lock these fins in an extended position when excited, thereby inflicting a dramatic sting if mishandled. Fragments of tissue and spine may remain in the wound. The venom contains dermonecrotic, vasoconstrictive, and other bioactive agents (57). Immediate severe pain, throbbing, and weakness occur. The pain usually radiates locally and proximally and generally resolves in 30 to 60 min, occasionally lasting for 48 h. Nausea, vomiting, respiratory distress, and mild hypotension may occur. Muscle fasciculations and local muscle spasms are common. The wound site may appear pale and bleed longer than expected. Cyanosis at the puncture site may occur, followed by local tissue necrosis or skin sloughing. Swelling of the extremity, a serous discharge, slow wound healing, and local lymphadenopathy may persist for weeks to months (321). Secondary infections are common, and gangrene has been reported. Envenomation by the oriental catfish (*Plotosus lineatus*) may produce more marked systemic symptoms (57).

Treatment is analogous to that for stingray envenomations, although the venom is not as potent (16). X rays should be obtained, as the radiopaque spines are frequently left in place. The wound should be thoroughly irrigated and debrided. Irrigation with permanganate, bicarbonate, acetic acid, or papain has not been shown to be of benefit. Tourniquets have no value (16). Updating of tetanus immunization, as in other marine puncture wounds, is essential. Antibiotics should be administered if the wound is dirty or complicated. Local wound care alone is probably adequate for properly treated clean wounds in healthy individuals (321).

INVERTEBRATE ENVENOMATIONS

Coelenterates

The phylum Cnidaria (formerly Coelenterata) is a massive group of marine invertebrates consisting of more than 9,000 species, of which at least 100 are hazardous to humans (17). The classes in this phylum are Scyphozoa (true jellyfish), Hydrozoa (fire coral, Portuguese man-of-war, and Pacific bluebottle), and Anthozoa (sea anemones and soft coral) (176). These species may contain millions of nematocysts (also known as "stinging capsules" or "nettle cells"), which are microscopic toxin-containing organs capable of injecting venom into their prey when triggered. Nematocysts are found along the outside of long streaming tentacles and near the mouth of the animal. Each nematocyst consists of a minute capsule (cnidoblast) that contains a spiral-coiled thread with a barbed end. Specialized triggers (cnidocils) on the capsule are capable of forcefully ejecting the venomous barbs at pressures of up to 2 to 5 lb/in^2, enough to penetrate a surgical glove (57). This produces a severe sting. The size of the barb and the potency of the venom vary among the different species. The cnidocil may be triggered by abrasion or freshwater contact. A single man-of-war envenomation may involve several hundred thousand nematocysts (16).

The human reactions to jellyfish toxin may be classified as systemic, local, chronic, or fatal (66). Local reactions include persistent or recurrent eruptions, eruptions distant to the site of envenomation, exaggerated local angioedema, papular urticaria, and contact dermatitis. Chronic reactions include keloid formation, pigmentation, fat atrophy, mononeuritis, autonomic nerve paralysis, gangrene, vascular spasm, and ataxia. Systemic reactions may include muscle cramps, nausea, vomiting, tachycardia, abdominal pain, and hypertension. Death may occur through cardiotoxic, central respiratory, or renal mechanisms. Anaphylaxis has been reported (440).

The potency and composition of the toxin vary among different species. After injection of large doses of toxin into human skin, a perivascular mononuclear cell infiltrate appears within the dermis. A cell-mediated and humoral immune response then occurs. Lymphokines and prostaglandins account for some of the cutaneous manifestations of jellyfish envenomation (65). Serotonin, histamine, or histamine-releasing agents are responsible for much of the burning pain and urticaria. High-molecular-weight toxins may inhibit nerve activity through altered ionic permeability. These protein and tetramine fractions have direct and indirect effects on the autonomic nervous system and end organs, particularly the vascular, cardiac, and central nervous systems. A destabilizing effect on the cell membrane appears to be mediated by the calcium channel. Verapamil may block this effect (57).

Fire corals (*Millepora* spp.) are not true corals. They are branching bottom dwellers which may attain heights of 1 to 2 m. They develop upright, clavate, bladelike, or branching calcareous growths that form encrustations over rocks, shellfish, other coral, and man-made objects. The white to yellow-green lime carbonate exoskeleton may become razor sharp. The nematocyst-bearing tentacles protrude from numerous minute surface gastropores (18). These stings account for the majority of coelenterate envenomations. An intense burning pain, with central radiation and reactive regional lymphadenopathy, follows envenomation (17).

The Portuguese man-of-war (*Physalia physalis*) (Fig. 4) and the Pacific bluebottle (*Physalia utriculus*) are not true jellyfish; they are colonial hydroids (176). These open-sea surface creatures are widely distributed in the Atlantic (*P. physalis*) and Pacific (*P. utriculus*) Oceans, although both are most commonly found in the semitropical Atlantic Ocean. They are composed of a large nitrogen and carbon monoxide-filled sail which may achieve lengths up to 30 cm across. Numerous nematocyst-laden tentacles (up to 750,000 nematocysts per tentacle) stream downward from the sail, attaining lengths of up to 30 m (*P. physalis*). The animal is carried along by wind and ocean currents. Fish and other objects may become entangled in the tentacles, which contract rhythmically in search of prey. Broken-off tentacle fragments may retain their potency for months (16).

Chironex fleckeri (the box jellyfish or sea wasp) is the most venomous sea creature known (16). Death may occur within 1 min of envenomation, and the overall mortality rate has been reported to be as high as 20%, although this number may be inflated, as evidenced by more recent studies (343). These creatures are found in the protected waters off the northern Australian coast. There have been 55 confirmed deaths to date due to stings from these creatures (326). A less lethal variety is found in the waters of the Chesapeake Bay (57). Up to 10 ml of venom may be injected during a "sting." They are small creatures (2 to 10 cm in diameter) capable of attaining speeds up to 2 knots in steady winds with swift currents. Factors

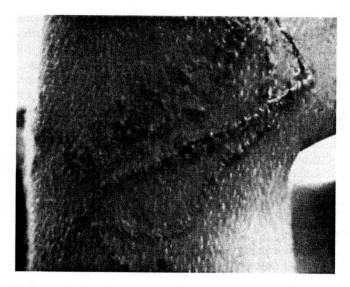

Figure 4. The sting of the Portuguese man-of-war is one of the most painful conditions known to afflict the skin. The wrapping of the tentacles typically results in linear circumferential stripes, which are caused by the deposition of urticariogenic and irritant substances and not by the force of the swing. Reprinted from reference 459a with permission.

determining the severity of envenomation include the length and width of the wheal, the length of the contact, the thickness of the skin, the percentage of nematocysts discharged, and the "venom load," which is related to recent feeding (284). A sheep-derived antivenin is available and is given intravenously or intramuscularly (20,000 U, or one vial, intravenously over 5 min or three vials intramuscularly) (284). Verapamil is contraindicated (435).

Sea anemones are sessile, multicolored, flowerlike anthozoans which may attain diameters of up to 0.5 m (16). They have fingerlike projections containing numerous modified nematocysts referred to as sporocysts. They are usually encountered by skin divers and waders.

The Irukundji syndrome may follow stings by a jellyfish (*Carukia barnesi*) of the class Cubozoa (66). A small but transient sting initiates this reaction. A severe, boring pain may develop in the abdomen or sacrum, with gradual spread to the thighs and chest, where the sensation is described as cramping. Severe, excruciating myalgia persists over the next 24 to 48 h. Other symptoms include tremor, anxiety, piloerection, hyperpnea, headache, nausea, vomiting, sweating, restlessness, tachycardia, blood-streaked sputum, and oliguria. A rapidly developing pulmonary edema leading to acute respiratory failure may develop (145). This syndrome, similar to excess catecholamine release, is assumed to represent a toxic reaction to the venom of the small jellyfish (66).

The person who has endured a coelenterate sting should immediately soak the area in 5% acetic acid (vinegar) (17). Isopropyl alcohol (40 to 70%) is a reasonable alternative, although some argue that this may cause further venom release. Other detoxicants of possible benefit include dilute ammonium hydroxide, sodium bicarbonate, olive oil, sugar, urine, and papain (unseasoned meat tenderizer). Fresh water should never be applied to the area, as this may trigger further nematocyst release. The area should be soaked for at least 30 min or until the pain disappears. The area should not be abraded or scrubbed. Any large tentacles or remaining fragments should be removed by a forceps with doubly gloved hands. Once cleaned, shaving cream should be applied and the area shaved gently.

Anaphylaxis should always be anticipated. After decontamination, corticosteroids or topical anesthetics can be used. Antibiotics are usually not needed; however, large open lesions should be cleaned daily and covered with a thin layer of nonsensitizing antiseptic ointment. Tetanus immunization should be current. Wounds should be checked by a physician for signs of infection 3 and 7 days after the injury.

Echinoderms

Sea urchins (Fig. 5) and starfish are found in the echinoderm group of marine animals. The venom contains many toxic substances, including steroid glycosides, serotonin, and acetylcholine-like substances. Certain sea urchins may produce potent neurotoxins (16).

Sea urchins are globular or flattened animals with a hard shell enclosing their vital organs (18). Regularly arranged spines and a triple-jawed seizing organ (pedicellariae) cover this shell. Spines may be venom bearing or not. The pedicel-

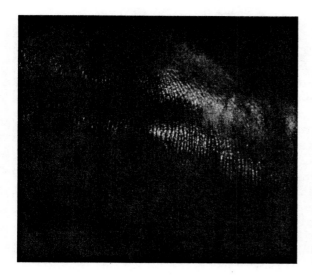

Figure 5. Wounds caused by a sea urchin. Sea urchins have spines that may be several inches long. When stepped upon by an unwary swimmer, the spines may be driven deep into the skin and break off, resulting in an extremely painful injury. Secondary infections are nearly inevitable if the spines are left in. Reprinted from reference 459a with permission.

lariae are dispersed among the spines and may grab hold with their pincerlike jaws. They also contain venom glands that release toxic material when they contract. The venom inflicts intense burning stings which may progress to muscular paralysis, respiratory distress, and occasionally death if numerous spines are involved. Hot water may provide relief. The pedicellariae and embedded spines should be removed with care because they are easily fractured. Residual spines may form granulomas (17).

Starfish are simple, free-living, stellate echinoderms covered with simple thorny spines of calcium carbonate crystals held erect by muscle tissue (18). Glandular tissue interspersed throughout or located beneath the integument produces a slimy, venomous substance that causes a contact dermatitis. Envenomation occurs when the victim contacts the thorny spines, some of which may grow to 6 cm in length. Envenomation can, rarely, induce systemic symptoms, including paresthesias, vomiting, and muscular paralysis. The dermatitis may be treated with hot water and topical calamine with 0.5% menthol.

Mollusks

Cone shells are potentially lethal gastropods that possess a sophisticated venom apparatus (16). At least 18 to 400 species have been implicated in human fatalities. They are nocturnal feeders and are found in the Indo-Pacific area. A set of minute harpoon-like radular teeth may contain venom which is injected from an extensible proboscis. The venom interferes with neuromuscular transmission in a manner analogous to curare. Initial symptoms include local ischemia, cyanosis, and numbness. More severe envenomations may induce paresthesias and generalized muscular paralysis with respiratory failure. Other symptoms include dysphagia, aphonia, weakness, diplopia, blurred vision, cerebral edema, disseminated intravascular coagulation, coma, and cardiovascular collapse. Death may occur in as little as 2 h. Therapy is largely supportive. Hot-water immersions may alleviate some of the pain.

Octopuses are cephalopods found in the warm waters of the intertidal zone (16). The Australian spotted (*Octopus maculosus*) and blue-ringed (*Octopus lunulatus*) octopuses have been implicated in human fatalities. The blue-ringed octopus is covered with poorly visible blue rings which become iridescent peacock blue when the octopus is angered. Parrot-like and powerful chitinous jaws are capable of penetrating through the dermis of the skin and into the muscle tissue. Venom is injected into the victim, who is usually a naive swimmer playing with what seems to be a harmless creature. The toxin blocks nerve conduction most likely by altering sodium conductance. Myocardial and respiratory depression are observed in animal models. Following the initial bite, an intense burning or throbbing with central radiation occurs. Within 30 min, marked local erythema, swelling, pruritus, and pain may occur. Severe envenomations include nausea, vomiting, paresthesias, blurred vision, aphonia, dysphagia, ataxia, myoclonus, flaccid paralysis, hypotension, and respiratory failure. Treatment is supportive, with wide excision of the involved area down to deep fascia. Closure may be primary or by a full-thickness skin graft. There is no effective antivenin available.

Dermatitis

Most cases of dermatitis in swimmers and beachgoers are the result of contact with the Coelenterata. In 1991, an outbreak of cercarial dermatitis was noted among 37 students frequenting a Delaware beach. In 1999, 63 confirmed cases of cercarial dermatitis were reported among 450 families swimming near a snail-infested beach near the city of Quebec, Canada (267). Cercarial dermatitis, or "swimmer's itch," is a cutaneous inflammation due to penetration of the skin by cercariae, which are the free-living larval stages of bird schistosomes (76). Hosts include migratory waterbirds, including shorebirds, ducks, and geese. Adult worms are carried in the bloodstream and produce eggs that are passed in the feces. Once exposed to the water, the eggs hatch to produce miracidia, which infect mollusks. The parasite develops in the snail to produce cercariae, which penetrate the skin of birds to complete the cycle. Humans are accidental hosts. The cercariae are able to penetrate the skin but do not develop further.

This dermatologic entity has a worldwide distribution. Symptoms include reddening and itching of exposed skin in the water or immediately after emerging and delayed onset of pruritic raised papules which may form vesicles. Previous exposure may elicit a more severe response upon reexposure. Treatment consists of antihistamines and topical antipruritic medications.

Cutaneous larva migrans is a dermatitis caused by invasion of the skin by larval nematodes (328). Most infections are due to the filariform larvae of the dog and cat hookworm, *Ancylostoma braziliense*, although several other larval nematodes may cause the disease, including *Ancylostoma caninum*, *Ancylostoma duodenale*, and *Necator americanus*. Adult *A. braziliense* inhabits the intestines of dogs and cats. It produces eggs which pass in the feces to hatch in the soil in 1 to 2 days. Within a week, the organisms become infective filariform larvae. Humans are inadvertent hosts when the larvae penetrate the skin, although they usually do not penetrate further than the epidermis. The disease has a worldwide distribution and is much more common in tropical and semitropical areas. People who frequent beaches are at increased risk (hence the synonym "sandworm").

Symptoms develop within a few hours of penetration into the skin. An itching red papule develops which may form a serpiginous track. The surrounding tissues become edematous and acutely inflamed. The tracks may become encrusted and secondarily infected. The pruritus may become extremely intense. Untreated, the larvae may persist in the skin for months. Treatment consists of thiabendazole administered orally or topically.

SWIMMER'S EAR

Swimmer's ear, or acute otitis externa, is the most common medical problem faced by swimmers (393). It begins initially not as an infection but as an eczema of the ear canal caused by retention of water in the ear following bathing, showering, or swimming (382). By the time medical attention is sought, the ear is usually secondarily infected. The normal external auditory canal is sterile bacteriologically in up to 30% of the population, with the remainder harboring mixed flora, including *Staphylococcus albus*, *Staphylococcus epidermidis*, diphtheroids, and to a lesser extent, *Staphylococcus aureus* and viridans group streptococci (31, 417). In external otitis media, cultures usually reveal mixed flora, with gram-negative bacteria predominating in up to three-quarters of affected individuals under the age of 21 years. *Pseudomonas* species, the most common offending organisms, are isolated in up to one-half of the cases (69). Other species include *Proteus vulgaris*, *E. coli*, *S. aureus*, *S. epidermidis*, streptococci, diphtheroids, *Enterobacter aerogenes*, *Klebsiella pneumoniae*, and *Citrobacter* spp. Approximately 40% of infected ears yield fungal isolates, with *Aspergillus* species representing the majority of such (393).

The pathogenesis of swimmer's ear is multifactorial, with cerumen playing a major role. Cerumen imparts an acid reaction to the external canal, lowering its pH to 5, thereby inhibiting bacterial and fungal growth. In addition, its lipid content provides a protective surface to the squamous epithelium and pilosebaceous elements of the canal. Cerumen, therefore, provides a chemical and mechanical barrier to infection. Excessive moisture in the external canal, which can occur during swimming, bathing, or excessive sweating, can lead to mechanical disruption of this barrier, with subsequent desquamation and maceration. In addition, the decrease in cerumen results in a raising of the pH to 7, which allows bacterial species to proliferate. As inflammation occurs, a purulent exudate forms which mixes with the dry skin, providing a wet environment suitable for bacterial growth.

The earliest symptom is usually itching, which often leads to manipulation (393). Trauma from cotton swabs or mechanical objects inserted into the canal can exacerbate the condition. A purulent discharge develops accompanied by progressive tenderness and pain. Hearing loss may result from canal skin edema and accumulation of debris. The diagnosis can be confirmed by manipulation of the tragus and pinna, which elicits a severe painful reaction. Attempts at otoscopic visualization may be hampered by the pain as well as the accumulation of debris. Regional lymphadenopathy and cellulitis of the external auricle can occasionally occur. Fungal otitis externa may be accompanied only by itching and a feeling of fullness. In these cases, hyphae may be visualized on microscopic examination, or in the case of *Aspergillus niger*, a grayish membrane may be noted in the external canal.

Initial treatment should begin with the recognition and elimination of specific precipitating factors, such as swimming or manipulation of the ear, until the disorder is corrected (393). Pain control may be necessary during the first 24 to 48 h of treatment (399). Severe cases may require narcotic analgesics or even hospitalization for intramuscular analgesics and intravenous antibiotics. Thorough irrigation and cleaning are essential to remove the purulent debris and allow penetration by topical antibiotics. Various cleansing solutions have been utilized, including 3% acetic acid, 70% alcohol, 3% boric acid–70% alcohol solution, and Burow's solution (393). Cleansing and irrigation may be required on a daily basis. In cases where the debris is too thick, an expanding cellulose wick may be implanted within the canal to allow antibiotic penetration.

Topical antibiotics are usually adequate in all but the most severe cases, which may require systemic agents. The most widely prescribed otic solutions contain the antibiotics neomycin and polymyxin, which are effective against most of the usual pathogens. Neomycin is effective against *Proteus* and *Staphylococcus* species; polymyxin is usually effective against *Pseudomonas*. Chloromycetin otic drops are available for less commonly encountered anaerobic infections. In the event of otitis externa due to *A. niger*, local application of amphotericin B, oxytetracycline and polymyxin, clioquinol, and nystatin may be effective (393). Candidal infections may be treated with topical nystatin. Most otic preparations also contain an acidifying agent(s) and a topical steroid to reduce the inflammation.

Individuals prone to otitis externa who are frequently exposed to water may benefit from any of several commercially available earplugs and other devices which prevent water from entering the canal. A recent comparison of seven different ear protectors used by a group of swimmers found the most effective plugs to be cotton wool coated in paraffin jelly (373). Prevention may be further enhanced by the use of acidifying drops and/or drying ear drops before and after swimming. Domeboro, Swim Ear, Aqua Ear, Ear Magic, and VoSol Otic drops are several such agents (393). Alternatively, the user may make his or her own preparation by mixing white vinegar with 70% alcohol. Controversy exists with regard to swimming with tympanostomy tubes in place (214, 280, 296). While some experts advocate the use of protective earplugs or avoidance of water immersion, others have recommended pre- and postexposure antibiotic otic drops. A third group utilizing data revealing that the incidence of otitis media was no greater in swimmers with tympanostomy tubes in place who swam without protection than in those without tympanostomy tubes has suggested that no ear protection or instillation of pre- and postexposure antibiotic drops is necessary (155, 214, 262, 280, 480). Until this matter is clarified, it may be prudent to advocate some means of protection against infection in prone individuals who are frequently exposed to water (393).

VIRAL HEPATITIS AND OTHER VIRUSES ASSOCIATED WITH WATER AND SHELLFISH

Marine samples of water have been estimated to yield between 5×10^6 and 15×10^6 total viruses per ml (33). Even though the majority of these viruses are non-pathogenic in humans, viral agents associated with hepatitis and gastroenteritis are known to be present in and capable of producing disease through contaminated water (111, 112). Samples of water taken off the Texas Gulf Coast have revealed the presence of enteroviruses such as coxsackievirus, echovirus, poliovirus, and hepatitis A virus (152). These enteroviruses were detected in over 40% of waters deemed safe for recreational use by fecal-coliform standards. Thirty-five percent of waters approved for shellfish harvesting yielded enteroviruses (152). Enteroviruses have been reported to survive for 2 to 130 days in seawater in laboratory studies (294) and possibly for up to 18 months (165). Temperature seems to be the most important factor, with many enteroviruses able to survive for months at temperatures below 10°C (153). Marine sediments also protect against virus inactivation, probably by reducing the rate of thermal inactivation (153).

Although controversy about their role exists, swimming areas have been suggested to be involved in the spread of some common viral illnesses (67, 388). In Wisconsin, a statistically significant increase was noted in the use of public beaches by children with documented enteroviral illness compared to children without enteroviral illness (67, 115, 388). Several other reports have similarly suggested increased enteroviral infections in swimmers using public swimming areas (58, 67, 71, 388; J. W. Mosely, presented at an international symposium on discharge of sewage from sea outfalls, 1974). A survey of oysters contaminated by enteroviruses in Japan found nearly identical viruses in sick children in the immediate area. The authors suggested that water and oyster contamination ultimately depends on the prevalence of enteric viral infections by local inhabitants (483). In addition to more common and less severe enteroviral illnesses, an outbreak of hepatitis A involving 20 campers in Louisiana was associated with swimming in a contaminated swimming pool (286).

Shellfish harvested from contaminated waters have been implicated in numerous outbreaks of food-borne illness (458). They spread disease by virtue of their ability to filter large amounts of water, retain filtered products in the gills and alimentary tract, and accumulate them in the liver. Shellfish have the ability to concentrate hepatitis A virus at up to 15 times the level in the immediate water (M. Hu, T. Li, and X. Hu, Abstr. IXth Int. Congr. Infect. Parasitic Dis., p. 688, 1986). Commercially harvested waters are monitored for contamination through the use of bacterial counts. Although this method effectively decreases the incidence of illness related to contaminated shellfish, there is not a reliable correlation between bacterial counts and the presence of pathogenic viruses (152). Several methods of detecting viruses or viral particles have been investigated, although the use of any one method of testing may not be sufficient to provide accurate measurements (483). Furthermore, viral testing has proven to be costly and time consuming (174). Control measures have included the regulation of drainage effluent into monitored areas, supervision of drainage from commercial fishing boats, frequent testing of water and shellfish from harvest areas for fecal coliforms and other bacteria, closing of contaminated waters, and removal of contaminated shellfish from markets (174). Depuration measures in which bacteria and viruses are removed by bathing in rapidly circulating salt water treated continuously by UV radiation for up to 72 h have decreased the incidence of food-borne outbreaks, although this process is not infallible (132, 462). Outbreaks of viral diseases have been attributed to depurated shellfish (182). Prevention of illness additionally relies on public education, particularly in regard to proper cooking of shellfish. It has been shown that it takes up to 6 min of steaming for the internal temperature of clams to reach that of the immediate surrounding (249). Clams open their shells in less than 1 min. Hepatitis A virus has been shown to be inactivated by heating at 85°C for 1 min and partially inactivated by heating at 60°C for 60 min (290, 395). Recent evidence suggests that microwaving may be beneficial in inactivating hepatitis A virus; however, further studies are needed (300).

Hepatitis A Virus

Hepatitis A was first linked to the ingestion of raw shellfish in Sweden in 1956; 629 oyster-associated cases were documented (377). The first cases of hepatitis A linked to raw-shellfish consumption in the United States occurred in 1961; both clams and oysters were involved (356). Hepatitis A virus caused less than 7% of the 224 recorded outbreaks of waterborne disease in the United States between 1971 and 1978; it caused none of the outbreaks recorded in 1981 (179, 364). From 1983 to 1988, the incidence of reported cases of hepatitis A increased from 9.2 to 10.9 cases per 100,000 population, which represented the first increase in hepatitis A in more than a decade (79, 80, 83, 84). In 1988, 26,600 cases of hepatitis A were reported in the United States, 7.3% of which were associated with food-borne or waterborne outbreaks (80, 84). In August 1988, 61 persons developed hepatitis A after having ingested oysters illegally harvested from coastal waters off Bay County, Fla. (78, 122, 123). That same year, the largest documented epidemic to date occurred in Shanghai, China, in which more than 288,000 people developed hepatitis A after ingesting raw or improperly cooked clams (174, 427).

Shellfish implicated in cases of hepatitis A include oysters, clams, cockles, and mussels (11). In addition, the illness has been traced to contaminated lettuce, raspberries, ice-slush beverages, and community water sources (78, 367, 379, 458). Sporadic cases also occur, and the disease is probably underreported. Restaurant-related outbreaks due to poor personal hygiene by infected food preparers have also been noted (11, 300). In many cases, a source for outbreaks is never determined (78, 300).

The incubation period ranges from 3 to 6 weeks. Presentation consists of a prodrome of fatigue, malaise, anorexia, nausea, and right upper quadrant discomfort. Dark urine subsequently develops, with liver enlargement and biochemical evidence of hepatitis. Icteric disease may be prolonged in adults, lasting 4 to 6 weeks; fulminant hepatic failure is rare, and chronic disease or a carrier state does not develop. Secondary cases in families may be seen. Attack rates vary, ranging from 10 to 97% with higher rates associated with increasing dose and age (140, 458). A vaccine is currently available for use in persons over 2 years of age (87).

Norwalk Virus

Norwalk virus is the most common infectious cause of acute gastroenteritis following shellfish ingestion (140). Named after the town in Ohio in which an outbreak of acute gastroenteritis occurred in 1968, this virus was not identified until 1972, by immune electron microscopy of bacterium-free stool isolates from the 1968 outbreak (128). The particles measured 27 nm and were noted to be more visible when present in clusters covered with antibody. They were also noted to aggregate with convalescent- but not acute-phase sera from patients with the gastroenteritis. A serum radioimmunoassay for IgM antibody to Norwalk virus or the demonstration of a fourfold rise in titers utilizing paired acute- and convalescent-phase sera is more sensitive and specific than electron microscopy (140, 171, 230). Using similar methods, Norwalk virus was identified as the cause of 42% of the 74 outbreaks of acute, nonbacterial gastroenteritis investigated by the CDC between 1976 and 1980 (111, 112, 179, 230). Six additional outbreaks involving more than 820 persons were noted between 1981 and 1983 (111, 112). Drinking water and recreational water used for swimming were the vehicles of transmission in most of these earlier outbreaks. Contamination by human sewage was the most likely explanation, although this was never proven. Shellfish-associated Norwalk virus illness was first recognized in Australia in 1978, when 2,000 people developed acute gastroenteritis after raw-oyster ingestion (322). Immune electron microscopy of 93 stool specimens revealed the 27-nm viral particle in 39% of those examined. An additional, as-yet-unclarified 22-nm viral particle was also identified in 50% of the specimens examined. In 1982, 103 well-documented outbreaks of oyster- and clam-associated illness involving 1,017 persons were attributed to Norwalk virus in New York State in 1982 (318). Seroconversion to Norwalk virus antibody or a positive response for IgM antibody to the virus (or both) was noted in five of seven outbreaks; radioimmunoassay revealed Norwalk virus antibody in four of six clam and oyster specimens examined, including clams and oysters from two of the outbreaks. Testing of the waters from which the shellfish were harvested showed that coliform levels were well within acceptable limits. In 2002, 21 outbreaks of acute gastroenteritis due to Norwalk virus occurred on 17 cruise ships, demonstrating how easily Norwalk virus can be transmitted from person to person in a closed environment (90).

Incubation times have ranged from 24 to 48 h in most recorded outbreaks, with a duration of illness ranging from 2 to 60 h (mean, 12 to 60 h). Symptoms have consisted of nausea, vomiting, diarrhea, abdominal cramps, and headache, with vomiting being more prominent than diarrhea in children and diarrhea being more common than vomiting in adults. Fever, myalgia, chills, and upper respiratory complaints, such as a sore throat, cough, and runny nose, were also noted on occasion. The disease is rarely severe enough to require hospitalization, and no fatalities have been recorded. Secondary spread is quite common.

The antibody response is not entirely understood. Antibody prevalence appears to peak within the first five decades of life, reaching a prevalence in the United States of 50%. Children tend to acquire antibody earlier in less developed countries. Individuals exposed to the Norwalk agent who do not become ill in volunteer studies have been shown to not develop an antibody response. When immunity develops, it is specific to the Norwalk virus and short-lived, lasting from 6 weeks to 2 months (128).

The mechanism by which Norwalk virus causes diarrhea is not known. Related agents include the Hawaii, Snow Mountain, and Taunton agents, named after the places where they were first described. Only the Snow Mountain agent has been associated with waterborne transmission. Illnesses caused by these Norwalk-like agents are indistinguishable from that due to the Norwalk agent. These other agents are antigenically distinct, and antibodies are not cross-protective (458).

Hepatitis E Virus

Hepatitis E virus is the only known cause of enterically transmitted non-A, non-B hepatitis. Hepatitis E virus is largely waterborne and has been responsible for epidemics of infectious hepatitis in parts of Asia, Indonesia, Africa, and Mexico (162). Previously known as enterically transmitted non-A, non-B hepatitis, illness due to hepatitis E virus was first documented in New Delhi, India, in 1955, when 29,000 cases of icteric hepatitis were identified following fecal contamination of the city's water supply (454). A similar epidemic occurred in 1975 in Ahmedabad, India, when the city's water supply became fecally contaminated as well (413). Both epidemics were thought to be due to hepatitis A virus until retrospectively analyzed paired serum samples from documented cases revealed in 1980 that neither hepatitis A nor hepatitis B virus was responsible for the epidemics (471). It now appears that in developing countries, more than 50% of acute viral hepatitis cases are caused by agents other than hepatitis A or B virus (53). Numerous epidemics of hepatitis E have been reported in Pakistan, Bangladesh, Nepal, Burma, Borneo, Algeria, Somalia, Sudan, Ivory Coast, Mexico, the People's Republic of China, Egypt, Ethiopia, and the former Soviet Union (162, 444). Imported cases have been reported in the United States (T. Bader, K. Krawczynski, and M. Favorov, Letter, *N. Engl. J. Med.* 325:1659, 1991). One case acquired in San Jose, Calif., has been described (254).

The incubation period appears to be 2 to 9 weeks, with an average of 6 weeks (53). Attack rates have been variable, with the highest rates noted in young to middle-aged adults (15 to 40 years old). The clinical presentation is that of a self-limiting disease resembling infection due to hepatitis A virus. Chronic liver disease or persistent viremia has not been reported. The mortality rate has been reported to be 0.5 to 3.0% in the general population. Women in the third trimester of pregnancy have an unusually high mortality rate, up to 20%, for unknown reasons. In contrast, pregnant women infected with hepatitis A virus have a mortality rate ranging from 3 to 8%.

The diagnosis of infection due to hepatitis E virus has primarily been based on identification of the virus in stool samples by immune electron microscopy. Hepatitis E virus is a spherical, nonenveloped virus 32 to 34 nm in size, with a genome consisting of a single strand of polyadenylated RNA (52, 53). Identification of viral particles in clinical samples has been inconsistent, possibly due to proteolytic degradation or susceptibility to freezing and pelleting (53). Cynomolgus monkeys, and more recently owl monkeys, have been shown to be promising animal models of the serologic response to infection by the hepatitis E virus (436). Radioimmunoassay and enzyme-linked immunoassay for hepatitis E antigen using acute- or convalescent-phase IgM or IgG have previously met with little success, possibly due to the lability of the virus (53). More recently, an enzyme-linked immunosorbent assay based on clonal recombinant hepatitis E antigen has been developed to detect hepatitis E IgG and IgM antibodies (162). Preliminary results are encouraging.

Rotavirus and Small Round Virus

Rotavirus is a common viral pathogen responsible for a large percentage of childhood diarrheal illnesses. Rotavirus may be responsible for up to 50% of all cases of diarrhea in hospitalized children and 10 to 20% of diarrhea cases in the community. By the third year of life, 90% of children have been exposed to rotavirus and develop antibody. Seventy percent of adults have antibody to rotavirus (476). Adult epidemics of diarrheal illness due to rotavirus in the absence of contact with children have been reported (46, 295). Waterborne transmission of rotavirus occurs and was first described in Africa in 1978 (364). In 1981, an outbreak of gastroenteritis due to waterborne transmission of rotavirus involving 1,761 cases occurred in Colorado (179).

Small round viruses are poorly understood uncultivable viruses which have been linked to shellfish-related epidemics of gastroenteritis (12, 157). They are morphologically distinct from other gastroenteritis viruses by electron microscopy and antigenically distinct from Norwalk and Norwalk-like viruses. Asymptomatic individuals have been shown to shed the virus in some instances.

REFERENCES

1. **Abbott, S. L., C. Powers, C. A. Kaysner, Y. Takeda, M. Ishibashi, S. W. Joseph, and J. M. Janda.** 1989. Emergence of a restricted bioserovar of *Vibrio parahaemolyticus* as the predominant cause of *Vibrio*-associated gastroenteritis on the West Coast of the United States and Mexico. *J. Clin. Microbiol.* **27:**2891–2893.
2. **Adams, W. N., and J. J. Miescier.** 1980. Commentary on AOAC method for paralytic shellfish poisoning. *J. Assoc. Off. Anal. Chem.* **63:**1336–1343.
3. **Aldova, E., K. Laznickova, and E. Stepankova.** 1968. Isolation of nonagglutinable vibrios from an enteritis outbreak in Czechoslovakia. *J. Infect. Dis.* **118:**25–31.
4. **Ali, M. B., and M. J. Raff.** 1990. Primary Vibrio vulnificus sepsis in Kentucky. *South. Med. J.* **83:**356–357.
5. **Anderson, D. M., J. J. Sullivan, and B. Reguera.** 1989. Paralytic shellfish poisoning in Northwest Spain: the toxicity of the dinoflagellate Gymnodinium catenatum. *Toxicon* **27:**665–674.
6. **Anonymous.** 1989. Case records of the Massachusetts General Hospital. Weekly clinicopathological exercises. Case 41-1989. A 65-year-old man with fever, bullae, erythema, and edema of the leg after wading in brackish water. *N. Engl. J. Med.* **321:**1029–1038.
7. **Anonymous.** 1991. Food safety. Paralytic shellfish poisoning. *Wkly. Epidemiol. Rec.* **66:**185–187.
8. **Anonymous.** 1988. Mycobacteria, p. 535–572. *In* E. W. Koneman, S. D. Allen, V. R. Dowell, Jr., W. M. Janda, H. M. Sommers, and W. C. Winn, Jr. (ed.), *Color Atlas and Textbook of Diagnostic Microbiology*, 3rd ed. J. B. Lippincott Co., Philadelphia, Pa.
9. **Anonymous.** 1990. Paralytic shellfish poisoning (red tide). *Epidemiol. Bull.* **11:**9.

10. **Anonymous.** 1990. Shuck your oysters with care. *Lancet* **336:**215–216.

11. **Appleton, H.** 1990. Foodborne viruses. *Lancet* **336:**1362–1364.

12. **Appleton, H., and M. S. Pereira.** 1977. A possible virus etiology in outbreaks of food-poisoning from cockles. *Lancet* **i:**780.

13. **Arita, M., T. Takeda, T. Honda, and T. Miwatani.** 1986. Purification and characterization of Vibrio cholerae non-O1 heat-stable enterotoxin. *Infect. Immun.* **52:**45–49.

14. **Aronson, J. D.** 1926. Spontaneous tuberculosis in saltwater fish. *J. Infect. Dis.* **39:**315–320.

15. **Asai, S., J. J. Krzanowski, and W. H. Anderson.** 1982. Effects of the toxin of red tide, Ptychodiscus brevis, on canine tracheal smooth muscle: a possible new asthma-triggering mechanism. *J. Allergy Clin. Immunol.* **69:**418–428.

16. **Auerbach, P. S.** 1984. Hazardous marine animals. *Emerg. Med. Clin. N. Am.* **2:**531–544.

17. **Auerbach, P. S.** 1991. Marine envenomations. *N. Engl. J. Med.* **325:**486–493.

18. **Auerbach, P. S., and B. Halstead.** 1982. Marine hazards: attacks and envenomations. *J. Emerg. Nurs.* **8:**115–122.

19. **Auerbach, P. S., and B. W. Halstead.** 1989. Hazardous aquatic life, p. 933–1028. *In* P. S. Auerbach and E. C. Geehr (ed.), *Management of Wilderness and Environmental Emergencies.* C. V. Mosby, St. Louis, Mo.

20. **Auerbach, P. S., D. M. Yajko, and P. S. Nassos.** 1987. Bacteriology of the marine environment: implications for clinical therapy. *Ann. Emerg. Med.* **16:**643–649.

21. **Baden, D. G.** 1983. Marine food-borne dinoflagellate toxins. *Int. Rev. Cytol.* **82:**99–150.

22. **Baden, D. G., and T. J. Mende.** 1982. Toxicity of two toxins from the Florida red tide marine dinoflagellate Ptychodiscus brevis. *Toxicon* **20:**457–461.

23. **Bagnis, R., F. Berglund, P. F. Elias, G. J. van Esch, B. W. Halstead, and K. Kojima.** 1970. Problems of toxicants in marine food products. 1. Marine biotoxins. *Bull. W. H. O.* **42:**69–88.

24. **Bagnis, R., S. Chanteau, and S. Chungue.** 1980. Origins of ciguatera fish poisoning: a new dinoflagellate, Gambierdiscus toxicus adachi and fukoyo, definitely involved as a causal agent. *Toxicon* **18:**199–208.

25. **Bagnis, R., T. Kuberski, and S. Laugier.** 1979. Clinical observations on 3,009 cases of ciguatera (fish poisoning) in the South Pacific. *Am. J. Trop. Med. Hyg.* **28:**1067–1073.

26. **Baker, J. A., and W. A. Hagan.** 1942. Tuberculosis of Mexican platyfish (Platypoecilus maculatus). *J. Infect. Dis.* **70:**248–252.

27. **Baldridge, H. D., and J. Williams.** 1969. Shark attack: feeding or fighting? *Mil. Med.* **134:**130–133.

28. **Barker, W. H., Jr.** 1974. Vibrio parahaemolyticus outbreaks in the United States. *Lancet* **i:**551–554.

29. **Bart, K. J., Z. Huq, and M. Khan.** 1970. Seroepidemiologic studies during a simultaneous epidemic of infection with El Tor, Ogawa and classical Inaba Vibrio cholerae. *J. Infect. Dis.* **12(Suppl.):**17–24.

30. **Baumann, L., A. L. Furniss, and J. V. Lee.** 1984. Genus I. *Vibrio* Pacini 1854, 411, p. 518–538. *In* N. R. Krieg and J. G. Holt (ed.), *Bergey's Manual of Systematic Bacteriology*, vol. 1. The Williams & Wilkins Co., Baltimore, Md.

31. **Becker, G. D., and G. J. Parell.** 1979. Otolaryngologic aspects of scuba diving. *Otolaryngol. Head Neck Surg.* **87:**569–572.

32. **Becker, K., K. Southwick, J. Reardon, R. Berg, and J. N. MacCormack.** 2001. Histamine poisoning associated with eating tuna burgers. *JAMA* **285:**1327–1330.

33. **Bergh, O., K. Y. Borsheim, G. Bratbak, and M. Heldal.** 1989. High abundance of viruses found in aquatic environments. *Nature* **340:**467–468.

34. **Binta, G. M., T. B. Tjaberg, P. N. Nyaga, and M. Vallard.** 1982. Market fish hygiene in Kenya. *J. Hyg.* **89:**47–52.

35. **Blake, P. A.** 1983. Vibrios on the half shell: what the walrus and the carpenter didn't know. *Ann. Intern. Med.* **99:**558–559.

36. **Blake, P. A., D. T. Allegra, J. D. Snyder, T. J. Barrett, L. McFarland, C. T. Caraway, J. C. Feeley, J. P. Craig, J. V. Lee, N. D. Puhr, and R. A. Feldman.** 1980. Cholera—a possible endemic focus in the United States. *N. Engl. J. Med.* **302:**305–309.

37. **Blake, P. A., M. H. Merson, and R. E. Weaver.** 1979. Disease caused by a marine vibrio: clinical characteristics and epidemiology. *N. Engl. J. Med.* **300:**1–5.

38. **Blake, P. A., R. E. Weaver, and D. G. Hollis.** 1980. Diseases of humans (other than cholera) caused by vibrios. *Annu. Rev. Microbiol.* **34:**341–367.

39. **Blakesley, M. L.** 1983. Scombroid poisoning: prompt resolution of symptoms with cimetidine. *Ann. Emerg. Med.* **12:**104–106.

40. **Blanc, M. H., A. Zwahlen, and M. Robert.** 1977. Symptoms of shellfish poisoning. *N. Engl. J. Med.* **296:**287–288.

41. **Bockemuhl, J., K. Roch, B. Wohlers, V. Aleksic, S. Aleksic, and R. Wokatsch.** 1986. Seasonal distribution of facultatively enteropathogenic vibrios (Vibrio cholerae, Vibrio mimicus, Vibrio parahaemolyticus) in the freshwater of the Elbe River at Hamburg. *J. Appl. Bacteriol.* **60:**435–442.

42. **Bode, R. B., P. R. Brayton, R. R. Colwell, F. M. Russo, and W. E. Bullock.** 1986. A new Vibrio species, Vibrio cincinnatiensis, causing meningitis: successful treatment in an adult. *Ann. Intern. Med.* **104:**55–56.

43. **Bolen, J. R., S. A. Zamiska, and W. B. Greenough.** 1974. Clinical features in enteritis due to Vibrio parahaemolyticus. *Am. J. Med.* **57:**638–641.

44. Reference deleted.

45. **Bonner, J. R., A. S. Coker, C. R. Berryman, and H. M. Pollock.** 1983. Spectrum of vibrio infections in a Gulf Coast community. *Ann. Intern. Med.* **99:**464–469.

46. **Bonsdorff, C. H., T. Hovi, and P. Makela.** 1978. Rotavirus infections in adults in association with acute gastroenteritis. *J. Med. Virol.* **2:**21–28.

47. **Borison, H. L., S. Ellis, and L. E. McCarthy.** 1980. Central respiratory and circulatory effects of Gymnodinium breve toxin in anaesthetized cats. *Br. J. Pharmacol.* **70:**249–256.

48. **Bowdre, J. H., J. H. Hull, and D. M. Cochetto.** 1983. Antibiotic efficacy against Vibrio vulnificus in the mouse: superiority of tetracycline. *J. Pharmacol. Exp. Ther.* **225:**595–598.

49. **Bower, D., R. Hart, P. Matthews, and M. Howden.** 1981. Nonprotein neurotoxins. *Clin. Toxicol.* **18:**813–863.

50. **Bowman, P.** 1984. Amitriptylline and ciguatera. *Med. J. Aust.* **143:**802.

51. **Braback, M., K. Riesbeck, and A. Forsgren.** 2002. Susceptibilities of *Mycobacterium marinum* to gatifloxacin, gemifloxacin, levofloxacin, linezolid, moxifloxacin, telithromycin, and quinupristin-dalfopristin (Synercid) compared to its susceptibilities to reference macrolides and quinolones. *Antimicrob. Agents Chemother.* **46:**1114–1116.

52. **Bradley, D., A. Andjaparidze, and E. H. Cook.** 1988. Aetiological agent of enterically transmitted non-A, non-B hepatitis. *J. Gen. Virol.* **69:**731–738.

53. **Bradley, D. W.** 1990. Enterically-transmitted non-A, non-B hepatitis. *Br. Med. Bull.* **46:**442–461.

54. **Brayton, P. R., R. B. Bode, R. R. Colwell, M. T. MacDonnell, H. L. Hall, D. J. Grimes, P. A. West, and T. N. Bryant.** 1986. *Vibrio cincinnatiensis* sp. nov., a new human pathogen. *J. Clin. Microbiol.* **23:**104–108.

55. **Brenner, D. J., F. W. Hickman-Brenner, J. V. Lee, A. G. Steigerwalt, G. R. Fanning, D. G. Hollis, J. J. Farmer III, R. E. Weaver, S. W. Joseph, and R. J. Seidler.** 1983. *Vibrio furnissii* (formerly aerogenic biogroup of *Vibrio fluvialis*), a new species isolated from human feces and the environment. *J. Clin. Microbiol.* **18:**816–824.

56. **Brennt, C. E., A. C. Wright, S. K. Dutta, and J. G. Morris, Jr.** 1991. Growth of Vibrio vulnificus in serum from alcoholics: association with high transferrin iron saturation. *J. Infect. Dis.* **164:**1030–1032.

57. **Brown, C. K., and S. M. Shepherd.** 1992. Marine trauma, envenomations, and intoxications. *Emerg. Med. Clin. N. Am.* **10:**385–408.

58. **Brown, J. M., E. A. Campbell, and A. D. Rickards.** 1987. Sewage pollution of bathing water. *Lancet* **ii:**1208–1209.

59. **Brown, J. W., III, and C. V. Sanders.** 1987. Mycobacterium marinum infections: a problem of recognition, not therapy? *Arch. Intern. Med.* **147:**817–818.

60. **Bruckner-Tuderman, L., and A. A. Blank.** 1985. Unusual cutaneous dissemination of a tropical fish tank granuloma. *Cutis* **36:**405–408.

61. **Bryan, F. L., H. W. Anderson, and O. D. Cook.** 1987. *Procedures to Investigate Foodborne Illness*, 4th ed., p. 67. International Association of Milk, Food, and Environmental Sanitarians, Ames, Iowa.

62. **Bryant, R. G.** 1983. Food microbiology update. Emerging foodborne pathogens. *Appl. Biochem. Biotechnol.* **8:**437–454.

63. **Buck, J. D., S. Spotte, and J. J. Gadbaw, Jr.** 1984. Bacteriology of the teeth from a great white shark: potential medical implications for shark bite victims. *J. Clin. Microbiol.* **20:**849–851.

64. Reference deleted.

65. **Burnett, J. W.** 1990. Some natural jellyfish toxins, p. 333–335. *In* S. Hall and G. Strichartz (ed.), *Marine Toxins. Origin, Structure, and Molecular Pharmacology.* American Chemical Society, Washington, D.C.

66. **Burnett, J. W., and G. J. Calton.** 1987. Jellyfish envenomation syndromes updated. *Ann. Emerg. Med.* **16:**1000–1005.

67. **Cabelli, V. J., A. P. DuFour, and L. J. McCabe.** 1982. Swimming associated gastroenteritis and water quality. *Am. J. Epidemiol.* **115:**606–616.

68. **Carson, R. L.** 1961. The changing year, p. 28–36. *In* R. L. Carson (ed.), *The Sea Around Us.* Oxford University Press, New York, N.Y.

69. **Cassissi, N., A. Cohn, and T. Davidson.** 1972. Diffuse otitis externa: clinical and microbiologic findings in the course of a multicenter study on a new otic solution. *Ann. Otol. Rhinol. Laryngol.* **86**(Suppl.):39.

70. **Center for Disease Control.** 1969. Follow-up outbreak of gastroenteritis during a tour of the orient–Alaska. *Morb. Mortal. Wkly. Rep.* **18:**168.

71. **Center for Disease Control.** 1979. Gastroenteritis associated with lake swimming. *Morb. Mortal. Wkly. Rep.* **28:**413.

72. **Center for Disease Control.** 1969. An outbreak of acute gastroenteritis during a tour of the orient– Alaska. *Morb. Mortal. Wkly. Rep.* **18:**150.

73. **Center for Disease Control.** 1978. Paralytic shellfish poisoning—Washington. *Morb. Mortal. Wkly. Rep.* **27:**416–417.

74. **Centers for Disease Control.** 1988. ACIP: cholera vaccine. *Morb. Mortal. Wkly. Rep.* **37:**617–624.

75. **Centers for Disease Control.** 1983. Annual mussel quarantine—California. *Morb. Mortal. Wkly. Rep.* **32:**281.

76. **Centers for Disease Control.** 1992. Cercarial dermatitis outbreak in a state park—Delaware, 1991. *Morb. Mortal. Wkly. Rep.* **41:**225–228.

77. **Centers for Disease Control.** 1991. Cholera—Peru, 1991. *Morb. Mortal. Wkly. Rep.* **40:**108–110.

78. **Centers for Disease Control.** 1990. Foodborne hepatitis A—Alaska, Florida, North Carolina, Washington. *Morb. Mortal. Wkly. Rep.* **39:**228–232.

79. **Centers for Disease Control.** 1987. Hepatitis surveillance report no. 51, p. 10–17. U.S. Department of Health and Human Services, Atlanta, Ga.

80. **Centers for Disease Control.** 1989. Hepatitis surveillance report no. 52, p. 19–21. U.S. Department of Health and Human Services, Atlanta, Ga.

81. **Centers for Disease Control.** 1991. Paralytic shellfish poisoning—Massachusetts and Alaska, 1990. *Morb. Mortal. Wkly. Rep.* **40:**157–161. (Erratum, **40:**242.)

82. **Centers for Disease Control.** 1986. Restaurant-associated scombroid fish poisoning—Alabama, Tennessee. *Morb. Mortal. Wkly. Rep.* **35:**264–265.

83. **Centers for Disease Control.** 1987. Summary of notifiable diseases, United States. *Morb. Mortal. Wkly. Rep.* **36:**54.

84. **Centers for Disease Control.** 1989. Table III. Cases of specified notifiable diseases, United States. *Morb. Mortal. Wkly. Rep.* **37:**803.

85. **Centers for Disease Control.** 1991. Update: cholera outbreak—Peru, Ecuador, and Colombia. *Morb. Mortal. Wkly. Rep.* **40:**108–110.

86. **Centers for Disease Control and Prevention.** 1995. Cholera associated with food transported from El Salvador—Indiana, 1994. *Morb. Mortal. Wkly. Rep.* **44:**385–386.

87. **Centers for Disease Control and Prevention.** 1997. Hepatitis A vaccination programs in communities with high rates of hepatitis A. *Morb. Mortal. Wkly. Rep.* **46:**600–603.

88. **Centers for Disease Control and Prevention.** 1993. Imported cholera associated with a newly described toxigenic Vibrio cholerae O139 strain—California, 1993. *Morb. Mortal. Wkly. Rep.* **42:**501–503.

89. **Centers for Disease Control and Prevention.** 1998. Outbreak of Vibrio parahaemolyticus infections associated with eating raw oysters—Pacific Northwest, 1997. *Morb. Mortal. Wkly. Rep.* **47:**457–462.

90. **Centers for Disease Control and Prevention.** 2002. Outbreaks of gastroenteritis associated with noroviruses on cruise ships—United States, 2002. *Morb. Mortal. Wkly. Rep.* **51:**1112–1115.

91. **Centers for Disease Control and Prevention.** 1996. Surveillance for foodborne-disease outbreaks—United States, 1988–1992. *Morb. Mortal. Wkly. Rep.* **45:**1–66.

92. **Centers for Disease Control and Prevention.** 2000. Surveillance for possible estuary-associated syndrome—six states, 1998–1999. *Morb. Mortal. Wkly. Rep.* **49:**372–373.

93. **Centers for Disease Control and Prevention.** 1996. Tetrodotoxin poisoning associated with eating puffer fish transported from Japan—California, 1996. *Morb. Mortal. Wkly. Rep.* **45:**389–391.

94. **Centers for Disease Control and Prevention.** 2002. Update: neurologic illness associated with eating Florida pufferfish, 2002. *Morb. Mortal. Wkly. Rep.* **51:**414–416.

95. **Centers for Disease Control and Prevention.** 1993. Vibrio vulnificus infections associated with raw oyster consumption—Florida, 1981–1992. *Morb. Mortal. Wkly. Rep.* **42:**405–407.

96. **Chatterjee, G. C., and S. K. Das.** 1965. Purification and some properties of Vibrio El Tor phospholipase B. *Enzyme* **28:**346–354.

97. **Cheng, H.-S., S. O. Chua, J.-S. Hung, and K.-K. Yip.** 1991. Creatine kinase MB elevation in paralytic shellfish poisoning. *Chest* **99:**1032–1033.

98. **Chow, S. P., F. K. Ip, J. H. K. Lau, R. J. Collins, K. D. Luk, Y. C. So, and W. K. Pun.** 1987. Mycobacterium marinum infection of the hand and wrist. Results of conservative treatment in twenty-four cases. *J. Bone Jt. Surg. Am. Vol.* **69A:**1161–1168.

99. **Chowdhury, M. A. R., K. M. S. Aziz, Z. Rahim, and B. A. Kay.** 1986. Toxigenicity and drug sensitivity of Vibrio mimicus isolated from fresh water prawns (Macrobrachium malcolmsonii) in Bangladesh. *J. Diarrhoeal Dis. Res.* **4:**237–240.

100. **Chowdhury, M. A. R., H. Yamanaka, S. Miyoshi, K. M. S. Aziz, and S. Shinoda.** 1989. Ecology of *Vibrio mimicus* in aquatic environments. *Appl. Environ. Microbiol.* **55:**2073–2078.

101. **Christenson, B., M. Soler, L. Nieves, and L. M. Souchet.** 1997. Septicemia due to a non-O:1, non-O:139 Vibrio cholerae. *Bol. Asoc. Med. P. R.* **89:**31–32.

102. **Clark, R. B., H. Spector, D. M. Friedman, K. J. Oldrati, C. L. Young, and S. C. Nelson.** 1990. Osteomyelitis and synovitis produced by *Mycobacterium marinum* in a fisherman. *J. Clin. Microbiol.* **28:**2570–2572.

103. **Coffey, J. A., Jr., R. L. Harris, M. L. Rutledge, M. W. Bradshaw, and T. W. Williams, Jr.** 1986. Vibrio damsela: another potentially virulent marine vibrio. *J. Infect. Dis.* **153:**800–802.

104. **Collins, C. H., J. M. Grange, W. C. Noble, and M. D. Yates.** 1985. Mycobacterium marinum infections in man. *J. Hyg. Camb.* **94:**135–149.

105. **Collins, C. H., and H. C. Uttley.** 1988. In-vitro activity of seventeen antimicrobial compounds against seven species of mycobacteria. *J. Antimicrob. Chemother.* **22:**857–861.

106. **Colwell, R. R., R. J. Seidler, J. Kaper, S. W. Joseph, S. Garges, H. Lockman, D. Maneval, H. Bradford, N. Roberts, E. Emmers, I. Huq, and A. Huq.** 1981. Occurrence of *Vibrio cholerae* serogroup O1 in Maryland and Louisiana estuaries. *Appl. Environ. Microbiol.* **41:**555–558.

107. **Colwell, R. R., P. A. West, D. Maneval, E. F. Remmers, E. L. Elliott, and N. E. Carlson.** 1984. Ecology of pathogenic vibrios in Chesapeake Bay, p. 367–387. *In* R. R. Colwell (ed.), *Vibrios in the Environment.* John Wiley & Sons, Inc., New York, N.Y.

108. **Connolly, J.** 1997. Foodborne illness from seafood appear to be increasing. *Infect. Dis. News* **10:**6, 10.

109. **Cook, J.** 1777. *A Voyage Towards the South Pole and Round the World,* vol. 2. Strahan and Cadell, London, England.

110. **Cover, T. L., B. E. Dunn, R. T. Ellison, and M. J. Blaser.** 1989. Vibrio cholerae wound infection acquired in Colorado. *J. Infect. Dis.* **160:**1083.

111. **Craun, G. F.** 1986. Introduction, p. 3–11. *In* G. F. Craun (ed.), *Waterborne Diseases in the United States.* CRC Press, Boca Raton, Fla.

112. **Craun, G. F.** 1986. Recent statistics of waterborne outbreaks (1981–1983), p. 161–168. *In* G. F. Craun (ed.), *Waterborne Diseases in the United States.* CRC Press, Boca Raton, Fla.

113. **Cunningham, L. W., R. A. Promisloff, and A. V. Cichelli.** 1991. Pulmonary infiltrates associated with Vibrio vulnificus septicemia. *J. Am. Osteopath. Assoc.* **91:**84–86.

114. **Dakin, W. P. H., D. J. Howell, R. G. A. Sutton, M. F. O'Keefe, and P. Thomas.** 1974. Gastroenteritis due to non-agglutinable (non-cholera) vibrios. *Med. J. Aust.* **2:**487–490.

115. D'Alessio, D. J., T. E. Minor, and C. I. Allen. 1981. A study of the proportions of swimmers among well controls and children with enterovirus-like illness shedding or not shedding an enterovirus. *Am. J. Epidemiol.* **113**:533–541.

116. Daniels, N., L. MacKinnon, and R. Bishop. 2000. Vibrio parahaemolyticus infections in the United States, 1973–1998. *J. Infect. Dis.* **181**:1661–1666.

117. Datta-Roy, K., K. Banerjee, S. P. De, and A. C. Ghose. 1986. Comparative study of expression of hemagglutinins, hemolysins, and enterotoxins by clinical and environmental isolates of non-O1 *Vibrio cholerae* in relation to their enteropathogenicity. *Appl. Environ. Microbiol.* **52**:875–879.

118. Davis, B. R., G. R. Fanning, J. M. Madden, A. G. Steigerwalt, H. B. Bradford, Jr., H. L. Smith, Jr., and D. O. Brenner. 1981. Characterization of biochemically atypical *Vibrio cholerae* strains and designation of a new pathogenic species, *Vibrio mimicus*. *J. Clin. Microbiol.* **14**:631–639.

119. Davis, J. W., and R. K. Sizemore. 1982. Incidence of *Vibrio* species associated with blue crabs (*Callinectes sapidus*) collected from Galveston Bay, Texas. *Appl. Environ. Microbiol.* **43**:1092–1097.

120. DeGerome, J. H., and M. T. Smith. 1974. Noncholera vibrio enteritis contracted in the United States by an American. *J. Infect. Dis.* **129**:587–589.

121. De Paola, A. 1981. Vibrio cholerae in marine foods and environmental waters: a literature review. *J. Food Sci.* **46**:66–70.

122. Desenclos, J. A., K. C. Klontz, L. E. Wolfe, and S. Hoecherl. 1991. The risk of vibrio illness in the Florida raw oyster eating population, 1981–1988. *Am. J. Epidemiol.* **134**:290–297.

123. Desenclos, J.-C. A., K. C. Klontz, and M. H. Wilder. 1991. A multistate outbreak of hepatitis A caused by the consumption of raw oysters. *Am. J. Public Health* **81**:1268–1272.

124. Dhar, R., M. A. Ghafoor, and A. Y. Nasralah. 1989. Unusual non-serogroup O1 Vibrio cholerae bacteremia associated with liver disease. *J. Clin. Microbiol.* **27**:2853–2855.

125. Dickey, R. W., G. A. Fryxell, H. R. Granade, and D. Roelke. 1992. Detection of the marine toxins okadaic acid and domoic acid in shellfish and phytoplankton in the Gulf of Mexico. *Toxicon* **30**:355–359.

126. DiGaetano, M., S. F. Ball, and J. G. Straus. 1989. Vibrio vulnificus corneal ulcer. *Arch. Ophthalmol.* **107**:323–324.

127. Dilmore, L. A., and M. A. Hood. 1986. Vibrios of some deep-water invertebrates. *FEMS Microbiol. Lett.* **35**:221–224.

128. Dolin, R., J. J. Treanor, and H. P. Madore. 1987. Novel agents of viral enteritis in humans. *J. Infect. Dis.* **155**:365–375.

129. Donta, S. T., P. W. Smith, R. E. Levitz, and R. Quintiliani. 1986. Therapy of mycobacterium marinum infections: use of tetracyclines vs rifampin. *Arch. Intern. Med.* **146**:902–904.

130. Doyle, M. P. 1985. Food-borne pathogens of recent concern. *Annu. Rev. Nutr.* **5**:25–41.

131. Reference deleted.

132. DuPont, H. L. 1986. Consumption of raw shellfish—is the risk now unacceptable? *N. Engl. J. Med.* **314**:707–708.

133. Eason, R. J., and E. Harding. 1987. Neurotoxic fish poisoning in the Solomon Islands. *P. N. G. Med. J.* **30**:49–52.

134. Eastaugh, J., and S. Shepherd. 1989. Infectious and toxic syndromes from fish and shellfish consumption. A review. *Arch. Intern. Med.* **149**:1735–1740.

135. Eng, R. H. K., H. Chmel, S. M. Smith, D. Haacker, and A. Grigoriu. 1988. Early diagnosis of overwhelming Vibrio vulnificus infections. *South. Med. J.* **81**:410–411.

136. English, V. L., and R. B. Lindberg. 1977. Isolation of Vibrio alginolyticus from wounds and blood of a burn patient. *Am. J. Med. Technol.* **43**:989–993.

137. Enzenauer, R. J., J. McKoy, and D. Vincent. 1990. Disseminated cutaneous and synovial Mycobacterium marinum infection in a patient with systemic lupus erythematosus. *South. Med. J.* **83**:471–474.

138. Etkind, P., M. E. Wilson, K. Gallagher, and J. Cournoyer. 1987. Bluefish-associated scombroid poisoning. *JAMA* **258**:3409–3410.

139. Eyles, M. J., G. R. Davey, and G. Arnold. 1985. Behavior and incidence of Vibrio parahaemolyticus in Sydney rock oysters (Crassostrea commercialis). *Int. J. Food Microbiol.* **1**:327–334.

140. Fang, G., V. Araujo, and R. L. Guerrant. 1991. Enteric infections associated with exposure to animals or animal products. *Infect. Dis. Clin. N. Am.* **5**:681–701.

141. **Farmer, J. J., F. W. Hickman-Brenner, and M. T. Kelly.** 1985. *Vibrio*, p. 282–301. *In* G. H. Lennette, A. Balows, W. J. Hausler, and H. J. Shadomy (ed.), *Manual of Clinical Microbiology*, 4th ed. American Society for Microbiology, Washington, D.C.

142. **Farmer, J. J., III.** 1979. Vibrio ("Beneckea") vulnificus, the bacterium associated with sepsis, septicemia and the sea. *Lancet* **ii:**903.

143. Reference deleted.

144. **Feldman, R. A., M. W. Long, and H. L. David.** 1974. Mycobacterium marinum: a leisure time pathogen. *J. Infect. Dis.* **129:**618–621.

145. **Fenner, P. J., J. A. Williamson, and J. W. Burnett.** 1988. The "Irukundji Syndrome" and acute pulmonary edema. *Med. J. Aust.* **149:**150–156.

146. **Field, M.** 1979. Modes of action of enterotoxins of Vibrio cholerae and Escherichia coli. *Rev. Infect. Dis.* **1:**918–921.

147. **Florescu, D. P., N. Nacescu, and C. Ciufecu.** 1981. Vibrio cholerae non group O:1 associated with middle ear infection. *Arch. Roum. Pathol. Exp. Microbiol.* **40:**369–372.

148. **Fonde, E. C., J. Britton, and H. Pollock.** 1984. Marine Vibrio sepsis manifesting as necrotizing fasciitis. *South. Med. J.* **77:**933–934.

149. **Franca, S. M. C., D. L. Gibbs, P. Samuels, and W. D. Johnson, Jr.** 1980. Vibrio parahaemolyticus in Brazilian coastal waters. *JAMA* **244:**587–588.

150. **Fuhrman, F. A.** 1986. Tetrodotoxin, tarichatoxin, and chiriquitoxins. Historical perspectives. *Ann. N. Y. Acad. Sci.* **479:**1–14.

151. **Furniss, A. L., J. V. Lee, and T. J. Donovan.** 1977. Group F, a new Vibrio? *Lancet* **ii:**565–566.

152. **Gerba, C. P., C. M. Goyal, and R. I. LaBelle.** 1979. Failure of indicator bacteria to reflect the occurrence of enteroviruses in marine waters. *Am. J. Public Health* **69:**1116–1119.

153. **Gerba, C. P., and S. M. Goyal.** 1986. Development of a qualitative pathogen risk assessment methodology for ocean disposal of municipal sludge. Publication ALAO-CIN-493. U.S. Environmental Protection Agency, Cincinnati, Ohio.

154. **Gessner, B., and M. Schloss.** 1996. A population-based study of paralytic shellfish poisoning in Alaska. *Alsk. Med.* **38:**54–58.

155. **Giannoni, C.** 2000. Swimming with tympanostomy tubes. *Arch. Otolaryngol. Head Neck Surg.* **126:**1507–1509.

156. **Gilbert, D., R. Moellering, and M. Sande.** 2002. *Sanford Guide to Antimicrobial Therapy*, 32nd ed. Antimicrobial Therapy, Inc., Hyde Park, Vt.

157. **Gill, O. N., W. D. Cubitt, and D. A. McSwiggan.** 1983. Epidemic of gastroenteritis caused by oysters contaminated with small round structured viruses. *Br. Med. J.* **287:**1532–1534.

158. **Gillespie, N. C., R. J. Lewis, and J. H. Pearn.** 1986. Ciguatera in Australia: occurrence, clinical features, pathophysiology, and management. *Med. J. Aust.* **145:**584–590.

159. **Gilman, R. H., W. M. Spira, G. H. Rabbani, and A. Al-Mahomod.** 1980. Invasive E. coli and V. parahaemolyticus a rare cause of dysentery in Dacca. *Trans. R. Soc. Trop. Med. Hyg.* **74:**688–689.

160. **Glasgow, H. J., J. Burkholder, D. Schmechel, P. Tester, and P. Rublee.** 1995. Insidious effects of a toxic estuarine dinoflagellate on fish survival and human health. *Toxicol. Environ. Health* **46:**501–522.

161. Reference deleted.

162. **Goldsmith, R., P. O. Yarbough, and G. R. Reyes.** 1992. Enzyme-linked immunosorbent assay for diagnosis of acute sporadic hepatitis E in Egyptian children. *Lancet* **339:**328–331.

163. **Gombert, M. E., E. L. C. Goldstein, and M. L. Corrado.** 1981. Disseminated Mycobacterium marinum infection after renal transplantation. *Ann. Intern. Med.* **94:**486–487.

164. **Gorbach, S. L., J. G. Banwell, N. F. Pierce, B. D. Chatterjee, and R. C. Mitra.** 1970. Intestinal microflora in a chronic carrier of Vibrio cholerae. *J. Infect. Dis.* **121:**383–390.

165. **Goyal, S. M.** 1984. Viral pollution of the marine environment. *Crit. Rev. Environ. Control* **14:**32.

166. **Grattan, L. M., D. Oldatch, T. M. Pearl, M. H. Lowitt, D. L. Matuszak, C. Dickson, C. Parrott, R. C. Shoemaker, C. L. Kauffman, M. P. Wasserman, J. R. Hebel, P. Charache, and J. G. Morris, Jr.** 1998. Learning and memory difficulties after environmental exposure to waterways containing toxin-producing Pfiesteria or Pfiesteria-like dinoflagellates. *Lancet* **352:**532–539.

167. **Gray, L. D., and A. S. Kreger.** 1986. Detection of anti-*Vibrio vulnificus* cytolysin antibodies in sera from mice and a human surviving V. vulnificus disease. *Infect. Immun.* **51:**964–965.

168. **Gray, L. D., and A. S. Kreger.** 1985. Purification and characterization of an extracellular cytolysin produced by *Vibrio vulnificus. Infect. Immun.* **48**:62–72.
169. **Greenough, W. B. I.** 1990. Vibrio cholerae, p. 1636–1646. *In* G. L. Mandell, R. G. Douglas, Jr., and J. E. Bennett (ed.), *Principles and Practice of Infectious Diseases*, 3rd ed. Churchill Livingstone, New York, N.Y.
170. **Grimes, D. J., J. Stemmler, and H. Hada.** 1984. Vibrio species associated with mortality of sharks held in captivity. *Microb. Ecol.* **10**:271–282.
171. **Gunn, R. A., H. T. Janowski, and S. Lieb.** 1982. Norwalk virus gastroenteritis following raw oyster consumption. *Am. J. Epidemiol.* **115**:348–351.
172. **Hackney, C. R., E. G. Kleeman, B. Ray, and M. L. Speck.** 1980. Adherence as a method for differentiating virulent and avirulent strains of *Vibrio parahaemolyticus. Appl. Environ. Microbiol.* **40**:652–658.
173. **Haddad, L. M., R. F. Lee, and O. McConnell.** 1983. Toxic marine life, p. 303–317. *In* L. M. Haddad and J. F. Winchester (ed.), *Clinical Management of Poisoning and Drug Overdose.* W. B. Saunders, Philadelphia, Pa.
174. **Halliday, M. L., L. Kang, and T. Zhou.** 1991. An epidemic of hepatitis A attributable to the ingestion of raw clams in Shanghai, China. *J. Infect. Dis.* **164**:852–859.
175. **Halstead, B. W.** 1965. *Poisonous and Venomous Marine Animals of the World*, vol. 1. *Invertebrates*, p. 59–61. U.S. Government Printing Office, Washington, D.C.
176. **Halstead, B. W.** 1987. Coelenterate (Cnidarian) stings and wounds. *Clin. Dermatol.* **5**:8–13.
177. **Halstead, B. W., and E. J. Schantz.** 1984. *Paralytic Shellfish Poisoning*, p. 1–59. WHO offset publication. World Health Organization, Geneva, Switzerland.
178. **Hare, P., T. Scott-Burden, and D. R. Woods.** 1983. Characterization of extracellular alkaline proteases and collagenase induction in Vibrio alginolyticus. *J. Gen. Microbiol.* **129**:1141–1147.
179. **Harris, J. R., M. L. Cohen, and E. C. Lippy.** 1981. Water-related disease outbreaks in the United States, 1981. *J. Infect. Dis.* **148**:759–762.
180. **Harrison, L. J.** 1991. Poisonous marine morsels. *J. Fla. Med. Assoc.* **78**:219–221.
181. **Heineman, H. S., S. Spitzer, and T. Pianphongsant.** 1972. Fish tank granuloma. A hobby hazard. *Arch. Intern. Med.* **130**:121–123.
182. **Heller, D., O. N. Gill, E. Raynham, T. Kirkland, P. M. Zadick, and R. Stanwell-Smith.** 1986. An outbreak of gastrointestinal illness associated with consumption of raw depurated oysters. *Br. Med. J.* **292**:1726–1727.
183. **Hemmert, W. H.** 1975. The public health implications of Gymnodinium breve red tides, a review of the literature and recent events, p. 489–497. *In* V. R. Locicero (ed.), *Proceedings of the First International Conference on Toxic Dinoflagellate Blooms.* Massachusetts Science and Technology Foundation, Boston.
184. **Herrington, D. A., R. H. Hall, G. Losonsky, J. J. Mekalanos, R. K. Taylor, and M. M. Levine.** 1988. Toxin, toxin-coregulated pili, and the toxR regulon are essential for Vibrio cholerae pathogenesis in humans. *J. Exp. Med.* **168**:1487–1492.
185. **Hessel, D. W., B. W. Halstead, and N. H. Peckham.** 1960. Marine biotoxins. 1. Ciguatera poison: some biological and chemical aspects. *Ann. N. Y. Acad. Sci.* **90**:788–797.
186. **Hickman, F. W., J. J. Farmer, D. G. Hollis, G. R. Fanning, A. G. Steigerwalt, R. E. Weaver, and D. J. Brenner.** 1982. Identification of *Vibrio hollisae* sp. nov. from patients with diarrhea. *J. Clin. Microbiol.* **15**:395–401.
187. **Hickman-Brenner, F. W., D. J. Brenner, and A. G. Steigerwalt.** 1984. *Vibrio fluvialis* and *Vibrio furnissii* isolated from a stool sample of one patient. *J. Clin. Microbiol.* **20**:125–127.
188. **Hill, M. K., and C. V. Sanders.** 1987. Localized and systemic infection due to Vibrio species. *Infect. Dis. Clin. N. Am.* **1**:687–707.
189. **Hirschhorn, N., J. L. Kinzie, and D. B. Sachar.** 1968. Decrease in net stool output during intestinal perfusion with glucose-containing solutions. *N. Engl. J. Med.* **279**:176.
190. **Hoashi, K., K. Ogata, H. Taniguchi, H. Yamashita, K. Tsuji, Y. Mizuguchi, and N. Ohtomo.** 1990. Pathogenesis of Vibrio parahaemolyticus: intraperitoneal and orogastric challenge experiments in mice. *Microbiol. Immunol.* **34**:355–366.
191. **Hoffman, T. J., B. Nelson, R. Darouiche, and T. Rosen.** 1988. Vibrio vulnificus septicemia. *Arch. Intern. Med.* **148**:1825–1827.

192. **Hoge, C. W., D. Watsky, R. N. Peeler, J. P. Libonati, E. Israel, and J. G. Morris, Jr.** 1989. Epidemiology and spectrum of Vibrio infections in a Chesapeake Bay community. *J. Infect. Dis.* **160:**985–993.

193. **Hollis, D. G., R. E. Weaver, C. N. Baker, and C. Thornsberry.** 1976. Halophilic *Vibrio* species isolated from blood cultures. *J. Clin. Microbiol.* **3:**425–431.

194. **Holmberg, S.** 1988. Vibrios and Aeromonas. *Infect. Dis. Clin. N. Am.* **2:**655–676.

195. **Holmgren, J., and A. Svennerholm.** 1977. Mechanisms of disease and immunity in cholerae. A review. *J. Infect. Dis.* **136**(Suppl):105–112.

196. Reference deleted.

197. **Honda, T., and R. A. Finkelstein.** 1979. Purification and characterization of a hemolysin produced by *Vibrio cholerae* biotype El Tor: another toxic substance produced by cholera vibrios. *Infect. Immun.* **26:**1020–1027.

198. **Honda, T., S. Taga, T. Takeda, M. A. Hasibuan, Y. Takeda, and T. Miwatani.** 1976. Identification of lethal toxin with the thermostable direct hemolysin produced by *Vibrio parahaemolyticus*, and some physicochemical properties of the purified toxin. *Infect. Immun.* **13:**133–139.

199. **Hood, M. A., G. E. Ness, and G. E. Rodrick.** 1981. Isolation of *Vibrio cholerae* serotype O1 from the eastern oyster, *Crassostrea virginica. Appl. Environ. Microbiol.* **41:**559–560.

200. **Howard, R. J., and S. Lieb.** 1988. Soft-tissue infections caused by halophilic marine Vibrios. *Arch. Surg.* **123:**245.

201. **Hoyt, R. E., J. E. Bryant, and S. F. Glessner.** 1989. M. marinum infections in a Chesapeake Bay community. *Va. Med. Mon.* **16:**467–470.

202. Reference deleted.

203. **Hughes, J. M.** 1979. Epidemiology of shellfish poisoning in the United States, 1971–1977, p. 23–28. *In* D. L. Taylor and H. H. Seliger (ed.), *Toxic Dinoflagellate Blooms.* Elsevier/North Holland, New York, N.Y.

204. **Hughes, J. M., D. G. Hollis, E. J. Gangarosa, and R. E. Weaver.** 1978. Non-cholera vibrio infections in the United States: clinical, epidemiologic, and laboratory features. *Ann. Intern. Med.* **88:**602–606.

205. **Hughes, J. M., and M. H. Merson.** 1976. Fish and shellfish poisoning. *N. Engl. J. Med.* **295:**1117–1120.

206. **Hughes, J. M., and M. E. Potter.** 1991. Scombroid-fish poisoning. From pathogenesis to prevention. *N. Engl. J. Med.* **324:**766–768.

207. **Hughes, J. M., and R. V. Tauxe.** 1990. Food-borne disease, p. 898. *In* G. L. Mandell, R. G. Douglas, and J. E. Bennett (ed.), *Principles and Practice of Infectious Diseases*, 3rd ed. Churchill Livingstone, New York, N.Y.

208. **Huminer, D., S. D. Pitlik, C. Block, L. Kaufman, S. Amit, and J. B. Rosenfeld.** 1986. Aquarium-borne Mycobacterium marinum skin infection: report of a case and review of the literature. *Arch. Dermatol.* **122:**698–703.

209. **Huq, A., S. A. Huq, D. J. Grimes, K. M. O'Brien, K. H. Chu, J. M. Capuzzo, and R. R. Colwell.** 1986. Colonization of the gut of the blue crab (*Callinectes sapidus*) by *Vibrio cholerae. Appl. Environ. Microbiol.* **52:**586–588.

210. **Huq, A., P. A. West, E. B. Small, M. I. Huq, and R. R. Colwell.** 1984. Influence of water temperature, salinity, and pH on survival and growth of toxigenic *Vibrio cholerae* serovar O1 associated with live copepods in laboratory microcosms. *Appl. Environ. Microbiol.* **48:**420–424.

211. **Huq, M. I., A. K. M. J. Alam, and D. J. Brenner.** 1980. Isolation of *Vibrio*-like group, EF-6, from patients with diarrhea. *J. Clin. Microbiol.* **11:**621–624.

212. **Hurst, L. C., P. C. Amadio, M. A. Badalamente, J. L. Ellstein, and R. J. Dattwyler.** 1987. Mycobacterium marinum infections of the hand. *J. Hand Surg.* **12A:**428–435.

213. **Izumi, A. K., C. W. Hanke, and M. Higaki.** 1977. Mycobacterium marinum infections treated with tetracycline. *Arch. Dermatol.* **113:**1067–1068.

214. **Jaffe, B. F.** 1981. Are water and tympanostomy tubes compatible? *Laryngoscope* **91:**563–564.

215. **Janda, J. M., R. Brenden, J. A. DeBenedetti, M. O. Constantino, and T. Robin.** 1986. Vibrio alginolyticus bacteremia in an immunocompromised patient. *Diagn. Microbiol. Infect. Dis.* **5:**337–340.

216. **Janda, J. M., C. Powers, R. G. Bryant, and S. L. Abbott.** 1988. Current perspectives on the epidemiology and pathogenesis of clinically significant *Vibrio* spp. *Clin. Microbiol. Rev.* **1:**245–267.

217. Jean-Jacques, W., K. R. Rajashekaraiah, J. J. Farmer III, F. W. Hickman, J. G. Morris, and C. A. Kallick. 1981. *Vibrio metschnikovii* bacteremia in a patient with cholecystitis. *J. Clin. Microbiol.* 14:711–712.

218. Johnston, J. M., W. A. Andes, and G. Glasser. 1983. Vibrio vulnificus: a gastronomic hazard. *JAMA* 249:1756–1757.

219. Johnston, J. M., S. F. Becker, and L. M. McFarland. 1986. Gastroenteritis in patients with stool isolates of Vibrio vulnificus. *Am. J. Med.* 80:336–338.

220. Johnston, J. M., S. F. Becker, and L. M. McFarland. 1985. Vibrio vulnificus: man and the sea. *JAMA* 253:2850–2853.

221. Johnston, J. M., D. L. Martin, J. Perdue, L. M. McFarland, C. T. Caraway, E. C. Lippy, and P. A. Blake. 1983. Cholera on a Gulf Coast oil rig. *N. Engl. J. Med.* 309:523–526.

222. Johnston, J. M., L. M. McFarland, H. C. Bradford, and C. T. Caraway. 1983. Isolation of nontoxigenic *Vibrio cholerae* O1 from a human wound infection. *J. Clin. Microbiol.* 17:918–920.

223. Jolly, H. W., and J. H. Seabury. 1972. Infections with Mycobacterium marinum. *Arch. Dermatol.* 106:32–36.

224. Jones, M. W., I. A. Wahid, and J. P. Matthews. 1988. Septic arthritis of the hand due to Mycobacterium marinum. *J. Hand Surg.* 13B:333–334.

225. Joseph, S. W., R. R. Colwell, and J. B. Kaper. 1983. Vibrio parahaemolyticus and related halophilic vibrios. *Crit. Rev. Microbiol.* 10:77–124.

226. Kan, S. K. P., N. Singh, and M. K. C. Chan. 1986. Oliva vidua fulminans, a marine mollusc, responsible for five fatal cases of neurotoxic food poisoning in Sabah, Malaysia. *Trans. R. Soc. Trop. Med. Hyg.* 80:64–65.

227. Kaneko, T., and R. R. Colwell. 1978. The annual cycle of Vibrio parahemolyticus in Chesapeake Bay. *Microb. Ecol.* 4:135–155.

228. Kaneko, T., and R. R. Colwell. 1973. Ecology of *Vibrio parahaemolyticus* in Chesapeake Bay. *J. Bacteriol.* 113:24–32.

229. Kaper, J. B., H. Lockman, and R. R. Colwell. 1979. Ecology, serology, and enterotoxin production of *Vibrio cholerae* in Chesapeake Bay. *Appl. Environ. Microbiol.* 37:91–103.

230. Kaplan, J. E., R. A. Goodman, and R. C. Baron. 1982. Epidemiology of Norwalk gastroenteritis and the role of Norwalk virus in outbreaks of acute nonbacterial gastroenteritis. *Ann. Intern. Med.* 96:756–761.

231. Karunasagar, I., I. Karunasagar, Y. Oshima, and T. Yasumoto. 1990. A toxin profile for shellfish involved in an outbreak of paralytic shellfish poisoning in India. *Toxicon* 28:868–870.

232. Karunasagar, I., I. Karunasagar, M. N. Venugopal, and C. N. Nagesha. 1987. Survival of Vibrio parahaemolyticus in estuarine and seawater and in association with clams. *Syst. Appl. Microbiol.* 9:316–319.

233. Karunasagar, I., M. N. Venugopal, I. Karunasagar, and K. Segar. 1987. Role of chitin in the survival of Vibrio parahaemolyticus at different temperatures. *Can. J. Microbiol.* 32:889–891.

234. Kat, M. 1983. Diarrhetic mussel poisoning in the Netherlands related to the dinoflagellate Dinophysis acuminata. *Antonie Leeuwenhoek* 49:417–427.

235. Kaye, J. J. 1990. Vibrio vulnificus infections in the hand. Report of three patients. *J. Bone Jt. Surg. Am.* 72-A:283–285.

236. Kaysner, C. A., M. M. Wekell, and C. Abeyta, Jr. 1990. Enhancement of virulence of two environmental strains of Vibrio vulnificus after passage through mice. *Diagn. Microbiol. Infect. Dis.* 13:285–288.

237. Kelly, M. T., and D. M. Avery. 1980. Lactose-positive *Vibrio* in seawater: a cause of pneumonia and septicemia in a drowning victim. *J. Clin. Microbiol.* 11:278–280.

238. Kelly, M. T., and E. M. D. Stroh. 1989. Urease-positive, Kanagawa-negative *Vibrio parahaemolyticus* from patients and the environment in the Pacific Northwest. *J. Clin. Microbiol.* 27:2820–2822.

239. Kerketta, J., A. Paul, V. Kirubakaran, M. Jesudason, and P. Moses. 2002. Non-O1 Vibrio cholerae septicemia and meningitis in a neonate. *Indian J. Pediatr.* 69:909–910.

240. Khan, M. V., and M. Shahidullah. 1982. Epidemiologic pattern of diarrhoea caused by nonagglutinating Vibrio (NAG) and EF-6 organisms in Dacca. *Trop. Geogr. Med.* 34:19–27.

241. King, A. J., J. A. Fairley, and J. E. Rasmussen. 1983. Disseminated cutaneous Mycobacterium marinum infection. *Arch. Dermatol.* 119:268–270.

242. **Klontz, K. C.** 1990. Fatalities associated with Vibrio parahaemolyticus and Vibrio cholerae non-O1 infections in Florida (1981 to 1988). *South. Med. J.* **83:**500–502.

243. **Klontz, K. C., and J.-C. A. Desenclos.** 1990. Clinical and epidemiological features of sporadic infections with Vibrio fluvialis in Florida, USA. *J. Diarrhoeal Dis. Res.* **8:**24–26.

244. **Klontz, K. C., S. Lieb, M. Schreiber, H. T. Janowski, L. M. Baldy, and R. A. Gunn.** 1988. Syndromes of Vibrio vulnificus infections. Clinical and epidemiologic features in Florida cases, 1981–1987. *Ann. Intern. Med.* **109:**318–323.

245. **Kobayashi, M., S. Kondo, T. Yasumoto, and Y. Ohizumi.** 1986. Cardiotoxic effects of maitotoxin, a principal toxin of seafood poisoning, on guinea pig and rat cardiac muscle. *J. Pharmacol. Exp. Ther.* **238:**1077–1083.

246. **Kodama, A. M., Y. Hokama, T. Yasumoto, M. Fukui, S. J. Manea, and N. Sutherland.** 1989. Clinical and laboratory findings implicating palytoxin as cause of ciguatera poisoning due to Decapterus macrosoma (mackerel). *Toxicon* **27:**1051–1053.

247. **Kodama, H., Y. Gyobu, N. Tokuman, I. Okada, H. Uetake, T. Shimada, and R. Sakazaki.** 1984. Ecology of non-O1 Vibrio cholerae in Toyama prefecture. *Microbiol. Immunol.* **28:**311–325.

248. **Kodama, M., T. Ogata, Y. Fukuyo, T. Ishimaru, S. Wisessang, K. Saitanu, V. Panichyakarn, and T. Piyakarnchana.** 1988. Protogonyaulax cohorticula, a toxic dinoflagellate found in the Gulf of Thailand. *Toxicon* **26:**707–712.

249. **Koff, R. S., and H. S. Sear.** 1967. Internal temperature of steamed clams. *N. Engl. J. Med.* **276:**737–739.

250. **Kothary, M. H., and S. H. Richardson.** 1987. Fluid accumulation in infant mice caused by *Vibrio hollisae* and its extracellular enterotoxin. *Infect. Immun.* **55:**626–630.

251. **Kreger, A., L. DeChatelet, and P. Shirley.** 1981. Interaction of Vibrio vulnificus with human polymorphonuclear leukocytes: association of virulence with resistance to phagocytosis. *J. Infect. Dis.* **144:**244–248.

252. **Kreger, A. S.** 1984. Cytolytic activity and virulence of *Vibrio damsela. Infect. Immun.* **44:**326–331.

253. **Krzanowski, J., Y. Sakamoto, and R. Duncan.** 1984. The mechanism of Ptychodiscus brevis toxin induced rat vas deferens contraction. *Pharmacologist* **26:**175.

254. **Kwo, P.** 1997. Acute hepatitis E by a new isolate acquired in the United States. *Mayo Clin. Proc.* **72:**1133–1136.

255. **Lacy, J. N., S. F. Viegas, J. Calhoun, and J. T. Mader.** 1989. Mycobacterium marinum flexor tenosynovitis. *Clin. Orthop. Relat. Res.* **238:**288–293.

256. **Lam, S., and E. Monteiro.** 1984. Isolation of mucoid *Vibrio parahaemolyticus* strains. *J. Clin. Microbiol.* **19:**87–88.

257. **Lam, S., and E. Monteiro.** 1981. Unusual Vibrio species found in diarrhoeal stools. *Singap. Med. J.* **22:**259–261.

258. **Lam, S., and M. Yeo.** 1980. Urease-positive *Vibrio parahaemolyticus* strain. *J. Clin. Microbiol.* **12:**57–59.

259. **Lam, S. Y. S., and L. T. Goi.** 1985. Isolations of "Group F Vibrios" from human stools. *Singap. Med. J.* **26:**300–302.

260. **Larsen, J. L., and J. F. Farid.** 1980. In vitro antibiotic sensitivity testing of Vibrio alginolyticus. *Acta Pathol. Microbiol. Scand.* **88:**307–310.

261. **Lawrence, D. N., M. B. Enriquez, R. M. Lumish, and A. Maceo.** 1980. Ciguatera fish poisoning in Miami. *JAMA* **244:**254–258.

262. **Lee, D., A. Youk, and N. Goldstein.** 1999. A meta-analysis of swimming and water precautions. *Laryngoscope* **109:**536–540.

263. **Lee, J. V., T. J. Donovan, and A. L. Furniss.** 1978. Characterization, taxonomy, and emended description of *Vibrio metschnikovii. Int. J. Syst. Bacteriol.* **28:**99–111.

264. **Lee, J. V., P. Shread, and A. L. Furniss.** 1981. Taxonomy and description of Vibrio fluvialis sp. nov. (synonym group F vibrios, group EF-6). *J. Appl. Bacteriol.* **50:**73–94.

265. **Lerke, P. A., S. B. Werner, S. L. Taylor, and L. S. Guthertz.** 1978. Scombroid poisoning: report of an outbreak. *West. J. Med.* **12:**381–386.

266. **Lessner, A. M., R. M. Webb, and B. Rabin.** 1985. Vibrio alginolyticus conjunctivitis. *Arch. Ophthalmol.* **103:**229–230.

267. **Levesque, B., P. Giovenazzo, P. Guerrier, D. Laverdiere, and H. Prud'Homme.** 2002. Investigation of an outbreak of cercarial dermatitis. *Epidemiol. Infect.* **129:**379–386.

268. **Levine, M. M., R. E. Black, M. L. Clements, D. R. Nalin, L. Cisneros, and R. A. Finkelstein.** 1981. Volunteer studies in development of vaccines against cholera and enterotoxigenic E. coli: a review, p. 443–459. *In* T. Holme, J. Holmgren, M. H. Merson, and R. Mollby (ed.), *Acute Enteric Infections in Children: New Prospects for Treatment and Prevention.* Elsevier/North Holland, Amsterdam, The Netherlands.

269. **Lewis, N.** 1986. Disease and development: ciguatera fish poisoning. *Soc. Sci. Med.* **23:**983–993.

270. **Limpert, G. H., and J. E. Peacock.** 1988. Soft tissue infections due to noncholera vibrios. *Am. Fam. Physician* **37:**193–198.

271. **Lin, F. Y., J. G. Morris, Jr., J. B. Kaper, T. Gross, J. Michalski, C. Morrison, J. B. Libonati, and E. Israel.** 1986. Persistence of cholera in the United States: isolation of Vibrio cholerae O1 from a patient with diarrhea in Maryland. *J. Clin. Microbiol.* **23:**624–626.

272. **Linell, F., and A. Norden.** 1954. Mycobacterium balnei: a new acid-fast bacillus occurring in swimming pools and capable of producing skin lesions in humans. *Acta Tuberc. Scand. Suppl.* **33:**1–84.

273. **Link, K., F. Counselman, J. Steele, and M. Caughey.** 1999. A new hazard for windsurfers: needlefish impalement. *J. Emerg. Med.* **17:**255–259.

274. **Lipp, E., and J. Rose.** 1997. The role of seafood in foodborne diseases in the United States of America. *Rev. Sci. Tech.* **16:**620–640.

275. **Ljungberg, B., B. Christensson, and R. Grubb.** 1987. Failure of doxycycline treatment in aquarium-associated Mycobacterium marinum infections. *Scand. J. Infect. Dis.* **19:**539–543.

276. **Lockwood, D. E., A. S. Kreger, and S. H. Richardson.** 1982. Detection of toxins produced by Vibrio fluvialis. *Infect. Immun.* **35:**702–708.

277. **Long, R. R., J. C. Sargent, and K. Hammer.** 1990. Paralytic shellfish poisoning: a case report and serial electrophysiologic observations. *Neurology* **40:**1310–1312.

278. **Lopez-Sabater, E., J. Rodriguez-Jerez, M. Hernandez-Herrero, and M. Mora-Ventura.** 1996. Incidence of histamine-forming bacteria and histamine content in scombroid fish species from retail markets in the Barcelona area. *Int. J. Food Microbiol.* **28:**411–418.

279. **Loria, P. R.** 1976. Minocycline hydrochloride treatment for atypical acid-fast infection. *Arch. Dermatol.* **112:**517–519.

280. **Lounsbury, B. F.** 1985. Swimming unprotected with long-shafted middle ear ventilation tubes. *Laryngoscope* **95:**340–343.

281. **Love, M., D. Teebken-Fisher, J. E. Hose, J. J. Farmer III, F. W. Hickman, and G. R. Fanning.** 1981. Vibrio damsela, a marine bacterium, causes skin ulcers on the damselfish Chromis punctipinnis. *Science* **214:**1139.

282. **Lowry, P. W., L. M. McFarland, B. H. Peltier, N. C. Roberts, H. B. Bradford, J. L. Herndon, D. F. Stroup, J. B. Mathison, P. A. Blake, and R. A. Gunn.** 1989. Vibrio gastroenteritis in Louisiana: a prospective study among attendees of a scientific congress in New Orleans. *J. Infect. Dis.* **160:**978–984.

283. **Lowry, P. W., L. M. McFarland, and H. K. Threefoot.** 1986. Vibrio hollisae septicemia after consumption of catfish. *J. Infect. Dis.* **154:**730–731.

284. **Lumley, J., J. A. Williamson, and P. J. Fenner.** 1988. Fatal envenomation by Chironex fleckeri, the north Australian box jellyfish: the continuing search for lethal mechanisms. *Med. J. Aust.* **148:**527–534.

285. **Magnusson, B., and J. Gulasekharam.** 1965. A lecithin-hydrolyzing enzyme which correlates with hemolytic activity in El Tor vibrio isolates. *Nature* **206:**728.

286. **Mahoney, F. J., T. A. Farley, and K. Y. Kelso.** 1992. An outbreak of hepatitis A associated with swimming in a public pool. *J. Infect. Dis.* **165:**613–618.

287. **Mazumder, D. N. G., A. K. Ghosh, S. P. De, and B. K. Sirkar.** 1977. Vibrio parahaemolyticus infection in man. *Indian J. Med. Res.* **66:**180–188.

288. **McCabe, M. J., W. M. Hammon, and B. W. Halstead.** 1978. A fatal brain injury caused by a needlefish. *Neuroradiology* **15:**137–139.

289. **McCollum, J. P. K., R. C. M. Pearson, and H. R. Ingham.** 1968. An epidemic of mussel poisoning in North-east England. *Lancet* **ii:**767–770.

290. **McCollum, R. W., and A. J. Zuckerman.** 1981. Viral hepatitis: report on a WHO informal consultation. *J. Med. Virol.* **8:**1–29.

291. **McGuigan, M.** 1981. Shellfish poisoning. *Clin. Toxicol. Rev.* **3:**12.

292. Mead, P., L. Slutsker, and V. Dietz. 1999. Food-related illness and disease in the United States. *Emerg. Infect. Dis.* **5:**1–20.

293. Reference deleted.

294. Melnick, J. L., and C. P. Gerba. 1980. The ecology of enteroviruses in natural waters. *Crit. Rev. Environ. Control* **10:**65–93.

295. Meurman, O. H., and M. J. Laine. 1977. Rotavirus epidemics in adults. *N. Engl. J. Med.* **296:**1298–1299.

296. Meyerhoff, W. L., T. Morizono, and C. G. Wright. 1983. Tympanostomy tubes and otic drops. *Laryngoscope* **93:**1022–1027.

297. Mhalu, F. S., A. M. Yusufali, J. Mbwana, and R. Nyambo. 1982. Cholera-like diseases due to Vibrio parahaemolyticus. *J. Trop. Med. Hyg.* **85:**169–171.

298. Miller, C. J., B. S. Drasar, and R. G. Feacham. 1984. Response of toxigenic Vibrio cholerae O1 to physico-chemical stresses in aquatic environments. *J. Hyg.* **93:**475–495.

299. Mills, A. R., and R. Passmore. 1988. Pelagic paralysis. *Lancet* **331:**161–164.

300. Mishu, B., S. C. Hadler, and V. A. Boaz. 1990. Foodborne hepatitis A: evidence that microwaving reduces risk. *J. Infect. Dis.* **162:**655–658.

301. Miyake, M., T. Honda, and T. Miwatani. 1989. Effects of divalent cations and saccharides on Vibrio metschnikovii cytolysin-induced hemolysis of rabbit erythrocytes. *Infect. Immun.* **57:**158–163.

302. Miyake, M., T. Honda, and T. Miwatani. 1988. Purification and characterization of Vibrio metschnikovii cytolysin. *Infect. Immun.* **56:**954–960.

303. Miyamoto, Y., Y. Obara, T. Nikkawa, S. Yamai, T. Kato, Y. Yamada, and M. Ohashi. 1980. Simplified purification and biophysicochemical characteristics of Kanagawa phenomenon-associated hemolysin of Vibrio parahaemolyticus. *Infect. Immun.* **28:**567–576.

304. Molenda, J. R., W. G. Johnson, M. Fishbein, B. Wentz, I. J. Mehlman, and T. A. Dadisman, Jr. 1972. Vibrio parahaemolyticus gastroenteritis in Maryland: laboratory aspects. *Appl. Microbiol.* **24:**444–448.

305. Mollohan, C. S., and M. S. Romer. 1961. Public health significance of swimming pool granuloma. *Am. J. Public Health* **51:**883–891.

306. Morgan, D. R., B. D. Ball, and D. G. Moore. 1985. Severe Vibrio cholerae sepsis and meningitis in a young infant. *Tex. Med.* **81:**37–38.

307. Morris, J. G., Jr. 1990. Ciguatera fish poisoning: barracuda's revenge. *South. Med. J.* **83:**371–372.

308. Morris, J. G., Jr. 1988. Vibrio vulnificus—a new monster of the deep? *Ann. Intern. Med.* **109:**261–263.

309. Morris, J. G., Jr., and R. E. Black. 1985. Cholera and other vibrioses in the United States. *N. Engl. J. Med.* **312:**343–350.

310. Morris, J. G., Jr., H. G. Miller, R. Wilson, C. O. Tacket, D. G. Hollis, F. W. Hickman, R. E. Weaver, and P. A. Blake. 1982. Illness caused by Vibrio damsela and Vibrio hollisae. *Lancet* **i:**1294–1297.

311. Morris, J. G., Jr., J. H. Tenney, and G. L. Drusano. 1985. In vitro susceptibility of pathogenic Vibrio species to norfloxacin and six other antimicrobial agents. *Antimicrob. Agents Chemother.* **28:**442–445.

312. Morris, J. G., Jr., R. Wilson, B. R. Davis, I. K. Wachsmuth, C. F. Riddle, H. G. Wathen, R. A. Pollard, and P. A. Blake. 1981. Non-O group 1 Vibrio cholerae gastroenteritis in the United States: clinical, epidemiologic, and laboratory characteristics of sporadic cases. *Ann. Intern. Med.* **94:**656–658.

313. Morris, J. G., Jr., P. Lewin, N. T. Hargrett, C. W. Smith, P. A. Blake, and R. Schneider. 1982. Clinical features of ciguatera fish poisoning: a study of the disease in the US Virgin Islands. *Arch. Intern. Med.* **142:**1090–1092.

314. Morris, J. G., Jr., J. L. Picardi, S. Lieb, J. V. Lee, A. Roberts, M. Hood, R. A. Gunn, and P. A. Blake. 1984. Isolation of nontoxigenic Vibrio cholerae O group 1 from a patient with severe gastrointestinal disease. *J. Clin. Microbiol.* **19:**296–297.

315. Morris, P. D., D. S. Campbell, and J. I. Freeman. 1990. Ciguatera fish poisoning: an outbreak associated with fish caught from North Carolina coastal waters. *South. Med. J.* **83:**379–382.

316. Morris, P. D., D. S. Campbell, T. J. Taylor, and J. I. Freeman. 1991. Clinical and epidemiological features of neurotoxic shellfish poisoning in North Carolina. *Am. J. Public Health* **81:**471–474.

317. Morrow, J. D., G. R. Margolies, J. Rowland, and L. J. Roberts II. 1991. Evidence that histamine is the causative toxin of scombroid-fish poisoning. *N. Engl. J. Med.* **324:**716–720.

318. **Morse, D. L., J. J. Guzewich, and J. P. Hanrahan.** 1986. Widespread outbreaks of clam- and oyster-associated gastroenteritis: role of Norwalk virus. *N. Engl. J. Med.* **314:**678–681.

319. Reference deleted.

320. **Mulder, G. D., T. M. Ries, and T. R. Beaver.** 1989. Nontoxigenic Vibrio cholerae wound infection after exposure to contaminated lake water *J. Infect. Dis.* **159:**809–810.

321. **Murphey, D. K., E. J. Septimus, and D. C. Waagner.** 1992. Catfish-related injury and infection: report of two cases and review of the literature. *Clin. Infect. Dis.* **14:**689–693.

322. **Murphy, A. M., G. S. Grohmann, P. J. Christopher, W. A. Lopez, G. R. Davey, and R. H. Millson.** 1979. An Australia-wide outbreak of gastroenteritis from oysters caused by Norwalk virus. *Med. J. Aust.* **2:**329–333.

323. **Murphy, E. B., K. A. Steidinger, and B. S. Roberts.** 1975. An explanation for the Florida East Coast Gymnodinium breve red tide of November 1972. *Limnol. Oceanogr.* **20:**481–486.

324. **Murray, C. K., G. Hobbs, and R. J. Gilbert.** 1982. Scombrotoxin and scombrotoxin-like poisoning from canned fish. *J. Hyg.* **88:**215–220.

325. **Nacescu, N., C. Ciufecu, and D. Florescu.** 1980. Vibrio alginolyticus enteritis. *Ann. Sclavo* **22:**169–172.

326. **Nataloni, R.** 1998. As more people pursue water sports, number of stings increase. *Infect. Dis. Child.* **11:**13–14.

327. **National Oceanic and Atmospheric Administration (NOAA).** 2002. *2001 Fisheries of the United States,* p. v. National Oceanic and Atmospheric Adminstration, Silver Spring, Md.

328. **Neafie, R. C., and W. M. Meyers.** 1991. Cutaneous larva migrans, p. 773–775. *In* G. T. Strickland (ed.), Hunter's *Tropical Medicine,* 7th ed. W. B. Saunders Co., Philadelphia, Pa.

329. **Nilsen, A., and O. Boe.** 1980. Fish tank granuloma. *Acta Dermatovenereol.* (Stockholm) **60:**451–452.

330. **Nip-Sakamoto, C. J., and F. D. Pien.** 1989. Vibrio vulnificus infection in Hawaii. *Int. J. Dermatol.* **28:**311–316.

331. **Nishibuchi, M., S. Doke, S. Toizumi, T. Umeda, M. Yoh, and T. Miwatani.** 1988. Isolation from a coastal fish of *Vibrio hollisae* capable of producing a hemolysin similar to the thermostable direct hemolysin of *Vibrio parahaemolyticus. Appl. Environ. Microbiol.* **54:**2144–2146.

332. **Nishibuchi, M., M. Ishibashi, Y. Takeda, and J. B. Kaper.** 1985. Detection of the thermostable direct hemolysin gene and related DNA sequences in *Vibrio parahaemolyticus* and other *Vibrio species* by the DNA colony hybridization test. *Infect. Immun.* **49:**481–486.

333. **Nishibuchi, M., and R. J. Seidler.** 1983. Medium-dependent production of extracellular enterotoxins by non-O1 *Vibrio cholerae, Vibrio mimicus,* and *Vibrio fluvialis. Appl. Environ. Microbiol.* **45:**228–231.

334. **Nishibuchi, M., R. J. Seidler, D. M. Rollins, and S. W. Joseph.** 1983. *Vibrio* factors cause rapid fluid accumulation in suckling mice. *Infect. Immun.* **40:**1083–1091.

335. **Obara, Y., S. Yamai, T. Nikkawa, Y. Miyamoto, M. Ohashi, and T. Shimada.** 1974. Histochemical changes in the small intestine of suckling mice challenged orally with purified hemolysin from *Vibrio parahaemolyticus,* p. 278–284. *In* T. Fujino, G. Sakaguchi, R. Sakazaki, and Y. Takeda (ed.), *International Symposium on Vibrio parahaemolyticus.* Saikon Publ. Co., Tokyo, Japan.

336. **Oberhofer, T. R., and J. K. Podgore.** 1982. Urea-hydrolyzing *Vibrio parahaemolyticus* associated with acute gastroenteritis. *J. Clin. Microbiol.* **16:**581–583.

337. **O'Brien, A. D., M. E. Chen, R. K. Holmes, J. Kaper, and M. M. Levine.** 1984. Environmental and human isolates of Vibrio cholerae and Vibrio parahaemolyticus produce a Shigella dysenteriae 1 (Shiga)-like cytotoxin. *Lancet* **i:**77–78.

338. **Ohashi, M., T. Shimada, and H. Fukumi.** 1972. In vitro production of enterotoxin and hemorrhagic principle by Vibrio cholerae, NAG. *Jpn. J. Med. Sci. Biol.* **25:**179–194.

339. **Oliver, J. D.** 1981. Lethal cold stress of *Vibrio vulnificus* in oysters. *Appl. Environ. Microbiol.* **41:**710–717.

340. **Oliver, J. D., R. A. Warner, and D. R. Cleland.** 1983. Distribution of *Vibrio vulnificus* and other lactose-fermenting vibrios in the marine environment. *Appl. Environ. Microbiol.* **45:**985–998.

341. **Oliver, J. D., J. E. Wear, M. B. Thomas, M. Warner, and K. Linder.** 1986. Production of extracellular enzymes and cytotoxicity by Vibrio vulnificus. *Diagn. Microbiol. Infect. Dis.* **5:**99–111.

342. **Opal, S. M., and J. R. Saxon.** 1986. Intracranial infection by *Vibrio alginolyticus* following injury in saltwater. *J. Clin. Microbiol.* **23:**373–374.

343. O'Reilly, G., G. Isbister, P. Lawrie, G. Treston, and B. Currie. 2001. Prospective study of jellyfish stings from tropical Australia, including the major box jellyfish Chironex fleckeri. *Med. J. Aust.* **175**:652–655.

344. Palafox, N., L. Jain, A. Pinano, T. Gulick, R. Williams, and I. Schatz. 1988. Successful treatment of ciguatera fish poisoning with intravenous mannitol. *JAMA* **259**:2740–2742.

345. Palasuntheram, C., and S. Selvarajah. 1981. Vibrio parahaemolyticus in Colombo environment. *Indian J. Med. Res.* **73**:13–17.

346. Park, S. D., H. S. Shon, and N. J. Joh. 1991. Vibrio vulnificus septicemia in Korea: clinical and epidemiologic findings in seventy patients. *J. Am. Acad. Dermatol.* **24**:397–403.

347. Park, S. D., H. S. Sohn, and J. W. Koh. 1986. Effect of hydrogen ions on the growth of Vibrio vulnificus. *Korean J. Dermatol.* **24**:354–357.

348. Pavia, A. T., J. A. Bryan, K. L. Maher, T. R. Hester, Jr., and J. J. Farmer III. 1989. Vibrio carchariae infection after a shark bite. *Ann. Intern. Med.* **111**:85–86.

349. Perl, T. M., L. Bedard, T. Kosatsky, J. C. Hockin, E. C. D. Todd, and R. S. Remis. 1990. An outbreak of toxic encephalopathy caused by eating mussels contaminated with domoic acid. *N. Engl. J. Med.* **322**:1775–1780.

350. Peterson, E. M., P. Jemison-Smith, L. M. de la Maza, and D. Miller. 1982. Cholecystitis: its occurrence with cholelithiasis associated with a non-O1 Vibrio cholerae. *Arch. Pathol. Lab. Med.* **106**:300–301.

351. Peterson, J. W., and L. G. Ochoa. 1989. Role of prostaglandins and cAMP in the secretory effects of cholera toxin. *Science* **245**:857–859.

352. Pien, F. D., K. S. Ang, N. T. Nakashima, D. G. Evans, J. A. Grote, M. L. Hefley, and E. A. Kubota. 1983. Bacterial flora of marine penetrating injuries. *Diagn. Microbiol. Infect. Dis.* **1**:229–232.

353. Plotkin, B. J., S. G. Kilgore, and L. McFarland. 1990. Polyvibrio infections: Vibrio vulnificus and Vibrio parahaemolyticus dual wound and multiple site infections. *J. Infect. Dis.* **161**:364–365.

354. Poli, M. A., R. J. Lewis, R. W. Dickey, S. M. Musser, C. A. Buckner, and L. G. Carpenter. 1997. Identification of Caribbean ciguatoxins as the cause of an outbreak of fish poisoning among U.S. soldiers in Haiti. *Toxicon* **35**:733–741.

355. Pool, M. D., and J. D. Oliver. 1978. Experimental pathogenicity and mortality in ligated ileal loop studies of the newly reported halophilic lactose-positive Vibrio sp. *Infect. Immun.* **20**:126–129.

356. Portnoy, B. L., P. A. Mackowiak, and C. T. Caraway. 1975. Oyster-associated hepatitis: failure of shellfish certification programs to prevent outbreaks. *JAMA* **233**:1065–1068.

357. Reference deleted.

358. Prevost, E., E. M. Walker, Jr., A. J. Kreutner, and J. Manos. 1982. Mycobacterium marinum infections: diagnosis and treatment. *South. Med. J.* **75**:1349–1352.

359. Prociv, P. 1978. Vibrio alginolyticus in Western Australia. *Med. J. Aust.* **2**:296.

360. Quilliam, M. A., and J. L. C. Wright. 1989. The amnesic shellfish poisoning mystery. *Anal. Chem.* **61**:1053–1059.

361. Rainer, M. D. 1972. Mode of action of ciguatoxin. *Fed. Proc.* **31**:1139–1145.

362. RaLonde, R. 1996. Paralytic shellfish poisoning; the Alaska problem. *Alsk. Mar. Resour.* **8**(2):1–20.

363. Reference deleted.

364. Ramia, S. 1985. Transmission of viral infections by the water route: implications for developing countries. *Rev. Infect. Dis.* **7**:180–188.

365. Rank, E. L., I. B. Smith, and M. Langer. 1988. Bacteremia caused by Vibrio hollisae. *J. Clin. Microbiol.* **26**:375–376.

366. Reichelt, J. L., P. Baumann, and L. Baumann. 1976. Study of genetic relationships among marine species of the genus Beneckea and Photobacterium by means of in vitro DNA/DNA hybridization. *Arch. Microbiol.* **110**:101–120.

367. Reid, T. M. S., and H. G. Robinson. 1987. Frozen raspberries and hepatitis A. *Epidemiol. Infect.* **98**:109–112.

368. Rhodes, J. B., D. Schweitzer, and J. E. Ogg. 1985. Isolation of non-O1 Vibrio cholerae associated with enteric disease of herbivores in western Colorado. *J. Clin. Microbiol.* **22**:572–575.

369. Rhodes, J. B., H. L. Smith, Jr., and J. E. Ogg. 1986. Isolation of non-O1 Vibrio cholerae serovars from surface waters in western Colorado. *Appl. Environ. Microbiol.* **51**:1216–1219.

370. Richards, C. A. 1998. Pfiesteria piscicida studies underway in six states. *Infect. Dis. News* **11**:14–15.

371. **Ries, K. M., G. L. White, Jr., and R. T. Murdock.** 1990. Atypical mycobacterial infection caused by Mycobacterium marinum. *N. Engl. J. Med.* **322:**633.

372. **Risk, M., K. Werrbach-Perez, and J. R. Perez-Polo.** 1979. Mechanism of action of the major toxin from Gymnodinium breve davis, p. 367–372. *In* D. L. Taylor and H. H. Seliger (ed.), *Toxic Dinoflagellate Blooms.* Elsevier/Holland, New York, N.Y.

373. **Robinson, A. C.** 1989. Evaluation for waterproof ear protectors in swimmers. *J. Laryngol. Otol.* **103:**1154–1157.

374. **Rodrick, G. E., M. A. Hood, and N. J. Blake.** 1982. Human vibrio gastroenteritis. *Med. Clin. N. Am.* **66:**665–673.

375. **Rodrigue, D. C., R. A. Etzel, S. Hall, E. de Porras, O. H. Velasquez, R. V. Tauxe, E. M. Kilbourne, and P. A. Blake.** 1990. Lethal paralytic shellfish poisoning in Guatemala. *Am. J. Trop. Med. Hyg.* **42:**267–271.

376. **Roland, F., R. Bertini, and J. Jhang.** 1985. Vibrio parahaemolyticus osteomyelitis of 12 years duration. *R. I. Med. J.* **68:**553–555.

377. **Roos, B.** 1956. Hepatitis epidemic transmitted by oysters. *Sven. Lak-Tidning* **53:**989–1003.

378. **Rosenberg, C. E.** 1962. *The Cholera Years: The United States in 1832, 1849, and 1866.* University of Chicago Press, Chicago, Ill.

379. **Rosenblum, L. S., I. R. Mirkin, and D. T. Allen.** 1990. A multifocal outbreak of hepatitis A traced to commercially distributed lettuce. *Am. J. Public Health* **80:**1075–1079.

380. **Rubin, L. G., J. Altman, L. K. Epple, and R. H. Yolken.** 1981. Vibrio cholerae meningitis in a neonate. *J. Pediatr.* **98:**940–942.

381. **Russell, F. E.** 1961. Injuries by venomous animals in the US. *JAMA* **177:**85.

382. **Ryan, A. J.** 1989. Nontraumatic medical problems, p. 391–414. *In* A. J. Ryan and F. L. Allman (ed.), *Sports Medicine,* 2nd ed. Academic Press, Inc., San Diego, Calif.

383. **Sacks-Berg, A., M. J. Strampfer, and B. A. Cunha.** 1987. Vibrio vulnificus bacteremia: report of a case and review of the literature. *Heart Lung* **16:**706–709.

384. **Safrin, S., J. G. Morris, Jr., M. Adams, V. Pons, R. Jacobs, and J. E. Conte, Jr.** 1988. Non-O:1 Vibrio cholerae bacteremia: case report and review. *Rev. Infect. Dis.* **10:**1012–1017.

385. **Sakamoto, Y., R. F. Lockey, and J. J. Krzanowski.** 1987. Shellfish and fish poisoning related to the toxic dinoflagellates. *South. Med. J.* **80:**866–872.

386. **Sakamoto, Y., J. J. Krzanowski, and R. Lockey.** 1985. The mechanism of Ptychodiscus brevis toxin induced contraction of rat vas deferens. *J. Allergy Clin. Immunol.* **76:**117–122.

387. **Sakazaki, R.** 1968. Proposal of Vibrio alginolyticus for the biotype 2 of Vibrio parahaemolyticus. *Jpn. J. Med. Sci. Biol.* **21:**359–362.

388. **Saliba, L. J., and R. Helmer.** 1990. Health risks associated with pollution of coastal bathing waters. *World Health Stat. Q.* **43:**177–187.

389. **Salmaso, S., D. Greco, B. Bonfiglio, M. Castellani-Pastoris, G. De Filip, A. Bracciotti, G. Sitzia, A. Congiu, G. Piu, G. Angioni, L. Barra, A. Zampieri, and W. B. Baine.** 1980. Recurrence of pelecypod-associated cholera in Sardinia. *Lancet* **ii:**1124–1127.

390. **Samadi, A. R., M. I. Huq, and N. S. Shahid.** 1983. Classical Vibrio cholerae biotype displaces El Tor in Bangladesh. *Lancet* **i:**805–807.

391. **Sanders, W. E., Jr.** 1987. Intoxications from the seas: ciguatera, scombroid, and paralytic shellfish poisoning. *Infect. Dis. Clin. N. Am.* **1:**665–676.

392. **Sarkar, B. L., G. B. Nair, A. K. Banerjee, and S. C. Pal.** 1985. Seasonal distribution of *Vibrio parahaemolyticus* in freshwater environs and in association with freshwater fishes in Calcutta. *Appl. Environ. Microbiol.* **49:**132–136.

393. **Sarnaik, A. P., M. P. Vohra, S. W. Sturman, and W. M. Belenky.** 1986. Medical problems of the swimmer. *Clin. Sports Med.* **5:**47–64.

394. **Schandevyl, P., E. Van Dyck, and P. Piot.** 1984. Halophilic *Vibrio* species from seafish in Senegal. *Appl. Environ. Microbiol.* **48:**236–238.

395. **Scheid, R., F. Deinhardt, and G. Frosner.** 1982. Inactivation of hepatitis A and B virus and risk of iatrogenic transmission, p. 627–628. *In* W. Szmuness, H. J. Alter, and H. E. Maynard (ed.), *Viral Hepatitis.* Franklin Institute Press, Philadelphia, Pa.

396. **Schiraldi, O., V. Benvestito, C. DiBari, R. Moschetta, and G. Pastore.** 1974. Gastric abnormalities in cholera: epidemiologic and clinical considerations. *Bull. W. H. O.* **51:**349–352.

397. **Schmidt, V., H. Chmel, and C. Cobbs.** 1979. *Vibrio alginolyticus* infections in humans. *J. Clin. Microbiol.* **10:**666–668.

398. **Schonherr, U., G. O. H. Naumann, G. K. Lang, and A. A. Bialasiewicz.** 1989. Sclerokeratitis caused by Mycobacterium marinum. *Am. J. Ophthalmol.* **108:**607–608.

399. **Schuller, D. E., and R. A. Bruce.** 1991. Ear, nose, throat, and eye, p. 189–203. *In* R. Strauss (ed.), *Sports Medicine,* 2nd ed. W. B. Saunders Co., Philadelphia, Pa.

400. **Seidler, R. J., D. A. Allen, and R. R. Colwell.** 1980. Biochemical characteristics and virulence of environmental group F bacteria isolated in the United States. *Appl. Environ. Microbiol.* **40:**715–720.

401. **Seidler, R. J., and T. M. Evans.** 1984. Computer-assisted analysis of Vibrio field data: four coastal areas, p. 411–426. *In* R. R. Colwell (ed.), *Vibrios in the Environment.* John Wiley & Sons, Inc., New York, N.Y.

402. **Shandera, W. X., J. M. Johnston, B. R. Davis, and P. A. Blake.** 1983. Disease from infection with Vibrio mimicus, a newly recognized Vibrio species: clinical characteristics and epidemiology. *Ann. Intern. Med.* **99:**169–171.

403. **Shirai, H., H. Ito, T. Hirayama, Y. Nakamoto, N. Nakabayashi, K. Kumagai, Y. Takeda, and M. Nishibuchi.** 1990. Molecular epidemiologic evidence for association of thermostable direct hemolysin (TDH) and TDH-related hemolysin of *Vibrio parahaemolyticus* with gastroenteritis. *Infect. Immun.* **58:**3568–3573.

404. **Simpson, L. M., and J. D. Oliver.** 1983. Siderophore production by *Vibrio vulnificus. Infect. Immun.* **41:**644–649.

405. **Sims, J. K., and D. C. Ostman.** 1986. Pufferfish poisoning: emergency diagnosis and management of mild human tetrodotoxication. *Ann. Emerg. Med.* **15:**1094–1098.

406. **Sims, J. K.** 1987. A theoretical discourse on the pharmacology of toxic marine ingestions. *Ann. Emerg. Med.* **16:**1006–1015.

407. **Singleton, F. L., R. Attwell, S. Jangi, and R. R. Colwell.** 1982. Effects of temperature and salinity on *Vibrio cholerae* growth. *Appl. Environ. Microbiol.* **44:**1047–1058.

408. **Singleton, F. L., R. W. Attwell, S. Jangi, and R. R. Colwell.** 1982. Influence of salinity and organic nutrient concentration on survival and growth of *Vibrio cholerae* in aquatic microcosms. *Appl. Environ. Microbiol.* **43:**1080–1085.

409. **Sircar, B. K., P. Dutta, S. P. De, S. N. Sikdar, B. C. Deb, and S. C. Pal.** 1981. ABO blood group distributions in diarrhoea cases including cholera in Calcutta. *Ann. Hum. Biol.* **8:**289–291.

410. **Smith, G. C., and J. R. Merkel.** 1982. Collagenolytic activity of *Vibrio vulnificus:* potential contribution to its invasiveness. *Infect. Immun.* **35:**1155–1156.

411. **Sodeman, W. A., Jr.** 1991. Venomous marine animals, p. 869–875. *In* G. T. Strickland (ed.), *Hunter's Tropical Medicine,* 7th ed. W. B. Saunders Co., Philadelphia, Pa.

412. **Soppe, G. G.** 1989. Marine envenomation and aquatic dermatology. *Am. Fam. Physician* **40:**97–106.

413. **Sreenivasan, M. A., K. Banerjee, and P. G. Pandya.** 1978. Epidemiologic investigations of an outbreak of infectious hepatitis in Ahmedabad City during 1975–76. *Indian J. Med. Res.* **67:**197–206.

413a.**Stafford-Deitsch, J.** 1991. *Reef: a Safari through the Coral World.* Sierra Club Books, San Francisco, Calif.

414. **Stahr, B., S. T. Threadgill, T. L. Overman, and R. C. Noble.** 1989. Vibrio vulnificus sepsis after eating raw oysters. *J. Ky. Med. Assoc.* **87:**219–222.

415. **Steidinger, K. A.** 1979. Collection, enumeration, and identification of free-living marine dinoflagellates, p. 435–442. *In* D. L. Taylor and H. H. Seliger (ed.), *Toxic Dinoflagellate Blooms.* Elsevier/North Holland, New York, N.Y.

416. **Steinkuller, P. G., M. T. Kelly, S. J. Sands, and J. C. Barber.** 1980. Vibrio parahaemolyticus endophthalmitis. *J. Pediatr. Ophthalmol. Strabismus* **17:**150–153.

417. **Stewart, J. P.** 1951. Chronic exudative otitis externa. *J. Laryngol. Otol.* **65:**24.

418. **Subba Rao, D. V., M. A. Quilliam, and R. Pocklington.** 1988. Domoic acid—a neurotoxic amino acid produced by the marine diatom Nitzschia pungens in culture. *Can. J. Fish. Aquat. Sci.* **45:**2076–2079.

419. **Sullivan, J. J., and W. T. Iwaoka.** 1983. High pressure liquid chromatographic determination of toxins associated with paralytic shellfish poisoning. *J. Assoc. Off. Anal. Chem.* **66:**297–303.

420. **Swerdlow, D. L., and A. A. Ries.** 1992. Cholera in the Americas. Guidelines for the clinician. *JAMA* **267:**1495–1499.

421. **Swift, S., and H. Cohen.** 1962. Granulomas of the skin due to Mycobacterium balnei after abrasions from a fish tank. *N. Engl. J. Med.* **267**:1244–1246.

422. **Tacket, C. O., T. J. Barrett, G. E. Sanders, and P. A. Blake.** 1982. Panophthalmitis caused by *Vibrio parahaemolyticus. J. Clin. Microbiol.* **16**:195–196.

423. **Tacket, C. O., F. Brenner, and P. A. Blake.** 1984. Clinical features and an epidemiological study of Vibrio vulnificus infections. *J. Infect. Dis.* **149**:558–561.

424. **Tacket, C. O., F. Hickman, and G. V. Pierce.** 1982. Diarrhea associated with *Vibrio fluvialis* in the United States. *J. Clin. Microbiol.* **16**:991–992.

425. **Tamplin, M., G. E. Rodrick, N. J. Blake, and T. Cuba.** 1982. Isolation and characterization of Vibrio vulnificus from two Florida estuaries. *Appl. Environ. Microbiol.* **44**:1466–1470.

426. **Tan, C. T. T., and E. J. D. Lee.** 1986. Paralytic shellfish poisoning in Singapore. *Ann. Acad. Med. Singap.* **15**:77–79.

427. **Tang, Y. W., J. X. Wang, Z. Y. Xu, Y. F. Guo, W. H. Qian, and J. X. Xu.** 1991. A serologically confirmed, case-control study, of a large outbreak of hepatitis A in China, associated with consumption of clams. *Epidemiol. Infect.* **107**:651–657.

428. **Taylor, R., M. McDonald, G. Russ, M. Carson, and E. Lukaczynski.** 1981. Vibrio alginolyticus peritonitis associated with ambulatory peritoneal dialysis. *Br. Med. J.* **283**:275.

429. **Taylor, S. L., J. E. Stratton, and J. A. Nordlee.** 1989. Histamine poisoning (scombroid fish poisoning): an allergy-like intoxication. *J. Toxicol. Clin. Toxicol.* **27**:225–240.

430. **Tefany, F. J., S. Lee, and S. Shumack.** 1990. Oysters, iron overload and Vibrio vulnificus septicaemia. *Australas. J. Dermatol.* **31**:27–31.

431. **Teitelbaum, J. S., R. J. Zatorre, S. Carpenter, D. Gendron, E. C. Evans, A. Gjedde, and N. R. Cashman.** 1990. Neurologic sequelae of domoic acid intoxication due to the ingestion of contaminated mussels. *N. Engl. J. Med.* **322**:1781–1787.

432. **Tester, P. A., P. K. Fowler, and J. T. Turner.** 1990. Gulf Stream transport of the toxic red tide dinoflagellate Ptychodiscus brevis from Florida to North Carolina, p. 349–358. *In* E. M. Cosper, E. J. Carpenter, and V. M. Bricelj (ed.), *Novel Phytoplankton Blooms: Causes and Impact of Recurrent Brown Tides and Other Unusual Blooms.* Springer-Verlag, Berlin, Germany.

433. **Thekdi, R. J., A. G. Lakhani, V. B. Rale, and M. V. Panse.** 1990. An outbreak of food poisoning suspected to be caused by Vibrio fluvialis. *J. Diarrhoeal. Dis. Res.* **8**:163–165.

434. **Thibaut, K., P. Van de Heying, and S. R. Pattyn.** 1986. Isolation of non-O1 Vibrio cholerae from ear tracts. *Eur. J. Epidemiol.* **2**:316–317.

435. **Tibballs, J., D. Williams, and S. K. Sutherland.** 1998. The effects of antivenom and verapamil on the haemodynamic actions of Chironex fleckeri (box jellyfish) venom. *Anaesth. Intensive Care* **26**:40–45.

436. **Ticehurst, J., L. L. J. Rhodes, and K. Krawczynski.** 1992. Infection of owl monkeys (Aotus trivirgatus) and cynomolgus monkeys (Macaca fascicularis) with hepatitis E virus from Mexico. *J. Infect. Dis.* **165**:835–845.

437. **Tison, D. L., and M. T. Kelly.** 1984. Vibrio species of medical importance. *Diagn. Microbiol. Infect. Dis.* **2**:263–276.

438. **Tison, D. L., and M. T. Kelly.** 1984. *Vibrio vulnificus* endometritis. *J. Clin. Microbiol.* **20**:185–186.

439. **Tison, D. L., M. Nishibuchi, R. J. Seidler, and R. J. Sieberling.** 1986. Isolation of non-O1 Vibrio cholerae serovars from Oregon coastal waters. *Appl. Environ. Microbiol.* **51**:444–445.

440. **Togias, A. G., J. W. Burnett, A. Kagey-Sobotka, and L. M. Lichtenstein.** 1985. Anaphylaxis after contact with a jellyfish. *J. Allergy Clin. Immunol.* **75**:672–675.

441. **Trestrail, J. H., III, and Q. M. al-Mahasneh.** 1989. Lionfish sting experiences of an inland poison center: a retrospective study of 23 cases. *Vet. Hum. Toxicol.* **31**:173–175.

442. **Tripuraneni, J., A. Koutsoris, L. Pestic, P. De Lanerolle, and G. Hecht.** 1997. The toxin of diarrheic shellfish poisoning, okadaic acid, increases intestinal epithelial paracellular permeability. *Gastroenterology* **112**:100–108.

443. **Truwit, J. D., D. B. Badesch, A. M. Savage, and M. Shelton.** 1987. Vibrio vulnificus bacteremia with endocarditis. *South. Med. J.* **80**:1457–1459.

444. **Tsega, E., K. Krawczynski, and B. G. Hansson.** 1991. Outbreak of hepatitis E virus infection among military personnel in Northern Ethiopia. *J. Med. Virol.* **34**:232–236.

445. **Tu, A. T.** 1987. Biotoxicology of sea snake venoms. *Ann. Emerg. Med.* **16**:1023–1028.

446. **Tu, A. T.** 1990. Neurotoxins from sea snake and other vertebrate venoms, p. 336–346. *In* S. Hall and G. Strichartz (ed.), *Marine Toxins. Origin, Structure, and Molecular Pharmacology.* American Chemical Society, Washington, D.C.

447. **Twedt, R. M.** 1989. Vibrio parahaemolyticus, p. 543–568. *In* M. P. Doyle (ed.), *Foodborne Bacterial Pathogens.* Marcel Dekker, New York, N.Y.

448. **Twedt, R. M., J. M. Madden, J. M. Hunt, D. W. Francis, J. T. Peeler, A. P. Duran, W. O. Herbert, S. G. McCay, C. N. Roderick, G. T. Spite, and T. J. Wazenski.** 1981. Characterization of *Vibrio cholerae* isolated from oysters. *Appl. Environ. Microbiol.* **41:**1475–1478.

449. **Vancouver, G.** 1798. *A Voyage of Discovery to the North Pacific Ocean and Round the World,* vol. 2, p. 284–286. Robinson, London, England.

450. **van der Sar, A.** 1982. Ciguatera poisoning and T-wave changes. *JAMA* **247:**1345.

451. **Van Dyke, J. J., and K. B. Lake.** 1975. Chemotherapy for aquarium granuloma. *JAMA* **233:**1380–1381.

452. **Vartian, C. V., and E. J. Septimus.** 1990. Osteomyelitis caused by Vibrio vulnificus. *J. Infect. Dis.* **161:**363.

453. **Vincenzi, C., F. Bardazzi, and A. Tosti.** 1992. Fish tank granuloma: report of a case. *Cutis* **49:**275–276.

454. **Viswanathan, R.** 1957. Infectious hepatitis in Delhi (1955–56): a critical study; epidemiology. *Indian J. Med. Res.* **45**(Suppl.)**:**1–30.

455. **Wagner, R. F., A. B. Tawil, A. J. Colletta, L. C. Hurst, and L. D. Yecies.** 1981. Mycobacterium marinum tenosynovitis in a Long Island fisherman. *N. Y. State J. Med.* **81:**1091–1094.

456. **Walker, S. T.** 1884. Fish mortality in the Gulf of Mexico. *Proc. U. S. Natl. Mus.* **6:**105–109.

457. **Wallace, C. K., N. F. Pierce, P. N. Anderson, T. C. Brown, G. W. Lewis, S. N. Sanyal, G. V. Segre, and R. H. Waldman.** 1967. Probable gallbladder infection in convalescent cholera patients. *Lancet* **1:**865–868.

458. **Wanke, C. A., and R. L. Guerrant.** 1987. Viral hepatitis and gastroenteritis transmitted by shellfish and water. *Infect. Dis. Clin. N. Am.* **1:**649–664.

459. **Watsky, D.** 1983. Vibrio fluvialis and Vibrio mimicus associated with terminal ileitis. *Clin. Microbiol. Newsl.* **5:**111.

459a. **Weinberg, S., N. Prose, and L. Kristal.** 1998. *Color Atlas of Pediatric Dermatology.* McGraw-Hill, New York, N.Y.

460. **Weissman, J. B., W. E. DeWitt, J. Thompson, C. N. Muchnick, B. L. Portnoy, J. C. Feeley, and E. J. Gangarosa.** 1975. A case of cholera in Texas, 1973. *Am. J. Epidemiol.* **100:**487–498.

461. **West, B., R. Silberman, and W. Otterson.** 1998. Acalculous cholecystitis and septicemia caused by non-O1 Vibrio cholerae: first reported case and review of biliary infections with Vibrio cholerae. *Diagn. Microbiol. Infect. Dis.* **30:**187–191.

462. **West, P. A.** 1986. Hazard Analysis Critical Control Point (HACCP) Concept: application to bivalve shellfish purification systems. *J. R. Soc. Health* **106:**133–140.

463. **West, P. A.** 1989. The human pathogenic vibrios—a public health update with environmental perspectives. *Epidemiol. Infect.* **103:**1–34.

464. **West, P. A., and J. V. Lee.** 1982. Ecology of Vibrio species, including Vibrio cholerae, in natural wares of Kent, England. *J. Appl. Bacteriol.* **52:**435–448.

465. **West, P. A., P. C. Wood, and M. Jacob.** 1985. Control of food poisoning risks associated with shellfish. *J. R. Soc. Health* **105:**15–21.

466. **Wickboldt, I. G., and C. V. Sanders.** 1983. Vibrio vulnificus infection: case report and update since 1970. *J. Am. Acad. Dermatol.* **9:**243–251.

467. **Williams, C. S., and D. C. Riordan.** 1973. Mycobacterium marinum (atypical acid-fast bacillus) infections of the hand: a report of six cases. *J. Bone Jt. Surg. Am. Vol.* **55A:**1042–1050.

468. **Williams, L. A., and P. A. La Rock.** 1985. Temporal occurrence of *Vibrio* species and *Aeromonas hydrophila* in estuarine sediments. *Appl. Environ. Microbiol.* **50:**1490–1495.

469. **Wilson, R., S. Lieb, A. Roberts, S. Stryker, H. Janowski, R. Gunn, B. Davis, C. F. Riddle, T. Barrett, J. G. Morris, Jr., and P. A. Blake.** 1981. Non-O group 1 Vibrio cholerae gastroenteritis associated with eating raw oysters. *Am. J. Epidemiol.* **114:**293–298.

470. **Withers, N. W.** 1982. Ciguatera fish poisoning. *Annu. Rev. Med.* **33:**97–111.

471. **Wong, D. C., R. H. Purcell, and M. A. Sreenivasan.** 1980. Epidemic and endemic hepatitis in India: evidence for a non-A, non-B hepatitis etiology. *Lancet* **ii:**876–879.

472. **World Health Organization.** 1986. *Environmental Health Criteria*, p. 73–75. World Health Organization, Geneva, Switzerland.
473. **World Health Organization.** 1980. Cholera and other vibrio-associated diarrhoeas. *Bull W. H. O.* **58**:353–374.
474. **World Health Organization.** 1969. Outbreak of gastroenteritis by non-agglutinable (NAG) vibrios. *WHO Wkly. Epidemiol. Rec.* **44**:10.
475. **World Health Organization.** 1970. *Principles and Practice of Cholera Control.* World Health Organization, Geneva, Switzerland.
476. **World Health Organization.** 1980. Rotavirus and other viral diarrhoeas. *Bull. W. H. O.* **58**:183–198.
477. **Wozniak, D. F., G. R. Stewart, J. P. Miller, and J. W. Olney.** 1991. Age-related sensitivity to kainate neurotoxicity. *Exp. Neurol.* **114**:250–253.
478. **Wright, A. C., L. M. Simpson, and J. D. Oliver.** 1981. Role of iron in the pathogenesis of *Vibrio vulnificus* infections. *Infect. Immun.* **34**:503–507.
479. **Wright, A. C., L. M. Simpson, J. D. Oliver, and J. G. Morris, Jr.** 1990. Phenotypic evaluation of acapsular transposon mutants of *Vibrio vulnificus. Infect. Immun.* **58**:1769–1773.
480. **Wright, D. N., and J. M. Alexander.** 1974. Effect of water on the bacterial flora of swimmer's ears. *Arch. Otolaryngol.* **99**:15–18.
481. **Yamamoto, K., Y. Ichinose, N. Nakasone, M. Tanabe, M. Nagahama, J. Sakurai, and M. Iwanaga.** 1986. Identity of hemolysins produced by *Vibrio cholerae* non-O1 and *V. cholerae* O1, biotype El Tor. *Infect. Immun.* **51**:927–931.
482. **Yamamoto, K., Y. Takeda, T. Miwatani, and J. P. Craig.** 1983. Evidence that a non-O1 *Vibrio cholerae* produces enterotoxin that is similar but not identical to cholera enterotoxin. *Infect. Immun.* **41**:896–901.
483. **Yamashita, T., K. Sakae, Y. Ishihara, and S. Isomura.** 1992. A 2-year survey of the prevalence of enteric viral infections in children compared with contamination in locally-harvested oysters. *Epidemiol. Infect.* **108**:155–163.
484. **Yasumoto, J.** 1985. Recent progress in the chemistry of dinoflagellate toxins, p. 259–270. *In* D. M. Anderson, A. W. White, and D. G. Baden (ed.), *Toxic Dinoflagellates.* Elsevier, New York, N.Y.
485. **Yasumoto, T., A. Inoue, and R. Bagnis.** 1979. Ecological survey of a toxic dinoflagellate associated with ciguatera, p. 221–224. *In* D. L. Taylor and H. H. Seliger (ed.), *Toxic Dinoflagellate Blooms.* Elsevier/North Holland, New York, N.Y.
486. **Yoh, M., T. Honda, and T. Miwatani.** 1986. Purification and partial characterization of a Vibrio hollisae hemolysin that relates to the thermostable direct hemolysin of Vibrio parahaemolyticus. *Can. J. Microbiol.* **32**:632–636.
487. **Yokoo, A.** 1950. Chemical studies on tetrodotoxin. Report III. Isolation of spheroidine. *J. Chem. Soc. Jpn.* **71**:591–592.
488. **Yoshida, S., M. Ogawa, and Y. Mizuguchi.** 1985. Relation of capsular materials and colony opacity to virulence of *Vibrio vulnificus. Infect. Immun.* **47**:446–451.
489. **Yoshii, Y., H. Nishino, K. Satake, and K. Umeyama.** 1987. Isolation of Vibrio fluvialis, an unusual pathogen in acute suppurative cholangitis. *Am. J. Gastroenterol.* **82**:903–905.
490. Reference deleted.
491. **Zen-yoji, H., Y. Kudoh, H. Igarashi, K. Ohta, and K. Fukai.** 1974. Purification and identification of enteropathogenic toxins "a" and "a'" produced by Vibrio parahaemolyticus and their biological and pathological activities, p. 237–243. *In* T. Fujino, G. Sakaguchi, R. Sakazaki, and Y. Takeda (ed.), *International Symposium on Vibrio parahaemolyticus.* Saikon Publishing Co., Tokyo, Japan.

Infections of Leisure, Third Edition
Edited by David Schlossberg
© 2004 ASM Press, Washington, D.C.

Chapter 2

Freshwater: from Lakes to Hot Tubs

Bertha Ayi and David Dworzack

This chapter focuses on infections acquired in nonmarine environments, including natural freshwater environments (lakes, ponds, rivers, and streams) and manmade aquatic environments (swimming pools, hot tubs, whirlpools, and spas). The discussion is limited to infections associated with immersion or other exposure to aquatic macro- or microenvironments. An appreciation of the wide variety of potential pathogens which occasionally cause problems for patients exposed to freshwater can be gained from Table 1.

These waterborne pathogens may enter the body through inhalation, aspiration, direct application to intact or injured skin, or invasion of respiratory or gastrointestinal mucosa. The pathogens may be native to the environments where infections are acquired, or they may proliferate there because of the influence of humans or their waste products. Infections produced by these pathogens are often merely nuisances. On occasion, however, they can be life threatening or cause severe long-term sequelae.

SKIN AND SOFT TISSUE INFECTIONS

Skin, soft tissue, and wound infections acquired in aquatic, nonmarine environments run the gamut from relatively benign conditions which resolve without specific therapy to life-threatening processes requiring intensive medical and surgical care. Infections caused by pyogenic bacteria, mycobacteria, parasites, and algae have all been reported (23).

Pseudomonas Dermatitis/Folliculitis

Pseudomonas dermatitis/folliculitis, a superficial infection which is usually recognized in cluster or localized outbreaks, was first reported in 1975 by McCausland and Cox (178). This original outbreak, like most others reported since, was

Bertha Ayi and David Dworzack • Department of Medical Microbiology and Immunology and Department of Internal Medicine, Section of Infectious Diseases, Creighton University Medical Center, Omaha, NE 68131.

Table 1. Infections associated with exposure to freshwater

Skin and soft tissue infections
  P. aeruginosa dermatitis/folliculitis
  P. aeruginosa hot-foot syndrome
  Acute diffuse otitis externa (swimmer's ear)
  Schistosome dermatitis (swimmer's itch, clam digger's itch)
  Nontuberculous mycobacterial infections (M. marinum, M. ulcerans, rapidly growing mycobacteria)
  Gram-negative bacilli (Aeromonas, Edwarsiella)
  Prototheca infection
  Cyanobacterium infection

Ocular infections
  Pharyngoconjunctival fever (swimming pool conjunctivitis)
  Amoebic keratitis (Acanthamoeba spp.)
  P. aeruginosa keratitis

Urinary tract infections
  P. aeruginosa infection

Pulmonary infections
  Legionella infection (pneumonia, Pontiac fever)
  P. aeruginosa pneumonia
  M. avium infection
  Pneumonia following near drowning
    Aerobic gram-negative bacteria (P. aeruginosa, Aeromonas spp., B. pseudomallei, Legionella spp.)
    S. pneumoniae
    Aspergillus spp.
    P. boydii

Disseminated infections
  Leptospirosis
  C. violaceum

Central nervous system infections
  PAM (N. fowleri)
  P. boydii brain abscess and meningitis
  Coxsackieviruses

associated with exposure to heated water in a hotel whirlpool (138, 214, 257, 265). Similar occurrences have followed the use of home spas (221) as well as swimming pools (42). The largest (265 cases of 650 exposed) and first outbreak involving exposure at a water slide was in Salt Lake City, Utah, in 1983 (39). Since then, more outbreaks involving water slides have been reported (77). More unusual are reports associated with the use of neoprene diving suits (149) and contaminated synthetic sponges used in bathing (170). These outbreaks may be more common in the summer, when outdoor activities are common (187).

In most outbreaks, faulty maintenance of water in man-made pools has been associated with overgrowth of *Pseudomonas aeruginosa*. Recommendations for treatment of pool water include maintaining the pH between 7.2 and 7.8 and free-chlorine levels greater than 0.5 mg/liter (40). In one outbreak, however, the pH and the chlorine content of contaminated water were found to be within these guidelines, suggesting that some strains of *P. aeruginosa* may be resistant to recommended chlorine concentrations (138). In another more recent outbreak where adequate chlorination had been maintained in swimming pool water, the source of the infection was traced to inflatables used by children (241). These inflatables serve as obstacle courses which are kept inflated by an air pump during use and deflated after use. Currently no guidelines exist on how to clean the inside and outside of these devices. Microorganisms can grow on these devices when they are kept outside the pool and not allowed to dry, or they can be contaminated from residual water inside the inflatable. Folliculitis occurs after skin contact with a contaminated inflatable.

There have been more outbreaks associated with whirlpools or spas than with swimming pools, indicating that the environment of the former is more conducive to the growth of organisms that cause folliculitis. In part, this appears to be related to the difficulty in maintaining a stable free-chlorine level in whirlpools compared to swimming pools because of the higher temperature of the water, mechanical agitation and aeration by pressurized jets, and a higher concentration of organic material due to the larger number of bathers per volume of water (205). For this reason, some have recommended higher concentrations of free chlorine (1 to 3 mg/liter) in whirlpool or spa water (37, 138, 224). The use of cyanuric acid to stabilize chlorine levels in indoor pools and hot tubs may also decrease the antimicrobial capacity of free chlorine (42). In addition to the predisposing environmental factors mentioned above, dilatation of skin pores because of the higher water temperature may facilitate entry of the *P. aeruginosa* organisms contained in the water (265).

Some outbreaks have been due to faulty chlorination systems (39, 42) in swimming pools. Occasionally a source of the organism is found. In one recent water slide outbreak (77), *P. aeruginosa* was isolated from the water butt used to draw water for games as well as the tank of the fire engine that supplied the water. Guidelines for swimming pools have been proposed (6, 40).

The source of *P. aeruginosa* infection in patients with diving suit-associated lesions was less clear. Although the suits were worn in salt water, which poorly supports the growth of *P. aeruginosa*, the microenvironment next to the skin was not salty, and the source might have been skin colonization (both patients were health care workers). Alternatively, freshwater used to rinse the suits after use may have contained *P. aeruginosa*. The use of synthetic sponges to bathe has given rise to family outbreaks as well as sporadic cases of folliculitis (145). It is hypothesized that the minor trauma of rubbing the skin with a contaminated sponge might favor entrance of the organism into the skin (170). Some outbreaks may occur at home, related to bath toys (114), infected bathroom faucets, wells (275), loofah sponges (26), or beauty aids (89). Sporadic cases after depilation of the legs have been traced to contaminated sponges (63) or cosmetics (202, 248; L. E. Moreno Amado, M. Rodriguez Garcia, M. D. Jimenez-Beatty Navarro, and C. Martinez Vazquez, Letter, *Rev. Clin. Esp.* **190**:103–104, 1992 [in Spanish]; S. Tomas Vecina and J. Torne Cachot, Letter, *Rev. Clin. Esp.* **190**:104, 1992 [in Spanish]). Loofah sponges must be allowed to dry after use or decontaminated intermittently (25).

Most outbreaks have been associated with serogroup O-11 *P. aeruginosa*, although other serogroups have been implicated occasionally, including O-1, O-3, O-4, O-6, O-7, O-8, O-9, O-10, and O-16 (39, 148, 199). An outbreak due to O-4 seemed to be associated with systemic symptoms. It is unclear whether this was due to higher pathogenicity.

Clinically, *P. aeruginosa* dermatitis/folliculitis presents after an incubation period which averages 48 h, with a range of 8 to 120 h. Younger patients (<20 years old) appear to be predisposed, as do those who are exposed to contaminated water longer or more frequently (103). Showering after exposure to *P. aeruginosa*-laden water does not appear to prevent development of infection, suggesting that the organism rapidly gains access to the deeper regions of the skin pores during water exposure (138). This has been confirmed in a recent outbreak (241). *P. aeruginosa* is not a component of normal skin flora (44); certain factors may predispose to colonization and multiplication (227). Initially, the infection is manifest as pruritic follicular papules 2 to 10 mm in diameter, generally located on the buttocks, thighs, arms, and axillae, with sparing of palms, soles, and mucous membranes (103). These are areas in which apocrine sweat glands are located, which open into hair follicles. Other skin areas can be involved as well. Women not infrequently develop a low-grade mastitis through infection of the glands of Montgomery (148). A greater intensity of rash in areas covered by tight bathing suits has been reported (148, 149, 211, 265). Application to the skin of felt pads wetted with water containing pseudomonads and covered with an occlusive dressing has been shown to induce a maculopustular rash on the superhydrated skin, similar to the eruptions described for patients (115). The face and scalp are generally not affected, as these parts of the body are typically not immersed when the patient is using a whirlpool or spa. With time, pinpoint pustules develop in the middle of the papules, and the rash generally heals within 2 to 5 days without scarring. Some may last for a week (22). Deeper infections with nodules have been noted (148). Hyperpigmentation may persist at the site of the papules for some time. In most patients this eventually resolves (148); however, a rare case of persistent hyperpigmentation and residual scarring has been noted despite the use of therapeutic UV light and tetracycline (120). Fever, if present at all, is usually low grade. Malaise and headache are uncommon; however, in some outbreaks headache, fatigue, muscle aches (42), and burning eyes have occurred in more than 30% of patients (39). Secondary infections involving friends or family members have not been documented, except for cases involving contaminated bath sponges (170).

Systemic or topical antibiotic therapy is not required, and topical corticosteroid therapy may delay resolution of folliculitis.

P. aeruginosa "Hot-Foot" Syndrome

The *Pseudomonas* "hot-foot" syndrome has recently been described (83). This is a condition characterized pathologically by perivascular and perieccrine neutrophilic infiltrates or microabscesses and clinically by painful erythematous plantar nodules and pustular lesions. In contrast to *Pseudomonas* folliculitis, these lesions are nodular and involve the soles of the feet, which may have been predisposed to invasion by the abrasive nature of the pool floor. Similar hot, tender, plantar nodules of this nature have been noted in past hot tub outbreaks (148, 198). The syndrome resolves without specific therapy.

Acute Diffuse Otitis Externa (Swimmer's Ear)

Acute diffuse otitis externa is also usually caused by *P. aeruginosa* and may be similar to *Pseudomonas* folliculitis in its pathogenesis. They may occur in the same patient (77, 104). Swimmer's ear has been seen more frequently in swimming pool users than in whirlpool and spa users, who usually keep their heads out of the water. However, an outbreak has been reported related to the use of redwood hot tubs (38). Clinical manifestations of swimmer's ear include discharge from a pruritic and painful external auditory canal that, on examination, is erythematous, edematous, and filled with debris. Usually systemic antibiotic therapy is unnecessary, as most cases resolve spontaneously without serious complications (21). However, one patient was reported to have developed purulent otitis externa with a temperature of 104°F, severe dermatitis, and axillary lymphadenopathy and required hospitalization and the use of intravenous antibiotic (39). Most mild infections respond to 2% acetic acid otic solution, which impairs the growth of *P. aeruginosa*. Ear drops containing topical steroids and antibiotics are also employed. Infection is often recurrent in swimmers.

Schistosome Dermatitis (Swimmer's Itch or Clam Digger's Itch)

Schistosome dermatitis is caused when the cercariae of schistosome parasites present in environmental water penetrate human skin, are unable to proceed any further, and are destroyed, causing a pruritic skin rash. Schistosomes are trematodes whose life cycle involves a definitive host (humans, other mammals, or birds) and an intermediate host, usually snails, from which cercariae are released into a body of water (5). Dermatitis can be seen occasionally in human schistosomiasis (*Schistosoma mansoni* and *Schistosoma haematobium*); however, this dermatitis is usually more severe and occurs more often when cercariae of nonhuman (usually waterfowl or nonprimate mammal) schistosomes penetrate human skin. The disease was first noted in the United States by Cort in 1928 among patients who had waded in Douglas Lake in Michigan (52). Since then, more than 20 species of cercariae from freshwater snails and at least four species from marine snails have been found to produce the illness. It has been described in North, Central, and South America, as well as Oceania, India, Europe, and Africa. More recently, an outbreak in Iceland has been reported (147). In the United States, the illness following swimming or wading in lakes in the north-central states has been most frequent. Marine outbreaks in Florida, southern California, and Hawaii have also been reported.

The association of 317 cases of schistosome dermatitis with the limnological characteristics of a northern Michigan lake has been investigated (160). Patients were more likely to have had exposure to lake water in the morning and to have been exposed in shallower water and in water with a high algal content. Dermatitis was most frequent during June and early July. These characteristics are related to the emergence and peak population of cercariae in water.

Clinical manifestations include an initial "prickling" sensation, typically felt when the film of water evaporates on the skin. This is followed by urticaria, which spontaneously subsides, usually within an hour, with persistence of pruritic macules. With time, these macules may evolve into papules or pustules, which reach their peak intensity in 48 to 72 h. The severity of the reaction varies markedly from person to person and appears to increase with repeated exposures, as the patient becomes sensitized. In most patients, symptoms subside in 4 to 7 days, but severely allergic individuals may be symptomatic for more than a week.

Histopathologically, the cercariae are unable to penetrate human skin, become walled off, and evoke an acute inflammatory response, with infiltration of lymphocytes, neutrophils, and eosinophils.

There is no specific antihelminthic therapy. The illness is treated with topical and systemic medications to control the pruritis. Prevention is largely keyed to control of the intermediate host by application of molluscicides, such as copper sulfate and copper carbonate, to the water. Newer methods under development to assist in identification of infested water bodies and to minimize parasitic exposure include traps impregnated with linoleic acid (101) to stimulate attachment of cercariae as well as PCR amplification (112) techniques to detect cercariae. The rash must be differentiated from sea bather's eruption (caused by *Linuche unguiculata* [thimble jellyfish]), which occurs under swimsuits after swimming in marine environments.

Skin and Soft Tissue Infections Caused by Nontuberculous Mycobacteria

Mycobacterium marinum is the most frequently identified mycobacterial species causing skin and subcutaneous infections associated with immersion. The organism is a photochromogen which grows best at 30 to 32°C and poorly at 37°C or more (94). It inhabits both fresh- and saltwater environments (including aquariums and swimming pools) as a free-living organism. It was first recognized as a pathogen in aquarium fish in 1926 by Aronson (12). Human infection was described definitely in 1954, when an outbreak of 80 cases of infection acquired in a swimming pool was reported. The responsible organism was initially identified as *Mycobacterium balnei*, later shown to be synonymous with *M. marinum* (163). Further swimming pool-related outbreaks were reported (182) prior to the institution of guidelines for swimming pool disinfection. *M. marinum* does not survive chlorine concentrations of ≥0.6 mg/liter. In one study it was repeatedly isolated from pool water when chlorine levels dropped to <0.2 mg/liter but could not be isolated at concentrations above 0.5 to 0.6 mg/liter (58). Better adherence to current guidelines for swimming pool disinfection (40) may explain why skin infections acquired in pools are now unusual (158). Currently, fish tank exposure has proven to be the most consistent risk factor for acquiring this infection (13, 35, 158), with 84% of the largest series of patients (total of 63) reporting fish tank exposure. Other recreational activities associated with this infection include skin diving, dolphin training, and boating activities (94).

Human infection is usually associated with trauma, such as abrasions, injuries from fish spines, or pricks from crustaceans or shellfish (13). The skin injury itself may be trivial, may have healed (128), or may be an open cutaneous lesion (158). Usually the infection is confined to cooler areas of the body, such as the extremities. The incubation period appears to be several weeks, although the mean time to diagnosis is 3 to 4 months (128), with initial lesions appearing as groups of small papules, a nodule, or a plaque with a verrucous surface (158). Often there is progression to shallow ulcerations (94). However, there is considerable pleomorphism in the appearance of infections, with "sporotrichoid" variants, in which nodules appear in the afferent lymphatics, simulating sporotrichosis. The latter has been found to be the more common presentation in certain studies (13, 35). Fewer than half of the patients experience pain, and systemic symptoms are uncommon (94). Adults are more commonly infected due to direct exposure to contaminated environmental water. Children who develop infections usually have fish tanks in their homes (30, 81, 228).

Involvement of deeper structures in the hand, such as the synovium, tendons, and bones, has been demonstrated (13). Dissemination in both immunosuppressed and immunocompetent patients has been reported (97, 143). Human immunodeficiency virus-associated *M. marinum* infections have also been reported, usually acquired from home aquariums. The use of rubber or plastic gloves to handle fish and to clean aquariums has been recommended for these patients (93) and may be useful for the general public as well, especially if preexisting skin lesions are present.

Diagnosis is made most readily from tissue biopsy. The specimen should be submitted for mycobacterial culture as well as histology, since the organism frequently cannot be identified microscopically in the biopsy sample. Growth of the organism in the laboratory is facilitated by incubation at 30 to 32°C. Pulsed-field gel electrophoresis and pattern restriction site analysis after PCR have enhanced the accuracy and speed of identification from culture (74, 273). A range of histopathological findings is possible, with some lesions showing suppuration and others showing granulomas with various degrees of organization. The tuberculin skin test may be positive (158).

Skin lesions caused by *M. marinum* can spontaneously resolve (94). This quality makes it difficult to judge the broad clinical applicability of anecdotal reports describing successful interventional drug or surgical therapy. Many smaller lesions are adequately resected at the time of biopsy and require no further therapy. Surgical debridement is sometimes required for infections of the hand, where closed spaces may be involved.

Of the antimicrobial agents commonly used to treat other mycobacteria, *M. marinum* is usually susceptible to rifampin, rifabutin, ethambutol, trimethoprim-sulfamethoxazole, tetracyclines, and amikacin. It is usually resistant to isoniazid and streptomycin (7, 212). Because antimicrobial therapy is felt to shorten the duration of this frequently painful illness, patients are usually given such therapy, especially if the lesion is on the hand.

Successes as well as failures have been reported with tetracyclines and trimethoprim-sulfamethoxazole (121). Rifampin, with or without ethambutol, has generally been reported to produce favorable results, even in cases where tetracycline has failed (65). Rifampin and rifabutin seem to be the most active agents in vitro, with MICs at which 90% of isolates are inhibited being 0.5 and 0.06 µg/ml, respectively (13, 14). Clarithromycin (191) with or without additional agents such as ethambutol has also shown clinical benefit in studies involving limited numbers of patients (24, 158, 159). This has been confirmed in a more recent study involving a larger series of patients (13). In addition to surgical therapy, clarithromycin was the agent endorsed by the American Thoracic Society (7) in 1997. Increasing experience with this antibiotic has led some authors to recommend it as a first-line agent in any combination therapy (158). Azithromycin, a newer macrolide, has recently been reported to produce clinical cure when used with ethambutol (246), even though in vitro MICs have been shown to be in the range of 8 to 128 µg/ml (14), higher than typical peak concentrations in serum. Quinolones have also been used successfully in the treatment of *M. marinum* infections (79). Moxifloxacin and sparfloxacin appear to be active in vitro, with MICs of 1 and 2 µg/ml, respectively (14). However, other in vitro studies have not shown newer quinolones to have superior activity to ciprofloxacin, with an order of decreasing activity as follows: ciprofloxacin = gatifloxacin = moxifloxacin > levofloxacin > gemifloxacin (28). Clinical use of the quinolones for these infections has been limited. Attainable peak concentrations in serum are close to measured MICs. Levofloxacin has been reported to be effective in a patient infected with a multidrug-resistant isolate (119), while a combination of rifabutin and ciprofloxacin was curative in a patient for whom six previous regimens had failed (159). Linezolid, an oxazolidinone, has been shown to have excellent in vitro antimicrobial activity, with a MIC of 0.5 to 4 µg/ml. These concentrations are below those usually achieved in serum and tissue at conventional dosages (28). Clinical experience with this agent is limited. In general, susceptibility testing with the agar dilution method or the E-test (86) may be used to guide therapy, although more recent reports have validated the better accuracy of the agar dilution method (14, 28). Combination therapy with two or three agents is associated with better cure rates (24, 69, 273). Monotherapy should probably be avoided especially in deep infections, due to a higher failure rate (13). The proper duration of therapy is uncertain, with most authors recommending 6 to 24 weeks (65, 94). However, the duration of therapy also depends on clinical response; some deep infections may require as long as 25 months of treatment (13).

Myobacterium ulcerans is a nontuberculous mycobacterium responsible for Buruli or Bairnsdale ulcer, a chronic cutaneous ulceration seen in parts of Africa, Australia, Papua New Guinea, Malaysia, Suriname, Mexico, Peru, Japan, and China (8, 235). Worldwide, this ulceration is the third most common mycobacterial disease after tuberculosis and leprosy. This infection has been associated with rivers and bodies of water used for recreation. Transmission is thought to be through minor trauma or skin abrasions (181). The lesions initially appear as painless plaques, papules, or nodules on the extremities and gradually develop into undermined ulcers. These lesions often heal with resultant severe contracture deformities as well as loss of organs such as the eye, breast, or genitalia. In earlier studies, isolation of the organism from water was difficult; however, recently the use of PCR has considerably improved the ability to detect *M. ulcerans* from bodies of water suspected to contain the organism (234, 235, 236). PCR techniques have also suggested a very close genetic relationship between *M. marinum* and *M. ulcerans* (237). *M. ulcerans* has not been isolated from skin lesions in the United States, although with frequent international travel, infections acquired abroad may be diagnosed in this country. It is found more commonly in children in poor communities who frequent contaminated water. No gender predilection has been noted, and there does not appear to be an increased risk in patients with human immunodeficiency virus infection. Most patients have a positive tuberculin skin test (229). Drugs with in vitro activity include clarithromycin, rifampin, rifabutin, streptomycin, and amikacin; however, antimicrobial treatment has been unsuccessful. Thus far, surgery is the only consistently effective management. Application of heat to affected areas has resulted in cure in a few cases (180).

It is unusual to encounter community-acquired skin and soft tissue infections caused by mycobacteria other than *M. marinum* and *M. ulcerans* in which immersion in freshwater is an epidemiological factor. A new species of mycobacterium with significant DNA sequence homology with *M. ulcerans, M. marinum,* and *Mycobacterium tuberculosis* has recently been isolated from the Chesapeake Bay in Maryland from fish with skin lesions (204). This may become a potential source of infection. Occasional infections by rapidly growing mycobacteria (*Mycobacterium fortuitum, Mycobacterium chelonae,* or *Mycobacterium abscessus*) have occurred following injuries in water, but far more common is a history of injury caused by objects contaminated with soil (15, 261). An outbreak of *M. fortuitum* furunculosis involving 110 patients occurred among customers of a nail salon who had used 10 different whirlpool footbaths. These infections were severe and protracted and resulted in scarring. The same strain of *M. fortuitum* was recovered from the footbaths and the tap water in the salon. The patients were more likely than controls to have shaved their legs with a razor before pedicure (269). Sporotrichoid lesions due to *M. abscessus* occurred in two women who worked at a public bath (155). The rapidly growing mycobacteria are resistant to most antituberculous agents but are often susceptible to amikacin, ciprofloxacin, cefoxitin, doxycycline, and rifampin (260). Extensive debridement, coupled with combination antimicrobial agent therapy, appears to offer the best chance of cure.

Soft Tissue Infections Caused by Gram-Negative Bacilli

Aeromonas species are ubiquitous gram-negative straight or curved bacilli found in freshwater (including fish tanks, swimming pools, and tap water) as well as brackish water worldwide. They have been known to cause infection in cold-blooded animals (fish, reptiles, and amphibians). Their pathogenicity for humans was noted in 1968 (258). They have been implicated as a cause of gastroenteritis, traumatic and surgical wound infections, myonecrosis, gangrene, osteomyelitis, and, rarely, lower respiratory tract and ocular infections. *Aeromonas hydrophila* is the species most commonly associated with soft tissue infections (126).

Traumatic wound infections in which *A. hydrophila* appears to have been acquired from contaminated freshwater or salt water have been reported frequently. These infections tend to occur on the lower extremities or hand and are often sustained while wading or swimming (95, 139). The spectrum of severity is broad ranging, from mild cellulitis to rapidly progressive, life-threatening myonecrosis with gangrene. Presumably, the virulence of the infecting strain, the severity of the injury, and the immune status of the patient are all factors determining this severity. Janda has provided an excellent review of *Aeromonas* virulence factors and pathogenicity (124).

Cases of cellulitis have been described related not only to injuries that occur while immersed in environmental water but also to an abrasion associated with a fish tank (264), to a boating accident (274), to an unusual football injury (62), to blunt trauma while diving (95), and to swimming in river water in which no injuries were sustained (E. Delbeke, M. J. Demarcq, C. Roubin, and B. Baleux, Letter, *Presse Med.* **14**:1292, 1985 [in French]). The incubation period may be as short as 8 h (62). The cellulitis is characterized by fever, pain, warmth, erythema, edema, and a foul "fishy" odor (95). Characteristic subcutaneous abscesses may form and were noted in 91% of patients in one series (95). The cellulitis is clinically indistinguishable from that due to beta-hemolytic streptococci. The infections have also been noted to occur in warm weather, emphasizing the role of water exposure (95). Burn wound infections have also been known to occur in patients following immersion in untreated water (141, 222). These may be complicated by rapidly evolving deep infection. Cellulitis "one step removed" from freshwater has been reported as a complication of the use of the medicinal freshwater leech *Hirudo medicinalis* for treatment of vascular congestion after surgical procedures. *A. hydrophila* is part of the normal gut flora of this annelid, and *Aeromonas* infections have occurred in up to 20% of patients treated with leeches, leading to use of prophylactic antibiotics at the time of leech application (162, 226). No definite aeromonad infections have been reported in cases of naturally acquired leech bites.

More severe aeromonad tissue infections, including myonecrosis with or without gas gangrene, have been reported. In a number of these cases, the original injury occurred in association with freshwater (126, 225). Some patients had underlying conditions associated with immune defects, such as diabetes or corticosteroid use (157, 219), while others appeared to be immunocompetent. The latter group included the case of a 19-year-old man whose leg was lacerated by a motorboat propeller and that of an 88-year-old woman who cut her hand on a fish bone (111, 225). Bacteremia may complicate these severe soft tissue infections, and it appears to significantly worsen the prognosis. Heckerling et al., in their case report and literature review, found no survivors among patients with *Aeromonas* myonecrosis complicated by bacteremia (111). In their article on human infections caused by *Aeromonas* species, Janda and Duffrey reviewed studies of patients with bacteremia previously reported in the literature; mortality ranged from 29 to 73%. Most of these bacteremic patients did not have associated severe soft tissue infections. In fact, the precipitating event was not apparent for many patients, although some had a history of contact with water. *Aeromonas* bacteremia may give rise to ecthyma gangrenosum, which has a clinical appearance identical to that seen in *P. aeruginosa* septicemia (126). In addition to traumatic injuries, hematologic malignancies, solid tumors, and hepatobiliary disorders all appear to predispose to *Aeromonas* bacteremia (139).

Aeromonas soft tissue infections, which complicate trauma in freshwater, can lead to contiguous osteomyelitis (95). Karam et al. reported two such cases occurring in immunologically normal patents (135).

In vitro, *A. hydrophila* is generally susceptible to broad-spectrum cephalosporins, chloramphenicol, trimethoprim-sulfamethoxazole, fluoroquinolones, aztreonam, and aminoglycosides. *Aeromonas sobria* tends to be more susceptible to cephalothin but is more variable in susceptibility to chloramphenicol and amikacin (213). Broad-based beta-lactam resistance may develop in *Aeromonas* species through stable depression of inducible beta-lactamases (17). Clinical reports have generally described therapy with combinations of antibiotics, often broad-spectrum cephalosporins combined with aminoglycosides. Surgical debridement is usually required and may lead to favorable outcomes even in situations where the initial antibiotic choice was not appropriate (62).

Edwarsiella tarda is a gram-negative bacterium that has been isolated from reptiles, fish, mammals, birds, and environmental water sources (47). It is a rare cause of human infections and is associated with gastroenteritis in >80% of cases. Soft tissue infections, the second most common infections caused by *E. tarda*, have been associated with injuries sustained in freshwater (125). They are more common in the warm-weather months (223). Clinically, these infections appear to be similar to *Aeromonas* cellulitis (47, 252). Coinfection with these organisms can occur, which emphasizes their common source (223). The cellulitis may be complicated by abscess formation and necrotizing fasciitis (177). The first case of cellulitis complicated by myonecrosis due to *E. tarda* was reported to occur in a man who sustained an injury while crab fishing (223). In one case of neonatal sepsis, a mother who was immersed in lake water during the sixth month of gestation also had vaginal and gastrointestinal colonization with the same strain of *E. tarda* (184). The organism is susceptible in vitro to ampicillin, chloramphenicol, aminoglycoside, cephalosporins, tetracyclines, fluoroquinolones, and trimethoprim-sulfamethoxazole (201).

Bacteria of the genus *Vibrio* can also cause extensive skin and soft tissue infection usually after exposure to brackish water. This is discussed elsewhere in this book (chapter 1).

Prototheca Skin and Soft Tissue Infections

Prototheca species are unicellular achlorophyllous algae. They are found in aquariums, freshwater or stagnant water, and other moist environments (239). Of the four identified species (*Prototheca wickerhamii*, *Prototheca zopfii*, *Prototheca filamenta*, and *Prototheca stagnora*), *P. wickerhamii* and *P. zopfii* are known to infect humans, with the former being a more common cause of infections (46). Since the first human infection was described by Davies et al. in 1964, about 108 cases have been described (61, 193). Several types of human infection have been described. The most frequent have been papulonodular or ulcerative skin lesions which have generally followed minor trauma or surgical incisions, particularly on the extremities or face (27). Often, patients with these wound infections report exposure to environments known to harbor this organism. Another type of infection is olecranon bursitis, usually following minor (even nonpenetrating) trauma. In the United States, most *Prototheca* infections have been reported from southern or central states (190). Immunosuppression appears to be a risk factor for both localized and disseminated infections and has been reported for over half the affected patients, although healthy patients may also be infected (43, 46). In a recent report of infection in an AIDS patient there was a history of bathing in an urban pond (193). Nasopharyngeal ulceration complicating prolonged endotracheal intubation (118), as well as meningitis in a patient with AIDS, has also been reported, but this was apparently not related to water exposure (133). Four other cases in association with AIDS were also cutaneous (34, 150, 194, 271).

Diagnosis is best established by biopsy and culture. Sporangia with symmetrically arranged endospores (spoked-wheel appearance) are characteristic. Microabscesses and granulomata are seen histologically. Fungal stains, such as Gomori methenamine-silver, will usually identify the organism in the biopsied tissue. Histologically, *Prototheca* species must be differentiated from *Coccidioides immitis, Cryptococcus neoformans, Rhinosporidium seeberi, Blastomyces dermatitidis,* and *Acanthamoeba* species, which may have similar clinical presentations. *Prototheca* grows on Sabouraud agar, producing whitish colonies (239).

Antimicrobial and/or surgical therapy is usually necessary; few lesions have resolved spontaneously. Amphotericin B and ketoconazole have been used in larger lesions; smaller ones can often be resected successfully (190). In more recent studies, itraconazole has appeared to be the most effective antimicrobial agent for these infections, although surgical intervention has been utilized as first-line management for olecranon bursitis. Fluconazole has also been used successfully (43, 46, 87, 134, 142).

Cyanobacterium (Blue-Green Alga) Infection

Both dermatologic (rash, pruritis, and blistering) and gastrointestinal (abdominal pain, nausea and vomiting, and diarrhea) symptoms have been statistically linked to domestic (showering or bathing) and recreational water use during periods of high concentrations of blue-green algae. These ill effects are thought to be caused by exposure to various toxins produced by these organisms. The organisms themselves are killed by chlorination, although the toxins appear to be unaffected (73).

OCULAR INFECTIONS

Pharyngoconjunctival Fever (Swimming Pool Conjunctivitis)

Pharyngoconjunctival fever, a pediatric and occasionally adult syndrome, has been associated with a number of adenoviruses, most commonly serotypes 3 and 7 in this country and serotype 4 in Asia and Latin America (259). Pharyngoconjunctival fever often occurs in outbreaks or small epidemics and has been reported as a hazard at children's summer camps (10, 59, 107).

The illness is characterized by fever as high as 38°C, bulbar and palpebral conjunctivitis, pharyngitis, and enlargement of the adenoids. Abdominal pain may occur (107). Usually, symptoms begin in one eye but ultimately involve both. Occasionally, symptoms other than conjunctivitis are lacking. The illness usually lasts 3 to 5 days, is not complicated by bacterial superinfections, and can be treated symptomatically (33, 259). Outbreaks can usually be terminated or prevented by adequate chlorination of pool water (>0.2 mg/liter) (59).

Amoebic Keratitis

Free-living amoebae of the genus *Acanthamoeba* have been responsible for several hundred reported cases of keratitis since the original description of a case in a Texas rancher in 1975 (256). This infection has proven difficult to treat, often resulting in severe impairment or loss of vision.

Acanthamoeba species are found in a variety of environmental settings, including soil, water, and air (172, 256). They have even been isolated from the respiratory tracts of healthy people. The species reported to cause keratitis in humans include *Acanthamoeba hatchetti, Acanthamoeba castellanii, Acanthamoeba polyphaga, Acanthamoeba culbertsoni,* and *Acanthamoeba rhysodes. Acanthamoeba* species exist in nature only in the trophozoite or cyst stage. Identifying markers of trophozoites include a diameter of 14 to 40 μm; a single nucleus containing a centrally placed, prominent nucleolus; and spinelike plasma membrane projections (acanthopodia). Motility is sluggish. Cysts are 12 to 16 μm in diameter and have a wrinkled, double-layered wall with pores (173).

Acanthamoeba species are capable of producing a granulomatous encephalitis in debilitated or immunosuppressed patients. By contrast, the keratitis that they produce can occur in healthy people as well as those with underlying diseases. Most, if not all, of these patients have been soft contact lens wearers (217). The illness has been associated with minor corneal trauma and exposure to contaminated water. A case control study of soft contact lens wearers found that patients with *Acanthamoeba* keratitis were more likely than controls to use homemade saline for rinsing and as a wetting agent and to wear their lenses while swimming. They also appear to disinfect their lenses less frequently than recommended by the manufacturers (231). Other authors remarked on the use of chemical rather than thermal disinfection of contact lenses as a risk factor (49). There is no gender predilection, and most cases have been reported in the United States (232).

Histologically, both trophozoites and cysts are found within the cornea in association with an acute inflammatory infiltrate. Giant cells may be present. Corneal neovascularization is variably present. Involvement of the posterior chamber of the eye in amoebic keratitis occurs only rarely (16).

Symptoms of amoebic keratitis generally begin with a sensation of a foreign body in the eye, followed by pain, photophobia, tearing, blepharospasm, and altered visual acuity. In isolated cases the infection may be painless (209, 240). The progression of symptoms is variable and may take place over several days to several months. Periods of remission are not unusual, and when these coincide with a change in therapy, an erroneous impression of the etiology may occur. Findings on examination in one-half or more of patients include iritis, a ring-shaped corneal infiltrate, and recurrent epithelial breakdown or cataracts. Less commonly found are hypopyon, increased intraocular pressure, or anterior nodular scleritis (16). The ring-shaped corneal infiltrate has been described as a characteristic finding in amoebic keratitis and is probably caused by the presence of antigen-antibody complexes in the cornea and resultant chemoattraction of neutrophils (16, 242). Although this ring-shaped infiltration has occasionally been reported to occur in other conditions, such as herpes simplex, fungal, or bacterial keratitis, its presence should signal the need for microbiological studies to determine if amoebae are present.

Elevated corneal epithelial lines also appear to be a clinical indication of *Acanthamoeba* infection. Histopathological examination of scrapings of these lines has revealed both trophozoites and cysts (85). Dendriform epithelial involvement has also been reported as an early finding in *Acanthamoeba* keratitis (161). The infection may be complicated by chorioretinitis as well as painful sclerokeratitis (152, 183).

The definitive diagnosis of amoebic keratitis requires a demonstration of *Acanthamoeba* in corneal scrapings, biopsy, or culture. Motile trophozoites can sometimes be identified in wet mounts of scrapings. Cysts and trophozoites can be identified in fixed material with several different stains, including hematoxylin-eosin, Wright, Giemsa, and periodic acid-Schiff (16). Calcofluor white, a chemofluorescent dye, has been reported to facilitate the identification of trophozoites in cysts in tissue (267). Routine culture methods are frequently misleading in the diagnosis of *Acanthamoeba* keratitis. Because of colonization of the corneal scrapings or contamination, culture may reveal potential bacterial pathogens. A nonnutrient agar with an *Escherichia coli* or *Aerobacter aerogenes* overlay has been shown to successfully grow *Acanthamoeba* from the majority of biopsy-positive specimens (16, 172). Cultures of contact lenses or lens solutions may also be helpful diagnostically (49). A variety of nonmorphological identification criteria have also been described, including restriction fragment length polymorphism analysis of mitochondrial or genomic DNA, PCR (189), and immunofluorescence (172).

Effective treatment of *Acanthamoeba* keratitis requires both surgical and medical components. Diagnosis early in the course can sometimes lead to successful management by employing debridement of abnormal epithelium in combination with topical medication for 3 to 4 weeks (116). In many cases, however, penetrating keratoplasty is necessary for pain relief and to improve vision (49). Deep lamellar keratectomy with corneal flap is a recent surgical approach that has been used with success in refractory cases (55). Topical medications that have been reported to be beneficial include the following:

1. A combination of 1% miconazole nitrate, 0.1% propamidine isethionate, and Neosporin (161)
2. A combination of 1% clotrimazole, 0.1% propamidine isethionate, and Neosporin (66)
3. 0.1% propamidine isethionate and 0.15% dibromopropamidine (272)
4. 0.02% polyhexamethylene biguanide (151)
5. 0.02% chlorhexidine (110)

Unfortunately, propamidine and dibromopropamidine, both analogs of stilbamidine, are not available commercially in the United States. Topical steroids are also frequently, but not universally, employed to inhibit neovascularization in the cornea. However, some experimental evidence suggests that when used for *Acanthamoeba* keratitis, steroids may not be effective for this purpose (130). The use of systemic steroids has appeared to be useful in *Acanthamoeba* sclerokeratitis, a painfully disabling complication of amoebic keratitis that may require enucleation (152). In vitro, *A. culbertsoni* and *A. polyphaga* are killed at relatively low concentrations of azithromycin, but there are no reports regarding the efficacy of macrolide therapy of amoebic keratitis (D. A. Place, S. D. Allen, and C. G. Culbertson, *Abstr. 34th Intersci. Conf. Antimicrob. Agents Chemother.*, abstr. 77, 1994).

Prevention of *Acanthamoeba* keratitis in contact lens wearers is possible. Microwave irradiation has been shown to effectively kill trophozoites and cysts in as little as 3 min without affecting the integrity of the lens (113). Heat disinfection of contact lenses is preferable to chemical disinfection (167). Homemade saline solutions should be avoided for lens cleaning and storage, and contact lenses should not be worn while swimming in freshwater (231).

P. aeruginosa Keratitis

P. aeruginosa keratitis usually occurs in contact lens wearers with no history of freshwater immersion. However, it has been reported in conjunction with *P. aeruginosa* folliculitis (120). A patient who had *P. aeruginosa* folliculitis during a whirlpool exposure outbreak developed a corneal ulcer that resolved with antibiotics.

URINARY TRACT INFECTIONS

P. aeruginosa Urinary Tract Infections

In addition to dermatitis/folliculitis, keratitis, and pneumonia, *P. aeruginosa* has been known to cause urinary tract infection in whirlpool users (210). Three previously healthy outpatients developed *Pseudomonas* urinary tract infection within 48 h after exposure to whirlpools. *P. aeruginosa* was later isolated from the whirlpool associated with each case.

PULMONARY INFECTIONS

Legionella

Members of the genus *Legionella* are fastidious, non-spore-forming, gram-negative bacilli. *Legionella pneumophila* is the major pathogen for humans and causes infections in healthy hosts as well as those with underlying disease. Nineteen other *Legionella* species have been isolated from humans, usually immunosuppressed patients (238). Most legionellae have been found growing naturally in a variety of freshwater habitats. *L. pneumophila* and other species have been isolated from flowing streams and rivers as well as lakes, thermal ponds, and groundwater. They can gain access to man-made water supplies, such as air conditioning cooling towers, potable-water systems, and whirlpools or spas. They tolerate water temperatures in excess of 60°C. Aerosols from both natural and man-made water sources appear to be the usual source for human respiratory tract infections investigated since the first identified outbreak in 1976. It has been thought that legionellae may be non-free-living microorganisms. There is some evidence that they live on the products of blue-green and thermophilic algae as well as other bacteria, such as *Pseudomonas* and *Flavobacterium*, which commonly share the same environment. In addition, legionellae are capable of intracellular survival and multiplication in free-living amoebae (70, 238).

L. pneumophila causes pneumonia, Pontiac fever (an influenza-like illness with less severe respiratory symptoms), and occasional soft tissue infections. Although most outbreaks of *Legionella* pneumonia or Pontiac fever have resulted from exposure to airborne bacteria from air conditioning systems, hospital potable-water systems, or machine tool grinding coolants, infections related to immersion have also been reported. A 1982 outbreak of Pontiac fever related to the use of a whirlpool spa was reported (169). Fourteen female members of a church group who used a health club whirlpool developed chills, fever, chest pain, cough, and nausea within 2 days. Most of these patients seroconverted to antigen from *L. pneumophila* serogroup 6. This organism was recovered from the whirlpool water. It was hypothesized that legionellae seeded the whirlpool from an air conditioner condensation pan with a blocked drain. The organism can reach high numbers in heated, agitated, and underchlorinated water. Whirlpool aerators produce droplets of 2 to 8 μm which are capable of reaching the alveolar air spaces when inhaled. Two similar outbreaks, one involving 34 cases of Pontiac fever and the other involving 7 cases of pneumonia, were reported in 1982, associated with a whirlpool at a Vermont inn (K. Spitalny, R. Vogt, L. Witherell, L. Ociari, L. Orrison, P. Etkind, and L. Novick, *Program Abstr. 22nd Intersci. Conf. Antimicrobial Agents Chemother.*, abstr. 87, 1982). Six college students on a ski trip to Vermont developed Pontiac fever (five cases) or Legionnaires' disease (one case) after using a whirlpool spa (D. L. Thomas, M. L. Mundy, and P. C. Tucker, *Program Abstr. 31st Intersci. Conf. Antimicrob. Agents Chemother.*, abstr. 310, 1991). Pontiac fever was confirmed in a mother and possibly occurred in her two children after similar exposure (245). In 1996, an outbreak was reported consisting of 50 confirmed or probable cases of Legionnaires' disease associated with exposure to whirlpool spas during a total of nine cruises on a single ship. Infection was associated not only with immersion but also with spending time in the area around the spas. Bacterium-laden aerosols generated from the spas presumably infected the latter patients. *L. pneumophila* serogroup 1 was isolated from the sand filter in the spa water treatment system. An isolate matching the spa strain by monoclonal antibody subtyping and arbitrarily primed PCR was recovered from one patient. It was felt that the brominator in the system did not adequately disinfect the spa water after it passed through the sand filter (127).

A hospital-associated wound infection caused by *L. pneumophila* serogroup 4 was related to immersion in a Hubbard tank (29). The pathogenic isolate and other *L. pneumophila* serogroups were grown from the Hubbard tank as well as a small whirlpool tank near it. Povidone iodine, which was use to disinfect the tank and was added to the water used to immerse the patients, was ineffective in killing

L. pneumophila at concentrations under 1,000 ppm. An outbreak of three cases of sternal wound infection caused by *L. pneumophila* and *Legionella dumoffii* has also been reported. The authors presented evidence that the infections were acquired from tap water baths in the intensive care unit. Both *Legionella* species were recovered from water taps in the intensive care unit (166).

Most patients with Pontiac fever have recovered from their illness without specific therapy. This holds true for those involved in the above-mentioned whirlpool-associated outbreaks. Before the advent of the newer macrolides, erythromycin, with frequent addition of rifampin in severe cases, was the therapy of choice for *L. pneumophila* pneumonia as well as infections caused by other species of *Legionella*. Azithromycin, a newer macrolide with more potent intracellular activity, better lung penetration, fewer side effects, and once-daily dosing, is currently the preferred agent. Tetracycline, trimethoprim-sulfamethoxazole, and ciprofloxacin have been used with success in smaller numbers of patients (45, 78). The newer quinolones, including levofloxacin and moxifloxacin, have also shown efficacy in vitro and have been used as monotherapy for patients with community-acquired pneumonia when *L. pneumophila* was considered to be a possible pathogen (71). Rifampin may be added to any of the macrolides or quinolones.

Disinfection of hospital water systems colonized by *Legionella* has been accomplished thermally, through hyperchlorination, and by use of silver copper ion generators (164). *Legionella* is relatively chlorine tolerant and even more resistant to bromine, which is used occasionally for whirlpool disinfection (169). Levels of residual chlorine of 2 to 6 ppm are effective but, as discussed earlier, difficult to maintain in whirlpools, spas, and hot tubs.

P. aeruginosa

Pneumonia caused by *P. aeruginosa* has been reported for a patient with a 50-year history of smoking but no other underlying medical problems who sat in a whirlpool spa for 90 min 1 day prior to the onset of respiratory symptoms (208). The sputum culture and the cultures of the spa water grew identical serogroups of *P. aeruginosa*. It was hypothesized that prolonged inhalation of the *P. aeruginosa*-laden aerosol from the spa was responsible for the development of pneumonia in this patient, whose pulmonary clearance mechanisms were probably impaired from heavy smoking. In this regard, the pathogenesis is similar to the development of nosocomial *P. aeruginosa* pneumonia after inhalation of contaminated humidified air during mechanical ventilation (99). *P. aeruginosa* has also been implicated in pneumonia associated with near drowning in hot tubs (247).

Mycobacterium avium Complex

A previously healthy young woman apparently developed widespread pulmonary infection with *M. avium* complex acquired from a hot tub. Isolates from the patient and the hot tub water had identical enzymatic profiles by multilocus enzyme electrophoresis. In addition, a high degree of relatedness of their insertion sequence, IS*1245*, was demonstrated by restriction fragment length polymorphism analysis (132).

Pneumonia following Near Drowning

The risk of pneumonia in submersion victims has been related to the severity of the pulmonary insult. Patients with abnormal lung examination results after submersion and those requiring ventilation have developed pneumonia more frequently than patients with milder lung injuries. A wide variety of respiratory pathogens have been recovered from these patients. However, in many cases, it has been difficult to differentiate pathogens acquired from the aquatic environment from those which colonized or infected the patients prior to the near drowning or later in the hospital setting.

Aerobic Gram-Negative Bacteria

Aeromonas species are found in both freshwater and brackish water. In addition to soft tissue infections associated with immersion, discussed earlier in this chapter, *Aeromonas* species can also cause pneumonia, usually complicated by septicemia, in the setting of near drowning (76). Several such cases have been reported, but it is difficult to discern whether there was actual pulmonary parenchymal infection in all cases (91, 200). Sometimes the patients' pulmonary findings have been more compatible with noncardiogenic pulmonary edema and the *Aeromonas* has been recovered only from blood cultures. Although *A. hydrophila* was identified as the species causing infection in most of the cases noted above, more recently differentiated *Aeromonas* species, such as *A. sobria*, *Aeromonas caviae*, and *Aeromonas veronii*, may have been responsible (124). The mortality of patients with *Aeromonas* pneumonia associated with near drowning has been reported to exceed 50% (75).

The antimicrobial susceptibility of *Aeromonas* species and the therapy of infections are discussed in "Skin and Soft Tissue Infections" above.

Burkholderia pseudomallei, the cause of melioidosis, has been associated with pneumonia related to near drowning in tropical Asian countries where the organism is endemic, including the Philippines (75), Thailand (1), Vietnam (102), and Taiwan (153). This agent is also associated with dissemination from the lungs and a high risk of mortality. The organism is usually susceptible to antipseudomonal penicillins, cefoperazone, ceftazidime, ampicillin-sulbactam, amoxicillin-clavulanate, chloramphenicol, and tetracyclines. Fluoroquinolone susceptibility is variable, and most isolates demonstrate resistance to trimethoprim-sulfamethoxazole and aminoglycosides (144).

Pneumonia definitely or probably associated with *Legionella* species has been associated with near drowning in a hot spring spa (220), in dirty swamp water (243), and in swimming pool water (51). Only one of the pathogens in these cases was identified as *L. pneumophila*.

Streptococcus pneumoniae

S. pneumoniae has been linked to pneumonia associated with near drowning in three fatal pediatric cases, two of which occurred in freshwater (253).

Aspergillus spp.

Invasive pulmonary aspergillosis has been reported following the near drowning of a 27-year-old man in a ditch after a motor vehicle accident (254). Preexisting bronchiectasis was present in this patient. He was successfully treated with amphotericin B and flucytosine. Of the newer antifungal therapies, voriconazole and caspofungin have been approved in the United States for the treatment of invasive aspergillosis that is refractory to other therapies and have been used successfully (131, 262).

Pseudallescheria boydii

P. boydii has been isolated from polluted water, sewage sludge (50), soil, and animal manure (18). This fungus has caused pulmonary infections in severely immunocompromised patients and, occasionally, in previously healthy individuals who have aspirated contaminated water (179, 251, 268). The organism appears to have a propensity for spreading from the initial site of infection in the lungs, often producing widespread metastasis, including brain abscesses (68). On one occasion, infected kidneys from a patient with a fatal disseminated case were transplanted into two recipients, both of whom developed *P. boydii* infections (251). Therapy with antifungal drugs has been disappointing overall. In vitro susceptibility tests usually indicate resistance to amphotericin B and flucytosine, with susceptibility to miconazole and, to a lesser extent, ketoconazole. The last two agents have been used successfully to treat human pulmonary and bone infections (68, 90). Itraconazole has been used successfully to treat a patient with *P. boydii* and *Aspergillus terreus* coinfection in the lungs (96). Voriconazole, a newer triazole antifungal agent, is approved for pulmonary infection due to *P. boydii*, having achieved some clinical success (122, 185, 262).

DISSEMINATED INFECTIONS

Leptospirosis

Leptospires are aerobic, motile, spiral, flexible microorganisms with hooked ends. They can be cultured in artificial media containing rabbit serum or bovine serum albumin and long-chain fatty acids, although the incubation time for optimal growth can range from a few days to a few weeks (156).

Two species are recognized as causes of disseminated infections. *Leptospira biflexa* is considered saprophytic and is found in surface and potable water. *Leptospira interrogans* is pathogenic and may be carried for prolonged periods in proximal renal tubular cells of many different mammalian species. Members of these two *Leptospira* species can be distinguished biochemically, but within each species members can be divided into serovars only on the basis of their agglutinogenic characteristics with rabbit antiserum. More than 210 serovars of *L. interrogans* are known (156). Mammals are affected year-round in the tropical regions and during warm and rainy seasons in temperate regions (80). From the site of infection in the kidney, leptospires are shed into the urine in variable numbers. With some serovars in some hosts, this excretion may be lifelong. With other host-serovar combinations, however, urine shedding may persist for only a few months (250).

Human leptospirosis is a zoonosis that has been found to be an occupational risk for cattle, dairy, or swine farmers; rice farmers; farmers in marshy areas; cray-fishers; veterinarians; and abattoir workers (60, 156). Humans can also be infected by exposure, such as when swimming or wading in water contaminated with animal urine (4, 54, 136). The first reported waterborne outbreak of leptospirosis occurred in 1939 (108). Since then, similar outbreaks and small epidemics have occurred regularly. Crawford et al. have reviewed 12 such outbreaks in the United States associated with swimming in natural freshwater pools, streams, and rivers. In several outbreaks, contamination of water with animal urine or offal was proven. They point out that sporadic cases of leptospirosis may occur as a result of various kinds of contact but that epidemics are usually associated with swimming or other types of water immersion (54). Tropical river rafting (Costa Rica and Thailand) was the apparent mode of transmission in two reported cases (41, 249). Infections related to water sports have also been reported (106). Human infections appear to be more common in tropical regions. Within the United States, Hawaii has been the state with the highest incidence (80).

Many human cases of leptospirosis are asymptomatic. Human illness varies in severity from a mild influenza-like syndrome to severe renal and hepatic failure accompanied by hemorrhage, shock, and confusion. The severe form of leptospirosis is called Weil's disease or Weil syndrome, after the initial describer of the illness.

Leptospires may enter the body through intact mucosal membranes, the conjunctiva, or abraded skin. They are rapidly disseminated hematogenously. The incubation period is usually 7 to 12 days. During the influenza-like septicemic phase of anicteric leptospirosis, the organism can be cultured from blood, cerebrospinal fluid, and other tissues. Despite its presence in spinal fluid, patients usually have no meningeal signs in this phase of the illness, although headache is usually present, as are fever, nausea, vomiting, anorexia, myalgia, and fatigue. The most common physical finding is conjunctival suffusion in the absence of purulent discharge. After 4 to 7 days, the illness resolves for a day or two, followed in many patients by an "immune" stage of the illness, which can last up to a month.

Circulating immunoglobulin M antibody can be detected, and patients may have meningismus, uveitis, and rash. Blood and cerebrospinal fluid cultures are usually negative during this phase, but the organism can be found in the urine and the aqueous humor of the eye. The meningitis in the immune stage, although sterile, is characterized by cerebrospinal fluid pleocytosis, a variably elevated protein level, and a normal glucose level. Eye findings of photophobia, ocular pain, and conjunctival hemorrhage are common (72, 80).

In icteric leptospirosis, there is less distinction between the septicemic and immune phases, although the renal and hepatic complications generally are not present before 3 to 7 days. The jaundice usually does not reflect hepatocellullar necrosis, and no residual hepatic dysfunction has been found in survivors. Elevation of liver enzymes is relatively modest. Creatine kinase levels are quite high, however. Renal failure usually does not progress to the point where the patient requires dialysis, and this dysfunction resolves completely (72, 80). Thrombocytopenia occurs in about one-half of patients and is correlated with renal failure. Death is usually related to vascular collapse, thought to be caused by vasculitis and hemorrhagic myocarditis, which occurs in about 50% of fatal cases.

Diagnosis may be established by serologic means or by culturing the organism from clinical specimens (usually blood, cerebrospinal fluid, or urine). Tween 80-albumin agar is usually commercially available and is used in clinical laboratories. Cultures are incubated for 5 to 6 weeks in the dark; growth is usually apparent by 2 weeks, however. Leptospires can also be identified in clinical specimens by dark-field examination and by immunostaining and can be faintly stained by Giemsa or Wright's stain. In tissue specimens, the organism can be detected by silver staining (80, 156).

Most diagnoses are made serologically. The microscopic agglutination test is used most frequently but is highly serovar specific and requires the use of a battery of antigens. Titers of ≥1:100 are considered significant. Macroscopic agglutination tests with single or pooled Formalin-fixed antigens are also available, as well as enzyme-linked immunosorbent assays and an indirect hemagglutination test (80). PCR assays for leptospiral DNA detection in clinical specimens afford rapid diagnosis, while the use of DNA primers may allow for rapid serovar identification (80).

Traditional antibiotic therapy for leptospirosis has been penicillin G or tetracycline. Evidence from humans indicates that therapy is effective even in severe disease treated after the initial septicemic period. Animal studies indicate that penicillins, tetracyclines, and some cephalosporins are effective, while other cephalosporins are not (3). Intravenous penicillin or ampicillin should be used for severe disease; oral ampicillin or doxycycline should be used for mild symptoms. Therapy should be given for 5 to 7 days. A recent prospective randomized control trial showed that the times to defervescence were the same for ceftriaxone and penicillin G (3 days), and the former can be used once daily; it suggested that it should be the preferred agent in regions of the world where it is affordable (188). Because of the year-round occurrence of leptospirosis and its relation to water immersion recreational activities, a proposal to give weekly prophylactic doxycycline to those travelers intending to participate in water sports has been made (106).

Chromobacterium violaceum

C. violaceum is a gram-negative, facultatively anaerobic, fermentative bacillus which is a normal inhabitant of soil and water and has caused human infections, primarily in tropical and subtropical areas. Most reports have not linked infection to freshwater exposure, but cases have been reported in which immersion appears to play a role. One case occurred in a 44-year-old woman who sustained a wasp sting while bathing in a Paraguayan lagoon. One month later, she developed septicemia in association with inflammation of the sting site and purplish ulcerating nodular lesions on her thigh, abdomen, and back. Blood and skin lesion cultures grew *C. violaceum*. She responded to mezlocillin and gentamicin therapy despite shock and renal failure. However, the infection recurred 2 weeks after the antibiotic course was completed, leading to her demise (137).

A second patient (a 53-year-old man), who nearly drowned in a Florida river, developed multiple liver abscesses, lung infiltrates, and a pustular skin rash 2 months after the accident. Blood and pustule cultures grew *C. violaceum*, and the patient responded to chloramphenicol, ampicillin, and carbenicillin (230).

Other fatal cases have been linked to exposure to stagnant water (195). The features of the disseminated infections in these patients were a long incubation period and skin lesions as well as hepatic and pulmonary abscesses.

This organism is usually susceptible to fluoroquinolones, trimethoprim-sulfamethoxazole, tetracyclines, aminoglycosides, extended-spectrum penicillins, and chloramphenicol (2).

CENTRAL NERVOUS SYSTEM INFECTIONS

PAM

Amoebic meningoencephalitis was first described in 1965 in Australia (88). It is caused by *Naegleria fowleri*, a thermophilic free-living amoeba that inhabits freshwater ponds, lakes, and rivers; minimally chlorinated pools; and hot springs throughout the world (175). Other free-living amoebae include *Acanthamoeba* and *Balamuthia*. These amphizoic amoebae, so called because they can exist as parasites or free-living organisms, may cause fulminant rapidly progressive central nervous system infection called primary amoebic meningoencephalitis (PAM) (due to *Naegleria fowleri*) or chronic slowly progressive disease called granulomatous amoebic encephalitis (GAE), primarily caused by several species of *Acanthamoeba* and by *Balamuthia mandrillaris*. PAM was so named to distinguish it from metastatic amoebic abscesses involving the brain caused by *Entamoeba histolytica*. PAM was originally thought to be caused by an *Acanthamoeba* species. Some *B. mandrillaris* meningitis cases were originally diagnosed as caused by *Acanthamoeba*, and the true cause of the disease was recognized only after death. GAE caused by *Acanthamoeba* species occurs in debilitated or immunosuppressed patients, while that due to *B. mandrillaris* occurs in healthy hosts (64). The pathogenesis of GAE does not appear to be related to immersion. Rather, the *Acanthamoeba* species reach the brain via the hematogenous route from a primary focus, usually thought to be the lungs or skin. It is hypothesized that these primary foci become infected by dusts, aerosols, or air containing the *Acanthamoeba* cysts.

N. fowleri is a small amoeba, measuring 10 to 35 μm. In unfavorable environments, it transforms into a pear-shaped biflagellate stage. The amoeba may also encyst. The cysts are spherical and smooth walled, have mucus-plugged pores, and measure 7 to 15 μm (256). *N. fowleri* is a thermophilic organism and tolerates water as warm as 45°C (105). It has worldwide distribution in naturally warm as well as thermally polluted waters (129). The concentration of amoebae in warm water frequently exceeds one organism per 25 ml (266). With its wide distribution in water frequently used for recreation, it is apparent that millions of people have been exposed. Human cases, however, number in the range of 150 to 200. Eighty-one cases had been reported in the United States as of 1 October 1996 (175). In 1998, four more cases were identified, and during the period from 1999 to 2000, four additional fatal cases were reported in the United States (154). These last patients were all less than 19 years old; three had exposure to recreational water, and the fourth fell into stagnant water during a jet ski accident. In 2002, six more U.S. cases were reported—two each in Texas, Arizona, and Florida. Only eight survivors of PAM have been documented in the literature to date (9, 11, 31, 67, 123, 165, 196, 216, 263). What factors provide immunity to *N. fowleri* in the majority of exposed individuals is uncertain. Most patients have been healthy prior to infection, although one case in a patient with AIDS has been reported (48). The majority of cases occur in children in the summer months (48). Antibody to the amoeba can be demonstrated in the human population, but its protective role is unclear (56, 129).

The organism is thought to enter the central nervous system via the nasal route. Amoebae from contaminated water are deposited on the olfactory mucosal epithelium and penetrate the submucosal nervous plexus and cribriform plate. Olfactory neuroepithelium is capable of active phagocytosis, and the amoebae travel to the terminus of the olfactory nerve in the olfactory bulb, which is in the subarachnoid space and surrounded by cerebrospinal fluid. Multiplication of the amoebae occurs in the meninges and in neural tissue, and eventually a diffuse hemorrhagic necrotic meningoencephalitis develops. Cortical gray matter is severely affected, with hemorrhage and edema, often leading to uncal or cerebellar herniation. Trophozoites can be identified in the necrotic olfactory bulbs as well as the adventitia and perivascular spaces of small to medium-sized arteries and cerebrospinal fluid. No cysts are found (129, 168). Tissue necrosis in response to *Naegleria* infections, seen in the nasal mucosa as well as in the neural tissue, has been ascribed to the release of lysosomal enzymes or cytopathic toxins by the amoebae or to enzymes on the surface of the organism (57, 82).

Unfortunately, there is little in the clinical picture of PAM to distinguish it from acute bacterial meningitis. As a result, clinicians often do not consider PAM in their initial differential diagnosis when a patient presents with purulent meningitis. The period between exposure and the onset of symptoms may vary from 2 to 14 days, although most cases have occurred within 5 days. The majority of cases have involved children and young adults. Initially, the patient may notice some alteration of taste or smell. This is rapidly followed by fever, headache, anorexia, nausea, vomiting, and meningismus. The majority of patients also exhibit confusion at the time of presentation. This progresses to coma, and the infection is usually fatal within a week (168, 244). Outside the central nervous system, focal myocarditis has been described to occur in fatal cases of PAM. The pathogenesis is unclear, however, since the amoebae have not been demonstrated in myocardial tissue (171).

PAM should be considered in any case of acute pyogenic meningitis which occurs in a patient with a history of swimming in water potentially contaminated with amoebae (172). Cerebrospinal fluid pressure is often elevated, and the fluid generally has an increased number of erythrocytes, sometimes sufficient to appear grossly hemorrhagic. Leukocyte counts in the cerebrospinal fluid can vary widely, but there is a predominance of neutrophils. Glucose levels may be normal or slightly reduced, with an elevated protein level (174). It is of paramount diagnostic importance to do a wet-mount microscopic examination of the spinal fluid to detect motile trophozoites. Phase-contrast or dark-field microscopy may aid in this detection (174). Trophozoites are not usually recognized on Gram stain because of disruption of the amoebae by the fixation process (168, 176). Cerebrospinal fluid can be examined by Giemsa or other stains after preparation of the sample by cytospinning and fixation (172, 255). Confirmation of the diagnosis requires cultures of clinical specimens (as mentioned earlier in the discussion of *Acanthamoeba* keratitis) or an indirect immunofluorescent-antibody test. A PCR assay has been described (203). Serologic tests may be positive for asymptomatic individuals and are not helpful in diagnosis of acute infections (206). Computed tomographic scanning studies have been reported for a few patients. Cerebral edema and diffuse-contrast enhancement of the gray matter have been reported (31, 176). Magnetic resonance imaging may show meningeal enhancement or ring enhancing lesions with a predilection for diencephalon, thalamus, brain stem, and posterior fossa structures (31, 123, 140).

A successful clinical outcome is related to early diagnosis and appropriate aggressive therapy. Amphotericin B is the drug that has shown the greatest clinical activity, and it has been employed in the therapy of all survivors. The drug is given in high doses both intravenously and intrathecally. Even when given within 24 h of admission, its use has not been universally successful (233). Rifampin has also been given in combination with amphotericin B to several survivors. Azithromycin has shown better activity than amphotericin B in vitro and in a mouse model (100). It may be a useful adjunct to therapy in human infections.

P. boydii

As noted earlier in this chapter, *P. boydii* can be found in polluted waters as well as other sources. Most central nervous system infections have been preceded by aspiration of potentially contaminated material in near drownings, often associated with loss of consciousness from closed head trauma and asphyxiation (68). Usually, but not always, pneumonia in which *P. boydii* is cultured from the sputum precedes the development of central nervous system infection (84). Both meningitis and brain abscesses have been reported, although most cases of meningitis have been associated with abscess formation. Rarely, meningitis has occurred alone in association with trauma and contiguous infection or spinal anesthesia (215, 270). Both solitary and multiple brain abscesses may occur, although patients who develop central nervous system infection after aspiration and pneumonia usually have multiple abscesses. That these abscesses are caused by fungemia is evidenced by the frequency of documented abscesses elsewhere in these patients (thyroid, kidney, heart, lungs, and skin) (20).

Surgical therapy appears to be effective in solitary or contiguous brain abscesses where adequate drainage can be performed. Indeed, one patient with a solitary abscess survived after drainage even though amphotericin B (to which the isolate was resistant in vitro) was used therapeutically (19). In addition to the feasibility of surgical drainage, factors which may improve survival include prolonged high-dose antifungal drug administration and avoidance of corticosteroid therapy (68). Most isolates have been resistant to amphotericin B and flucytosine and somewhat more susceptible to miconazole than to ketoconazole. The survival of two patients who developed multiple brain abscesses (as well as other foci of infection) was reported following prolonged, high-dose intravenous miconazole therapy (up to 90 mg/kg of body weight/day). One of these patients also had probable meningitis and was treated intrathecally with miconazole as well. It was noted for both patients that frequent dosage increases were necessary in order to keep blood drug levels above the MICs for the isolates (68). Miconazole is extensively metabolized by hepatic enzymes, and it is possible that with prolonged dosing this metabolism is facilitated (32). Unfortunately, miconazole is no longer available in the United States and cannot be obtained even for compassionate use (186). As mentioned earlier in this chapter, itraconazole has been used successfully in pulmonary *P. boydii* infections. However, there is no information regarding its efficacy in central nervous system infections. Fluconazole has good central nervous system penetration but does not appear to be active in vitro. The newer azoles have shown promise in the treatment of disseminated infections due to *P. boydii*. In a mouse model of disseminated infection with *P. boydii*, posiconazole at high doses was found to be more effective than itraconazole in preventing death and clearing the organisms from tissues (98). Voriconazole, a triazole antifungal, has proven effective in the therapy of disseminated infections in immunosuppressed and immunocompetent patients (36, 92, 186, 197, 262; J. Torre-Cisneros, A. Gonzalez-Ruiz, M. R. Hodges, and I. Lutsar, *Program Abstr. 38th Annu. Meet. Infect. Dis. Soc. Am.*, abstr. 305, 2000). It has been approved by the Food and Drug Administration for patients with *P. boydii* infections that are intolerant or refractory to other agents (131). Of all tested antifungal agents, it appears to have the lowest MIC for *P. boydii* (131, 197, 218). It is available in both intravenous and oral forms, has 90% bioavailability, and achieves concentrations in cerebrospinal fluid and the brain that are 50 and 200% of that in serum (131). In vitro data also suggest good activity by the echinocandins, but more data are needed (192).

Coxsackieviruses

Coxsackieviruses are members of the genus *Enterovirus*, along with polioviruses, echovirus, and enteroviruses 68 to 71. Coxsackieviruses are divided into groups A and B based on their infection patterns in mice and growth in primate cells. Twenty-three serotypes of group A and six serotypes of group B have been recognized (207).

Most infections caused by coxsackieviruses either are asymptomatic or take the form of undifferentiated febrile illness. Aseptic meningitis, encephalitis, paralysis, myopericarditis, pleurodynia, conjunctivitis, exanthema, enanthema, pharyngitis, and lower respiratory tract infections are additional infection patterns that can be caused by various coxsackievirus serotypes.

Apparent waterborne infections caused by coxsackieviruses B_5 and A_{16} have been described. Hawley et al. reported a summer outbreak of illness caused by coxsackievirus B_5 at a boys' camp on Lake Champlain in Vermont. The illness included conjunctivitis, meningitis, and/or gastroenteritis. The virus was also recovered from a roped-off swimming area in the lake adjacent to the camp (109).

Denis et al. reported an illness which consisted of fever, vomiting, anorexia, diarrhea, and myalgia in five children who had swum in a lake in France. Coxsackievirus A_{16} was cultured from a patient and from the lake water. The two boys tested both had increased titers of antibody to this virus (F. A. Denis, E. Blanchouin, A. de Lignieres, and P. Flamen, Letter, *JAMA* **228**:1370-1371, 1974).

Enteroviruses are thought to be transmitted between humans mostly by the fecal-oral route. Coxsackieviruses are often shed simultaneously from both the upper respiratory and gastrointestinal tracts (146). Coxsackievirus A_{21}, which causes upper respiratory tract infections, is thought to be spread additionally by the respiratory-oral route (53). Urban sewage sampling, especially in summer months, commonly shows enteroviruses, and it may be that outbreaks of freshwater coxsackievirus infection are caused by contamination with sewage or the presence of infected swimmers who are spreading the virus (117).

REFERENCES

1. **Achana, V., K. Silpapojakul, W. Thininta, and S. Kalnaowakul.** 1985. Acute *Pseudomonas pseudomallei* pneumonia and septicemia following aspiration of contaminated water: a case report. *Southeast Asian J. Trop. Med. Public Health* **16**:500–504.
2. **Aldridge, K. E., G. T. Valainis, and C. V. Sanders.** 1988. Comparison of the *in vitro* activity of ciprofloxacin and 24 other antimicrobial agents against clinical strains of *Chromobacterium violaceum*. *Diagn. Microbiol. Infect. Dis.* **10**:31–39.
3. **Alexander, A. D., and P. L. Rule.** 1986. Penicillins, cephalosporins, and tetracyclines in treatment of hamsters with fatal leptospirosis. *Antimicrob. Agents Chemother.* **30**:835–839.
4. **Alston, J. M., and J. C. Broom.** 1958. *Leptospirosis in Man and Animals.* E. and S. Livingstone, Edinburgh, Scotland.
5. **Amer, M.** 1994. Cutaneous schistosomiasis. *Dermatol. Clin.* **12**:713–717.
6. **American Public Health Association.** 1981. Public swimming pools: recommended regulations for design and construction, operation and maintenance. American Public Health Association, Washington, D.C.
7. **American Thoracic Society.** 1997. Diagnosis and treatment of disease caused by nontuberculous mycobacteria. *Am. J. Respir. Crit. Care Med.* **156**:S1–S25.
8. **Amofah, G., F. Bonsu, C. Tetteh, J. Okrah, K. Asamoa, K. Asiedu, and J. Addy.** 2002. Buruli ulcer in Ghana: results of a national case search. *Emerg. Infect. Dis.* **8**:167–170.
9. **Anderson, K., and A. Jamieson.** 1972. Primary amoebic meningoencephalitis. *Lancet* i:902–903.
10. **Anonymous.** 1992. Outbreak of pharyngoconjunctival fever at a summer camp—North Carolina, 1991. *Infect. Control Hosp. Epidemiol.* **13**:499–500.
11. **Apley, J., S. K. Clarke, A. P. Roome, S. A. Sandry, G. Saygi, B. Silk, and D. C. Warhurst.** 1970. Primary amoebic meningoencephalitis in Britain. *Br. Med. J.* **1**:596–599.
12. **Aronson, J. D.** 1926. Spontaneous tuberculosis in saltwater fish. *J. Infect. Dis.* **39**:315–319.
13. **Aubry, A., O. Chosidow, E. Caumes, J. Robert, and E. Cambau.** 2002. Sixty-three cases of *Mycobacterium marinum* infection: clinical features, treatment, and antibiotic susceptibility of causative isolates. *Arch. Intern. Med.* **162**:1746–1752.
14. **Aubry, A., V. Jarlier, S. Escolano, C. Truffot-Pernot, and E. Cambau.** 2000. Antibiotic susceptibility pattern of *Mycobacterium marinum*. *Antimicrob. Agents Chemother.* **44**:3133–3136.

15. **Aubuchon, C., J. J. Hill, Jr., and D. R. Graham.** 1986. Atypical mycobacterial infection of soft tissue associated with use of a hot tub. A case report. *J. Bone Jt. Surg. Am. Vol.* **68:**766–768.

16. **Auran, J. D., M. B. Starr, and F. A. Jakobiec.** 1987. *Acanthamoeba* keratitis. A review of the literature. *Cornea* **6:**2–26.

17. **Bakken, J. S., C. C. Sanders, R. B. Clark, and M. Hori.** 1988. Beta-lactam resistance in *Aeromonas* spp. caused by inducible beta-lactamases active against penicillins, cephalosporins, and carbapenems. *Antimicrob. Agents Chemother.* **32:**1314–1319.

18. **Bell, R. G.** 1976. The development in beef cattle manure of *Petriellidium boydii* (Shear) Malloch, a potential pathogen for man and cattle. *Can. J. Microbiol.* **22:**552–556.

19. **Bell, W. E., and M. G. Myers.** 1978. *Allescheria (Petriellidium) boydii* brain abscess in a child with leukemia. *Arch. Neurol.* **35:**386–388.

20. **Berenguer, J., J. Diaz-Mediavilla, D. Urra, and P. Munoz.** 1989. Central nervous system infection caused by *Pseudallescheria boydii:* case report and review. *Rev. Infect. Dis.* **11:**890–896.

21. **Berger, R. S., and M. R. Seifert.** 1990. Whirlpool folliculitis: a review of its cause, treatment, and prevention. *Cutis* **45:**97–98.

22. **Bhatia, A., and R. T. Brodell.** 1999. 'Hot tub folliculitis.' Test the waters—and the patient—for *Pseudomonas. Postgrad. Med.* **106:**43–46.

23. **Bisno, A. L.** 1984. Cutaneous infections: microbiologic and epidemiologic considerations. *Am. J. Med.* **76:**172–179.

24. **Bonnet, E., D. Debat-Zoguereh, N. Petit, I. Ravaux, and H. Gallais.** 1994. Clarithromycin: a potent agent against infections due to *Mycobacterium marinum. Clin. Infect. Dis.* **18:**664–666.

25. **Bottone, E. J., and A. A. Perez II.** 1993. *Pseudomonas aeruginosa* folliculitis acquired through use of a contaminated loofah sponge: an unrecognized potential public health problem. *J. Clin. Microbiol.* **31:**480–483.

26. **Bottone, E. J., A. A. Perez II, and J. L. Oeser.** 1994. Loofah sponges as reservoirs and vehicles in the transmission of potentially pathogenic bacterial species to human skin. *J. Clin. Microbiol.* **32:**469–472.

27. **Boyd, A. S., M. Langley, and L. E. King, Jr.** 1995. Cutaneous manifestations of *Prototheca* infections. *J. Am. Acad. Dermatol.* **32:**758–764.

28. **Braback, M., K. Riesbeck, and A. Forsgren.** 2002. Susceptibilities of *Mycobacterium marinum* to gatifloxacin, gemifloxacin, levofloxacin, linezolid, moxifloxacin, telithromycin, and quinupristin-dalfopristin (Synercid) compared to its susceptibilities to reference macrolides and quinolones. *Antimicrob. Agents Chemother.* **46:**1114–1116.

29. **Brabender, W., D. R. Hinthorn, M. Asher, N. J. Lindsey, and C. Liu.** 1983. *Legionella pneumophila* wound infection. *JAMA* **250:**3091–3092.

30. **Brady, R. C., A. Sheth, T. Mayer, D. Goderwis, and M. R. Schleiss.** 1997. Facial sporotrichoid infection with *Mycobacterium marinum. J. Pediatr.* **130:**324–326.

31. **Brown, R. L.** 1991. Successful treatment of primary amebic meningoencephalitis. *Arch. Intern. Med.* **151:**1201–1202.

32. **Brugmans, J. P., J. Van Cutsem, J. Heyksnts, V. Scheurmans, and D. Thierpont.** 1972. Systemic antifungal potential, safety, biotransport and transformation of miconazole nitrate. *Eur. J. Clin. Pharmacol.* **5:**93–102.

33. **Caldwell, G. G., N. J. Lindsey, H. Wulff, D. D. Donnelly, and F. N. Bohl.** 1974. Epidemic of adenovirus type 7 acute conjunctivitis in swimmers. *Am. J. Epidemiol.* **99:**230–234.

34. **Carey, W. P., Y. Kaykova, J. C. Bandres, G. S. Sidhu, and N. Brau.** 1997. Cutaneous protothecosis in a patient with AIDS and a severe functional neutrophil defect: successful therapy with amphotericin B. *Clin. Infect. Dis.* **25:**1265–1266.

35. **Casal, M., and M. M. Casal.** 2001. Multicenter study of incidence of *Mycobacterium marinum* in humans in Spain. *Int. J. Tuberc. Lung Dis.* **5:**197–199.

36. **Castiglioni, B., D. A. Sutton, M. G. Rinaldi, J. Fung, and S. Kusne.** 2002. *Pseudallescheria boydii* (anamorph *Scedosporium apiospermum*). Infection in solid organ transplant recipients in a tertiary medical center and review of the literature. *Medicine* (Baltimore) **81:**333–348.

37. **Centers for Disease Control.** 1981. *Suggested Health and Safety Guidelines for Public Spas and Hot Tubs.* DHHS publication no. 99–960. U.S. Department of Health and Human Services, Public Health Service, Washington, D.C.

38. **Centers for Disease Control.** 1982. Otitis due to *Pseudomonas aeruginosa* serotype O–10 associated with mobile redwood hot tub system—North Carolina. *Morb. Mortal. Wkly. Rep.* **31:**541–542.

39. **Centers for Disease Control.** 1983. An outbreak of *Pseudomonas* folliculitis associated with a waterslide—Utah. *Morb. Mortal. Wkly. Rep.* **32:**425–427.

40. **Centers for Disease Control.** 1988. *Swimming Pools: Safety and Disease Control through Proper Design and Operation.* DHHS publication no. (CDC)888319. U.S. Department of Health and Human Services, Public Health Service, Washington, D.C.

41. **Centers for Disease Control and Prevention.** 1997. Outbreak of leptospirosis among white-water rafters—Costa Rica, 1996. *Morb. Mortal. Wkly. Rep.* **46:**577–579.

42. **Centers for Disease Control and Prevention.** 2000. *Pseudomonas* dermatitis/folliculitis associated with pools and hot tubs—Colorado and Maine, 1999–2000. *Morb. Mortal. Wkly. Rep.* **49:**1087–1091.

43. **Chao, S. C., M. M. Hsu, and J. Y. Lee.** 2002. Cutaneous protothecosis: report of five cases. *Br. J. Dermatol.* **146:**688–693.

44. **Chiller, K., B. A. Selkin, and G. J. Murakawa.** 2001. Skin microflora and bacterial infections of the skin. *J. Investig. Dermatol. Symp. Proc.* **6:**170–174.

45. **Ching, W. T., and R. D. Meyer.** 1987. *Legionella* infections. *Infect. Dis. Clin. N. Am.* **1:**595–614.

46. **Cho, B. K., S. H. Ham, J. Y. Lee, and J. H. Choi.** 2002. Cutaneous protothecosis. *Int. J. Dermatol.* **41:**304–306.

47. **Clarridge, J. E., D. M. Musher, V. Fainstein, and R. J. Wallace, Jr.** 1980. Extraintestinal human infection caused by *Edwardsiella tarda. J. Clin. Microbiol.* **11:**511–514.

48. **Clavel, A., L. Franco, S. Letona, J. Cuesta, A. Barbera, M. Varea, J. Quilez, F. Javier Castillo, and R. Gomez-Lus.** 1996. Primary amebic meningoencephalitis in a patient with AIDS: unusual protozoological findings. *Clin. Infect. Dis.* **23:**1314–1315.

49. **Cohen, E. J., C. J. Parlato, J. J. Arentsen, G. I. Genvert, R. C. Eagle, Jr., M. R. Wieland, and P. R. Laibson.** 1987. Medical and surgical treatment of *Acanthamoeba* keratitis. *Am. J. Ophthalmol.* **103:**615–625.

50. **Cooke, W. B., and P. Kabler.** 1955. Isolation of potentially pathogenic fungi from polluted water and sewage. *Public Health Rep.* **70:**689–694.

51. **Cordes, L. G., H. W. Wilkinson, G. W. Gorman, B. J. Fikes, and D. W. Fraser.** 1979. Atypical *Legionella*-like organisms: fastidious water-associated bacteria pathogenic for man. *Lancet* **ii:**927–930.

52. **Cort, W. W.** 1928. Schistosome dermatitis in the United States (Michigan). *JAMA* **90:**1027–1029.

53. **Couch, R. B., R. G. Douglas, Jr., K. M. Lindgren, P. J. Gerone, and V. Knight.** 1970. Airborne transmission of respiratory infection with coxsackievirus A type 21. *Am. J. Epidemiol.* **91:**78–86.

54. **Crawford, R. P., J. M. Heinemann, W. F. McCulloch, and S. L. Diesch.** 1971. Human infections associated with waterborne *Leptospires*, and survival studies on serotype pomona. *J. Am. Vet. Med. Assoc.* **159:**1477–1484.

55. **Cremona, G., M. A. Carrasco, A. Tytiun, and M. J. Cosentino.** 2002. Treatment of advanced *Acanthamoeba* keratitis with deep lamellar keratectomy and conjunctival flap. *Cornea* **21:**705–708.

56. **Cursons, R. T., T. J. Brown, and E. A. Keys.** 1977. Immunity to pathogenic free-living amoebae. *Lancet* **ii:**875–876.

57. **Cursons, R. T., T. J. Brown, and E. A. Keys.** 1978. Virulence of pathogenic free-living amebae. *J. Parasitol.* **64:**744–745.

58. **Dailloux, M., P. Hartemann, and J. Beurey.** 1980. Study on the relationship between isolation of mycobacteria and classical microbiological and chemical indicators of water quality in swimming pools. *Zentbl. Bakteriol. Mikrobiol. Hyg. Ser. B* **171:**473–486.

59. **D'Angelo, L. J., J. C. Hierholzer, R. A. Keenlyside, L. J. Anderson, and W. J. Martone.** 1979. Pharyngoconjunctival fever caused by adenovirus type 4: report of a swimming pool-related outbreak with recovery of virus from pool water. *J. Infect. Dis.* **140:**42–47.

60. **Dastis-Bendala, C., E. de Villar-Conde, I. Marin-Leon, L. Manzanares-Torne, M. J. Perez-Lozano, G. Cano-Fuentes, J. Vargas-Romero, and T. Pumarola-Sune.** 1996. Prospective serological study of leptospirosis in southern Spain. *Eur. J. Epidemiol.* **12:**257–262.

61. **Davies, R. R., H. Spencer, and P. O. Wakelin.** 1964. A case of human protothecosis. *Trans. R. Soc. Trop. Med. Hyg.* **58:**448–451.

62. **Davis, P. J., and A. J. Stirling.** 1993. *Aeromonas hydrophila* wound infection associated with water immersion: an unusual football injury. *Injury* **24:**633–634.

63. De La Cuadra, J., P. Gil-Mateo, and R. Llucian. 1996. *Pseudomonas aeruginosa* folliculitis after depilation. *Ann. Dermatol. Venereol.* **123**:268–270. (In French.)

64. Denney, C. F., V. J. Iragui, L. D. Uber-Zak, N. C. Karpinski, E. J. Ziegler, G. S. Visvesvara, and S. L. Reed. 1997. Amebic meningoencephalitis caused by *Balamuthia mandrillaris*: case report and review. *Clin. Infect. Dis.* **25**:1354–1358.

65. Donta, S. T., P. W. Smith, R. E. Levitz, and R. Quintiliani. 1986. Therapy of *Mycobacterium marinum* infections. Use of tetracyclines vs. rifampin. *Arch. Intern. Med.* **146**:902–904.

66. Driebe, W. T., Jr., G. A. Stern, R. J. Epstein, G. S. Visvesvara, M. Adi, and T. Komadina. 1988. *Acanthamoeba* keratitis. Potential role for topical clotrimazole in combination chemotherapy. *Arch. Ophthalmol.* **106**:1196–1201.

67. Duma, R. J. 1989. Diseases caused by free-living amoeba. *Infect. Dis. Newsl.* **8**:25–32.

68. Dworzack, D. L., R. B. Clark, W. J. Borkowski, Jr., D. L. Smith, M. Dykstra, M. P. Pugsley, E. A. Horowitz, T. L. Connolly, D. L. McKinney, and M. K. Hostetler. 1989. *Pseudallescheria boydii* brain abscess: association with near-drowning and efficacy of high-dose, prolonged miconazole therapy in patients with multiple abscesses. *Medicine* (Baltimore) **68**:218–224.

69. Edelstein, H. 1994. *Mycobacterium marinum* skin infections. Report of 31 cases and review of the literature. *Arch. Intern. Med.* **154**:1359–1364.

70. Edelstein, P. H. 1985. Environmental aspects of *Legionella*. *ASM News* **51**:460–467.

71. Edelstein, P. H., M. A. Edelstein, K. H. Lehr, and J. Ren. 1996. In-vitro activity of levofloxacin against clinical isolates of *Legionella* spp., its pharmacokinetics in guinea pigs, and use in experimental *Legionella pneumophila* pneumonia. *J. Antimicrob. Chemother.* **37**:117–126.

72. Edwards, G. A., and B. M. Domm. 1960. Human leptospirosis. *Medicine* (Baltimore) **39**:117–156.

73. el Saadi, O. E., A. J. Esterman, S. Cameron, and D. M. Roder. 1995. Murray River water, raised cyanobacterial cell counts, and gastrointestinal and dermatological symptoms. *Med. J. Aust.* **162**:122–125.

74. Ena, P., L. A. Sechi, P. Saccabusi, M. Molicotti, M. P. Lorrai, M. Siddi, and S. Zanetti. 2001. Rapid identification of cutaneous infections by nontubercular mycobacteria by polymerase chain reaction-restriction analysis length polymorphism of the hsp65 gene. *Int. J. Dermatol.* **40**:495–499.

75. Ender, P. T., and M. J. Dolan. 1997. Pneumonia associated with near-drowning. *Clin. Infect. Dis.* **25**:896–907.

76. Ender, P. T., M. J. Dolan, D. Dolan, J. C. Farmer, and G. P. Melcher. 1996. Near-drowning-associated *Aeromonas* pneumonia. *J. Emerg. Med.* **14**:737–741.

77. Evans, M. R., E. J. Wilkinson, R. Jones, K. Mathias, and P. Lenartowicz. 2003. Presumed *Pseudomonas* folliculitis outbreak in children following an outdoor games event. *Commun. Dis. Public Health* **6**:18–21.

78. Fang, G. D., V. L. Yu, and R. M. Vickers. 1989. Disease due to the *Legionellaceae* (other than *Legionella pneumophila*). Historical, microbiological, clinical, and epidemiological review. *Medicine* (Baltimore) **68**:116–132.

79. Farooqui, M. A., C. Berenson, and J. W. Lohr. 1999. *Mycobacterium marinum* infection in a renal transplant recipient. *Transplantation* **67**:1495–1496.

80. Farr, R. W. 1995. Leptospirosis. *Clin. Infect. Dis.* **21**:1–6; quiz, 7–8.

81. Feddersen, A., J. Kunkel, D. Jonas, V. Engel, S. Bhakdi, and M. Husmann. 1996. Infection of the upper extremity by *Mycobacterium marinum* in a 3-year-old boy—diagnosis by 16S-rDNA analysis. *Infection* **24**:47–48.

82. Feldman, M. R. 1977. *Naegleria fowleri*: fine structural localization of acid phosphatase and heme proteins. *Exp. Parasitol.* **41**:283–289.

83. Fiorillo, L., M. Zucker, D. Sawyer, and A. N. Lin. 2001. The *Pseudomonas* hot-foot syndrome. *N. Engl. J. Med.* **345**:335–338.

84. Fisher, J. F., S. Shadomy, J. R. Teabeaut, J. Woodard, J. E. Michaels, M. A. Newman, E. White, P. Cook, A. Seagraves, F. Yaghman, and P. J. Rissing. 1992. Near-drowning complicated by brain abscess due to *Petriellidium boydii*. *Arch. Neurol.* **39**:511–513.

85. Florakis, G. J., R. Folberg, J. H. Krachmer, D. T. Tse, T. J. Roussel, and M. P. Vrabec. 1988. Elevated corneal epithelial lines in Acanthamoeba keratitis. *Arch. Ophthalmol.* **106**:1202–1206.

86. **Flynn, C. M., C. M. Kelley, M. S. Barrett, and R. N. Jones.** 1997. Application of the E-test to the antimicrobial susceptibility testing of *Mycobacterium marinum* clinical isolates. *J. Clin. Microbiol.* **35**:2083–2086.

87. **Follador, I., A. Bittencourt, F. Duran, and M. G. das Gracas Araujo.** 2001. Cutaneous protothecosis: report of the second Brazilian case. *Rev. Inst. Med. Trop. Sao Paulo* **43**:287–290.

88. **Fowler, M., and R. F. Carter.** 1965. Acute pyogenic meningitis probably due to *Acanthamoeba* sp.: a preliminary report. *Br. Med. J.* **ii**:740–742.

89. **Frenkel, L. M.** 1993. *Pseudomonas* folliculitis from sponges promoted as beauty aids. *J. Clin. Microbiol.* **31**:2838.

90. **Galgiani, J. N., D. A. Stevens, J. R. Graybill, D. L. Stevens, A. J. Tillinghast, and H. B. Levine.** 1984. *Pseudallescheria boydii* infections treated with ketoconazole. Clinical evaluations of seven patients and in vitro susceptibility results. *Chest* **86**:219–224.

91. **Genoni, L., and G. Domenighetti.** 1982. Near-drowning in an adult: favorable course after a 20–minute submersion. *Schweiz. Med. Wochenschr.* **112**:867–870. (In German.)

92. **Girmenia, C., G. Luzi, M. Monaco, and P. Martino.** 1998. Use of voriconazole in treatment of *Scedosporium apiospermum* infection: case report. *J. Clin. Microbiol.* **36**:1436–1438.

93. **Glaser, C. A., F. J. Angulo, and J. A. Rooney.** 1994. Animal-associated opportunistic infections among persons infected with the human immunodeficiency virus. *Clin. Infect. Dis.* **18**:14–24.

94. **Gluckman, S. J.** 1995. *Mycobacterium marinum. Clin. Dermatol.* **13**:273–276.

95. **Gold, W. L., and I. E. Salit.** 1993. *Aeromonas hydrophila* infections of skin and soft tissue: report of 11 cases and review. *Clin. Infect. Dis.* **16**:69–74.

96. **Goldberg, S. L., D. J. Geha, W. F. Marshall, D. J. Inwards, and H. C. Hoagland.** 1993. Successful treatment of simultaneous pulmonary *Pseudallescheria boydii* and *Aspergillus terreus* infection with oral itraconazole. *Clin. Infect. Dis.* **16**:803–805.

97. **Gombert, M. E., E. J. Goldstein, M. L. Corrado, A. J. Stein, and K. M. Butt.** 1981. Disseminated *Mycobacterium marinum* infection after renal transplantation. *Ann. Intern. Med.* **94**:486–487.

98. **Gonzalez, G. M., R. Tijerina, L. K. Najvar, R. Bocanegra, M. G. Rinaldi, D. Loebenberg, and J. R. Graybill.** 2003. Activity of posaconazole against *Pseudallescheria boydii:* in vitro and in vivo assays. *Antimicrob. Agents Chemother.* **47**:1436–1438.

99. **Goodison, R. R.** 1980. *Pseudomonas* cross-infection due to contaminated humidifier water. *Br. Med. J.* **281**:1288.

100. **Goswick, S. M., and G. M. Brenner.** 2003. Activities of azithromycin and amphotericin B against *Naegleria fowleri* in vitro and in a mouse model of primary amebic meningoencephalitis. *Antimicrob. Agents Chemother.* **47**:524–528.

101. **Graczyk, T. K., and C. J. Shiff.** 2000. Recovery of avian schistosome cercariae from water using penetration stimulant matrix with an unsaturated fatty acid. *Am. J. Trop. Med. Hyg.* **63**:174–177.

102. **Greenawald, K. A., G. Nash, and F. D. Foley.** 1969. Acute systemic melioidosis. Autopsy findings in four patients. *Am. J. Clin. Pathol.* **52**:188–198.

103. **Gregory, D. W., and W. Schaffner.** 1987. *Pseudomonas* infections associated with hot tubs and other environments. *Infect. Dis. Clin. N. Am.* **1**:635–648.

104. **Gustafson, T. L., J. D. Band, R. H. Hutcheson, Jr., and W. Schaffner.** 1983. *Pseudomonas* folliculitis: an outbreak and review. *Rev. Infect. Dis.* **5**:1–8.

105. **Gyori, E.** 2003. December 2002: 19–year old male with febrile illness after jet ski accident. *Brain Pathol.* **13**:237–239.

106. **Haake, D. A., M. Dundoo, R. Cader, B. M. Kubak, R. A. Hartskeerl, J. J. Sejvar, and D. A. Ashford.** 2002. Leptospirosis, water sports, and chemoprophylaxis. *Clin. Infect. Dis.* **34**:e40–e43.

107. **Harley, D., B. Harrower, M. Lyon, and A. Dick.** 2001. A primary school outbreak of pharyngoconjunctival fever caused by adenovirus type 3. *Commun. Dis. Intell.* **25**:9–12.

108. **Havens, W. P., C. J. Buchner, and H. A. Reinmann.** 1941. Leptospirosis: a public health hazard. Report of a small outbreak of Weil's disease in bathers. *JAMA* **116**:289–291.

109. **Hawley, H. B., D. P. Morin, M. E. Geraghty, J. Tomkow, and C. A. Phillips.** 1973. Coxsackievirus B epidemic at a boy's summer camp. Isolation of virus from swimming water. *JAMA* **226**:33–36.

110. **Hay, J., C. M. Kirkness, D. V. Seal, and P. Wright.** 1994. Drug resistance and *Acanthamoeba* keratitis: the quest for alternative antiprotozoal chemotherapy. *Eye* **8**(part 5):555–563.

111. **Heckerling, P. S., T. M. Stine, J. C. Pottage, Jr., S. Levin, and A. A. Harris.** 1983. *Aeromonas hydrophila* myonecrosis and gas gangrene in a nonimmunocompromised host. *Arch. Intern. Med.* **143:**2005–2007.

112. **Hertel, J., J. Hamburger, B. Haberl, and W. Haas.** 2002. Detection of bird schistosomes in lakes by PCR and filter-hybridization. *Exp. Parasitol.* **101:**57–63.

113. **Hiti, K., J. Walochnik, C. Faschinger, E. M. Haller-Schober, and H. Aspock.** 2001. Microwave treatment of contact lens cases contaminated with acanthamoeba. *Cornea* **20:**467–470.

114. **Hogan, P. A.** 1997. *Pseudomonas* folliculitis. *Australas. J. Dermatol.* **38:**93–94.

115. **Hojyo-Tomoka, M. T., R. R. Marples, and A. M. Kingman.** 1973. *Pseudomonas* infection in super-hydrated skin. *Arch. Dermatol.* **107:**723–727.

116. **Holland, G. N., and P. B. Donzis.** 1987. Rapid resolution of early *Acanthamoeba* keratitis after epithelial debridement. *Am. J. Ophthalmol.* **104:**87–89.

117. **Horstmann, D. M., J. Emmons, L. Gimpel, T. Subrahmanyan, and J. T. Riordan.** 1973. Enterovirus surveillance following a community-wide oral poliovirus vaccination program: a seven-year study. *Am. J. Epidemiol.* **97:**173–186.

118. **Iacoviello, V. R., P. C. DeGirolami, J. Lucarini, K. Sutker, M. E. Williams, and C. A. Wanke.** 1992. Prototothecosis complicating prolonged endotracheal intubation: case report and literature review. *Clin. Infect. Dis.* **15:**959–967.

119. **Iijima, S., J. Saito, and F. Otsuka.** 1997. *Mycobacterium marinum* skin infection successfully treated with levofloxacin. *Arch. Dermatol.* **133:**947–949.

120. **Insler, M. S., and H. Gore.** 1986. *Pseudomonas* keratitis and folliculitis from whirlpool exposure. *Am. J. Ophthalmol.* **101:**41–43.

121. **Izumi, A. K., C. W. Hanke, and M. Higaki.** 1977. *Mycobacterium marinum* infections treated with tetracycline. *Arch. Dermatol.* **113:**1067–1068.

122. **Jabado, N., J. L. Casanova, E. Haddad, F. Dulieu, J. C. Fournet, B. Dupont, A. Fischer, C. Hennequin, and S. Blanche.** 1998. Invasive pulmonary infection due to *Scedosporium apiospermum* in two children with chronic granulomatous disease. *Clin. Infect. Dis.* **27:**1437–1441.

123. **Jain, R., S. Prabhakar, M. Modi, R. Bhatia, and R. Sehgal.** 2002. *Naegleria* meningitis: a rare survival. *Neurol. India* **50:**470–472.

124. **Janda, J. M.** 1991. Recent advances in the study of the taxonomy, pathogenicity, and infectious syndromes associated with the genus *Aeromonas*. *Clin. Microbiol. Rev.* **4:**397–410.

125. **Janda, J. M., and S. L. Abbott.** 1993. Infections associated with the genus *Edwardsiella*: the role of *Edwardsiella tarda* in human disease. *Clin. Infect. Dis.* **17:**742–748.

126. **Janda, J. M., and P. S. Duffrey.** 1988. Mesophilic aeromonads in human disease: current taxonomy, laboratory identification, and infectious disease spectrum. *Rev. Infect. Dis.* **10:**980–997.

127. **Jernigan, D. B., J. Hofmann, M. S. Cetron, C. A. Genese, J. P. Nuorti, B. S. Fields, R. F. Benson, R. J. Carter, P. H. Edelstein, I. C. Guerrero, S. M. Paul, H. B. Lipman, and R. Breiman.** 1996. Outbreak of Legionnaires' disease among cruise ship passengers exposed to a contaminated whirlpool spa. *Lancet* **347:**494–499.

128. **Jernigan, J. A., and B. M. Farr.** 2000. Incubation period and sources of exposure for cutaneous *Mycobacterium marinum* infection: case report and review of the literature. *Clin. Infect. Dis.* **31:**439–443.

129. **John, D. T.** 1982. Primary amebic meningoencephalitis and the biology of *Naegleria fowleri*. *Annu. Rev. Microbiol.* **36:**101–123.

130. **John, T., J. Lin, D. Sahm, and J. H. Rockey.** 1991. Effects of corticosteroids in experimental *Acanthamoeba* keratitis. *Rev. Infect. Dis.* **13**(Suppl. 5)**:**S440–S442.

131. **Johnson, L. B., and C. A. Kauffman.** 2003. Voriconazole: a new triazole antifungal agent. *Clin. Infect. Dis.* **36:**630–637.

132. **Kahana, L. M., J. M. Kay, M. A. Yakrus, and S. Waserman.** 1997. *Mycobacterium avium* complex infection in an immunocompetent young adult related to hot tub exposure. *Chest* **111:**242–245.

133. **Kaminski, Z. C., R. Kapila, L. R. Sharer, P. Kloser, and L. Kaufman.** 1992. Meningitis due to *Prototheca wickerhamii* in a patient with AIDS. *Clin. Infect. Dis.* **15:**704–706.

134. **Kantrow, S. M., and A. S. Boyd.** 2003. Prototothecosis. *Dermatol. Clin.* **21:**249–255.

135. **Karam, G. H., A. M. Ackley, and W. E. Dismukes.** 1983. Posttraumatic *Aeromonas hydrophila* osteomyelitis. *Arch. Intern. Med.* **143:**2073–2074.

136. **Kaufman, A. F.** 1976. Epidemiological trends of leptospirosis in the United States 1965–1974, p. 177–189. *In* R. C. Johnson (ed.), *The Biology of Parasitic Spirochetes*. Academic Press, New York, N.Y.

137. **Kaufman, S. C., D. Ceraso, and A. Schugurensky.** 1986. First case report from Argentina of fatal septicemia caused by *Chromobacterium violaceum*. *J. Clin. Microbiol.* **23:**956–958.

138. **Khabbaz, R. F., T. W. McKinley, R. A. Goodman, A. W. Hightower, A. K. Highsmith, K. A. Tait, and J. D. Bandin.** 1983. *Pseudomonas aeruginosa* O:9. New cause of whirlpool-associated dermatitis. *Am. J. Med.* **74:**73–77.

139. **Khardori, N., and V. Fainstein.** 1988. *Aeromonas* and *Plesiomonas* as etiologic agents. *Annu. Rev. Microbiol.* **42:**395–419.

140. **Kidney, D. D., and S. H. Kim.** 1998. CNS infections with free-living amebas: neuroimaging findings. *AJR Am. J. Roentgenol.* **171:**809–812.

141. **Kienzle, N., M. Muller, and S. Pegg.** 2000. *Aeromonas* wound infection in burns. *Burns* **26:**478–482.

142. **Kim, S. T., K. S. Suh, Y. S. Chae, and Y. J. Kim.** 1996. Successful treatment with fluconazole of protothecosis developing at the site of an intralesional corticosteroid injection. *Br. J. Dermatol.* **135:**803–806.

143. **King, A. J., J. A. Fairley, and J. E. Rasmussen.** 1983. Disseminated cutaneous *Mycobacterium marinum* infection. *Arch. Dermatol.* **119:**268–270.

144. **Kiska, D. L., and P. H. Gilligan.** 2003. *Pseudomonas*, p. 719–728. *In* P. R. Murray, E. J. Baron, J. H. Jorgensen, M. A. Pfaller, and R. H. Yolken (ed.), *Manual of Clinical Microbiology*, 8th ed. American Society for Microbiology, Washington, D.C.

145. **Kitamura, M., S. Kawai, and T. Horio.** 1998. *Pseudomonas aeruginosa* folliculitis: a sporadic case from use of a contaminated sponge. *Br. J. Dermatol.* **139:**359–360.

146. **Kogon, A., I. Spigland, T. E. Frothingham, L. Elveback, C. Williams, C. E. Hall, and J. P. Fox.** 1969. The virus watch program: a continuing surveillance of viral infections in metropolitan New York families. VII. Observations on viral excretion, seroimmunity, intrafamilial spread and illness association in coxsackie and echovirus infections. *Am. J. Epidemiol.* **89:**51–61.

147. **Kolarova, L., K. Skirnisson, and P. Horak.** 1999. Schistosome cercariae as the causative agent of swimmer's itch in Iceland. *J. Helminthol.* **73:**215–220.

148. **Kosatsky, T., and J. Kleeman.** 1985. Superficial and systemic illness related to a hot tub. *Am. J. Med.* **79:**10–12.

149. **Lacour, J. P., P. el Baze, J. Castanet, D. Dubois, M. Poudenx, and J. P. Ortonne.** 1994. Diving suit dermatitis caused by *Pseudomonas aeruginosa*: two cases. *J. Am. Acad. Dermatol.* **31:**1055–1056.

150. **Laeng, R. H., C. Egger, T. Schaffner, B. Borisch, and E. Pedrinis.** 1994. Protothecosis in an HIV-positive patient. *Am. J. Surg. Pathol.* **18:**1261–1264.

151. **Larkin, D. F., S. Kilvington, and J. K. Dart.** 1992. Treatment of *Acanthamoeba* keratitis with polyhexamethylene biguanide. *Ophthalmology* **99:**185–191.

152. **Lee, G. A., T. B. Gray, J. K. Dart, C. E. Pavesio, L. A. Ficker, D. F. Larkin, and M. M. Matheson.** 2002. *Acanthamoeba* sclerokeratitis: treatment with systemic immunosuppression. *Ophthalmology* **109:**1178–1182.

153. **Lee, N., J. L. Wu, C. H. Lee, and W. C. Tsai.** 1985. *Pseudomonas pseudomallei* infection from drowning: the first reported case in Taiwan. *J. Clin. Microbiol.* **22:**352–354.

154. **Lee, S. H., D. A. Levy, G. F. Craun, M. J. Beach, and R. L. Calderon.** 2002. Surveillance for waterborne-disease outbreaks—United States, 1999–2000. *MMWR Surveill. Summ.* **51:**1–47.

155. **Lee, W. J., T. W. Kim, K. B. Shur, B. J. Kim, Y. H. Kook, J. H. Lee, and J. K. Park.** 2000. Sporotrichoid dermatosis caused by *Mycobacterium abscessus* from a public bath. *J. Dermatol.* **27:**264–268.

156. **Levett, P. N.** 2003. *Leptospira* and *Leptonema*, p. 929–936. *In* P. R. Murray, E. J. Baron, J. H. Jorgensen, M. A. Pfaller, and R. H. Yolken (ed.), *Manual of Clinical Microbiology*, 8th ed. American Society for Microbiology, Washington, D.C.

157. **Levin, M. L.** 1973. Gas-forming *Aeromonas hydrophila* infection in a diabetic. *Postgrad. Med.* **54:**127–129.

158. **Lewis, F. M., B. J. Marsh, and C. F. von Reyn.** 2003. Fish tank exposure and cutaneous infections due to *Mycobacterium marinum*: tuberculin skin testing, treatment, and prevention. *Clin. Infect. Dis.* **37:**390–397.

159. **Liang, R. B., P. J. Flegg, B. Watt, and C. L. Leen.** 1997. Antimicrobial treatment of fishtank granuloma. *J. Hand Surg.* (Br. vol.) **22**:135–137.
160. **Lindblade, K. A.** 1998. The epidemiology of cercarial dermatitis and its association with limnological characteristics of a northern Michigan lake. *J. Parasitol.* **84**:19–23.
161. **Lindquist, T. D., N. A. Sher, and D. J. Doughman.** 1988. Clinical signs and medical therapy of early *Acanthamoeba* keratitis. *Arch. Ophthalmol.* **106**:73–77.
162. **Lineaweaver, W. C., M. K. Hill, G. M. Buncke, S. Follansbee, H. J. Buncke, R. K. Wong, E. K. Manders, J. C. Grotting, J. Anthony, and S. J. Mathes.** 1992. *Aeromonas hydrophila* infections following use of medicinal leeches in replantation and flap surgery. *Ann. Plast. Surg.* **29**: 238–244.
163. **Linell, F., and A. Nordin.** 1954. *Mycobacterium blanei:* a new acid-fast bacillus occurring in swimming pools and capable of producing skin lesions in humans. *Acta Tuberc. Pneumol. Scand.* **33**(Suppl.):1–5.
164. **Liu, Z., J. E. Stout, M. Boldin, J. Rugh, W. F. Diven, and V. L. Yu.** 1998. Intermittent use of copper-silver ionization for *Legionella* control in water distribution systems: a potential option in buildings housing individuals at low risk of infection. *Clin. Infect. Dis.* **26**:138–140.
165. **Loschiavo, F., T. Ventura-Spagnolo, E. Sessa, and P. Bramanti.** 1993. Acute primary meningoencephalitis from entamoeba *Naegleria fowleri.* Report of a clinical case with a favourable outcome. *Acta Neurol.* (Naples) **15**:333–340.
166. **Lowry, P. W., R. J. Blankenship, W. Gridley, N. J. Troup, and L. S. Tompkins.** 1991. A cluster of *Legionella* sternal-wound infections due to postoperative topical exposure to contaminated tap water. *N. Engl. J. Med.* **324**:109–113.
167. **Ludwig, I. H., D. M. Meisler, I. Rutherford, F. E. Bican, R. H. Langston, and G. S. Visvesvara.** 1986. Susceptibility of *Acanthamoeba* to soft contact lens disinfection systems. *Investig. Ophthalmol. Vis. Sci.* **27**:626–628.
168. **Ma, P., G. S. Visvesvara, A. J. Martinez, F. H. Theodore, P. M. Daggett, and T. K. Sawyer.** 1990. *Naegleria* and *Acanthamoeba* infections: review. *Rev. Infect. Dis.* **12**:490–513.
169. **Mangione, E. J., R. S. Remis, K. A. Tait, H. B. McGee, G. W. Gorman, B. B. Wentworth, P. A. Baron, A. W. Hightower, J. M. Barbaree, and C. V. Broome.** 1985. An outbreak of Pontiac fever related to whirlpool use, Michigan 1982. *JAMA* **253**:535–539.
170. **Maniatis, A. N., C. Karkavitsas, N. A. Maniatis, E. Tsiftsakis, V. Genimata, and N. J. Legakis.** 1995. *Pseudomonas aeruginosa* folliculitis due to non-O:11 serogroups: acquisition through use of contaminated sponges. *Clin. Infect. Dis.* **21**:437–439.
171. **Markowitz, S. M., A. J. Martinez, R. J. Duma, and F. O. Shiel.** 1974. Myocarditis associated with primary amebic (*Naegleria*) meningoencephalitis. *Am. J. Clin. Pathol.* **62**:619–628.
172. **Marshall, M. M., D. Naumovitz, Y. Ortega, and C. R. Sterling.** 1997. Waterborne protozoan pathogens. *Clin. Microbiol. Rev.* **10**:67–85.
173. **Martinez, A. J.** 1983. Free-living amoeba: pathogenic aspects. A review. *Protozool. Abstr.* **7**:293–305.
174. **Martinez, A. J.** 1993. Free-living amebas: infection of the central nervous system. *Mt. Sinai J. Med.* **60**:271–278.
175. **Martinez, A. J., and G. S. Visvesvara.** 1997. Free-living, amphizoic and opportunistic amebas. *Brain Pathol.* **7**:583–598.
176. **Martinez, J. A.** 1985. *Free Living Amoebas: Natural History, Prevention, Diagnosis, Pathology and Treatment of Disease.* CRC Press, Boca Raton, Fla.
177. **Matsushima, S., S. Yajima, T. Taguchi, A. Takahashi, M. Shiseki, K. Totsuka, and T. Uchiyama.** 1996. A fulminating case of *Edwardsiella tarda* septicemia with necrotizing fasciitis. *Kansenshogaku Zasshi* **70**:631–636. (In Japanese.)
178. **McCausland, W. J., and P. J. Cox.** 1975. *Pseudomonas* infection traced to motel whirlpool. *J. Environ. Health* **37**:455–459.
179. **Meadow, W. L., M. A. Tipple, and J. W. Rippon.** 1981. Endophthalmitis caused by *Petriellidium boydii. Am. J. Dis. Child.* **135**:378–380.
180. **Meyers, W. M., W. M. Shelly, and D. H. Connor.** 1974. Heat treatment of *Mycobacterium ulcerans* infections without surgical excision. *Am. J. Trop. Med. Hyg.* **23**:924–929.
181. **Meyers, W. M., W. M. Shelly, D. H. Connor, and E. K. Meyers.** 1974. Human *Mycobacterium ulcerans* infections developing at sites of trauma to skin. *Am. J. Trop. Med. Hyg.* **23**:919–923.

182. **Mollohan, C. S., and M. S. Romer.** 1961. Public health significance of swimming pool granuloma. *Am. J. Public Health* **51:**883–891.

183. **Moshari, A., I. W. McLean, M. T. Dodds, R. E. Damiano, and P. L. McEvoy.** 2001. Chorioretinitis after keratitis caused by *Acanthamoeba:* case report and review of the literature. *Ophthalmology* **108:**2232–2236.

184. **Mowbray, E. E., G. Buck, K. E. Humbaugh, and G. S. Marshall.** 2003. Maternal colonization and neonatal sepsis caused by *Edwardsiella tarda. Pediatrics* **111:**e296–e298.

185. **Munoz, P., M. Marin, P. Tornero, P. Martin Rabadan, M. Rodriguez-Creixems, and E. Bouza.** 2000. Successful outcome of *Scedosporium apiospermum* disseminated infection treated with voriconazole in a patient receiving corticosteroid therapy. *Clin. Infect. Dis.* **31:**1499–1501.

186. **Nesky, M. A., E. C. McDougal, and J. E. Peacock, Jr.** 2000. *Pseudallescheria boydii* brain abscess successfully treated with voriconazole and surgical drainage: case report and literature review of central nervous system pseudallescheriasis. *Clin. Infect. Dis.* **31:**673–677.

187. **Palmer, A.** 1991. Summer and *Pseudomonas. Aust. Fam. Physician* **20:**1039.

188. **Panaphut, T., S. Domrongkitchaiporn, A. Vibhagool, B. Thinkamrop, and W. Susaengrat.** 2003. Ceftriaxone compared with sodium penicillin G for treatment of severe leptospirosis. *Clin. Infect. Dis.* **36:**1507–1513.

189. **Pasricha, G., S. Sharma, P. Garg, and R. K. Aggarwal.** 2003. Use of 18S rRNA gene-based PCR assay for diagnosis of *Acanthamoeba* keratitis in non-contact lens wearers in India. *J. Clin. Microbiol.* **41:**3206–3211.

190. **Pegram, P. S., Jr., F. T. Kerns, B. L. Wasilauskas, K. D. Hampton, M. Scharyj, and J. G. Burke.** 1983. Successful ketoconazole treatment of protothecosis with ketoconazole-associated hepatotoxicity. *Arch. Intern. Med.* **143:**1802–1805.

191. **Peters, D. H., and S. P. Clissold.** 1992. Clarithromycin. A review of its antimicrobial activity, pharmacokinetic properties and therapeutic potential. *Drugs* **44:**117–164.

192. **Pfaller, M. A., F. Marco, S. A. Messer, and R. N. Jones.** 1998. In vitro activity of two echinocandin derivatives, LY303366 and MK-0991 (L-743, 792), against clinical isolates of *Aspergillus, Fusarium, Rhizopus,* and other filamentous fungi. *Diagn. Microbiol. Infect. Dis.* **30:**251–255.

193. **Piyophirapong, S., R. Linpiyawan, P. Mahaisavariya, C. Muanprasat, A. Chaiprasert, and P. Suthipinittharm.** 2002. Cutaneous protothecosis in an AIDS patient. *Br. J. Dermatol.* **146:**713–715.

194. **Polk, P., and D. Y. Sanders.** 1997. Cutaneous protothecosis in association with the acquired immunodeficiency syndrome. *South. Med. J.* **90:**831–832.

195. **Ponte, R., and S. G. Jenkins.** 1992. Fatal *Chromobacterium violaceum* infections associated with exposure to stagnant waters. *Pediatr. Infect. Dis. J.* **11:**583–586.

196. **Poungverin, N., and P. Jarya.** 1991. The fifth nonlethal case of PAM. *J. Med. Assoc. Thail.* **74:**112–115.

197. **Poza, G., J. Montoya, C. Redondo, J. Ruiz, N. Vila, J. L. Rodriguez-Tudela, A. Ceron, and E. Simarro.** 2000. Meningitis caused by *Pseudallescheria boydii* treated with voriconazole. *Clin. Infect. Dis.* **30:**981–982.

198. **Rasmussen, J. E., and W. H. Graves III.** 1982. *Pseudomonas aeruginosa,* hot tubs, and skin infections. *Am. J. Dis. Child.* **136:**553–554.

199. **Ratnam, S., K. Hogan, S. B. March, and R. W. Butler.** 1986. Whirlpool-associated folliculitis caused by *Pseudomonas aeruginosa:* report of an outbreak and review. *J. Clin. Microbiol.* **23:**655–659.

200. **Reines, H. D., and F. V. Cook.** 1981. Pneumonia and bacteremia due to *Aeromonas hydrophila. Chest* **80:**264–267.

201. **Reinhardt, J. F., S. Fowlston, J. Jones, and W. L. George.** 1985. Comparative in vitro activities of selected antimicrobial agents against *Edwardsiella tarda. Antimicrob. Agents Chemother.* **27:**966–967.

202. **Reparaz Padros, J.** 1990. *Pseudomonas aeruginosa* folliculitis after skin depilation. *Enferm. Infecc. Microbiol. Clin.* **8:**393–394. (In Spanish.)

203. **Reveiller, F. L., P. A. Cabanes, and F. Marciano-Cabral.** 2002. Development of a nested PCR assay to detect the pathogenic free-living amoeba *Naegleria fowleri. Parasitol. Res.* **88:**443–450.

204. **Rhodes, M. W., H. Kator, S. Kotob, P. van Berkum, I. Kaattari, W. Vogelbein, F. Quinn, M. M. Floyd, W. R. Butler, and C. A. Ottinger.** 2003. *Mycobacterium shottsii* sp. nov., a slowly growing species isolated from Chesapeake Bay striped bass (*Morone saxatilis*). *Int. J. Syst. Evol. Microbiol.* **53:**421–424.

205. **Rinke, C. M.** 1983. Hot tub hygiene. *JAMA* **250:**2031.
206. **Rivera, V., D. Hernandez, S. Rojas, G. Oliver, J. Serrano, M. Shibayama, V. Tsutsumi, and R. Campos.** 2001. IgA and IgM anti-*Naegleria fowleri* antibodies in human serum and saliva. *Can. J. Microbiol.* **47:**464–466.
207. **Romero, J. R., and H. A. Rotbart.** 2003. Enteroviruses, p. 1427–1438. *In* P. R. Murray, E. J. Baron, J. H. Jorgensen, M. A. Pfaller, and R. H. Yolken (ed.), *Manual of Clinical Microbiology,* 8th ed. American Society for Microbiology, Washington, D.C.
208. **Rose, H. D., T. R. Franson, N. K. Sheth, M. J. Chusid, A. M. Macher, and C. H. Zeirdt.** 1983. *Pseudomonas* pneumonia associated with use of a home whirlpool spa. *JAMA* **250:**2027–2029.
209. **Roters, S., S. Aisenbrey, M. Severin, W. Konen, H. M. Seitz, and G. K. Krieglstein.** 2001. Painless *Acanthamoeba* keratitis. *Klin. Monatsbl. Augenheilkd.* **218:**570–573. (In German.)
210. **Salmen, P., D. M. Dwyer, H. Vorse, and W. Kruse.** 1983. Whirlpool-associated *Pseudomonas aeruginosa* urinary tract infections. *JAMA* **250:**2025–2026.
211. **Saltzer, K. R., P. J. Schutzer, J. M. Weinberg, I. A. Tangoren, and E. M. Spiers.** 1997. Diving suit dermatitis: a manifestation of *Pseudomonas* folliculitis. *Cutis* **59:**245–246.
212. **Sanders, W. J., and E. Wolinsky.** 1980. In vitro susceptibility of *Mycobacterium marinum* to eight antimicrobial agents. *Antimicrob. Agents Chemother.* **18:**529–531.
213. **San Joaquin, V. H., R. K. Scribner, D. A. Pickett, and D. F. Welch.** 1986. Antimicrobial susceptibility of *Aeromonas* species isolated from patients with diarrhea. *Antimicrob. Agents Chemother.* **30:**794–795.
214. **Sausker, W. F., J. L. Aeling, J. E. Fitzpatrick, and F. N. Judson.** 1978. *Pseudomonas* folliculitis acquired from a health spa whirlpool. *JAMA* **239:**2362–2365.
215. **Schiess, R. J., M. F. Coscia, and G. A. McClellan.** 1984. *Petriellidium boydii* pachymeningitis treated with miconazole and ketoconazole. *Neurosurgery* **14:**220–224.
216. **Seidel, J. S., P. Harmatz, G. S. Visvesvara, A. Cohen, J. Edwards, and J. Turner.** 1982. Successful treatment of primary amebic meningoencephalitis. *N. Engl. J. Med.* **306:**346–348.
217. **Sharma, S., M. Srinivasan, and C. George.** 1990. *Acanthamoeba* keratitis in non-contact lens wearers. *Arch. Ophthalmol.* **108:**676–678.
218. **Sheehan, D. J., C. A. Hitchcock, and C. M. Sibley.** 1999. Current and emerging azole antifungal agents. *Clin. Microbiol. Rev.* **12:**40–79.
219. **Shilkin, K. B., D. I. Annear, L. R. Rowett, and B. H. Laurence.** 1968. Infection due to *Aeromonas hydrophila. Med. J. Aust.* **1:**351–353.
220. **Shiota, R., K. Takeshita, K. Yamamoto, K. Imada, E. Yabuuchi, and L. Wang.** 1995. *Legionella pneumophila* serogroup 3 isolated from a patient of pneumonia developed after drowning in bathtub of a hot spring spa. *Kansenshogaku Zasshi* **69:**1356–1364. (In Japanese.)
221. **Silverman, A. R., and M. L. Nieland.** 1983. Hot tub dermatitis: a familial outbreak of *Pseudomonas* folliculitis. *J. Am. Acad. Dermatol.* **8:**153–156.
222. **Skoll, P. J., D. A. Hudson, and J. A. Simpson.** 1998. *Aeromonas* hydrophila in burn patients. *Burns* **24:**350–353.
223. **Slaven, E. M., F. A. Lopez, S. M. Hart, and C. V. Sanders.** 2001. Myonecrosis caused by *Edwardsiella tarda:* a case report and case series of extraintestinal *E. tarda* infections. *Clin. Infect. Dis.* **32:**1430–1433.
224. **Smith, G. L.** 1982. Methods for preventing *Pseudomonas* folliculitis. *Cutis* **29:**378, 381.
225. **Smith, J. A.** 1980. *Aeromonas hydrophila:* analysis of 11 cases. *Can. Med. Assoc. J.* **122:**1270–1272.
226. **Snower, D. P., C. Ruef, A. P. Kuritza, and S. C. Edberg.** 1989. *Aeromonas hydrophila* infection associated with the use of medicinal leeches. *J. Clin. Microbiol.* **27:**1421–1422.
227. **Solomon, S. L.** 1985. Host factors in whirlpool-associated *Pseudomonas aeruginosa* skin disease. *Infect. Control* **6:**402–406.
228. **Speight, E. L., and H. C. Williams.** 1997. Fish tank granuloma in a 14–month-old girl. *Pediatr. Dermatol.* **14:**209–212.
229. **Stanford, J. L., W. D. Revill, W. J. Gunthorpe, and J. M. Grange.** 1975. The production and preliminary investigation of Burulin, a new skin test reagent for *Mycobacterium ulcerans* infection. *J. Hyg.* **74:**7–16.
230. **Starr, A. J., L. S. Cribbett, J. Poklepovic, H. Friedman, and E. H. Ruffolo.** 1981. *Chromobacterium violaceum* presenting as a surgical emergency. *South. Med. J.* **74:**1137–1139.

231. **Stehr-Green, J. K., T. M. Bailey, F. H. Brandt, J. H. Carr, W. W. Bond, and G. S. Visvesvara.** 1987. *Acanthamoeba* keratitis in soft contact lens wearers. A case-control study. *JAMA* **258**:57–60.

232. **Stehr-Green, J. K., T. M. Bailey, and G. S. Visvesvara.** 1989. The epidemiology of *Acanthamoeba* keratitis in the United States. *Am. J. Ophthalmol.* **107**:331–336.

233. **Stevens, A. R., S. T. Shulman, T. A. Lansen, M. J. Cichon, and E. Willaert.** 1981. Primary amoebic meningoencephalitis: a report of two cases and antibiotic and immunologic studies. *J. Infect. Dis.* **143**:193–199.

234. **Stinear, T., J. K. Davies, G. A. Jenkin, J. A. Hayman, F. Oppedisano, and P. D. R. Johnson.** 2000. Identification of *Mycobacterium ulcerans* in the environment from regions in southeast Australia in which it is endemic with sequence capture-PCR. *Appl. Environ. Microbiol.* **66**:3206–3213.

235. **Stinear, T., J. K. Davies, G. A. Jenkin, F. Portaels, B. C. Ross, F. Oppedisano, M. Purcell, J. A. Hayman, and P. D. Johnson.** 2000. A simple PCR method for rapid genotype analysis of *Mycobacterium ulcerans*. *J. Clin. Microbiol.* **38**:1482–1487.

236. **Stinear, T., B. C. Ross, J. K. Davies, L. Marino, R. M. Robins-Browne, F. Oppedisano, A. Sievers, and P. D. R. Johnson.** 1999. Identification and characterization of IS*2404* and IS*2606*: two distinct repeated sequences for detection of *Mycobacterium ulcerans* by PCR. *J. Clin. Microbiol.* **37**:1018–1023.

237. **Stinear, T. P., G. A. Jenkin, P. D. Johnson, and J. K. Davies.** 2000. Comparative genetic analysis of *Mycobacterium ulcerans* and *Mycobacterium marinum* reveals evidence of recent divergence. *J. Bacteriol.* **182**:6322–6330.

238. **Stout, J. E., J. D. Rih, and V. L. Yu.** 2003. *Legionella*, p. 809–823. *In* P. R. Murray, E. J. Baron, J. H. Jorgensen, M. A. Pfaller, and R. H. Yolken (ed.), *Manual of Clinical Microbiology*, 8th ed. American Society for Microbiology, Washington, D.C.

239. **Sudman, M. S.** 1974. Prototothecosis. A critical review. *Am. J. Clin. Pathol.* **61**:10–19.

240. **Tabin, G., H. Taylor, G. Snibson, A. Murchison, A. Gushchin, and S. Rogers.** 2001. Atypical presentation of *Acanthamoeba* keratitis. *Cornea* **20**:757–759.

241. **Tate, D., S. Mawer, and A. Newton.** 2003. Outbreak of *Pseudomonas aeruginosa* folliculitis associated with a swimming pool inflatable. *Epidemiol. Infect.* **130**:187–192.

242. **Theodore, F. H., F. A. Jakobiec, K. B. Juechter, P. Ma, R. C. Troutman, P. M. Pang, and T. Iwamoto.** 1985. The diagnostic value of a ring infiltrate in acanthamoebic keratitis. *Ophthalmology* **92**:1471–1479.

243. **Thomason, B. M., P. P. Harris, M. D. Hicklin, J. A. Blackmon, W. Moss, and F. Matthews.** 1979. A *Legionella*-like bacterium related to WIGA in a fatal case of pneumonia. *Ann. Intern. Med.* **91**:673–676.

244. **Thong, Y. H.** 1980. Primary amoebic meningoencephalitis: fifteen years later. *Med. J. Aust.* **1**:352–354.

245. **Tolentino, A., S. Ahkee, and J. Ramirez.** 1996. Hot tub legionellosis. *J. Ky. Med. Assoc.* **94**:393–394.

246. **Torres, F., T. Hodges, and M. R. Zamora.** 2001. *Mycobacterium marinum* infection in a lung transplant recipient. *J. Heart Lung Transplant.* **20**:486–489.

247. **Tron, V. A., V. J. Baldwin, and G. E. Pirie.** 1985. Hot tub drownings. *Pediatrics* **75**:789–790.

248. **Trueb, R. M., P. Elsner, and G. Burg.** 1993. *Pseudomonas aeruginosa* folliculitis after depilation. *Hautarzt* **44**:103–105.

249. **van Crevel, R., P. Speelman, C. Gravekamp, and W. J. Terpstra.** 1994. Leptospirosis in travelers. *Clin. Infect. Dis.* **19**:132–134.

250. **Van der Hoeden, J.** 1958. Epizootiology of leptospirosis. *Adv. Vet. Sci.* **4**:277–339.

251. **van der Vliet, J. A., G. Tidow, G. Kootstra, H. F. van Saene, R. A. Krom, M. J. Sloof, J. J. Weening, A. M. Tegzess, S. Meijer, and W. P. van Boven.** 1980. Transplantation of contaminated organs. *Br. J. Surg.* **67**:596–598.

252. **Vartian, C. V., and E. J. Septimus.** 1990. Soft-tissue infection caused by *Edwardsiella tarda* and *Aeromonas hydrophila*. *J. Infect. Dis.* **161**:816.

253. **Vernon, D. D., W. Banner, Jr., G. P. Cantwell, B. H. Holzman, R. G. Bolte, and J. M. Dean.** 1990. *Streptococcus pneumoniae* bacteremia associated with near-drowning. *Crit. Care Med.* **18**:1175–1176.

254. **Vieira, D. F., H. K. Van Saene, and D. R. Miranda.** 1984. Invasive pulmonary aspergillosis after near-drowning. *Intensive Care Med.* **10**:203–204.

255. **Visvesvara, G. S.** 1993. Epidemiology of infections with free-living amebas and laboratory diagnosis of microsporidiosis. *Mt. Sinai J. Med.* **60**:283–288.

256. **Visvesvara, G. S.** 1995. Pathogenic and opportunistic free living amoeba, p. 1196–1203. *In* P. R. Murray, E. J. Baron, M. A. Pfaller, F. C. Tenover, and R. H. Yolken (ed.), *Manual of Clinical Microbiology*, 6th ed. American Society for Microbiology, Washington, D.C.

257. **Vogt, R., D. LaRue, M. F. Parry, C. D. Brokopp, D. Klaucke, and J. Allen.** 1982. *Pseudomonas aeruginosa* skin infections in persons using a whirlpool in Vermont. *J. Clin. Microbiol.* **15**:571–574.

258. **Von Graevenitz, A., and A. H. Mensch.** 1968. The genus *Aeromonas* in human bacteriology: report of 30 cases and review of the literature. *N. Engl. J. Med.* **278**:245–249.

259. **Wadell, G.** 1988. *Adenoviridae:* the adenoviruses, p. 284–300. *In* E. H. Lennette, P. Halonen, and F. A. Murray (ed.), *Laboratory Diagnosis of Infectious Diseases*, vol. II. Springer-Verlag, New York, N.Y.

260. **Wallace, R. J., Jr., J. M. Swenson, V. A. Silcox, and M. G. Bullen.** 1985. Treatment of nonpulmonary infections due to *Mycobacterium fortuitum* and *Mycobacterium chelonei* on the basis of in vitro susceptibilities. *J. Infect. Dis.* **152**:500–514.

261. **Wallace, R. J., Jr., J. M. Swenson, V. A. Silcox, R. C. Good, J. A. Tschen, and M. S. Stone.** 1983. Spectrum of disease due to rapidly growing mycobacteria. *Rev. Infect. Dis.* **5**:657–679.

262. **Walsh, T. J., I. Lutsar, T. Driscoll, B. Dupont, M. Roden, P. Ghahramani, M. Hodges, A. H. Groll, and J. R. Perfect.** 2002. Voriconazole in the treatment of aspergillosis, scedosporiosis and other invasive fungal infections in children. *Pediatr. Infect. Dis. J.* **21**:240–248.

263. **Wang, A., R. Kay, W. S. Poon, and H. K. Ng.** 1993. Successful treatment of amoebic meningoencephalitis in a Chinese living in Hong Kong. *Clin. Neurol. Neurosurg.* **95**:249–252.

264. **Warrier, R. P., R. Ducos, S. Azeemuddin, and A. Ruff.** 1984. *Aeromonas* infection in an infant with aplastic anemia. *Pediatr. Infect. Dis.* **3**:491.

265. **Washburn, J., J. A. Jacobson, E. Marston, and B. Thorsen.** 1976. *Pseudomonas aeruginosa* rash associated with a whirlpool. *JAMA* **235**:2205–2207.

266. **Wellings, F. M., P. T. Amuso, S. L. Chang, and A. L. Lewis.** 1977. Isolation and identification of pathogenic *Naegleria* from Florida lakes. *Appl. Environ. Microbiol.* **34**:661–667.

267. **Wilhelmus, K. R., M. S. Osato, R. L. Font, N. M. Robinson, and D. B. Jones.** 1986. Rapid diagnosis of *Acanthamoeba* keratitis using calcofluor white. *Arch. Ophthalmol.* **104**:1309–1312.

268. **Wilichowski, E., H. J. Christen, H. Schiffmann, W. Schulz-Schaeffer, and W. Behrens-Baumann.** 1996. Fatal *Pseudallescheria boydii* panencephalitis in a child after near-drowning. *Pediatr. Infect. Dis. J.* **15**:365–370.

269. **Winthrop, K. L., M. Abrams, M. Yakrus, I. Schwartz, J. Ely, D. Gillies, and D. J. Vugia.** 2002. An outbreak of mycobacterial furunculosis associated with footbaths at a nail salon. *N. Engl. J. Med.* **346**:1366–1371.

270. **Wolf, A., R. Benham, and L. Mount.** 1948. Maduramycotic meningitis. *J. Neuropathol. Exp. Neurol.* **7**:112–113.

271. **Woolrich, A., E. Koestenblatt, P. Don, and W. Szaniawski.** 1994. Cutaneous protothecosis and AIDS. *J. Am. Acad. Dermatol.* **31**:920–924.

272. **Wright, P., D. Warhurst, and B. R. Jones.** 1985. *Acanthamoeba* keratitis successfully treated medically. *Br. J. Ophthalmol.* **69**:778–782.

273. **Wu, T. S., C. H. Chiu, L. H. Su, J. H. Chia, M. H. Lee, P. C. Chiang, A. J. Kuo, T. L. Wu, and H. S. Leu.** 2002. *Mycobacterium marinum* infection in Taiwan. *J. Microbiol. Immunol. Infect.* **35**:42–46.

274. **Young, D. F., and R. J. Barr.** 1981. *Aeromonas hydrophila* infection of the skin. *Arch. Dermatol.* **117**:244.

275. **Zichichi, L., G. Asta, and G. Noto.** 2000. *Pseudomonas aeruginosa* folliculitis after shower/bath exposure. *Int. J. Dermatol.* **39**:270–273.

Infections of Leisure, Third Edition
Edited by David Schlossberg
© 2004 ASM Press, Washington, D.C.

Chapter 3

The Camper's Uninvited Guests

Richard F. Jacobs and Gordon E. Schutze

Venturing into wilderness environments can be exhilarating, and each year millions of people take time off to enjoy this pastime. During this relaxing endeavor the majority of adventurers will come into contact with different species of biting arthropods. Ticks, mosquitoes, lice, fleas, mites, bees, wasps, scorpions, and spiders can make time spent outdoors unpleasant, and they are potential carriers of disease. These biting arthropods may identify humans not only as enemies but also as potential sources of food. Biting, therefore, can be an act of feeding, probing, or defending. Contact with the host can be transient (mosquito) or prolonged (tick) and may result in the inoculation of salivary fluids or the regurgitation of digestive tract contents. Organisms present in these fluids are able to cause many different diseases in their human hosts.

In the United States the majority of illnesses attributed to biting arthropods are due to ticks and mosquitoes. Although potentially serious, the majority of bites from bees, wasps, scorpions, and spiders are simply painful. Physicians should consider arthropod-transmitted diseases during all seasons, but suspicions should be heightened during the summer, when arthropods are most abundant. Children are especially prone to encounter ticks due to their frequent contact with animals and tick habitats. The spectrum of disease caused by these arthropods is broad and can be confusing for the clinician. A history of rural travel, travel to areas where arthropod-borne diseases are endemic, tick bites, or wilderness exposure may aid in obtaining a diagnosis.

Many an adventurer attempts to avoid these uninvited guests by seeking refuge in lakes or streams. These bodies of water, especially those contaminated by wild animals such as beavers, are themselves not without risk of disease. Although the biting arthropods may be avoided, other uninvited guests, such as *Giardia lamblia*, have the potential to make a vacation equally unpleasant.

Richard F. Jacobs • Department of Pediatrics, UAMS College of Medicine, and Pediatric Infectious Diseases, Arkansas Children's Hospital, Little Rock, AR 72202. *Gordon E. Schutze* • Departments of Pediatrics and Pathology, UAMS College of Medicine, and Pediatric Infectious Diseases, Arkansas Children's Hospital, Little Rock, AR 72202.

TICKS

The major diseases in the United States which are transmitted to humans by ticks include Lyme disease, human monocytic (HME) and granulocytic (HGE) ehrlichiosis, Rocky Mountain spotted fever (RMSF), and tularemia (Table 1). Each of these disorders has a causative agent that is passed from a specific tick to the host. The two types of ticks usually encountered are the soft (argasid) tick and the hard (ixodid) tick. The hard ticks are of greater concern, since they are more frequently encountered, are difficult to remove, and are more likely to transmit disease to humans.

Nonspecific Fever

Recent data from areas of endemicity evaluated for nonspecific fever without a rash in northwest Wisconsin identified 27% ($n = 62$) of eligible patients with laboratory evidence of tick-borne infection (2). In a recent reevaluation of the military experience in Fort Chaffee, Ark., 162 of 1,067 persons (15.2%) had antibodies to one or more tick-borne pathogens following training exercises and contact with wooded areas (38). Finally, two recent seroprevalence surveys of children (aged 1 to 17 years) in the southeast United States found seropositivity rates of 2 to 20% for antibodies to RMSF and HME in randomly selected blood specimens (35, 36). These recent findings indicate the potential risk for a myriad of possibilities from symptomatic to classic presentations for tick-borne infections.

Lyme Disease

Lyme disease is considered by some experts to be the leading vector-borne disease in the United States (11). This multisystem inflammatory disease is caused by the spirochetal organism *Borrelia burgdorferi*. This spirochete was identified in the stomach of the main tick vector (*Ixodes scapularis*) and subsequently recognized as the causative agent for the disease (54). Other ticks implicated in transmission of the disease include *Ixodes pacificus*, *Ixodes cookei*, and *Amblyomma americanum* (the

Table 1. Infectious diseases transmitted by ticks

Disease	Agent
Lyme disease	*B. burgdorferi*
Ehrlichiosis	
HME	*E. chaffeensis*
HGE	*A. phagocytophilum*
RMSF	*R. rickettsii*
Tularemia	*F. tularensis*
Colorado tick fever	Arbovirus
Babesiosis	*Babesia* species
Fièvre boutonneuse	*Rickettsia conorii*
Siberian tick typhus	*Rickettsia sibirica*
Queensland tick typhus	*Rickettsia australis*
Powassan encephalitis	Flavivirus

Lone Star tick) (32, 48). Even when engorged, these *Ixodes* ticks are quite small, and therefore histories of tick bites are infrequently obtained. Lyme disease has been reported in most states, but cases remain concentrated in well-established areas in the northeastern, north-central, and Pacific Coast states. Approximately 95% of reported cases come from 12 states in these regions (6).

The clinical presentation of Lyme disease is divided into three stages. These stages are defined by the chronological relationship to the original tick bite (Table 2). The major manifestation of the first stage of the disease is the localized skin rash termed erythema migrans, which is present in up to 80% of patients (Fig. 1) (45). This rash usually begins anywhere from 4 to 21 days after the tick bite and consists of an erythematous papule which gradually enlarges to form a large plaque-like annular lesion (5 cm or more in diameter, with a median of 15 cm; sometimes with partial central clearing). The average duration of the untreated lesion is approximately 3 weeks. If appropriate antibiotics are given, the rash may resolve in several days. Patients in this stage of disease may also have fever, regional adenopathy, or other minor constitutional symptoms (55, 56).

The second stage of Lyme disease is the result of dissemination by the spirochete into the circulation. Although the potential clinical manifestations of this dissemination are extensive, the major characteristics are seen in the skin and the

Table 2. Major clinical manifestations of Lyme disease[a]

Stage and symptoms
Stage 1 (early infection)
Erythema migrans
Headache
Arthralgias
Regional lymphadenopathy
Stage 2 (disseminated disease)
Recurrent erythema migrans
Migratory bone and joint pain
Meningitis
Bell's palsy
Peripheral radiculoneuropathy
Atrioventricular block
Myocarditis
Pancarditis
Conjunctivitis
Mild hepatitis
Hematuria and proteinuria
Malaise and fatigue
Stage 3 (late disease)
Acrodermatitis chronica atrophicans
Prolonged arthritis
Chronic neurological syndromes
Keratitis

[a]Data are from references 43 and 47.

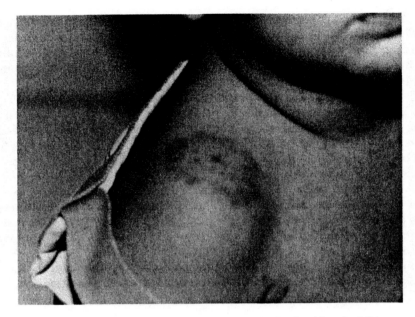

Figure 1. Annular lesion of erythema migrans on the shoulder of a child.

nervous and musculoskeletal systems. Patients in this stage may appear quite ill, with debilitating malaise and fatigue as the major symptoms. A secondary annular skin lesion may occur in approximately one-half of the patients. The musculoskeletal discomfort is generally migratory in joints, bursae, tendons, muscle, and bone, lasting only a few hours or days in one location (57). Disease of the nervous system is found in approximately 15% of the reported cases and usually begins approximately 4 weeks after the tick bite. The characteristic triad of findings includes meningitis, cranial nerve palsies, and a peripheral radiculoneuropathy (53). The most common manifestation of meningitis is usually a headache and a stiff neck, which is not generally associated with a Kernig's or Brudzinski's sign. Unilateral or bilateral facial nerve involvement (Bell's palsy) is the most common nerve palsy and may represent the only neurological abnormality (7). Other cranial nerves may also be involved. Cardiac involvement is limited to less than 10% of patients, with problems ranging from atrioventricular block to myopericarditis and left ventricular dysfunction (41). The length of cardiac involvement can be as brief as 3 days.

The third stage is highlighted by chronic complaints of arthritis. Although present very early in children, episodes of arthritis in adults become longer during the second and third years of illness, lasting months instead of weeks or days. Large joints, often those that were very close to the initial rash, are most commonly involved. The knee is the principal joint that is involved in the majority of patients (14). The involved joints tend to become swollen, warm, and painful but rarely red. Other clinical manifestations of the third stage of the disease include acrodermatitis chronica atrophicans, which is a progressive dermatologic condition that develops with increasing erythema and pigmentation changes of the skin surfaces. Chronic neurological complications, keratitis, and fatigue may also be seen. Late disease is uncommon in children who are treated with antibiotics in the early stages of disease (51).

Physicians remained concerned that pregnant women could be at risk for transplacental passage of *B. burgdorferi* to their fetuses. No causal relationship between Lyme disease in pregnancy and abnormalities or congenital disease has been confirmed. No evidence exists that Lyme disease can be transmitted via breast milk. The risk of an adverse outcome is quite low (34).

Lyme disease can be easily diagnosed if erythema migrans is present. Without this characteristic rash, a broad range of diseases should be considered. The primary rash is sometimes confused with staphylococcal or streptococcal cellulitis, erythema multiforme, or erythema marginatum. Other forms of arthritis that can be confused with Lyme disease include pauciarticular juvenile rheumatoid arthritis; Reiter syndrome; psoriatic arthritis; gonococcal arthritis; reactive arthritis due to *Salmonella*, *Shigella*, or *Yersinia*; parvovirus B19 arthritis; postinfectious (streptococcal) arthritis; and septic arthritis.

The specific diagnosis is made with clinical and epidemiological data and can be established early if erythema migrans is present. Otherwise, serologic studies will be needed to establish the diagnosis. Antibodies may not rise until 2 or 3 weeks after the infection and may be aborted with antimicrobial therapy (44). Antibodies are not detected in most patients with erythema migrans. Routine serologic tests are not recommended for children with typical signs and symptoms. These factors make the serologic diagnosis very difficult. Most untreated patients with long-standing disease will have positive antibody titers. Both an indirect fluorescent-antibody test and an enzyme-linked immunosorbent assay (ELISA) are available, but these prepackaged kit tests are 26 to 57% sensitive, with mean specificities ranging from 12 to 60%. Therefore, test results will vary depending on the expertise of the laboratory. The use of Western immunoblotting may aid in identifying those patients with false-positive ELISAs (46). In some centers, PCR testing for detection of borrelia DNA can be performed. However, non-research laboratory tests have not been shown to be sufficiently accurate to be clinically useful.

For patients with stage 1 disease (early infection), isolated Bell's palsy, arthritis, or mild carditis, oral antimicrobial therapy is recommended (44). For those patients over 9 years of age, tetracycline, doxycycline, or amoxicillin is recommended. Children less than 9 years of age should receive amoxicillin or penicillin. Erythromycin can be substituted when treating patients who are allergic to penicillin, but it may be less effective. The oral regimens are given until the patients demonstrate a clinical response, which is usually after a total of between 10 and 30 days of therapy. For those patients with persistent arthritis, severe carditis, meningitis, or encephalitis, parenteral medications should be used. Penicillin G, ceftriaxone, or cefotaxime for 14 to 21 days is recommended as the medication of choice. The risk of Lyme disease following a tick bite is low, and prophylactic antibiotic treatment is not routinely recommended for children even in areas of endemicity.

Animal studies indicate that prolonged attachment (>36 h) by infected ticks is required to transmit *B. burgdorferi*. Although a single dose of doxycycline (200 mg) is effective in preventing erythema migrans after a deer tick attachment of >72 h in adults from areas of hyperendemicity, this regimen is not recommended for children (51). There is currently no vaccine available for prevention.

Ehrlichiosis

Ehrlichiosis is a tick-borne disease that is caused by *Ehrlichia chaffeensis* (HME) or *Anaplasma phagocytophilum* (HGE). These organisms are intraleukocytic rickettsiae spread from a tick bite to the human host. Ehrlichiosis has been recognized as a disease in dogs since 1935, but human disease caused by this organism in the United States has been recognized only since 1986 (1, 13, 18, 31). The tick vector for canine *Ehrlichia* has been identified as *Rhipicephalus sanguineus*, but the principal vector for its spread to humans has not yet been confirmed. The canine vector is unlikely to transmit the disease, since this tick rarely feeds on humans (40).

Although HME and HGE were previously described in 19 states, with a substantial male predominance (74%) (61), more recent reports show activity in all states. Cases have been described for people of all ages, and nearly half of the patients are over 50 years old. One-half of reported cases have occurred in May or June, and approximately 80% of infected individuals have a history of tick exposure (4, 61). The incubation period required for human infection after a tick bite averages 10 to 14 days (range, 1 to 3 weeks) (17, 58).

The most commonly encountered clinical manifestations of HME are fever and headache (Table 3) (17, 22, 34, 49, 50). Fever (range, 38 to 41°C) is seen in almost 100% of patients during the first week of illness. Headaches in this disorder are usually quite severe. Other commonly encountered symptoms include chills or rigors, myalgias, nausea, anorexia, and malaise (49, 50). Rashes are found in up to

Table 3. Manifestations of *E. chaffeensis* infection

Feature	Children with feature[a] (%)
Fever	37/37 (100)
Tick attachment	28/34 (82)
Rash	21/32 (66)
Headache	15/24 (63)
Myalgia	17/27 (63)
Anorexia or nausea	17/30 (57)
Hepatosplenomegaly	9/22 (41)
Heart murmur	7/21 (33)
Aspartate aminotransferase (>55 U/liter)	25/28 (89)
Thrombocytopenia (<150 × 10^9/liter [150,000/mm^3])	27/33 (82)
Lymphopenia (<1.5 × 10^9/liter [1,500/mm^3])	24/30 (80)
Leukopenia (<4.0 × 10^9/liter [4,000/mm^3])	24/35 (69)
Hyponatremia (<135 mmol/liter [135 meq/liter])	13/20 (65)
Anemia (hematocrit, <0.30 [30%])	11/29 (38)

[a]Number of patients with positive results per number for whom data are available.

50% of patients but are more prominent in children. The classic rash is macular and is usually discovered upon presentation. The skin abnormalities usually start on the extremities but do not progress as does the rash of RMSF (17, 49, 50). Other physical abnormalities include cough, diarrhea, pharyngitis, arthralgia, weight loss, lymphadenopathy, dyspnea, abdominal pain, diaphoresis, splenomegaly, hepatomegaly, jaundice, meningismus, pulmonary edema, and pedal edema.

Hematologic abnormalities are present in the majority of patients. Leukopenia, frequently associated with lymphopenia, is the most common abnormality (34, 49). Lymphocyte counts are often below 1,500 per mm^3. Thrombocytopenia (a thrombocyte count of <150,000 per mm^3) and anemia can be encountered as well as hyponatremia, elevated liver function, hypoalbuminemia, and cerebrospinal fluid pleocytosis (19, 49, 50). Infections with *Ehrlichia* cause clinical symptoms similar to those of RMSF, except for a decreased frequency of rash and a more profound pancytopenia. Differential diagnosis should also include the other tick-borne diseases, such as tularemia, Colorado tick fever, Lyme disease, and meningococcemia (28).

The laboratory test for HME is an indirect fluorescent-antibody technique in which *E. chaffeensis* is used as an antigen (10). A titer of more than 1:80 provides a presumptive diagnosis of HME; however, paired acute- and convalescent-phase sera should be submitted. A fourfold rise or fall in the paired sera is considered diagnostic.

Treatment for all children with HME and HGE should include a tetracycline (preferably doxycycline) given orally for 10 to 14 days.

HGE has similar epidemiology, clinical presentation, and treatment requirements. The highest concentration of cases has been localized to the northeastern and upper midwestern states. A limited number of HGE cases have been reported to occur in children. Specific diagnosis is determined by antibody assays with a combination of related *Ehrlichia* antigens. In areas of endemicity, HGE and HME present with similar spectra of clinical and laboratory findings and should be presumptively treated with doxycycline.

RMSF

RMSF is the most important and severe disease in the spotted-fever group (37). This disease is caused by *Rickettsia rickettsii*, which is an organism transmitted by the bite of a tick. The wood tick (*Dermacentor andersoni*) in the West, the dog tick (*Dermacentor variabilis*) in the East, and the Lone Star tick (*A. americanum*) in the Southwest are all natural vectors of the disease. This disorder is most commonly seen in the spring and summer, with the majority of cases occurring between May and June. The peak incidence of RMSF is found in the 5- to 9-year age group (5).

The incubation period is short, with an average of 5 to 7 days after the tick bite (range, 3 to 12 days). Fever, headache, rash, toxicity, mental confusion, and myalgias are the major clinical symptoms of RMSF (Table 4) (3, 23). The fever that accompanies RMSF tends to remain relatively high (40°C) and is associated with an intense headache that is not easily relieved with medications. The rash seen with

Table 4. Signs and symptoms of RMSF[a]

Symptom	% of patients showing symptom
Fever	94
Rash	85
Headache	80
Myalgia	71
Tick exposure	60
Triad: fever, rash, headache	48

[a]Data are from references 3, 6, 21, and 26.

RMSF can be pathognomonic for the disorder. The skin lesions begin as small erythematous papules, which blanch with pressure. They progress and rapidly become maculopapular, then petechial, and occasionally hemorrhagic. A regular occurrence with this rash is the involvement of the palms of the hands and the soles of the feet (Fig. 2). When the rash becomes ecchymotic, it may be mistaken for meningococcemia. Patients may appear to be irritable, restless, or apprehensive and may rapidly progress to mental confusion and delirium.

The diagnosis of RMSF is based upon clinical features (30). In the spring-summer season, an illness with fever and a rash may be enough justification to start empirical therapy against this rickettsial infection, especially if the patient is from an area where the disease is endemic. Patients with this disorder can be confused with those suffering from meningococcemia and measles. Immunization and exposure histories can aid in diagnosis.

Specific antibody can be demonstrated in patients from 5 to 10 days after the onset of illness. Early serologic testing is negative in a large percentage of patients and never excludes the diagnosis. The serologic diagnosis is made by demonstrating a fourfold rise in specific antibody. Currently, ELISA and a microimmunofluorescence assay are available commercially for serologic diagnosis. A screening latex agglutination assay is now available. Other laboratory abnormalities that may aid in the diagnosis are leukopenia, thrombocytopenia, and hyponatremia.

Tetracycline and doxycycline are the antibiotics that have been proven to be effective against RMSF. Tetracycline and doxycycline are now recommended regardless of age (3). New data from the Centers for Disease Control and Prevention suggest that chloramphenicol is inferior to tetracyclines. A more detailed evaluation of tetracycline use has demonstrated that the tooth discoloration described for children may be due to multiple courses of administration. Therefore, it is felt that children less than 9 years of age may be treated safely with one course of medication. Recently, the quinolones have shown activity against rickettsial agents, but there are no data for children. Quinolones should be used cautiously in children and only after effectiveness has been proven compared to tetracycline treatment (21). Mortality and morbidity are increased if treatment is delayed more than 5 days from the onset of signs and symptoms. The total duration of therapy is usually between 7 and 10 days.

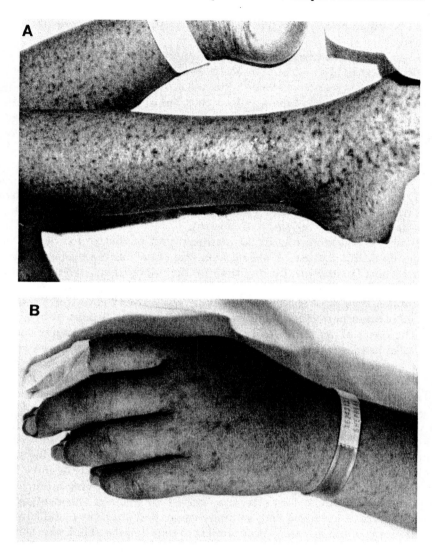

Figure 2. Maculopapular rash of RMSF on the legs (A) and hand (B).

Tularemia

Tularemia is a bacterial infection caused by *Francisella tularensis*. This acute febrile illness is a zoonotic disease for which humans are susceptible hosts. There are over 100 species in the animal kingdom that carry this bacterium (24). The organism is usually associated with lagomorphs (hares and rabbits) but is quite commonly found among rodents, raccoons, opossums, and cats. The infection is transmitted to humans by ingestion of infected animal tissue or direct contact with infected animals or through the bite of infected animals, ticks, or other

arthropods, inhalation of infected vapors, or consumption of water that is contaminated.

Two types of *F. tularensis* have been recognized. Biovar tularensis, also called
Jellison type A, has been isolated in North America, whereas biovar palaearctica,
or Jellison type B, is found wherever tularemia is found. Biovar tularensis is highly
virulent in humans, while biovar palaearctica has always been considered to be
less virulent. However, there has been more human disease attributed to biovar
palaearctica recently, and it may be that the extent of disease caused by this type is
not fully understood (60).

F. tularensis is a highly infectious bacterium, with as few as 10 organisms required to produce systemic disease in humans. The organism will gain access to
the body through the skin, oropharynx, conjunctiva, respiratory tract, or gastrointestinal tract. After the organism gains entry into the body, further dissemination
may occur via the blood or lymphatic system.

Ticks are the major vectors in the southern part of the United States for the
transmission of this disease. *A. americanum* (the Lone Star tick), *D. andersoni* (the
wood tick), and *D. variabilis* (the dog tick) are the principal tick vectors known not
only to transmit but also to serve as reservoirs for this disease. Other vectors, such
as fleas, mites, deer flies, and mosquitoes, are also known to transmit the disease.

The incubation period for this disorder is usually 3 to 4 days (range, 1 to 21
days). The onset of symptoms is usually quite abrupt; the symptoms consist of
fever, chills, headache, myalgias, vomiting, and photophobia. Children are more
likely to suffer from adenopathy and fever than adults. Six forms of the disease
have been described. The most common is the ulceroglandular form; the others
are the glandular, oculoglandular, oropharyngeal, typhoidal, and pneumonic
forms (Table 5) (26, 27).

In the ulceroglandular form of the disease, the organisms gain entry through
the skin via an embedded tick. After approximately 2 days, patients will complain
of tender, swollen lymph nodes, most commonly in the axillary or inguinal regions in adults and the cervical nodes in children (60). At the site of entry, there is
often a painful, swollen papule. This papule will rupture, leaving a punched-out
ulcer with raised borders. This ulcer may persist for months. The swollen lymph
node may become inflamed and, in many cases, will suppurate and drain. The
glandular form of the disease is very similar, except that the skin lesion is lacking.

Table 5. Common forms of tularemia[a]

Form	% of patients with form
Ulceroglandular	50
Glandular	9
Oculoglandular	1
Oropharyngeal	2
Typhoidal	8
Pneumonic	15
Unclassified	15

[a]Data are from references 24 and 25.

The conjunctival space is thought to be the portal of entry in the oculoglandular form of tularemia. The eye becomes involved, due to contact with infected secretions, most often from rubbing the eyes. The eyelids become edematous, inflamed, and extremely painful. Occasionally, multiple small, yellowish nodules or ulcers will appear on the palpebral conjunctiva or sclera (Fig. 3). Preauricular, submaxillary, and cervical adenopathy may also be evident.

In oropharyngeal tularemia, the organisms are introduced to the oropharyngeal mucosa through contaminated food and water. Complaints of a sore throat are usually out of proportion to the pharyngitis seen on examination. Cervical adenopathy may also be present (25).

The typhoidal form of tularemia often presents as an acute septicemia. The onset is usually quite abrupt, with fever, myalgias, and vomiting. Patients often have meningitis, delirium, and pulmonary involvement. In children, in whom typhoidal tularemia can be the result of the ingestion of the organism, necrotic lesions may be present throughout the bowel (12).

The pneumonic form of tularemia is uncommon, but when it presents, it is quite severe. This disorder has been limited to laboratory workers in the past (42). Pneumonia, however, may occur in up to 15% of cases of ulceroglandular disease and 80% of typhoidal tularemia cases.

The overall mortality rate for tularemia is approximately 2% (59). Patients with a poor outcome are more likely to have electrolyte or renal abnormalities, pneumonia and pleural effusion, rhabdomyolysis with elevated serum creatine phosphokinase, and *F. tularensis* bacteremia (43).

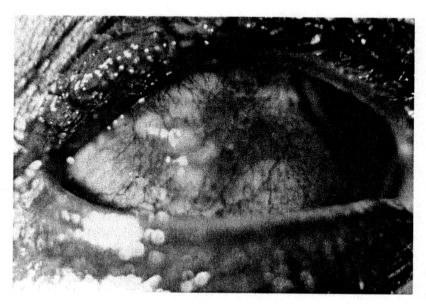

Figure 3. Small nodules on palpebral conjunctiva and sclera of a patient with oculoglandular tularemia.

The diagnosis of tularemia is established based upon history, physical examination, and serology. The agglutination test is the usual method employed for diagnosing tularemia. Antibody usually develops in the second week of illness. A titer of ≥1:160 is a presumptive diagnostic test, which suggests a current or past infection, while a fourfold rise in the convalescent-phase serum, with titers in the range of 1:1,280 to 1:2,560, is an easy way to document a current infection. Cultures for *F. tularensis* should not be attempted in the routine clinical laboratory due to the risk of infecting the workers.

The differential diagnosis of ulceroglandular and glandular tularemia includes diseases caused by routine pathogens, such as *Streptococcus* and *Staphylococcus*, and also diseases due to *Mycobacterium tuberculosis*, atypical *Mycobacterium*, and *Bartonella henselae* (cat scratch disease) as well as sporotrichosis and infectious mononucleosis. Typhoidal tularemia can be confused with acute bacterial sepsis. Tularemia pneumonia can resemble pneumonia that is caused by a number of organisms, including *Mycoplasma*, *Legionella*, *Chlamydia*, *Coxiella*, and *Mycobacterium*, and those of fungal and viral etiology.

Streptomycin was previously the drug of choice for tularemia. Gentamicin, however, has become the principal medication due to side effects and manufacturing problems with streptomycin. Although tetracycline and chloramphenicol have been demonstrated to cause a prompt response in patients with tularemia, a relatively high rate of relapse makes these medications less desirable. After institution of appropriate medication (gentamicin at 2.5 mg/kg of body weight three times daily or 5.0 mg/kg twice daily), patients demonstrate improvement within 24 to 48 h. The duration of treatment is usually 7 to 10 days, with at least four afebrile days prior to discontinuing the medication. Recent uncontrolled series have demonstrated the quinolone ciprofloxacin to be effective treatment. Some experts recommend ciprofloxacin treatment of tularemia in adults. Its use in children has the continuing issues of quinolone use in patients less than 18 years of age.

Prevention

A proper wardrobe is essential in preventing tick-transmitted diseases. Protective clothing that covers the arms, legs, and other usually exposed areas, ankle-high footwear, and pant legs that cinch at the ankles or are worn tucked into the socks can help protect the wilderness adventurer from unwanted travel companions. Permethrin can be sprayed on clothing to prevent tick attachment, and insect repellents that employ N,N-diethyl-*m*-toluamide (DEET) can be applied to the skin for further protection. Concentrations of more than 35% DEET should also be avoided, since they are not proven to be more effective than the lower concentrations and have a greater risk for complications due to overdose (20). DEET repels a variety of mosquitoes, chiggers, ticks, fleas, and biting flies. In the United States, DEET is available in formulations of 5 to 40% and 100% (52). DEET at 20% provides complete protection for 1 to 3 h. Higher concentrations provide longer-lasting protection (up to 12 h), but protection plateaus at concentrations over 50%. A long-acting product (EDTIAR; Ultrathon-3M) contains 25 or 33% DEET in a long-acting polymer formulation, which prevents loss from skin surfaces. This product provided more than 95% protection against mosquito bites for 6 to 12 h. One new product, picaridin, a piperidine derivative, will soon be marketed in the United States and may be as effective as DEET.

Close and regular inspections of all body parts are essential for the adventurer. Adult ticks are usually on the body for 1 to 2 h prior to attachment. The duration of tick feeding may be directly related to disease transmission (8). If ticks are discovered, they should be removed. The recommended method for tick removal is to grasp the tick as close to the skin as possible with tweezers or protected fingers and then pull the tick straight out with steady even pressure. Care should be taken to avoid twisting or jerking the tick, as this might cause mouthparts to break off and be left in the skin. Crushing or puncturing the body of the tick is also not suggested, since the body fluids may contain infective agents. After the tick is removed, the bite site should be disinfected (39). Traditional methods of tick removal, such as the application of fingernail polish or isopropyl alcohol to the tick or the use of a hot match, may induce the tick to salivate or regurgitate into the wound, thus spreading its infected secretions. The empirical use of antimicrobial agents after a tick bite to prevent the acquisition of tick-borne disease has been demonstrated not to be useful (8).

MOSQUITOES, LICE, FLEAS, AND MITES

There are many diseases transmitted by mosquitoes around the world, but very few are encountered in the United States (Table 6). The use of proper clothing can help prevent these diseases. Items that should be considered include long-sleeve shirts, protective facial netting, and mosquito netting for sleeping. These garments and nets should be used in areas with large mosquito populations. Insect repellents that employ DEET will also aid in the battle against these biting arthropods (20).

Lice are the main vectors for epidemic typhus. This disease, which is rarely reported in North America, is caused by *Rickettsia prowazekii*. Louse-borne disease is especially prominent in areas of poverty, overcrowding, and poor sanitation. The disease in the United States has been attributed to contact with flying squirrels in Virginia, West Virginia, and North Carolina (15). The disease is characterized by an influenza-like illness with headache, fever, and malaise. A rash begins

Table 6. Mosquito-borne infections

Disease	Agent
Western equine encephalitis	Alphavirus
Eastern equine encephalitis	Alphavirus
St. Louis encephalitis	Flavivirus
California virus encephalitis	Bunyavirus
Dengue	Flavivirus
Venezuelan encephalitis	Alphavirus
Tularemia	*F. tularensis*
West Nile fever	Flavivirus

approximately 4 to 7 days into the illness. This rash usually begins on the trunk and then spreads to involve the extremities. Illness usually varies from moderate to fatal and, if left untreated, will last approximately 2 weeks. Epidemic typhus is treated with tetracycline or chloramphenicol.

A second zoonotic infection transmitted by the flea is murine (endemic) typhus. This disorder is caused by the organism *Rickettsia typhi* and is transmitted from rats to humans by the rat flea. Fever, headache, malaise, and rash are the common clinical symptoms of this disease. Typhus is endemic in the southwestern regions of the United States and is treated with tetracycline (16).

Infections due to mites have been recognized for many years. The larval form of the mite is commonly referred to as the chigger and is responsible for many of these diseases. Scabies, rickettsialpox, and scrub typhus are all transmitted by mites. In the wilderness, most humans have trouble only with the bite of the chigger. Within 24 to 48 h, these bites become intensely pruritic and may develop small hemorrhagic papules or nodules. The inflammation is proportional to the host's hypersensitivity to the oral secretions of the mite. These bites may persist for 5 to 6 days and occur mostly on the lower legs or other exposed regions.

OTHER ARTHROPODS

Some other arthropod envenomations may be particularly severe. Stings of hymenopteran insects (bees, wasps, hornets, and ants) are the most common cause of envenomation, especially in children. They usually produce local pain, swelling, and erythema. If a stinger remains after the envenomation, it should be removed by carefully brushing it away. Grasping the stinger to remove it may squeeze the remaining venom into the wound (33). The application of ice or cool compresses often helps to reduce the pain and swelling. In older children, the use of oral antihistamines may provide relief. Early signs of generalized pruritus, urticaria, angioedema, or bronchospasm necessitate a medical evaluation emergently. If the patient cannot be evaluated, epinephrine is the drug of choice for systemic reactions and should be given in the field (20).

Although lethal scorpion bites are a serious problem throughout the world, in the United States the only dangerous species encountered is *Centruroides exilicauda*. This scorpion is found mostly in the desert climate of the Southwest. Symptoms are usually limited to local pain, but children younger than 2 years of age may demonstrate multisystem organ failure (9). The brown recluse (*Loxosceles reclusus*) and black widow (*Latrodectus mactans*) spiders may also cause painful bites. If signs of systemic envenomation develop, the victim requires medical evaluation. Antivenin is available for black widow and *C. exilicauda* bites.

GIARDIA

In certain high-risk regions or populations *G. lamblia* is an important cause of diarrhea. Travelers to the Rocky Mountains or consumers of contaminated water are at high risk for this parasite (45). Infection may occur after ingestion of only 10 to 100 cysts contained in only a few micrograms of stool (62). These cysts are very hardy and may be viable for up to 3 months in moist environments. Person-to-person transmission is the most common route of infection.

After the organisms are ingested, patients will demonstrate varied responses. They may be asymptomatic or develop an acute infectious diarrhea that has a sudden onset. This diarrhea is associated with watery, foul-smelling, explosive stools. Flatulence, abdominal distention, nausea, and anorexia are often present as well. Patients may also develop chronic diarrhea, with persistent gastrointestinal symptoms that last for months.

The diagnosis of *Giardia* can be made by examination of a fresh stool. Duodenal biopsy is believed to be the most sensitive method of detection, but it is expensive and not readily available. Certain medications, such as antibiotics, antacids, and antidiarrheal compounds, may interfere with the morphology of the organism and prevent identification (47). Patients should not receive these compounds for 48 to 72 h prior to stool examination. Immunofluoresence assays and ELISAs for detection of *Giardia* antigens in the stool are now widely available (29). These tests can be used on stool specimens or rectal swabs. Examinations such as these will alleviate problems due to intermittent shedding or low numbers of parasites, which make the diagnosis difficult.

Treatment of patients with acute diarrhea due to *Giardia* is recommended. Currently, acceptable medications include furazolidone, quinacrine, and metronidazole. The optimal period of treatment is 5 to 7 days. Other household members with symptoms should also be evaluated and treated.

REFERENCES

1. **Abramson, J. S., and L. B. Givner.** 1990. Should tetracycline be contraindicated for therapy of presumed Rocky Mountain spotted fever in children less than 9 years of age? *Pediatrics* **86:**123–124.
2. **Belongia, E. A., K. D. Reed, P. D. Mitchell, N. Mueller-Rizner, M. Vandermause, M. F. Finkel, and J. Kazmierczak.** 2001. Tickborne infections as a cause of nonspecific febrile illness in Wisconsin. *Clin. Infect. Dis.* **32:**1434–1439.
3. **Buckingham, S. C.** 2002. Rocky Mountain spotted fever: a review for the pediatrician. *Pediatr. Ann.* **31:**163–168.
4. **Centers for Disease Control.** 1990. Rocky Mountain spotted fever and human ehrlichiosis—United States, 1989. *Morb. Mortal. Wkly. Rep.* **39:**281–284.
5. **Centers for Disease Control.** 1991. Rocky Mountain spotted fever—United States, 1990. *Morb. Mortal. Wkly. Rep.* **40:**451–454.
6. **Centers for Disease Control and Prevention.** 2002. Lyme disease—United States, 2000. *Morb. Mortal. Wkly. Rep.* **51:**29–31.
7. **Clark, J. R., R. D. Carlson, C. T. Sasaki, A. R. Pachner, and A. C. Steere.** 1985. Facial paralysis in Lyme disease. *Laryngoscope* **95:**1341–1345.
8. **Costello, C. M., A. C. Steere, R. E. Pinkerton, and H. M. Feder, Jr.** 1989. A prospective study of tick bites in an endemic area for Lyme disease. *J. Infect. Dis.* **159:**136–139.
9. **Craft, J. C.** 1982. Giardia and giardiasis in childhood. *Pediatr. Infect. Dis. J.* **1:**196–211.
10. **Dawson, J. E., D. B. Fishbein, T. R. Eng, M. A. Redus, and N. R. Green.** 1990. Diagnosis of human ehrlichiosis with the indirect fluorescent antibody test: kinetics and specificity. *J. Infect. Dis.* **162:**91–95.
11. **Dennis, D. T.** 1991. Lyme disease: tracking an epidemic. *JAMA* **266:**1269–1270.
12. **Dienst, F. T.** 1963. Tularemia: a perusal of three hundred thirty-nine cases. *J. La. State Med. Soc.* **115:**114–127.

13. **Donatien, A., and F. Lestoquard.** 1935. Existence en algerie d'une *Rickettsia* du chien. *Bull. Soc. Pathol. Exot.* **28:**418–419.
14. **Doughty, R. A.** 1984. Lyme disease. *Pediatr. Rev.* **6:**20–25.
15. **Duma, R. J., D. E. Sonenshine, F. M. Bozeman, J. M. Veazey, Jr., B. L. Elisberg, D. P. Chadwick, N. I. Stocks, T. M. McGill, G. B. Miller, Jr., and J. N. MacCormack.** 1981. Epidemic typhus in the United States associated with flying squirrels. *JAMA* **245:**2318–2323.
16. **Dumler, J. S., J. P. Taylor, and D. H. Walker.** 1991. Clinical and laboratory features of murine typhus in south Texas, 1980 through 1987. *JAMA* **266:**1365–1370.
17. **Eng, T. R., J. R. Harkess, D. B. Fishbein, J. E. Dawson, C. N. Greene, M. A. Redus, and F. T. Satalowich.** 1990. Epidemiologic, clinical, and laboratory findings of human ehrlichiosis in the United States, 1988. *JAMA* **264:**2251–2258.
18. **Fishbein, D. B., L. A. Sawyer, C. J. Holland, E. B. Hayes, W. Okoroanyanwu, D. Williams, K. Sikes, M. Ristic, and J. E. McDade.** 1987. Unexplained febrile illness after exposure to ticks: infection with an *Ehrlichia*? *JAMA* **257:**3100–3104.
19. **Fishbein, D. B., A. Kemp, J. E. Dawson, N. R. Greene, M. A. Redus, and D. H. Fields.** 1989. Human ehrlichiosis: prospective active surveillance in febrile hospitalized patients. *J. Infect. Dis.* **160:**803–809.
20. **Gentile, D. A., and B. C. Kennedy.** 1991. Wilderness medicine for children. *Pediatrics* **88:**967–981.
21. **Guchiol, F., R. Pallares, J. Carratala, F. Bolao, J. Arita, G. Rufi, and P. F. Viladrich.** 1989. Randomized double-blind evaluation of ciprofloxacin and doxycycline for Mediterranean spotted fever. *Antimicrob. Agents Chemother.* **33:**987–988.
22. **Harkess, J. R., S. A. Ewing, T. Brumit, and C. R. Mettry.** 1991. Ehrlichiosis in children. *Pediatrics* **87:**199–203.
23. **Helmick, C. G., K. W. Bernard, and L. J. D'Angelo.** 1984. Rocky Mountain spotted fever: clinical, laboratory, and epidemiological features of 262 cases. *J. Infect. Dis.* **150:**480–488.
24. **Hopla, C. E.** 1974. The ecology of tularemia. *Adv. Vet. Sci. Comp. Med.* **18:**25–53.
25. **Hughes, W. T., and J. N. Etteldof.** 1957. Oropharyngeal tularemia. *J. Pediatr.* **51:**363–372.
26. **Jacobs, R. F., Y. M. Condrey, and T. Yamauchi.** 1985. Tularemia in adults and children: a changing presentation. *Pediatrics* **76:**818–822.
27. **Jacobs, R. F., and J. P. Narain.** 1983. Tularemia in children. *Pediatr. Infect. Dis. J.* **2:**487–491.
28. **Jacobs, R. F.** 2002. Human monocytic ehrlichiosis: similar to Rocky Mountain spotted fever but different. *Pediatr. Ann.* **31:**180–184.
29. **Johnston, S. P., M. M. Ballard, M. J. Beach, L. Causer, and P. P. Wilkins.** 2003. Evaluation of three commercial assays for detection of *Giardia* and *Cryptosporidium* organisms in fecal specimens. *J. Clin. Microbiol.* **41:**623–626.
30. **Linnemann, C. C., and P. J. Janson.** 1978. The clinical presentations of Rocky Mountain spotted fever: comments on recognition and management based on a study of 63 patients. *Clin. Pediatr.* **17:**673–679.
31. **Maeda, K., N. Markowitz, R. C. Hawley, M. Ristic, D. Cox, and J. E. McDade.** 1987. Human infection with *Ehrlichia canis*, a leukocytic *Rickettsia*. *N. Engl. J. Med.* **316:**853–856.
32. **Magnarelli, L. A., and R. K. Swihart.** 1991. Spotted fever group rickettsiae or *Borrelia burgdorferi* in *Ixodes cookei* (*Ixodidae*) in Connecticut. *J. Clin. Microbiol.* **29:**1520–1522.
33. **Maguire, J. F., and R. S. Geha.** 1986. Bee, wasp, and hornet stings. *Pediatr. Rev.* **8:**5–11.
34. **Markowitz, L. E., A. C. Steere, J. L. Benach, J. D. Slade, and C. V. Broome.** 1986. Lyme disease during pregnancy. *JAMA* **255:**3394–3396.
35. **Marshall, G. S., R. F. Jacobs, G. E. Schutze, H. Paxton, S. C. Buckingham, J. P. DeVincenzo, M. A. Jackson, V. H. San Joaquin, S. M. Standaert, and C. R. Woods for the Tick–Borne Infections in Children Study Group.** 2002. *Ehrlichia chaffeensis* seroprevalence among children in the southeast and south-central regions of the United States. *Arch. Pediatr. Adolesc. Med.* **156:**166–170.
36. **Marshall, G. S., G. G. Stout, R. F. Jacobs, G. E. Schutze, H. Paxton, S. C. Buckingham, J. P. DeVincenzo, M. A. Jackson, V. H. San Joaquin, S. M. Standaert, C. R. Woods, and the Tick-Borne Infections in Children Study (TICS) Group.** 2003. Antibodies reactive to *Rickettsia rickettsii* among children living in the southeast and south central regions of the United States. *Arch. Pediatr. Adolesc. Med.* **157:**443–448.

37. **Masters, E. J., G. S. Olson, S. J. Weiner, and C. D. Paddock.** 2003. Rocky Mountain spotted fever. *Arch. Intern. Med.* **163:**769–774.

38. **McCall, C. L., A. T. Curns, L. D. Roz, J. A. Singleton, T. A. Treadwell, J. A. Comer, W. L. Nicholson, J. G. Olson, and J. E. Childs.** 2001. Fort Chaffee revisited: the epidemiology of tick-borne rickettsial and ehrlichial diseases at a natural focus. *Vector Borne Zoonotic Dis.* **1:**119–127.

39. **Needham, G. R.** 1985. Evaluation of five popular methods for tick removal. *Pediatrics* **75:**997–1002.

40. **Nelson, V. A.** 1969. Human parasitism by the brown dog tick. *J. Econ. Entomol.* **62:**710–712.

41. **Olson, L. J., E. C. Okafor, and I. P. Clements.** 1986. Cardiac involvement in Lyme disease: manifestations and management. *Mayo Clin. Proc.* **61:**745–749.

42. **Overholt, E. L., W. D. Tigertt, P. J. Kadull, M. K. Ward, N. D. Charkes, R. M. Rene, T. E. Salzman, and M. Stephens.** 1961. An analysis of forty-two cases of laboratory acquired tularemia. Treatment with broad-spectrum antibiotics. *Am. J. Med.* **30:**785–806.

43. **Penn, R. L., and G. T. Kinasewitz.** 1987. Factors associated with a poor outcome in tularemia. *Arch. Intern. Med.* **147:**265–268.

44. **Plotkin, S. A., G. Peter, J. G. Easton, et al.** 1991. Treatment of Lyme borreliosis. *Pediatrics* **88:**176–179.

45. **Rendtorff, R. C.** 1954. The experimental transmission of human intestinal protozoan parasites. II. *Giardia lamblia* cysts given in capsules. *Am. J. Hyg.* **59:**209–220.

46. **Rose, C. D., P. T. Fawcett, B. H. Singsen, S. B. Dubbs, and R. A. Doughty.** 1991. Use of Western blot and enzyme-linked immunosorbent assays to assist in the diagnosis of Lyme disease. *Pediatrics* **88:**465–470.

47. **Rosoff, J. D., C. A. Sanders, S. S. Sonnad, P. R. De Lay, W. K. Hadley, F. F. Vincenzi, D. M. Yajko, and P. D. O'Hanley.** 1989. Stool diagnosis of giardiasis using a commercially available enzyme immunoassay to detect *Giardia*-specific antigen 65 (GSA-65). *J. Clin. Microbiol.* **27:**1997–2002.

48. **Schulze, T. L., G. S. Bowen, E. M. Bosler, M. F. Lakat, W. E. Parkin, R. Altman, B. G. Ormiston, and J. K. Shisler.** 1984. *Amblyomma americanum*: a potential vector of Lyme disease in New Jersey. *Science* **224:**601–603.

49. **Schutze, G. E., and R. F. Jacobs.** 1997. Human monocytic ehrlichiosis in children. *Pediatrics* **100:**e10.

50. **Schutze, G. E., and R. F. Jacobs.** 1997. Ehrlichiosis in children. *J. Pediatr.* **131:**184–192.

51. **Shapiro, E. D., and M. A. Gerber.** 2002. Lyme disease: fact versus fiction. *Pediatr. Ann.* **31:**170–177.

52. **Staub, D., M. Debrunner, L. Amsler, and R. Steffen.** 2002. Effectiveness of a repellent containing DEET and EBAAP for preventing tick bites. *Wilderness Environ. Med.* **13:**12–20.

53. **Stechenberg, B. W.** 1988. Lyme disease: the latest great imitator. *Pediatr. Infect. Dis. J.* **7:**402–409.

54. **Steere, A. C., R. L. Grodzicki, A. N. Kornblatt, J. E. Craft, A. G. Barbour, W. Burgdorfer, G. P. Schmid, E. Johnson, and S. E. Malawista.** 1983. The spirochetal etiology of Lyme disease. *N. Engl. J. Med.* **308:**733–740.

55. **Steere, A. C., N. H. Bartenhagen, J. E. Craft, G. J. Hutchinson, J. H. Newman, D. W. Rahn, L. H. Sigal, P. N. Spieler, K. S. Stenn, and S. E. Malawista.** 1983. The early clinical manifestations of Lyme disease. *Ann. Intern. Med.* **99:**76–82.

56. **Steere, A. C., E. Taylor, M. L. Wilson, J. F. Levine, and A. Spielman.** 1986. Longitudinal assessment of the clinical and epidemiological features of Lyme disease in a defined population. *J. Infect. Dis.* **154:**295–300.

57. **Steere, A. C.** 1989. Lyme disease. *N. Engl. J. Med.* **321:**586–596.

58. **Taylor, J. P., T. G. Betz, D. B. Fishbein, M. A. Roberts, J. Dawson, and M. Ristic.** 1988. Serological evidence of possible human infection with *Ehrlichia* in Texas. *J. Infect. Dis.* **158:**217–220.

59. **Taylor, J. P., G. R. Istre, T. C. McChesney, F. T. Satalowich, R. L. Parker, and L. M. McFarland.** 1987. Epidemiologic characteristics of human tularemia in the Southwest-Central States, 1981–1987. *Am. J. Epidemiol.* **133:**1032–1038.

60. **Uhari, M., H. Syrjala, and A. Salminen.** 1990. Tularemia in children caused by *Francisella tularensis* biovar *palaearctica*. *Pediatr. Infect. Dis. J.* **9:**80–83.

61. **Walker, D. H., and D. B. Fishbein.** 1991. Epidemiology of rickettsial diseases. *Eur. J. Epidemiol.* **7:**237–245.

62. **Wolfe, M. S.** 1978. Giardiasis. *N. Engl. J. Med.* **298:**319–321.

Infections of Leisure, Third Edition
Edited by David Schlossberg
© 2004 ASM Press, Washington, D.C.

Chapter 4

Infections in the Garden

Burke A. Cunha and Diane H. Johnson

Although there are many infections that one may acquire in the garden, people have gardened for years without becoming infected, yet others may become ill after a rather limited time in the garden. Being in the garden presents a series of complex possibilities from an infectious disease standpoint, and the likelihood of one acquiring an infectious disease while gardening depends upon many factors. Gardens are usually near the home and may be the closest that many people get to being in the great outdoors, especially in urban or suburban environments. The time spent in the garden is not nearly as important as the age and nature of the gardener, his friends, or his family (2, 6, 7, 12, 20).

Gardening may be a salutary experience for the well, but it is conceivably more dangerous to a patient with impaired immunity than to healthy individuals. For example, if a compromised host should contract coccidioidomycosis, histoplasmosis, or the organism responsible for cat scratch fever, he or she would be at increased risk for dissemination. Elderly patients are fortunately relatively well-off in terms of acquiring diseases in the garden. While elderly individuals can still acquire a variety of infections from the soil, animals, or animal-related insect bites, as a group they are not at increased risk for acquiring disorders solely on account of their age. Of course, if excavations are taking place, or there was construction nearby, and the area had *Legionella,* and if the wind was right, then an elderly person would be more likely to acquire or have a more severe case of Legionnaires' disease than their younger gardening counterparts.

Since many gardens are an extension of the home, children of various ages may frequent the garden or the land close to the house alone or with gardening adults. Many infectious diseases acquired in the garden are age specific; e.g., small children are more likely than adults to get *Strongyloides* or hookworm infections in the appropriate locale. The garden not only is inhabited by plants and visited by humans but also may be a stopping point or refuge for birds and animals. Because of its proximity to the house, household pets frequently wander freely throughout

Burke A. Cunha and Diane H. Johnson • Infectious Disease Division, Winthrop-University Hospital, Mineola, NY 11501, and State University of New York School of Medicine, Stony Brook, NY 11790.

the backyard and the garden. Even if you do not have pets, it is not uncommon that pets from the neighborhood will spend various lengths of time and perform various bodily functions while passing through your garden. Therefore, if dogs, cats, or rodents are in the area, it is wise to consider that your garden and yard present the potential for contact with these animals or their excreta. *Toxocara* organisms may be picked up by your dog or cat by ingestion and later transmitted via petting to children, for example. A stray neighborhood cat giving birth in or near your garden immediately sets the stage for the possibility of Q fever. The possibilities are almost endless. Birds may fly over, nest above, or be found sick or dead in the garden. Due to bird droppings in wood stacked for winter, or in nests near the soil, the potential for histoplasmosis or blastomycosis exists. Lastly, we come to the soil and plants themselves, which are, after all, the purpose of having a garden. What potential pathogens soil contains is largely a function of the animal life in the area as well as the particular location of the garden. For example, if the garden is located near moist, humid environments, along riverbanks in the South, then blastomycosis becomes a diagnostic consideration. In contrast, if the garden is in the Southwest, then coccidiomycosis and even plague, if an appropriately infected rodent is in the area, also become diagnostic possibilities. Rosebush thorn or sphagnum moss contact should immediately suggest the possibility of sporotrichosis. In the southeastern United States, where soil in moist areas may be contaminated with hookworm or *Strongyloides* larvae, these worms add to the potential diseases that can be acquired by contact of unprotected skin with the soil alone. The *Ixodes* ticks that transmit Lyme disease, babesiosis, and ehrlichiosis in areas of endemicity may be found in the lawn grass adjacent to the garden, so Lyme disease, babesiosis, and/or ehrlichiosis may literally be acquired in your own backyard or garden. Therefore, the soil, by the nature of the organisms that normally reside in specific locations, e.g., spores of coccidioidomycosis or larvae of hookworm, presents infectious disease hazards that need to be reckoned with, in addition to the contributions made by various animals to the soil either by their presence or by contamination with their body fluids. One can easily appreciate the large array of infectious diseases that confront a person simply slipping out of the house and walking across the yard to do a little gardening!

THE DIAGNOSTIC APPROACH

In trying to analyze diagnostic possibilities for someone who has become ill and has spent time in the garden, it is necessary to consider the diagnosis from three different perspectives. Firstly, one should consider the potential nature of contact, either passive or active, that the individual has had with sources of infection. If there has been extensive soil contact, then sporotrichosis is a diagnostic possibility. If piles of stacked or old moldy wood have been moved in association with wood gardening, then blastomycosis and histoplasmosis become additional possibilities. Nearby excavations with aerosolization of soil and water may suggest the possibility of Legionnaires' disease. If the particular location of the patient is one where Lyme disease (Table 1), babesiosis, or ehrlichiosis is endemic, then these diagnoses should be considered with the appropriate clinical presentation.

Table 1. Clinical picture of Lyme disease[a]

Stage	Dermatologic	Neurological	Rheumatology	Cardiac
1	ECM[b]	Possible headache, myalgias	Arthralgias Arthralgias	None None
2	Multiple and/ or recurrent ECM	Meningoencephalitis, peripheral neuritis	Arthralgias	Carditis
3	Acrodermatitis chronica atrophicans	Chronic encephalopathies	Chronic arthritis	Cardiomyopathy

[a]Adapted from reference 10a.
[b]ECM, erythema chronicum migrans.

Similarly, as mentioned in the introduction, specific locations suggest specific soil organisms, e.g., hookworm, *Coccidioides*, *Histoplasma*, etc. Additionally, potential animal contact needs to be considered from a variety of standpoints. The person's own pets and their interaction with insect vectors and other animals in the area should be carefully ascertained and considered. In addition to the gardener's own pets, one needs to consider the pets in the neighborhood as well as any wild animals interacting with the gardener or the gardener's pets. One should inquire specifically about dead birds or other animals that the gardener may have found and buried in the garden. Specific inquiry should be made as to the potential for contact with rodents or rabbits in the wild or runaway pets in the area. Only rarely is a disease actively transmitted from an animal to a human, and the situations are usually found to be straightforward if the proper question is asked. As has been mentioned previously, some infectious diseases may be acquired actively or passively; for example, sporotrichosis may be acquired by simple handling of sphagnum moss or may be actively acquired as the result of a puncture wound from the thorn of a rose. The epidemiological associations with infectious diseases acquired from plants, soil, or animal vectors are presented in Table 2.

The next step in the diagnostic process is to determine end organ involvement by the infectious disease process to limit diagnostic possibilities and suggest specific disease entities. For example, if the patient presents with lymphadenopathy and a history of garden contact, then diagnostic possibilities are narrowed to toxoplasmosis, cat scratch fever, sporotrichosis, and occasionally Lyme disease. Cat contact increases the likelihood that these lesions are due to cat scratch fever or toxoplasmosis, whereas nodular lymphangitis immediately suggests sporotrichosis. Obviously, there are many causes of adenopathy that have nothing to do with gardening or being in the garden, and the clinician must always be careful not to fail to consider the usual causes of lymph node involvement. However, if the adenopathy is most likely associated with gardening, then diagnostic possibilities are greatly reduced. If there are other associated findings, this also helps to limit diagnostic possibilities. It is a good diagnostic principle in infectious disease as well as in internal medicine to combine two diagnostic findings, even if they are nonspecific, to increase diagnostic specificity. For example, if the patient with a history of gardening and axillary adenopathy has in addition a mild nonexudative pharyngitis and a few atypical

Table 2. Epidemiological considerations in the garden

Focus/vector	Infectious disease or organism	
	Passively acquired[a]	Actively acquired
Soil/plants	Sporotrichosis Blastomycosis Histoplasmosis Strongyloidosis Hookworm Nocardiosis	Sporotrichosis Legionnaires' disease Nocardiosis
Animals		
Cats	Toxoplasmosis Q fever Tularemia CLM (*Ancylostoma*) VLM (*Toxocara cati*) *Strongyloides* *Campylobacter* Giardiasis *Yersinia* *Salmonella* Dermatophytes	Cat scratch fever *Pasteurella multocida* Rabies
Dogs	Group A streptococci VLM (*Toxocara canis*) CLM (*Ancylostoma*) Leptospirosis Brucellosis *Cryptosporidium* *Dirofilaria immitis* *Salmonella* Giardiasis *Campylobacter* RMSF (via tick bite) *Listeria* Dermatophytes	*P. multocida* DF-2 Rabies
Birds	Blastomycosis Histoplasmosis Cryptococcosis Q fever	
Rabbits	Tularemia Brucellosis	Tularemia
Rats	Leptospirosis	Rat-bite fever
Other rodents	Plague (via flea bite) Relapsing fever (via tick bite) Lyme disease (white-footed mouse) Leptospirosis *Salmonella* LCM (hamsters)	

[a]CLM, cutaneous larva migrans; RMSF, Rocky Mountain spotted fever; LCM, lymphocytic choriomeningitis.

lymphocytes, then the likelihood of acquired toxoplasmosis is enhanced. Similarly, the likelihood of Lyme disease being present in a patient with lymph node enlargement is enhanced if the patient has a facial nerve palsy. The more variables that one can combine, the easier it is to arrive at a definitive diagnosis. For example, if a patient presented with an ill-defined infiltrate on chest X ray, with abdominal pain and a cough, accompanied by mental confusion and some diarrhea, then the chances of that individual having Legionnaires' disease are very great. These would not be the findings in a patient with an other atypical pneumonia, i.e., Q fever, psittacosis, or *Mycoplasma pneumonia*. The diagnosis of worms producing cough or pneumonitis during their pulmonary migration phase may be a much more challenging diagnostic problem. Once again, by looking for associated features, one can increase diagnostic specificity and limit the differential diagnosis. For example, if a nonspecific pulmonary infiltrate was associated with eosinophilia, then strongyloidiasis becomes a very likely explanation for the patient's problem. Mental confusion, especially in a young child, with persistent eosinophilia, may suggest visceral larval migrans (VLM), especially if there has been a history of cat or dog contact. The differential diagnosis of infectious diseases by organ involvement is presented in Fig. 1. The clinician should remember that other diseases may produce similar end organ dysfunction and clinical manifestations, but Fig. 1 is particularly helpful if gardening is an important epidemiological factor to consider in assessing the patient's problem.

Laboratory tests represent the last approach to making the diagnosis. With all of the diseases potentially acquired by working in the garden, the clinician needs to establish a working diagnosis as described above and then arrive at a definitive diagnosis by ordering the appropriate specific tests. Aside from the specific laboratory tests needed to make a diagnosis, the clinician needs to have some clues that suggest the proper tests to be ordered for the individual patient. Therefore, nonspecific tests are most helpful when applied in the appropriate clinical context and combined with epidemiological and/or characteristic end organ manifestations. For example, anemia in a small child from a rural area of the southeastern United States should immediately prompt a search for hookworm or *Strongyloides*. The liver is involved in many infectious disease processes, and therefore the finding of abnormal liver function is an important clue to a whole range of infectious diseases. With respect to the gardening population, an increased bilirubin count in a patient with pneumonitis may suggest Legionnaires' disease, and in a patient with conjunctival suffusion it should suggest leptospirosis. Mild increases in the alkaline phosphatase or the serum transaminases may occur with dissimilar diseases such as toxoplasmosis and Rocky Mountain spotted fever (Table 3). If the patient has an atypical pneumonia, i.e., an ill-defined infiltrate and mild to moderately abnormal liver function tests, then diagnostic possibilities are quickly narrowed to Legionnaires' disease, psittacosis, and Q fever. Once again, it is important not to interpret diagnostic tests in a vacuum but rather to combine them with some other factor in the history of physical diagnosis that quickly limits the diagnostic possibilities and provides the rationale for the working diagnosis (Fig. 2).

SKIN
Cutaneous larva migrans
Lyme disease
RMSF
Dermatophytes
Histoplasmosis (erythema nodosum)
Tularemia
P. multocida
Group A streptococci
Strongyloides

LUNGS
Legionnaires' disease
Q fever
Psittacosis
Dirofilaria
Helminths

LYMPH NODES
Toxoplasmosis
Cat scratch fever
Sporotrichosis (nodular)
Lyme disease

EYE

Fundi	Cranial Nerve Abnormalities	Conjunctival Suffusion
Ocular larva migrans		RMSF
Toxoplasmosis	Lyme disease	Leptospirosis
		Relapsing fever

CENTRAL NERVOUS SYSTEM
Lyme disease
Visceral larva migrans
Toxoplasmosis
Cat scratch fever
Legionnaires' disease

PHARYNX
Toxoplasmosis
Cat scratch fever
Lyme disease

GASTROINTESTINAL TRACT
Dirofilaria
Strongyloides
Cryptosporidium
Campylobacter
Yersinia
Giardia

LIVER
Legionnaires' disease
RMSF
Q fever
Psittacosis
Lyme disease
Leptospirosis
Histoplasmosis
Cat scratch fever
Ehrlichia

SPLEEN
Q fever
Lyme disease
Psittacosis
Histoplasmosis

Figure 1. Infectious disease diagnostic considerations by organ involvement. RMSF, Rocky Mountain spotted fever.

SPECIFIC INFECTIOUS DISEASES

Sporotrichosis

The classic fungus associated with the soil is *Sporothrix schenckii. S. schenckii* is a dimorphic fungus which on culture produces conidia arranged in a "daisy" cluster on top of a conidiophore. In tissue the organism assumes an oval or cigar-shaped yeast form. The organism may be introduced into the skin via a minor abrasion such as a thorn or splinter, resulting in the development of a suppurative lymphangitis of the skin and subcutaneous tissues, although rarely hematogenous dissemination to the lungs, bones, and joints does occur. Alcoholics seem particularly prone to developing sporotrichosis, so this diagnostic point should be kept in mind when assessing patients who work in gardens and consume alcohol. The skin lesions of sporotrichosis usually begin as a small, gradually enlarging papular nodule which may become pustular and eventually ulcerates. Spread is distal to proximal along the lymphatics, and the lesions are characteristically not painful. While other diseases, such as tularemia, may resemble sporotrichosis, the

Table 3. Differential diagnosis of Rocky Mountain spotted fever[a]

Signs and symptoms	RMSF[b]	Meningococcal meningitis	Dengue	Leptospirosis	Atypical measles
Mental confusion	±	±	−	±	−
Headache	+++	+++	++	+++	−
Photophobia	+	+	+	−	−
Myalgia/arthralgia	+++	++	+	+++	+
Nausea/vomiting	+	+	−	−	−
Abdominal pain	±	−	−	±	−
Rash	Petechial— ankles, wrists, palms, soles	"Palpable" petechiae	Petechial	Maculo- papular, truncal	Urticarial, maculopapular, truncal
Jaundice	±	−	−	±	−
Splenomegaly	+ (50%)	−	±	±	−
Periorbital edema	++	−	−	−	−
Conjunctival suffusion	±	−	−	+	−
Abnormal LFTs	±	−	−	+++	−
Eosinophilia	±	−	−	−	+++
Chest film	−	−	−	−	+

[a]Adapted from reference 10b. Symbols: +, present; −, absent; ±, variable.
[a]RMSF, Rocky Mountain spotted fever.

indolent course of the illness along the lymphatic distribution with bridges of normal skin between painless lesions is highly suggestive of sporotrichosis. Diagnosis of sporotrichosis is made by culturing the organism from the affected tissue; however, repeat cultures may need to be performed. Direct examination of tissue for the presence of the yeast form may be helpful, but the organisms are generally rare. Serologic testing may help in the diagnosis of disseminated sporotrichosis (3, 14, 17).

Histoplasmosis

Histoplasmosis is caused by the dimorphic fungus *Histoplasma capsulatum*, which has a wide geographic distribution but is most heavily concentrated in North America along the Ohio and Mississippi river valleys. The organism has been associated with the presence of birds or bats and survives well in warm, moist soil contaminated by their droppings. Excavation, cleaning, or demolition of fecally contaminated organic material usually results in inhalation followed by acute pneumonitis in an nonimmune individual. Obviously the use of bird droppings as fertilizer enhances the likelihood of acquiring acute pulmonary histoplasmosis in nonimmune individuals. Acute pulmonary histoplasmosis manifests as a flu-like illness with cough and headache. Rarely, patients may have arthralgias or erythema nodosum. Infants, the elderly, or immunosuppressed persons may be predisposed to disseminated disease. Manifestations

↑WBC
  Group A streptococci

↑PLATELETS
  Rocky Mountain spotted fever

ATYPICAL LYMPHS
  Toxoplasmosis

EOSINOPHILIA
  Strongyloides
  Visceral larva migrans
  Group A streptococci
  Ascariasis
  Hookworm

ANEMIA
  Hookworm
  Strongyloides
  Histoplasmosis
  Babesiosis

ALKALINE PHOSPHATASES/TRANSAMINASES
  Legionnaires' disease
  Rocky Mountain spotted fever
  Q fever
  Leptospirosis
  Toxoplasmosis

↑BILIRUBIN
  Legionnaires' disease
  Leptospirosis

CHEST X-RAY
  Infiltrates
    Q fever
    Legionnaires' disease
    Histoplasmosis
    Blastomycosis
    Ascariasis
    Tularemia
  Coin Lesion
    Dirofilaria

ABNORMAL BRAIN CT SCAN
  Visceral larva migrans

ABNORMAL URINALYSIS
  Legionnaires' disease
  Leptospirosis
  Brucellosis

ABNORMAL CSF
  Toxoplasmosis
  Lyme disease
  LCM
  Cat scratch fever
  Visceral larva migrans
  Leptospirosis
  Rocky Mountain spotted fever
FECES
  Giardia
  Campylobacter
  Yersinia
  Ascariasis
  Hookworm
  Strongyloides
  Salmonella
  Cryptosporidium

Figure 2. Infectious disease considerations by lab and roentgen findings. WBC, white blood cell; CT, computed tomography; CSF, cerebrospinal fluid, LCM, lymphocytic choriomeningitis.

include fever, hepatosplenomegaly, and pancytopenia. Patients with chronic lung disease may develop chronic histoplasmosis, the symptoms of which resemble tuberculosis. In persons infected with human immunodeficiency virus (HIV), preexisting histoplasmosis can reactivate and present with a septicemia-like picture, with hepatic and renal involvement that may progress to a shock-like state. Persons with HIV should take particular care to avoid gardening situations in which exposure to *H. capsulatum* is likely. Definitive diagnosis is made by culturing the organism or identifying the yeast phase of the organism in tissue or through serologic techniques (4, 9, 16, 21, 30–32) (Fig. 3 and Table 4).

Other fungi are very uncommon or only distantly associated with gardening per se. Blastomycosis and cryptococcosis are unusual and are associated with typical clinical findings which should lead one to the diagnosis (Table 4).

Hematologic
  Thrombocytopenia
  Anemia
  Leukopenia
  Pancytopenia
  Splenomegaly
  Generalized adenopathy
  Eosinophilia

Pulmonary
  "Thick-walled" cavities
  Apical infiltrates
  Coin lesions
  Histoplasmosis
  Hilar adenopathy
  "Buckshot" calcifications
  Miliary calcifications
  "Marching cavities"
  Mediastinal fibrosis
  Obstruction of pulmonary/artery vein*
  Obstruction of superior vena cava*

Ear, Nose, and Throat
  Nose ulcers
  Lip ulcers
  Gum ulcers
  Mouth ulcers
  Tongue ulcers
  Laryngeal ulcers

Dermatologic
  Erythema nodosum
  Erythema multiforme
  Skin ulcers

Cardiac
  Endocarditis
  Pericarditis
    acute
    subacute
    fibrinous

Neurologic
  Chronic meningitis
  Focal cerebritis
  Spinal cord compression*

Gastrointestinal
  Esophageal obstruction*
  Granulomatous hepatitis
  Diarrhea
  Intestinal ulceration

Other
  Addison's disease

Figure 3. Clinical spectrum of histoplasmosis. *, secondary to lymph node compression or mediastinal fibrosis. Adapted from reference 9.

Blastomycosis

Blastomyces dermatitidis is the dimorphic fungus responsible for the development of blastomycosis. This organism has proven difficult to isolate from environmental sources; however, exposure to organically rich warm, moist soil appears to be a risk factor for the development of infection. Blastomycosis is endemic in the southeastern and midwestern United States and has been classically associated with the Ohio and Mississippi river valley regions. The fungus enters via the lungs and can result in asymptomatic disease, acute infection that mimics a bacterial pneumonia, or chronic pulmonary infection which may be confused clinically with tuberculosis. *B. dermatitidis* often disseminates hematogenously, with the skin being the most frequent site of extrapulmonary infection. The skin lesions are characteristically verrucous or ulcerative in nature.

Osteomyelitis due to *B. dermatitidis* occurs as well. Genitourinary tract involvement manifests as prostatitis and/or epididymo-orchitis in males, but involvement of the female genitourinary tract is rare. Central nervous system infection resulting in meningitis or a brain abscess is seen most commonly in immunocompromised individuals, especially in persons with AIDS (1, 5, 28).

The diagnosis of blastomycosis is confirmed by isolating the organism in culture or from a biopsy specimen where the fungus appears in its yeast phase. The organism may also be observed on KOH preps of clinical specimens such as sputum, pus, or prostatic secretions. Serologic testing remains unreliable and should be used only in conjunction with isolation of the organism.

Table 4. Differential diagnosis of histoplasmosis[a]

Factor	Histoplasmosis	Tuberculosis	Blastomycosis
Fever (double quotidian)	−	±	−
Laboratory tests			
Pancytopenia	+[b]	+	−
Hypergammaglobulinemia	−	−	−
Leukemoid reaction	−	+	−
Chest X ray			
Miliary calcification	+	±	−
Hilar ademopathy	+	−	−
Pleural effusion	−	+	−
Abdominal X ray (liver/splenic calcification)	+	−	−
Organ involvement			
Meningitis	+[b]	+	−
Oropharyngeal ulcers	+[b]	±	−
Pulmonary infiltrates	+	+	±
Endocarditis	+	−	−
Addison's disease	+[b]	+	−
Granulomatous hepatitis			
Splenomegaly	+[b]	±	±
Generalized adenopathy	+	±	−
Intestinal ulcers	+[b]	±	−
Bone/joint lesions		+	+
Glomerulonephritis	−	−	−
Epididymo-orchitis	−	+	+
Granulomatous prostatitis	+	−	+
Skin ulcers	+[b]	±	+
Erythema nodosum	+	+	±

[a]Adapted from reference 9. Symbols: +, present; −, absent; ±, variable.
[b]Only in disseminated histoplasmosis.

Legionnaires' Disease

Legionnaires' disease can be acquired in the garden only if the organism is in soil that is being excavated nearby and there is airborne spread of the organism in the garden area. Legionnaires' disease is varied in its distribution; some areas have a relatively high incidence of Legionnaires' disease, while the disease is unheard of in other locations. *Legionella* is most common in the late spring and early fall, and infection may begin with a flu-like illness. The course may be subacute or fulminant, and usually the illness most typically presents as a pneumonia. However, a nonpulmonary form, i.e., Pontiac fever, is a manifestation of *Legionella* infection without associated pneumonitis. Legionnaires' disease should be considered in the diagnosis of all community-acquired pneumonias, and specific diagnostic features should be looked for to arrive at a working diagnosis. The clue to all of the atypical pneumonias lies in their extrapulmonary manifestations, since they are all systemic infections. With *Legionella* infection, the patient's extrapulmonary manifestations commonly include changes in mental status, nonspecific abdominal pain, or diarrhea. In contrast with *Mycoplasma* pneumonia, Legionnaires' disease is not associated with otitis or pharyngitis. If the patient has a temperature in excess of 102°F on presentation to the physician, and the patient does not have an arrhythmia, does not have a pacemaker, or is not on beta-blockers, then a pulse-temperature deficit provides the single most important clue to the diagnosis. Relative bradycardia is present in virtually all patients with *Legionella* presenting with a temperature of >102°F, and if the pulse is charted with a temperature, a pulse-temperature deficit is readily seen by simple inspection. However, if one desires to calculate if there is relative bradycardia present, then one takes the temperature in degrees Fahrenheit, takes the last digit, decreases it by 1, multiplies that number by 10, and adds that number to 100. For example, if the temperature is 105°F, the 5 is reduced to 4 and multiplied by 10 to get 40, and this is added to 100 to get 140. Therefore, any pulse of <140 in a patient with a 105°F temperature indicates a pulse-temperature deficit even if the patient is "tachying along" at 120 beats/min.

The chest X ray is not characteristic, but it usually "behaves" in a typical way. Legionnaires' disease on chest X-ray is characterized by a rapidly progressive asymmetrical infiltrate(s). While not all *Legionella* infection behaves in this fashion, it is nevertheless the most typical roentgen manifestation. In terms of laboratory tests, a decreased serum phosphate level, when present, is a most helpful finding. A decreased serum sodium level appears to be more commonly associated with Legionnaires' disease than other pneumonias, but it is not specific for *Legionella* infections. A decrease in sodium on the basis of syndrome of inappropriate secretion of antidiuretic hormone may occur with any pulmonary process, whether it is infectious, inflammatory, or neoplastic. In contrast, a depressed serum phosphate level is uniquely associated with Legionnaires' disease. An elevated bilirubin count in association with an atypical pneumonia is more helpful and limits diagnostic possibilities to pneumococcal pneumonia and *Legionella*. The serum transaminases are almost always modestly elevated in patients with *Legionella pneumophila* pneumonia, and this is also true for other *Legionella* species. This is another important laboratory clue to the presence of an atypical pneumonia, since only *Legionella* pneumonia, Q fever, and psittacosis are frequently associated with abnormal liver function tests, in contrast to *Mycoplasma* pneumonia. Therefore, a working diagnosis can be readily obtained by combining the aforementioned features, while a definitive diagnosis depends upon demonstrating the organism with direct fluorescent-antibody assay of sputum or pleural fluid, urinary antigen testing, or indirect fluorescent-antibody assay serologic methods. The organism may also be cultured directly from sputum or appropriate samples of lung or pleural fluid. The differential diagnostic features of *Legionella* are presented in Table 5 (8, 10, 15, 22, 23, 25).

Table 5. Diagnostic features of atypical pneumonias[a]

Manifestations	*Mycoplasma* pneumonia	Legionnaires' disease	Psittacosis	Q fever	Tularemia
Symptoms					
Mental confusion	−	+	±	−	−
Headache	±	+	+	+	−
Meningismus	−	−	+	+	−
Myalgias	+	+	+	+	−
Ear pain	±	−	−	−	−
Pleuritic pain	±	+	±	±	−
Abdominal pain	−	+	−	−	−
Diarrhea	±	+	±	±	−
Hoarseness	−	−	−	−	−
Signs					
Rash	± (erythema multiforme)	−	±	± (Horders's spots)	±
Raynaud's phenomenon	±	−	−	−	−
Nonexudative pharyngitis	+	−	−	−	−
Hemoptysis	−	+	+	−	−
Lobar consolidation	−	±	±	±	±
Cardiac involvement	±	±	±	±	−
Splenomegaly	−	−	+	−	−
Relative bradycardia	−	+	+	+	−
Chest film findings					
Infiltrate	Patchy	Patchy/consolidation	Patchy/consolidation	Pleura-based oval infiltrates	Ovoid bodies
Bilateral hilar adenopathy	−	−	−	−	+
Pleural effusion	± (small)	±	±	−	+ (bloody)
Laboratory findings					
White blood cell count	→	→	Normal	Normal	Normal
Hypophosphatemia[b]	−	+	−	−	−
Increase in SGOT/SGPT[b]	−	+	+	+	−
Cold agglutinins	+	−	−	−	−
Microscopic hematuria	−	+	−	−	−

[a] Adapted from reference 10. Symbols: +, present; −, absent; ±, variable.
[b] SGOT/SGPT, serum glutamic oxalacetic transaminase/serum glutamic pyruvic transaminase.

Hookworm

Hookworm disease is caused by two intestinal nematodes, *Ancylostoma duodenale* and *Necator americanus*. The environmental conditions of the southeastern United States, with its warmth, high humidity, and heavy rainfall, are ideal for the life cycle of these nematodes. In contaminated soil, the eggs hatch in approximately 24 h and become rhabditiform larvae. The rhabditiform larvae incubate in the warm moist soil for 5 to 10 days, developing into the infectious filariform larvae. This form can survive for up to 1 month in the soil. Human infection occurs when the filariform larvae penetrate exposed skin, usually through bare feet. When *N. americanus* is involved, there is often a local skin reaction consisting of erythema and a pruritic papular or vesicular eruption near the entry site. This is less commonly seen with *A. duodenale*. These larvae enter the venous circulation, where they are carried to the lungs. Pulmonary complaints such as cough or wheezing or pulmonary infiltrates can be seen at this time. The filariform larvae then migrate into the pharynx, where they are swallowed. They mature into adult worms in the small intestine, where they attach and feed on the blood of the host and liberate more eggs. Symptoms at this time generally consist of nonspecific abdominal complaints such as pain, bloating, or nausea, or symptoms attributable to anemia. Laboratory findings may consist of a hypochromic, microcytic anemia, the degree of which is a function of the worm burden and consequent blood loss, eosinophilia, and hypoproteinuria. Diagnosis of hookworm disease is made by finding the characteristic oval eggs in a direct stool smear. Infections with light worm burdens require stool concentration techniques. Fresh stools should be examined immediately since eggs may hatch into rhabditiform larvae resembling the rhabditiform larvae of *Strongyloides* (13).

Strongyloides

Strongyloidiasis, or threadworm infection, results from infection with the nematode *Strongyloides stercoralis*. It is less commonly encountered than hookworm infection, and the threadworm is unique among the nematodes in its ability to cause autoinfection due to its peculiar triphasic life cycle. The filariform larvae of *Strongyloides* penetrate the skin in a manner analogous to that of the hookworm. A pruritic maculopapular eruption or larva currens, which is a migrating serpiginous linear rash, may be seen at that time. The filariform larvae are carried by the venous circulation to the lungs. In the healthy host, this pulmonary migration is usually asymptomatic, but in the immunocompromised host, cough, wheezing, dyspnea, and fleeting pulmonary infiltrates accompanied by peripheral eosinophilia may provide a clue to the diagnosis. The filariform larvae ascend and are swallowed to complete their life cycle within the small intestine of the host, where the presence of the nematode may cause abdominal pain, diarrhea, and weight loss. Autoinfection occurs when, while still in the intestine, the rhabditiform larvae develop into infectious filariform larvae, which in turn penetrate the colonic mucosa or perirectal skin, reinfecting the host. In immunocompromised individuals, a hyperinfection syndrome may be seen, which occurs when there is widespread dissemination of the filariform larvae via the bloodstream. Secondary bacterial infections are common in this condition due to large numbers of filariform larvae migrating from the intestine. Mortality associated with hyperinfection syndrome is quite high.

The diagnosis of strongyloidiasis is made by demonstrating the rhabditiform larvae in concentrated stool specimens or duodenal fluid. Peripheral eosinophilia is generally present in immunocompetent (but not immunocompromised) individuals, and total immunoglobulin E may be evaluated. The filariform larvae are also occasionally present in the urine or sputum of immunocompromised persons (19, 24, 29).

Nocardiosis

Nocardia species are soilborne aerobic actinomycetes that can cause localized or disseminated infection in humans. *Nocardia asteroides* is most frequently implicated in human illness, followed by *Nocardia brasiliensis* or *Nocardia otitidiscaviarum*. Although other species are now being recovered in increasing numbers, these organisms are recovered throughout the world from warm moist soil as well as from other environmental sources. Clinical infection with *Nocardia* occurs most commonly in immunocompromised individuals such as transplant recipients or persons with collagen vascular disease, lymphoreticular malignancies, or chronic pulmonary disease. Persons infected with HIV are also at risk for nocardiosis. The organism enters the body via inhalation into the lungs, although the portal is occasionally the gastrointestinal tract, or through traumatic implantation.

Pulmonary infection is characterized by the formation of multiple suppurative abscesses. The clinical symptoms of pulmonary nocardiosis are similar to those of tuberculosis, with fever, malaise, cough, weight loss, and night sweats. Sinus tract formation from the lungs can occur. Radiographically, the infiltrates of nocardiosis may present as consolidation, alveolar, or reticular infiltrates. Cavitation and pleural involvement are common, and empyema occurs in about one-quarter of patients. Pulmonary *Nocardia* infection can have a protracted course, but it may also remit spontaneously or have an acute self-limited course. Hematogenous spread of *Nocardia* from the lungs to distant sites can occur. Concurrent pulmonary symptoms may be absent at the time of discovery. The central nervous system is a common site of dissemination. The clinical picture is generally that of a brain abscess or tumor, with fever, headache, nausea, vomiting, and focal neurological deficits. There is frequent dissemination of the pathogen to the eyes, kidneys, heart, bones, and subcutaneous tissues. Dissemination can occur in the absence of pulmonary involvement. Cutaneous or subcutaneous manifestations are seen after traumatic inoculation through the skin. When subcutaneous abscesses form, they are generally discrete, firm, nonindurated nodules, which, in contrast to those of actinomycosis, do not form draining fistulas. One exception to this is when *Nocardia* species are the causative agent in maduromycosis; in these cases, draining of sinus tracts occurs.

The diagnosis of nocardiosis is made by isolation of the organism from a clinical specimen. A Gram stain should be performed on pus or sputum. When *Nocardia* organisms are present, they appear as weakly gram positive, branching, filamentous rods, often looking "beaded." Many species of *Nocardia* are acid-fast. *Nocardia* species grow well on standard laboratory media; however, growth may take longer than 48 h when the organisms are present in mixed culture. They grow poorly on routinely used fungal media. No useful serologic tests are available at present (11, 18, 26, 27).

CONCLUSIONS

Gardening is a wonderful pastime, and the garden is a very peaceful place to enjoy one's vocation. However, the garden may be a treacherous place for very young compromised hosts when one takes into account the infectious potential residing in the soil, as well as the insect vectors on plants and animals. The location of the garden and the characteristics of the soil play a part in determining its infectious potential. The most important factor making the garden an infectious and dangerous place is the number and interaction of animals, whether they are pets or in the wild, that temporarily use the garden as part of their daily activities. The clinician should always ask about garden exposure, which will help in eliminating the diagnostic possibilities for the patient. The diagnostic approach is to utilize epidemiological principles in concert with clinical clues, which together should suggest a reasonable list of diagnostic possibilities. Organ involvement and specific laboratory tests will help further narrow the differential diagnosis and will determine the specific tests necessary to make a definitive diagnosis.

REFERENCES

1. **Bradsher, R. W., S. W. Chapman, and P. G. Pappas.** 2003. Blastomycosis. *Infect. Dis. Clin. N. Am.* **17:** 21–40.
2. **Braude, A. I. (ed.).** *Infectious Diseases and Medical Microbiology,* 2nd ed. W. B. Saunders Company, Philadelphia, Pa.
3. **Centers for Disease Control.** 1988. Multistate outbreak of sporotrichosis in seedling handlers, 1988. *Morb. Mortal. Wkly. Rep.* **37:**652.
4. **Centers for Disease Control and Prevention.** 2001. Update: outbreak of acute febrile respiratory illness among college students—Acapulco, Mexico, March 2001. *Morb. Mortal. Wkly. Rep.* **50:**359–360.
5. **Chapman, S. W., R. W. Bradsher, Jr., G. D. Campbell, Jr., P. G. Pappas, and C. A. Kauffman.** 2000. Practice guidelines for the management of patients with blastomycosis. *Clin. Infect. Dis.* **30:**679–683.
6. **Cohen, J., and W. G. Powderly.** 2004. *Infectious Diseases,* 2nd ed. Mosby, New York, N.Y.
7. **Cook, G. C., and A. I. Zumia (ed.).** 2003. *Manson's Tropical Diseases,* 21st ed. Elsevier Science, Ltd., Edinburgh, Scotland.
8. **Cotton, E. M., M. J. Strampfer, and B. A. Cunha.** 1987. *Legionella* and *Mycoplasma* pneumonia—a community hospital experience with atypical pneumonias. *Clin. Chest Med.* **8:**441–453.
9. **Cunha, B. A.** 1986. Histoplasmosis. *Infect. Dis. Pract.* **9:**1–8.
10. **Cunha, B. A.** 1991. Atypical pneumonias. *Postgrad. Med.* **90:**89–101.
10a.**Cunha, B. A.** 1991. It's Lyme disease season. *Emerg. Med.* **23:**101–115.
10b.**Cunha, B. A.** 1988. Rocky Mountain spotted fever. *Emerg. Med.* **20:**129–138.
11. **Dorman, S. E., S. V. Guide, P. S. Conville, E. S. DeCarlo, H. L. Malech, J. I. Gallin, F. G. Witebsky, and S. M. Holland.** 2002. *Nocardia* infection in chronic granulomatous disease. *Clin. Infect. Dis.* **35:**390–394.
12. **Gorbach, S. L., J. G. Bartlett, and N. R. Blacklow (ed.).** 2003. *Infectious Diseases,* 3rd ed. W. B. Saunders Company, Philadelphia, Pa.

13. **Grencis, R. K., and E. S. Cooper.** 1996. Enterobius, Trichuris, Capillaria, and hookworm including Ancylostoma caninum. *Gastroenterol. Clin. N. Am.* **25:**579–597.
14. **Hajjeh, R., S. McDonnell, S. Reef, C. Licitra, M. Hankins, B. Toth, A. Padhye, L. Kaufman, L. Pasarell, C. Cooper, L. Hutwagner, R. Hopkins, and M. McNeil.** 1997. Outbreak of sporotrichosis among tree nursery workers. *J. Infect. Dis.* **176:**499–504.
15. **Johnson, R. D., M. Raff, and J. van Arsdall.** 1984. Neurologic manifestations of legionnaires' disease. *Medicine* (Baltimore) **63:**303.
16. **Karimi, K., L. J. Wheat, P. Connolly, G. Cloud, R. Hajjeh, E. Wheat, K. Alves, C. da Silva Lacaz, and E. Keath.** 2002. Differences in histoplasmosis in patients with acquired immunodeficiency syndrome in the United States and Brazil. *J. Infect. Dis.* **186:**1655–1660.
17. **Kauffman, C. A., R. Hajjeh, and S. W. Chapman for the Mycoses Study Group.** 2000. Practice guidelines for the management of patients with sporotrichosis. *Clin. Infect. Dis.* **30:**684–687.
18. **Lerner, P. I.** 1996. Nocardiosis. *Clin. Infect. Dis.* **22:**891–903.
19. **Mahmoud, A. A.** 1996. *Strongyloides. Clin. Infect. Dis.* **23:**949–952.
20. **Mandell, G. L., J. E. Bennett, and R. Dolin (ed.).** 2000. *Principles and Practice of Infectious Diseases,* 5th ed. Churchill Livingstone, Philadelphia, Pa.
21. **Medeiros, A. A., S. D. Marty, F. E. Tosh, and T. D. Y. Chin.** 1966. Erythema nodosum and erythema multiforme as clinical manifestations of histoplasmosis in a community outbreak. *N. Engl. J. Med.* **274:**415.
22. **Murdoch, D. R.** 2003. Diagnosis of Legionella infection. *Clin. Infect. Dis.* **36:**64–69.
23. **Murray, H. W., and C. Tuazon.** 1980. Atypical pneumonias. *Med. Clin. N. Am.* **64:**507.
24. **Siddiqui, A. A., and S. L. Berk.** 2001. Diagnosis of *Strongyloides stercoralis* infection. *Clin. Infect. Dis.* **33:**1040–1047.
25. **Stout, J. E., and V. L. Yu.** 1997. Legionellosis. *N. Engl. J. Med.* **337:**682–687.
26. **Threlkeld, S. C, and D. C. Hooper.** 1997. Update on management of patients with *Nocardia* infections. *Curr. Clin. Top. Infect. Dis.* **17:**1–23.
27. **Van Burik, J. A., R. C. Hackman, S. Q. Nadeem, J. W. Hiemenz, M. H. White, M. E. Flowers, and R. A. Bowden.** 1997. Nocardiosis after bone marrow transplantation: a retrospective study. *Clin. Infect. Dis.* **24:**1154–1160.
28. **Wallace, J.** 2002. Pulmonary blastomycosis: a great masquerader. *Chest* **121:**677–679.
29. **Wehner, J. H, and C. M. Kirsch.** 1997. Pulmonary manifestations of strongyloidiasis. *Semin. Respir. Infect.* **12:**122–129.
30. **Wheat, J.** 1997. Histoplasmosis. Experience during outbreaks in Indianapolis and review of the literature. *Medicine* (Baltimore) **76:**339–354.
31. **Wheat, J., G. Sarosi, D. McKinsey, R. Hamill, R. Bradsher, P. Johnson, J. Loyd, and C. Kauffman.** 2000. Practice guidelines for the management of patients with histoplasmosis. *Clin. Infect. Dis.* **30:**688–696.
32. **Wheat, L. J., and C. A. Kauffman.** 2003. Histoplasmosis. *Infect. Dis. Clin. N. Am.* **17:**1–19.

Infections of Leisure, Third Edition
Edited by David Schlossberg
© 2004 ASM Press, Washington, D.C.

Chapter 5

With Man's Best Friend

Sofia Sherman-Weber, Todd Levin, and Bennett Lorber

The relationship between humans and dogs is an ancient one. The dog has been our workmate, protector, guide, and companion. No one would question the merit of the long history of valuable service the dog has provided to humans; it is the stuff of legend and literature. We even have evidence that a dog companion is good for our physical health (35). Occasionally, however, pathogens may be transmitted from dogs to human beings, resulting in problems ranging from a trivial rash to life-threatening bacteremia. These infections are reviewed in this chapter.

Considering that there are an estimated 68 million pet dogs in the United States (14a, 31), physicians need to be familiar with the potential illnesses that can result from canine exposure. An inquiry into animal contact is an important part of the medical history. Some clinical conditions, along with etiologies to be considered, in persons with a canine exposure are listed in Table 1.

LOCAL INFECTIONS FOLLOWING DOG BITES

Epidemiology

Animal bites are a major public health problem and account for about 0.5 to 1% of emergency room visits; dogs are responsible for 75 to 90% of reported bites (31, 45, 110). Almost 5 million persons in the United States suffer a dog bite each year, and approximately 15% of these require medical attention. In most instances the dog belongs to the bite victim, a friend, or a neighbor (64). Most bites occur in warm-weather months, and bites are located most frequently on the hand and upper extremity. One-half to two-thirds of bites occur in children, with a peak incidence in those 5 to 9 years of age; in adult life, letter carriers, veterinarians, and animal control officers have a high incidence (14a, 111).

Sofia Sherman-Weber and Todd Levin • Section of Infectious Diseases, Temple University Hospital, Philadelphia, PA 19140. *Bennett Lorber* • Section of Infectious Diseases, Temple University School of Medicine and Hospital, Philadelphia, PA 19140.

Table 1. Etiologies to consider in patients with canine exposure

Clinical picture	Pathogen
Skin and soft tissue	
Local infection after a bite	
Less than 24 h	*Pasteurella multocida*
More than 24 h	*Streptococcus* spp., *Pasteurella* spp.
	Staphylococcus spp., anaerobes
Chronic	*Blastomyces dermatitidis*
Dermatitis (tinea, ringworm)	*Microsporum canis*
Creeping eruption	*Ancylostoma* species
Erythema migrans	*Borrelia burgdorferi*
Lymph nodes (regional lymphadenopathy)	*Bartonella henselae* (cat scratch)
	Francisella tularensis
	Yersinia pestis
Respiratory	
Pharyngitis	*Streptococcus pyogenes*[a]
Pneumonitis	*Toxocara canis*
	Coxiella burnetii
Pulmonary embolism	*Dirofilaria immitis*
Solitary pulmonary nodule	*Dirofilaria immitis*
Gastrointestinal	
Diarrhea	*Campylobacter jejuni*
	Salmonella enterica serovar Enteritidis
	Cryptosporidium species
	Isospora belli
	Giardia lamblia[a]
	Trichuris vulpis
	Dipylidium caninum
Pruritus ani	*Dipylidium caninum*
Hepatitis	*Leptospira interrogans*
Hepatomegaly	*Toxocara canis*
Articular (arthritis)	*Borrelia burgdorferi*[a]
Neurological	
Aseptic meningitis	*Leptospira interrogans*
	Borrelia burgdorferi[a]
Pyogenic meningitis	*Capnocytophaga canimorsus* (DF-2)
	Pasteurella multocida
	Bergeyella (formerly *Weeksella*) *zoohelcum* (IIj)
Visual disturbances	*Toxocara canis*
Encephalitis	Rabies virus
Systemic	
Septicemia (shock, DIC)	*Capnocytophaga canimorsus*
	Pasteurella multocida
Endocarditis	*Brucella canis*
	Capnocytophaga canimorsus
	Pasteurella multocida
	Staphylococcus aureus

Table 1. *Continued*

Clinical picture	Pathogen
Systemic *(continued)*	
Fever and rash.............................	*Rickettsia rickettsii*
Fever without localizing symptoms	*Salmonella enterica* serovar Enteritidis
	Brucella canis
	Ehrlichia species[a]
	Leptospira interrogans
Other	
Visceral mass.............................	*Echinococcus granulosus*
Eosinophilia.............................	*Toxocara canis*

[a]Transmission from dogs is controversial or unproved.

The risk of infection following a dog bite is considerably lower than with cat bites and is generally reported in the 5% range (110). Suturing does not seem to increase the risk of subsequent infection (1).

Microbiology

The oral flora of the dog is complex, plentiful, and made up of many aerobic and anaerobic species. Uninfected bite wounds should not be cultured, since they will typically grow multiple species and initial cultures show little correlation with later cultures from bites that become infected (31, 110).

Most infections following a dog bite are polymicrobial, typically yielding 2.5 to 4 species on wound culture. Common organisms are streptococcal species, staphylococcal species, anaerobes, and *Pasteurella* species, including *Pasteurella canis* and *Pasteurella multocida* (43, 102). *P. multocida* is less common in dog bite infections than in cat bites or scratches. Rarely, chronic cutaneous infection with the fungus *Blastomyces dermatitidis* has been reported after a dog bite injury from an infected dog (42).

Initial Bite Management

Wounds should be irrigated with large amounts of sterile saline using a large syringe and 18-gauge needle to create a high-pressure jet (110). Standard recommendations for rabies and tetanus prophylaxis should be adhered to. Suturing may be used when needed; deep puncture wounds should probably not be sutured.

Antibiotic Prophylaxis

Controlled studies have not shown a beneficial effect of antibiotics in preventing infection (30), but these studies were small and may be subject to statistical error since infection rates following canine bites are low to begin with. Many authorities recommend prophylactic antibiotics for wounds of the hands and face, deep puncture wounds that cannot be irrigated adequately, and immunocompromised persons, particularly postsplenectomy (1). There is no consensus regarding drug choice. Amoxicillin-clavulanate at 250 mg per os (p.o.) three times a day is a reasonable choice, with tetracycline at 500 mg p.o. four times a day as an alternative for penicillin-allergic individuals.

Treatment of Infection

There are really no good large-scale trials evaluating antibiotic treatment of infected dog bite wounds. Most infections are polymicrobial, and treatment should be adequate for staphylococci, streptococci, *P. canis*, *P. multocida*, and anaerobes. Those persons whose infection began more than 24 h following the bite should have therapy guided by Gram stain and culture when possible (31). Amoxicillin-clavulanate, ciprofloxacin or levofloxacin plus clindamycin, trimethoprim-sulfamethoxazole (TMP-SMX) plus clindamycin, or moxifloxacin alone is a reasonable therapeutic choice. Infections which manifest (pain, erythema) within a few hours to 24 h of the bite are usually due to *P. multocida*; penicillin is the drug of choice, with tetracycline, TMP-SMX, or a quinolone as alternatives in penicillin-allergic persons.

Prevention of Dog Bites

Large breeds of dogs (shepherds) and guard dogs account for a disproportionate percentage of bites. Children should not be left unattended with large dogs, should be educated never to startle feeding or sleeping dogs of any size, and should be encouraged to avoid unfamiliar animals entirely.

LIFE-THREATENING SYSTEMIC INFECTIONS

Capnocytophaga canimorsus (Dog Bite Septicemia)

C. canimorsus, formerly DF-2 (dysgonic fermenter 2), is a fastidious gram-negative rod which can cause serious systemic illness following a dog bite. Since it was first reported about 20 years ago, more than 60 human cases have been described (14). The bacterium has been isolated from the normal gingival flora of 16% of dogs (110).

Eighty percent of patients have had a predisposing condition, most commonly splenectomy (35%), alcohol abuse (35%), and evidence of immune dysfunction (17%) (due to steroid therapy, hematologic malignancy, or autoimmune disease). More than 75% of cases involved previous exposure to a dog, through either ownership or a direct bite (75).

The clinical illness is typically one of a severe septicemia; shock and disseminated intravascular coagulation are common. Manifestations of *C. canimorsus* septicemia include cellulitis, gangrene, arthritis, endocarditis, meningitis, brain abscess, rash, hemolytic-uremic syndrome, thrombotic thrombocytopenic purpura, purpura fulminans, adrenal hemorrhage (Waterhouse-Friderichsen syndrome), myocardial infarction (with normal coronary arteries and without evidence of endocarditis), and mononeuropathy by occlusion of vasa nervorum and infarction of the nerve. The mortality rate has been about 27% (7, 29, 53, 74–76).

C. canimorsus infection must be considered in a febrile, severely ill patient with a history of a dog bite or dog exposure (cats may also transmit this infection). Diagnosis depends on isolation of the organism from blood, other fluids, or tissues. Organisms may be seen in buffy coat smears, particularly for splenectomized patients.

Penicillin is thought to be the drug of choice. The bacterium is also susceptible to piperacillin, imipenem, erythromycin, vancomycin, clindamycin, expanded-spectrum cephalosporins, chloramphenicol, rifampin, TMP-SMX, ciprofloxacin, and tetracyclines. Resistance to aminoglycosides has been demonstrated (75).

Patients who have had splenectomies should be warned about this rare but devastating infection and advised to take prophylactic antibiotics following a dog bite or contamination of an open wound with dog saliva.

Endocarditis

In addition to rare instances of endocarditis due to *C. canimorsus*, endocarditis has been reported rarely as a complication of infection with *Brucella canis* and *P. multocida*. One instance of *Staphylococcus aureus* endocarditis was reported to occur in a dog breeder after minor bite trauma without evidence of infection at the bite site (12).

Rabies

The important problem of rabies and its ancient association with dog bites is considered in chapter 10.

BACTERIAL ZOONOTIC INFECTIONS

Bacterial zoonoses transmissible from dogs to human beings include campylobacteriosis, salmonellosis, leptospirosis, and brucellosis.

Campylobacteriosis

Campylobacteriosis is found throughout the world and is an important cause of human bacterial diarrhea, being as common as or more common than salmonellosis and shigellosis. The vast reservoir of *Campylobacter* in animals is probably the ultimate source for most human enteric infections; a number of outbreaks have followed ingestion of raw milk. *Campylobacter jejuni* is a cause of canine diarrhea (114). Investigations of healthy pet dogs below 1 year of age have revealed carrier rates of 20 to 25%. One study found that 29% of healthy puppies were colonized with *Campylobacter* spp. (47). Isolation rates are higher in puppies than in mature dogs and higher in kennel populations than among household dogs (9).

Several case studies have shown an association between human *Campylobacter* enteritis and a history of close contact with sick puppies (10, 87). Epidemiological investigation of these cases revealed that the only common factor was exposure to sick puppies. Young children have particularly close exposure to puppies and are, therefore, more susceptible to fecal-oral transmission.

The clinical picture of *Campylobacter* enteritis is usually one of abrupt onset with fever, abdominal pain, and diarrhea, sometimes with malaise, headache, myalgia, arthralgia, nausea, and vomiting. A history of grossly bloody stools is common, and many patients have at least one day of illness with eight or more bowel movements (11). Severe abdominal pain before the onset of diarrhea can mimic appendicitis (84). Most patients recover within a week. Nonsuppurative complications of *C. jejuni* enteritis include reactive arthritis and Guillain-Barré syndrome (58, 63).

Confirmation of the diagnosis of *C. jejuni* infection is based upon positive stool cultures, which must be placed on special selective media. Serologic testing can be done, but a low titer may reflect previous infection (9).

Fluid and electrolyte replacement is an important therapy in any diarrheal illness. *Campylobacter* enteritis is largely self-limiting and only in cases with severe prolonged symptoms are antibiotics warranted. *C. jejuni* is sensitive to a wide variety of antibiotics, including erythromycin, tetracyclines, and quinolones. Erythromycin remains the treatment of choice for *C. jejuni* infections. The newer macrolides (azithromycin, clarithromycin) are also effective, but they are more expensive and have no proven advantage over erythromycin. Unlike for *Salmonella* infection, treatment with antimicrobial agents does not prolong carriage of *C. jejuni*; on the contrary, erythromycin eliminates carriage within 72 h in most patients. Even though erythromycin does not alter the clinical course of infection, therapy has been suggested, in some instances, to prevent person-to-person transmission (3). The emerging resistance of organisms to fluoroquinolones has diminished their usefulness. Fluoroquinolones may be the best choice when bacterial gastroenteritis is suspected but no organisms have yet been isolated (2).

Salmonellosis

Nontyphoidal *Salmonella* species are relatively common inhabitants of the canine intestinal tract (114). In one study 27.6% of rectal swabs from dogs were positive for *Salmonella* (36). Younger dogs may have higher prevalence than older dogs. Despite this high prevalence and evidence that dogs may act as a reservoir for human infection with transmission through the fecal-oral route (20, 91), transmission to humans is rare.

The clinical features of canine infection vary with virulence of the strain, inoculum size, and host factors. Most dogs shedding *Salmonella* in their stools are asymptomatic. The common clinical presentation of canine salmonellosis consists of fever, vomiting, and diarrhea (varying from watery to mucoid to bloody). Abortion and stillbirth may occur and have epidemiological importance, as the meconium, membranes, and discharge contain the organism.

Humans that have acquired salmonellosis have similar clinical findings, with fever, nausea, vomiting, colicky abdominal pain, and diarrhea (with or without mucus and blood).

Diagnosis is confirmed by isolation of the organism from stool or blood.

Clinical management should be based upon severity of disease. Human *Salmonella* gastroenteritis is self-limiting and requires treatment only in special cases (the very young, the very old, and the immunocompromised). TMP-SMX, fluoro-quinolones, and expanded-spectrum cephalosporins can be used as initial therapy in high-risk patients or those suspected to be bacteremic, although a recent increase in TMP-SMX resistance has been noted (78). The intracellular nature of salmonellae may occasionally create discrepancies between in vitro sensitivity and clinical response.

With regard to public health risk, infected dogs typically shed *Salmonella* for 20 to 40 days, but sometimes up to 100 days. If one or more family members have confirmed salmonellosis without a known focus of exposure, the family pet should be tested regardless of symptoms. A thorough investigation should attempt to identify a common source for both human and pet.

Leptospirosis

Leptospires are finely coiled, motile spirochetes that are unique among other pathogenic spirochetes in that they can be cultivated readily on artificial media. Pathogenic leptospires belong to the species *Leptospira interrogans*, which has over 200 serovars.

Leptospirosis is a common zoonosis of livestock, pet animals, and wildlife in the United States and other parts of the world. Humans are accidental hosts, becoming infected through close contact with these animals or their urine. Dogs are important vectors of human illness. In one study of 223 dogs, 57% had antibodies to leptospires, with a higher seroprevalence in males and in animals older than 1 year (86). Infected canines may be asymptomatic or have fever, jaundice, conjunctivitis, and hemoglobinuria (34).

Infection of humans can occur (i) directly from urine or tissue of affected animals or (ii) indirectly through contact with water or soil that has been contaminated. Most human infections occur through exposed mucous membranes or abrasions of the skin (28). Leptospirosis can occur at all ages and in all seasons, but it is primarily a disease of young adults, of hot weather, and of males. Optimal factors that determine length of survival of leptospires in the environment are acid urine, neutral or slightly alkaline environment, temperature of 22°C or higher, and aqueous or wet soil. Given these conditions the leptospire may survive for several weeks.

Canine shedder or carrier states develop after infection; leptospires can survive in the distal convoluted tubules of the host kidney after they have disappeared from the host tissues. In the carrier state the host may have leptospiruria for months or for the remainder of its life. Humans do not develop a carrier state.

Most humans will have a subclinical infection or anicteric febrile disease and may initially be misdiagnosed as having a viral syndrome or aseptic meningitis. Leptospirosis may follow a biphasic illness after an incubation of 7 to 12 days, initially characterized by clinical manifestations of an acute systemic infection (septicemic phase) with fever, headache, myalgia, conjunctival suffusion, leptospiremia, and proteinuria. This terminates after 4 to 7 days. During this phase, leptospires can be isolated from blood, cerebrospinal fluid, and most tissues. The second phase is immunologically mediated and is manifested by meningitis, recurrent fever, uveitis, myositis, and leptospiruria. A detailed description of individual organ manifestations can be found in the review by Edwards and Domm (28). The severe form of leptospirosis is known as Weil's disease and is characterized by hepatic and renal dysfunction, hemorrhage, and circulatory collapse (44).

There are several vaccines available to prevent leptospirosis in dogs, and they appear to be effective in preventing clinical illness. However, there have been isolated case reports of dogs that have had leptospires isolated from their urine despite vaccination within the previous year (34).

Definitive diagnosis requires isolation of leptospires from a clinical specimen or demonstration of seroconversion. Leptospires can be isolated from the blood, cerebrospinal fluid, or tissue in the first 10 days of infection and identified by dark-phase microscopy or culture. Growth may be very slow, and cultures should be incubated in the dark for 6 weeks at 30°C (44). The laboratory diagnosis is usually made on the basis of serologic tests. A specific diagnosis is usually based on the demonstration of a fourfold rise in antibody titer. Agglutinins appear between the 6th and 12th days of illness. A variety of other testing methods have been used, including enzyme-linked immunosorbent assays (ELISAs) (69) and dot ELISAs (93, 100) along with indirect hemagglutination and immunofluorescent-antibody tests and gold immunoblot and PCR assays (24). Identification of the serotype may supply important epidemiological information (serotype Canicola, dogs; serotype Icterohaemorrhagiae, rats).

Treatment of leptospirosis remains controversial, as it is usually a nonfatal, self-limiting disease. Some studies suggest that penicillin G or doxycycline may shorten the duration of fever and reduce complications, but only if started before the fourth day of illness (69). In moderate to severe cases, most authorities would recommend penicillin G or ampicillin even if the patient has been ill for several days (44). The Jarisch-Herxheimer reaction is frequently observed during treatment (93).

Controlled studies of U.S. troops training in a high-risk environment in Panama demonstrated a significant decrease in the attack rate of leptospirosis in a doxycycline prophylaxis group (200 mg weekly) compared to a group receiving a placebo (100). Human vaccines have been used for some overseas populations, but no licensed preparation is available for use in the United States.

Brucellosis

Dogs infected with *B. canis*, which is transmitted during mating, may have disease manifested by spontaneous abortion, orchitis, epididymitis, fever, and lymphadenopathy. Infected dogs characteristically have prolonged bacteremia (23).

Human infection due to *B. canis* is rare, but like other forms of brucellosis, it may be protean in its manifestations (83). Patients may have a nonspecific febrile illness with headache and myalgias or may demonstrate findings consistent with focal infection. Endocarditis, osteomyelitis, and epidural abscess have been described (82).

The combination of potential exposure, consistent clinical features, and raised levels of *Brucella* agglutinins (with or without positive cultures of blood or tissue) confirms the diagnosis of brucellosis (88). Since antibodies to *B. canis* do not react with the standard antigens used when testing for *B. abortus*, *B. suis*, and *B. meliten-*

sis, specific serology for *B. canis* must be performed when infection with this organism is suspected (83). Cultures of blood and bone marrow are positive in 50 to 70% of cases. It may be necessary to hold culture bottles for up to 6 weeks.

Single-agent therapy and relatively short courses (less than 8 weeks) of combination treatments are associated with a high incidence of failure and relapse. The combination of doxycycline and an aminoglycoside (streptomycin, gentamicin, or netilmicin) for 4 weeks followed by the combination of doxycycline and rifampin for 4 to 8 weeks is the most effective regimen (48). It may be difficult to eradicate canine infection, and some authorities have recommended euthanasia for infected dogs.

Ehrlichiosis

Ehrlichiosis is a zoonotic infection caused by small, obligately intracellular, gram-negative bacteria of the family *Rickettsiaceae* and the genus *Ehrlichia*. *Ehrlichia canis* infection was first described for Algerian dogs in 1935 and is the known etiologic agent of canine monocytic ehrlichiosis. *Ehrlichia* species are capable of infecting human granulocytes and monocytes. Ticks are the likely vectors, and deer are the likely reservoirs. Ehrlichiae are known to reside and proliferate intracellularly within cytoplasmic phagosomes (5, 26, 27).

Human ehrlichiosis is manifested by acute onset of fever, malaise, and headache; rash is absent. Laboratory features include leukopenia, thrombocytopenia, and liver function abnormalities (5, 70). Most patients have a history of tick bite, and diagnosis has been established serologically. Doxycycline has been reported to be effective therapy. Studies (4, 24, 81, 96) indicate that human ehrlichiosis is caused by a species distinct from *E. canis*. A definite association with domestic dogs has not been shown (103).

Q Fever

Q fever is a zoonosis caused by *Coxiella burnetii*. Worldwide, cattle, sheep, and goats are the most common reservoirs for *C. burnetii* (89). A dog-related outbreak of Q fever was reported in which *C. burnetii* pneumonia developed in all three members of one family 8 to 12 days following exposure to an infected parturient dog (13).

Cat Scratch Disease

Cat scratch disease, reviewed in chapter 6, rarely has been reported following dog bites or scratches.

Streptococcosis

Group A beta-hemolytic *Streptococcus* (*Streptococcus pyogenes*) is a common cause of pharyngitis in children and adults. There are reports of dogs acting as reservoirs for this organism.

In one study, a family of four had recurrent group A streptococcal pharyngitis which was not eradicated until the family dog was treated (68).

Canine reservoirs for human streptococcal pharyngitis are probably exceedingly rare; that they occur at all is controversial (116). Nevertheless, it is probably prudent to consider a canine source in families with recurrent hemolytic streptococcal infection and a pet dog.

Two case reports identify infection with the group G streptococcus *Streptococcus canis* secondary to dog exposure. In one case the patient was inoculated through a bite wound on the thigh and was treated twice for recurrent bacteremia (101); in the other, bacteremia occurred following presumed entrance through venostasis ulcerations of the legs (8).

PARASITIC INFECTIONS

Many dogs harbor intestinal parasites; autopsy data have shown that more than 50% are infested with one or more such parasites (50). Some of these canine parasites may be transmitted to human beings, in whom they may produce symptomatic illness.

Cryptosporidiosis and Isosporiasis

Cryptosporidium is a ubiquitous coccidian protozoan parasite of the gastrointestinal tract, related to *Isospora* and *Toxoplasma,* that has been identified in a large variety of animals. It has six major developmental stages that all occur within a single host.

The parasite is acquired by the ingestion of fecally contaminated material, such as from the water supply, swimming pool water, food, fomites, and sexual activities that favor fecal-oral inoculation (18). In 1993, *Cryptosporidium* was responsible for a massive waterborne diarrheal outbreak that affected more than 400,000 individuals in Milwaukee, Wis. The source was a contaminated public water supply (103). Dogs can act as reservoirs for this organism (18, 22, 33, 51). The disease seems to be limited to puppies, but one study showed antibodies to cryptosporidia in 80% of all dogs tested (109).

Human cryptosporidiosis is characterized by watery diarrhea and cramping abdominal pain; fever is not prominent. The importance of this organism as a cause of human disease was recognized in AIDS patients, in whom it causes protracted wasting diarrheal illness; in immunocompetent hosts it produces a self-limiting illness of 1 to 2 weeks (21).

To date there are no documented cases of transmission from adult dogs or puppies to humans. However, considering the prevalence of this organism and the similarity in the mode of transmission to other pathogens, it seems likely that it will be noted in time. Outbreaks involving veterinary students suggest that human *Cryptosporidium* infection may be acquired from dogs and/or cats (32).

Diagnosis is made by microscopic identification of the organism in a fresh stool sample; leukocytes and blood are absent. After diagnosis, treatment of immunocompetent individuals may not be necessary. For immunocompromised patients, who are unable to clear the infection on their own, treatment has been frustrating and unsuccessful in most cases (22), although paromomycin sulfate has had limited success. Azithromycin has been found to be effective in animal models and is undergoing further study (103). More recently, nitazoxanide has been shown to reduce the duration of diarrhea compared to placebo (85).

The Centers for Disease Control and Prevention and the U.S. Public Health Service have issued guidelines for prevention of opportunistic infections, including cryptosporidiosis, in persons with human immunodeficiency virus (15). To prevent cryptosporidial infection, contact with human and animal feces should be avoided, and it is prudent to use disposable gloves for or immediately wash hands after contact with human feces (for example, changing diapers). Pet handling, gardening, or other contact with soil warrants similar precautions. Newly acquired puppies should be more than 6 months old, should not have diarrhea, and should not be stray. Human immunodeficiency virus-infected persons who wish to acquire a puppy younger than 6 months of age should have the puppy's stool examined for *Cryptosporidium* before contact.

The related protozoan *Isospora belli* causes clinical illness similar to that caused by *Cryptosporidium* and is diagnosed by identification of oocysts in fecal specimens. The size and shape (large and ovoid) of *Isospora* distinguish it from *Cryptosporidium*, which is round and smaller; both are acid-fast.

Isospora infection is common in dogs; one study (99) showed 9% of puppies from Atlanta, Ga., pet stores to harbor the parasite. Transmission to humans has not been proved. Treatment of humans with a week of oral TMP-SMX is curative; AIDS patients have a high frequency of recurrence but respond to retreatment.

Giardiasis

The flagellated enteric protozoan *Giardia lamblia* is an important worldwide cause of waterborne diarrhea in humans. Fecal-oral spread may also occur, particularly in daycare settings, in custodial institutions, and among sexually active male homosexuals.

Human infection is manifested initially by watery diarrhea without fever. Cramps, bloating, flatulence, and sulfuric belching are common. Later in the illness, stools may become greasy and foul smelling and may float.

Giardia may cause diarrhea in dogs, but their role in transmission of giardiasis to human beings has not been defined (31). Studies have shown carriage prevalence rates of 4 to 25% in dogs (38). *Giardia* species were identified in 34% of puppies in Atlanta pet stores (99). Compared with other sources, however, the risk of direct zoonotic transmission is small (38).

Giardiasis should be considered in all patients with prolonged diarrhea or malabsorptive symptoms. Diagnosis is achieved by seeing cysts or trophozoites in stool specimens or by sampling duodenal contents. The treatment of choice is metronidazole for 7 days. Quinacrine is also effective but is no longer available (production in the United States was discontinued in 1992). Furazolidone or metronidazole can be used in children. A recent study indicated that a 3-day course of nitazoxanide is equivalent to a 5-day course of metronidazole in the treatment of giardiasis in children (79).

Dirofilariasis

The dog heartworm, *Dirofilaria immitis* (L. *dirus*, evil; *filum*, thread), is found worldwide in warm climates. In the United States, canine and human dirofilariasis is most prevalent along the East Coast, Gulf Coast, Great Lakes, and Mississippi River Valley (19).

Mosquito vectors transmit the microfilarial form of the parasite from dog to dog and from dog to human being. In the canine host the adult worm lives in the right ventricle and pulmonary artery. Infected dogs are often asymptomatic but may have hemoptysis or evidence of heart failure secondary to right ventricular outflow obstruction.

In humans, larvae cannot develop into adults; most die before reaching the heart. Occasionally, a larva may reach the right ventricle, die, and embolize to the lung. Symptoms are rare but, when present, may mimic thromboembolic pulmonary embolism (pleuritic pain, fever, hemoptysis) (25, 107). The granulomatous lung reaction to the embolized larva produces the roentgenographic finding of a solitary pulmonary nodule (49, 71). Human infection is confirmed only when larvae are identified histologically following resection of a solitary pulmonary nodule. Eosinophilia is rarely noted. Other *Dirofilaria* species (*Dirofilaria repens* from dogs) may cause subcutaneous or conjunctival nodules in humans that are also impossible to diagnose until biopsy (57, 67).

Canine infection is diagnosed by demonstrating microfilariae in smears of peripheral blood. The ELISA has excellent sensitivity and specificity (103). Treatment of dogs and prophylaxis in areas of endemicity should be under veterinary supervision. Human infection should be considered in the differential diagnosis of a solitary lung nodule or a subcutaneous or conjunctival nodule; diagnosis is established following resection, and further treatment is unnecessary.

Toxocariasis

Toxocara canis is a roundworm that infects most puppies and many adult dogs in the United States, and it is the primary cause of visceral larva migrans (VLM) in humans.

Adult worms live for an average of 4 months in the proximal small intestine of dogs. By the time a dog has aged 6 months the majority of worms have been expelled. During that time, however, an adult female can produce 200,000 eggs per day. Eggs are then passed in the feces but are unembryonated and therefore uninfective. Embryonation occurs in the expelled feces over approximately a 2-week period; depending on temperature and moisture of the environment, eggs can remain viable for months.

Infection in adult dogs follows ingestion of embryonated eggs, ingestion of larvae in other infected hosts, or ingestion of larvae or immature adults from the vomitus or feces of infected pups. After hatching in the stomach, the larvae penetrate the intestinal mucosa, enter lymph and blood vessels, reach the liver within 24 h, and pass to the heart and lungs. From the lungs some of the larvae pass through the bronchioles to the trachea and pharynx, where they are swallowed and can complete their life cycle; they develop into adults in the intestine

(41). There larvae, as in human infections, rarely complete their life cycle. This results in the somatic migration of larvae which become encysted in various tissues. Hormonal changes in a pregnant bitch stimulate the larvae, resulting in transplacental migration of the larvae to the litter or passage of larvae in the bitch's milk (91).

Transmission to humans may occur by ingestion of eggs from the soil or from contaminated hands and fomites. Children 1 to 6 years of age are most prone to infection, particularly those with a history of pica and exposure to puppies. Twenty to 60% of soil samples recovered from backyards of residences, public parks, and children's sandboxes are contaminated with *T. canis* eggs (39, 80). Despite uniformly high levels of toxocariasis in dogs throughout the United States, the diagnosis of VLM in children is made most frequently in the south-central and south-eastern regions.

Human infection begins following ingestion of the infective egg; hatching occurs in the small intestine, releasing the larvae (40). The larvae penetrate the mucosa, migrate to the liver via the portal system, follow vascular channels to the lungs, and enter the systemic circulation. Larvae are stopped when the diameter of the blood vessel becomes too small to allow passage. They then bore through the vessel wall and migrate aimlessly. In humans, larvae migrate most frequently to the liver, but virtually any tissue can be invaded, and larvae can become dormant and may remain viable for many years. At a later time, they may reactivate and resume their migration.

Light infections are generally asymptomatic and probably occur most frequently; eosinophilia may be the only indicator of infection. In three human subjects who received 100 to 200 larvae as a single dose, moderate eosinophilia lasted for more than a year but there were no other signs or symptoms of disease (91).

Common signs and symptoms include cough, wheeze, pallor, malaise, irritability, and weight loss. Pruritic eruptions may occur, especially over the trunk and lower extremities. Pulmonary involvement is common, with approximately half of the patients developing transient infiltrates which are visible on chest radiograph. Patients may present with bronchitis, asthma, pneumonitis, or any combination of these signs.

Leukocyte counts ranging from 30,000 to 100,000 per mm^3, with 30% or more eosinophils, are not unusual. Eosinophilia may persist for months or years, even after other manifestations of the disease have abated.

In a study by Huntley et al. (55) of 51 patients with VLM, the most common symptoms were cough (80%) and wheezing (63%); fever (80%), hepatomegaly (65%), rales, and malnutrition were the most common physical findings.

The question of whether *Toxocara* is responsible for neurological disease in children has been raised. Skin testing for *Toxocara* in healthy individuals and those with epilepsy showed positive tests for 2.1 and 7.5%, respectively. Twenty-eight percent of the patients in the study by Huntley et al. had a history of seizures. Testing by Glickman and Schantz in 1979 (41) showed significantly higher *Toxocara* titers in epileptic children than in nonepileptic controls. Children with *Toxocara* are more likely to have lead poisoning than noninfected children; the two groups have the same risk factors, pica and lower socioeconomic status. Further studies are necessary to define the significance of *T. canis* in children with respect to neurological function and distinguish the effects from those of lead (39).

Ocular larva migrans is caused by the larvae of *Toxocara* entering the eye; it is typically a unilateral disease but occasionally occurs bilaterally. Presenting complaints are varied, and there is no pathognomonic pattern. Patients may complain of failing vision, strabismus, leukocoria, eye pain, fixed pupil, or red eye. Fundoscopic exam findings may vary from a solitary posterior pole lesion or peripheral granuloma in an asymptomatic eye to severe exudative endophthalmitis with retinal detachment. Generally, ocular cases differ from VLM in several important aspects. Ocular cases are more frequently reported for adults and are usually seen in the absence of visceral symptoms; unlike with VLM, a history of pica is infrequent.

A diagnosis of systemic toxocariasis should be considered in any child with persistent eosinophilic leukocytosis, especially given a history of pica. Laboratory and clinical findings are generally nonspecific and must be differentiated from other conditions with eosinophilia.

Ocular toxocariasis should be considered in any child with unilateral white or gray lesions in the fundus and needs to be differentiated from retinoblastoma, congenital and developmental abnormalities, exudative retinitis, and other causes of uveitis.

Diagnostic confirmation is based on demonstration of the larvae in pathological specimens (biopsy or autopsy). Stool samples are not useful, as the larvae rarely, if ever, mature in human beings. Percutaneous liver biopsy infrequently yields evidence of the larvae; laparoscopic biopsy may be more useful. Serologic tests using ELISA have been reported to be 91% sensitive and 86% specific (56).

The disease is usually self-limiting and only in rare instances have there been fatalities resulting from an exaggerated immune response in the heart, central nervous system, or lungs. Glucocorticoids may be employed to reduce inflammatory complications. Available antihelminthic drugs, including diethylcarbamazine, mebendazole, and albendazole, have not been shown conclusively to alter the course of larva migrans. Treatment of ocular disease is unsatisfactory, and the role of glucocorticoids or antihelmintic drugs in the management of ocular disease is controversial (65).

The best treatment may be to increase prevention by reducing the frequency of accidental ingestion of infective eggs. This can be accomplished by reducing the exposure of children to infected dogs and puppies, treating of infected dogs, and removing children with pica from environments thought to be contaminated. Dogs should also be prohibited from access to children's game areas, and sand in public parks should be turned over frequently (54).

Cutaneous Larva Migrans

The dog intestinal hookworms, *Ancylostoma caninum* and *Ancylostoma braziliense*, are the nematodes which cause human cutaneous larva migrans (creeping eruption). Larvae enter human skin after direct contact in areas contaminated with canine feces, such as beaches and playgrounds. The larvae do not possess the enzymes necessary to penetrate the dermis and remain confined to the epidermis. About 2 weeks after exposure, skin eruptions occur manifested by serpiginous, pruritic, red tunnels which spread a few millimeters per day. The skin appearance is diagnostic, and infection is self-limiting but may last for several weeks.

Treatment is best accomplished either through freezing with ethyl chloride spray directed at the advancing aspect of the track or through topical use of thiabendazole (112). Thiabendazole is also effective orally (59). Ivermectin is an alternative systemic agent. A rare eosinophilic enteritis syndrome due to *A. caninum* and manifested by abdominal pain may be treated with mebendazole (57).

Trichuriasis

Human infection with the dog whipworm, *Trichuris vulpis*, has been reported (27a). In this case, a 49-year-old woman with previous surgery for duodenal ulcer disease developed diarrhea, abdominal pain, and nausea. Ova of the dog whipworm were seen on stool exam, and her symptoms responded to mebendazole treatment. She owned five dogs.

Echinococcosis

Echinococcus granulosus is a small tapeworm whose definitive host is the dog. The adult cestode is found in the small intestine of dogs and wolves; gravid segments release eggs which are shed in the stool and may remain viable for up to a year. Once ingested by a human or other suitable intermediate host, the eggs make their way to the upper small intestine, where they hatch and oncospheres are released.

The released oncospheres penetrate the intestinal mucosa and obtain passage to the liver via portal veins. Here, most of the oncospheres are trapped; however, a few may pass through the liver and arrest in the lung. Those embryos that reach the systemic circulation may seed any organ. Wherever the parasite rests it either is destroyed by an inflammatory reaction or develops into a hydatid cyst, the latter being the culmination of a successful infection of the intermediate host. Cysts contain multiplying larvae and enlarge slowly over many years.

Upon death of the intermediate host, the larval hydatid may be eaten by a dog or another definitive host, whereupon the released scolices attach to the small intestinal mucosa. These scolices mature over a period of 6 to 8 weeks into an adult tapeworm 3 to 6 mm long, completing the life cycle (46, 92).

Humans act as intermediate hosts, but the prevalence of human echinococcosis is dependent upon the direct association of humans with infected canines. The frequency of infection is much higher in those regions where livestock is a major industry, especially in sheep-raising areas, where dogs feed on uncooked offal (46). The two epidemiological patterns that have been established are domestic (or pastoral) and sylvatic (or wild). The sylvatic cycle is seen in the tundra zones and in the coniferous forests of northern Alaska and Canada; intermediate hosts are reindeer and caribou (115).

The more common cycle is adapted to domesticated dogs, which become infected when they eat the contaminated viscera of sheep, cattle, or pigs. The cycle of transmission continues when the eggs passed in the dogs' feces are consumed by the herbivorous intermediate host. Human echinococcosis in the United States is found in sheep ranchers in California, Arizona, New Mexico, and Utah.

The majority of infections with *E. granulosus* are asymptomatic. Echinococcal cyst disease is indolent, and cysts enlarge slowly over many years. Some of the cysts die, shrink, become heavily calcified, and remain asymptomatic (90).

Symptomatic infections present with features of a space-occupying lesion and can involve almost any organ. Typical anatomical distribution is indicated by 1,802 cysts recorded in the Australasian Hydatid Registry: liver, 63%; lung, 25%; muscles, 5%; bone, 3%; kidney, 2%; spleen and brain, 1%; and heart, thyroid, breast, prostate, parotid, and pancreas, all less than 1% (46).

The most important complications of hydatid cysts are rupture, infection, and problems caused by compression. Leaking cysts can precipitate a wide range of reactions, from urticaria to anaphylaxis. Scolices that are released may lead to the establishment of secondary or metastatic hydatid infections elsewhere in the body. Bacterial infection of a cyst resembles an abscess of that organ (46, 90).

A geographic history must be taken when suspecting hydatid disease, since the diagnosis is more likely in an area of the world where the disease is prevalent.

Plain X rays of the abdomen may show calcification of the cyst rim. The chest film usually shows a round, uniformly dense lesion 1 to 20 cm in diameter, but calcification rarely occurs in lung cysts.

Skin testing for diagnosis has a poor yield, and false positives are quite common. ELISA, complement fixation, and indirect hemagglutination tests are better, but not all carriers have antibodies (90% with liver cysts; 75% with lung cysts). Aspiration of the cyst for diagnosis is not recommended, since leakage of contents or rupture of the cyst can lead to secondary infection or an anaphylactic reaction. Computerized axial tomography appears to be more helpful than ultrasound for pulmonary and extrahepatic cysts (90). The demonstration of intracystic septations, suggesting daughter cysts, is diagnostic of hydatid disease. Eosinophil counts or liver function tests may or may not be abnormal and should not be relied upon.

Therapy for echinococcosis is based on consideration of the size, location, and manifestations of cysts and the overall health of the patient. Surgery, when feasible, is the principal method of treatment having the potential to remove cysts, leading to complete cure (77). Risks at surgery from leakage of fluid include anaphylaxis and dissemination of infection. The latter complication has been minimized by the instillation of scolicidal solutions such as hypertonic saline or ethanol, which may cause hypernatremia, intoxication, or sclerosing cholangitis (95). Preoperative chemotherapy with albendazole or mebendazole may reduce the risk of secondary echinococcosis and should be given at least 4 days before surgery and for 1 month (albendazole) or 3 months (mebendazole) postoperatively. Operative mortality varies from 0.5 to 4%.

Ultrasound-guided cyst puncture, which was introduced in 1986, has diagnostic and therapeutic potential; however, diagnostic puncture should be used only if other diagnostic methods have failed.

The introduction of chemotherapy and of puncture-aspiration-injection-reaspiration (PAIR) offers alternatives for treatment, especially for inoperable cysts and for cases with a high surgical risk or those who refuse surgery. It has been used for the treatment of echinococcal cysts in the liver and for cysts in the abdominal cavity, spleen, kidney, and bones, but it should not be used for lung cysts. Four days of treatment with benzimidazoles before PAIR is mandatory and should last for 1 month (albendazole) or 3 months (mebendazole) after the procedure. PAIR is minimally invasive and less risky than surgery. It confirms the diagnosis and removes a large number of protoscolices and antigens with the aspirated cyst fluid (108). In a recent controlled trial (60), the safety and efficacy of percutaneous drainage were compared with those of surgical cystectomy. All patients undergoing percutaneous drainage were treated with albendazole, administered orally in a dose of 10 mg/kg of body weight/day for 8 weeks. Percutaneous drainage was performed on the 10th day of the drug regimen, with careful monitoring. Percutaneous drainage, combined with albendazole therapy, was found to be an effective and safe alternative to surgery for the treatment of uncomplicated hydatid cysts of the liver. The efficacy of percutaneous drainage is similar to that of standard treatment with cystectomy. The advantages of percutaneous drainage include a significantly shorter hospital stay and a lower complication rate (60). The data from this study and others have shown that percutaneous drainage is effective for both univesicular and multivesicular cysts (61, 62).

Treatment with chemotherapy alone is not yet satisfactory. Over a thousand well-documented cases of echinococcosis have been treated with benzimidazoles (albendazole, mebendazole). When evaluated for up to 12 months, 30% of patients show cyst disappearance (cure), 30 to 50% show degeneration of cysts and/or significant size reduction (improvement), but 20 to 40% exhibit no morphological changes (i.e., failure). Chemotherapy is indicated for inoperable patients with primary liver or lung echinococcosis and for patients with multiple cysts in two or more organs and peritoneal cysts. Another important indication for chemotherapy is the prevention of secondary echinococcosis. The presurgical use of benzimidazoles (albendazole, mebendazole) can reduce the risk of reoccurrence of cystic echinococcosis and/or facilitate the operation by reduction of intracystic pressure (106). Concomitant chemotherapy is also recommended for PAIR (113). Albendazole, which is better absorbed after oral administration, is preferable to mebendazole. Praziquantel has also been used for therapy. It has been shown to have effective protoscolicidal activity, and it may be more effective than albendazole in vitro. Praziquantel (40 mg/kg p.o. once a week) has been used alone and in combination with albendazole. A few reports suggest that the combination of albendazole and praziquantel as medical therapy or as postspillage prophylaxis is more effective than either therapy alone (72, 104).

Dipylidiasis

Dipylidium caninum is a common tapeworm of dogs. Larval cysticercoids of *D. caninum* develop in fleas and biting lice, which are the obligate intermediate hosts; dogs usually acquire this infection while nipping fleas. The ingested cysticercoid requires only 2 to 3 weeks to develop into an adult, proglottid shedding worm residing in the host intestine. Therefore, control of this parasite must include eradication of fleas and lice in addition to human antihelminthic therapy (37).

Human beings are infrequently parasitized, and most *Dipylidium* infections occur in children younger than 8 years, with one-third occurring in infants less than 6 months of age (6, 17, 66, 73, 108). Human infection begins when a flea or louse is accidentally ingested by a child while in contact with its pet. Symptoms are usually absent, but abdominal discomfort (6) or diarrhea and pruritis may occur (31). One case report describes a history of colic and feeding difficulties associated with dipylidiasis (108).

Diagnosis is made by isolating the proglottids from the feces or perineum. The parent usually notices the motile cucumber-seed-shaped proglottids resembling maggots in the stool. They can also migrate from the anus, which can cause a misdiagnosis of pinworms by history.

Treatment consists of praziquantel or niclosamide as a single dose. Human infection can be prevented by keeping pets free from fleas or tapeworms (103).

SUPERFICIAL FUNGAL INFECTIONS (DERMATOPHYTOSIS)

Dermatophytosis is a common superficial fungal infection of dogs, cats, and humans. Zoophilic dermatophytes are occasionally transmitted to humans, causing tinea or ringworm. Dermatophytes rarely invade the skin and produce disease by releasing allergens and creating an inflammatory reaction.

The most common fungi causing dermatophytosis in dogs are species of *Epidermophyton*, *Microsporum*, and *Trichophyton*. The cutaneous signs are variable and not characteristic for a specific dermatophyte. By far, the most common organism of dogs to cause skin infections of humans is *Microsporum canis*.

Diagnosis is established based on history, physical examination, Wood's lamp examination, KOH preparation, skin biopsy, and fungal culture. Fungal culture is the most accurate way of confirming the diagnosis. Ten to 30% of human cases of tinea corporis (ringworm), in urban settings, are estimated to be of animal origin (31).

Effective eradication of the infection should include treatment of the source animal as well as the human patient with topical agents, such as clotrimazole, miconazole, and ketoconazole. In severe cases, treatment with oral ketoconazole, fluconazole, or itraconazole is effective. The living environment, which may retain animal hair or dander, should be thoroughly cleansed (103).

An intensive care nursery outbreak due to *Malassezia pachydermatis* has been well documented; the organism caused fungemia, urinary tract infection, meningitis, and asymptomatic colonization in infants. The organism was introduced into the intensive care nursery on a health care worker's hands after they were colonized from pet dogs at home (16).

ECTOPARASITE-ASSOCIATED ILLNESS

Dogs that frequent the out-of-doors may disseminate the flea and tick vectors responsible for such serious human diseases as plague, Rocky Mountain spotted fever, tularemia, and Lyme disease. Thus, a pet owner need not leave home to be exposed to these infections; his or her dog can bring the vectors right into the living room.

Other canine ectoparasites (mites, fleas) may cause vexing dermatoses in humans. The most common ectoparasite-induced dermatoses of dogs are scabies, cheyletiellosis, and fleas. It has been estimated that over 5% of the cases presenting to human dermatology clinics are directly attributable to animal ectoparasites (52).

Canine Scabies

Sarcoptes scabiei var. *canis* causes canine scabies (sarcoptic mange), a nonseasonal pruritic transmissible infestation of the skin of dogs which is transmissible to humans. The adult female mite penetrates to the level of the stratum granulosum, where she feeds. She deposits her eggs in a burrow; the eggs hatch and give rise to the larval form. The larvae migrate to the surface and molt through nymphal and adult forms. Eggs develop into adult mites in 10 to 21 days.

Canine scabies has no age, sex, or breed preferences and is characterized by intense pruritis which is followed by an erythematous, nonfollicular papular dermatitis. These lesions, frequently found on the pinnae, face, limbs, and ventrolateral trunk, become excoriated and crusted. In the absence of early diagnosis or treatment, extension of these lesions may involve the entire animal, with accompanying alopecia (105). It is thought that prolonged skin to skin exposure is important for transmission to take place from a dog to a human being; 30 to 50% of human contacts of a canine case may be affected.

Hypersensitivity appears to play a role in canine and human scabies. In both species, dermatologic manifestations are out of proportion to the number of mites present. There is significant evidence that the immune system participates in the pathogenesis of this disease (94).

Diagnosis is generally established by history, clinical findings, or response to scabicides, since human skin scrapings frequently fail to demonstrate scabietic mites. Canine scrapings are more often positive, but in one study only 51% of canine scrapings were positive for ova or mites (94).

There is no correlation between the severity and duration of the canine disease and transmission to humans. The lesions in humans consist of vesicles, erythematous papules, wheals, crusts, and excoriations occurring in areas of pet contact. Therefore, it is seen especially on the arms, legs, abdomen, and chest. Unlike with human scabies, there are no burrows and no involvement of the hands, finger webs, or genitalia. Human infestation often occurs in small epidemics (97).

The severity of the eruption and its extent and duration can vary considerably. Generally the lesions are self-limiting without treatment after the infected animal has been separated. Human scabies and papular urticaria are the main conditions to be differentiated from canine scabies in humans. The history of exposure to an infested pet, the different distribution pattern, the lack of burrows, and demonstration of the causative organism on examination of the pet will aid in making the diagnosis.

Canine scabies is easily treated with weekly application of scabicidal dips (especially lindane or lime sulfur) until 2 weeks after clinical cure is achieved (94). All dogs in a household or in-contact dogs should be treated. In addition, a single washing of fomites in hot water and detergent is recommended.

Although many authors feel that human infestation is a self-limiting disease, there have been some reports indicating that this may not be the case (94). Successful treatment of humans has been achieved with a 24-h application of γ-benzene hexachloride cream. Permethrin is highly effective and relatively nontoxic. Orally administered ivermectin appears to be effective as a scabicide. Alternative scabicides, including benzyl benzoate, crotamine cream, and sulfur ointment, may be preferred for infants, pregnant women, or unsupervised mass treatments (98). Steroids are of value in those patients with severe inflammatory reactions, and antibiotics are indicated for those who develop secondary bacterial infections.

Cheyletiellosis

Cheyletiella dermatitis ("walking dandruff") is a nonseasonal, variably pruritic, transmissible infestation of the skin of dogs and cats caused by mites. In general, *C. yasguri* is considered the species affecting dogs.

These mites do not burrow but live in skin surface keratin. They move about rapidly but occasionally pierce the skin with their hooks and become engorged with tissue fluids (94).

Like with scabies, there is no apparent predilection for breed or sex. Pruritus is a variable finding, but there is usually some degree of dorsal scaling, crusting, and dermatitis (94). Adult dogs can be symptomatic carriers of mites, but puppies are most often clinically affected.

Skin lesions produced by *Cheyletiella* mites in human beings have been reported, with human involvement occurring in 20 to 80% of canine cases. In humans, the lesions begin as single or grouped erythematous macules which rapidly evolve into papules; these lesions frequently become vesicular or pustular. Old lesions develop a very characteristic central necrosis, which is of diagnostic significance. The pruritus may be intense and involve any portion of the body, but rarely the face. Other eruptions that may be produced by these mites include bullae, urticaria, erythema multiforme, and generalized pruritus without dermatitis.

Diagnosis is based on historical and physical findings, positive skin scrapings or Scotch tape preparations, and response to miticidal agents. Skin scrapings from humans are rarely positive.

Human infestations are self-limiting; *Cheyletiella* mites are unable to complete their life cycle on humans. The source of mites must be removed or treated with topical miticides. Dogs in contact with affected animals must be treated, and their environment must be vigorously cleaned. The human dermatoses should resolve in 3 weeks without specific treatment.

Fleas

Fleas can cause asymptomatic infestation or severe hypersensitivity skin disease in dogs and humans. In the United States, the genera of most importance are

Ctenocephalides and *Pulex* (94). Although flea bites in humans are generally trivial and not more than a nuisance, they may play a role in the transmission of systemic disease such as *Bartonella henselae* infection (103).

Hypersensitivity to flea salivary antigens plays a critical role in dermatoses. The typical lesion on human beings is an urticarial papule. Lesions favor exposed distal extremities and are extremely pruritic.

In diagnosing human flea bites, it is important to demonstrate fleas in the environment. This is often done by having the patient walk through infested areas wearing white knee socks to better visualize the fleas.

Treatment involves flea control measures as well as topical or systemic anti-inflammatory medication (if reaction is severe). Effective flea control requires treatment of the affected pets, their areas, and other animal contacts. Flea bombs or sprays are needed to kill larval forms and prevent reinfection. Pets should not be allowed to forage in areas where *Yersinia pestis* is prevalent.

MEASURES TO MINIMIZE DOG-ASSOCIATED ILLNESS

- Children should not be left unattended with dogs, unfamiliar dogs should be avoided, and feeding or sleeping dogs should not be startled.
- Dogs should be vaccinated for rabies and possibly for leptospirosis.
- Prophylaxis for dirofilariasis should be given in areas of endemicity.
- Newly acquired puppies should be treated for intestinal parasites before being taken into the home.
- Dogs should not be permitted to defecate on beaches or playgrounds, and animal feces on lawns should be removed at least weekly. Sand in public parks should be turned over frequently.
- Feces should not be used as fertilizer.
- Dogs should not be allowed to eat offal.
- Hands should be washed after animals are handled, and diarrhea in pets should cause increased attention to hygiene.
- Animals should be regularly inspected for fleas and ticks.

REFERENCES

1. **Aghababian, R. V., and J. E. Conte, Jr.** 1980. Mammalian bite wounds. *Ann. Emerg. Med.* **9:**79–83.
2. **Allos, B. M., and M. J. Blaser.** 2002. Campylobacter species, p. 157–168. *In* V. L. Yu, R. Weber, and D. Raoult (ed.), *Antimicrobial Therapy and Vaccines,* 2nd ed., vol. 1. Apple Trees Productions, LLC, New York, N.Y.
3. **Anders, B. J., B. A. Lauer, J. W. Paisley, and L. B. Reller.** 1982. Double-blind placebo controlled trial of erythromycin for treatment of Campylobacter enteritis. *Lancet* **i:**131–132.
4. **Anderson, B. E., J. E. Dawson, D. L. Jones, and K. H. Wilson.** 1991. Ehrlichia chaffeensis, a new species associated with human ehrlichiosis. *J. Clin. Microbiol.* **29:**2838–2842.
5. **Bakken, J. S., and J. S. Dumler.** 2000. Human granulocytic ehrlichiosis. *Clin. Infect. Dis.* **31:**554–560.

6. **Bartsocas, C. S., A. Von Graevenitz, and F. Blodgett.** 1966. *Dipylidium* infection in 6-month-old infant. *J. Pediatr.* **69:**814–815.

7. **Benerjee, T. K., W. Grubb, C. Otero, M. McKee, B. O. Brady, and N. W. Barton.** 1993. Musculocutaneous mononeuropathy complicating *Capnocytophaga canimorsus* infection. *Neurology* **43:** 2411–2412.

8. **Bert, F., and N. Lambert-Zechovsky.** 1997. Septicemia caused by *Streptococcus canis* in a human. *J. Clin. Microbiol.* **35:**777–779.

9. **Blaser, M. J., D. N. Taylor, and R. A. Feldman.** 1983. Epidemiology of *Campylobacter jejuni* infections. *Epidemiol. Rev.* **5:**157–176.

10. **Blaser, M. J., J. Cravens, B. W. Powers, and W. L. Wang.** 1978. Campylobacter enteritis associated with canine infection. *Lancet* **ii:**979–981.

11. **Blaser, M. J., and L. B. Reller.** 1981. Campylobacter enteritis. *N. Engl. J. Med.* **305:**1444–1452.

12. **Bradshaw, S.** 2003. Endocarditis due to *Staphylococcus aureus* after minor dog bite. *South. Med. J.* **96:**407–409.

13. **Buhariwalla, F., B. Cann, and T. J. Marrie.** 1996. A dog-related outbreak of Q fever. *Clin. Infect. Dis.* **23:**753–755.

14. **Butler, T.** 1998. Borrelia species and Spirillum minus, p. 1946–1952. *In* S. L. Gorbach, J. G. Bartlett, and N. R. Blacklow (ed.), *Infectious Diseases*, 2nd ed. W. B. Saunders Company, Philadelphia, Pa.

14a.**Centers for Disease Control and Prevention.** 2003. Nonfatal dog bite-related injuries treated in hospital emergency departments—United States, 2001. *Morb. Mortal. Wkly. Rep.* **52:**605–610.

15. **Centers for Disease Control and Prevention.** 2002. Guidelines for preventing opportunistic infections among HIV-infected persons—2002. *Morb. Mortal. Wkly. Rep.* **51:**1–46.

16. **Chang, H. J., H. L. Miller, N. Watkins, M. J. Arduino, D. A. Ashford, G. Midgley, S. M. Aguero, R. Pinto-Powell, F. Von Reyn, W. Edwards, M. M. McNeil, and W. R. Jarvis.** 1998. An epidemic of *Malassezia pachydermatis* in an intensive care nursery associated with colonization of health care workers' pet dogs. *N. Engl. J. Med.* **338:**706–711.

17. **Chappell, C. L., and H. M. Penn.** 1990. *Dipylidium caninum*, an underrecognized infection in infants and children. *Pediatr. Infect. Dis. J.* **9:**745–747.

18. **Chen, X. M., J. S. Keithly, C. V. Paya, and N. F. LaRusso.** 2002. Cryptosporidiosis. *N. Engl. J. Med.* **1346:**1723–1731.

19. **Ciferri, F.** 1982. Human pulmonary dirofilariasis in the United States: a critical review. *Am. J. Trop. Med. Hyg.* **31:**302–303.

20. **Cook, G. C.** 1989. Canine-associated zoonoses: an unacceptable hazard to human health. *Q. J. Med.* **70:**5–26.

21. **Current, W. L., N. C. Reese, J. V. Ernest, W. S. Bailey, M. B. Heyman, and W. M. Weinstein.** 1983. Human cryptosporidiosis in immunocompetent and immunodeficient persons. *N. Engl. J. Med.* **308:**1252–1286.

22. **Current, W. L.** 1988. The biology of *Cryptosporidium*. *ASM News* **54:**605–611.

23. **Currier, R. W., W. F. Raithel, R. J. Martin, and M. E. Potter.** 1982. Canine brucellosis. *J. Am. Vet. Med. Assoc.* **180:**132–133.

24. **Dawson, J. E., B. E. Anderson, D. B. Fishbein, J. L. Sanchez, C. S. Goldsmith, K. H. Wilson, and C. W. Duntley.** 1991. Isolation and characterization of an *Ehrlichia* sp. from a patient diagnosed with human ehrlichiosis. *J. Clin. Microbiol.* **29:**2741–2745.

25. **Dayal, Y., and R. C. Neafie.** 1975. Human pulmonary dirofilariasis: a case report and review of the literature. *Am. Rev. Respir. Dis.* **112:**437–443.

26. **Dumler, J. S., and J. S. Bakken.** 1995. Ehrlichial diseases of humans: emerging tick-borne infections. *Clin. Infect. Dis.* **20:**1102–1110.

27. **Dumler, J.S., and J. S. Bakken.** 1998. Human ehrlichiosis: newly recognized infections transmitted by ticks. *Annu. Rev. Med.* **49:**201–213.

27a.**Dunn, J. J., S. T. Columbus, W. E. Aldeen, M. Davis, and K. C. Carroll.** 2002. *Trichuris vulpis* recovered from a patient with chronic diarrhea and five dogs. *J. Clin. Microbiol.* **40:**2703–2704.

28. **Edwards, G. A., and B. M. Domm.** 1960. Human leptospirosis. *Medicine* (Baltimore) **39:**117–156.

29. **Ehrbar, H. U., J. Gubler, S. Harbarth, and B. Hirschel.** 1996. *Capnocytophaga canimorsus* sepsis complicated by myocardial infarction in two patients with normal coronary arteries. *Clin. Infect. Dis.* **23:**335–336.

30. **Elenbaas, R. M., W. K. McNabney, and W. A. Robinson.** 1981. Prophylactic antibiotics and dog bite wounds. *JAMA* **246:**833–834.

31. **Elliot, D. L., S. W. Tolle, L. Goldberg, and J. B. Miller.** 1985. Pet-associated illness. *N. Engl. J. Med.* **313:**985–995.

32. **Fang, G., V. Araujo, and R. L. Guerrant.** 1991. Enteric infections associated with exposure to animals or animal products. *Infect. Dis. Clin. N. Am.* **5:**681–700.

33. **Fayer, R., and B. L. P. Ungar.** 1986. *Cryptosporidium* spp. and cryptosporidiosis. *Microbiol. Rev.* **50:**458–483.

34. **Feigin, R. D., L. A. Lober, D. Anderson, and L. Pickering.** 1973. Human leptospirosis from immunized dogs. *Ann. Intern. Med.* **79:**777–785.

35. **Friedmann, E., A. H. Katcher, J. J. Lynch, and S. A. Thomas.** 1980. Animal companions and one-year survival of patients after discharge from a coronary care unit. *Public Health Rep.* **95:**307–312.

36. **Galton, M. M., J. E. Scatterday, and A. V. Hardy.** 1952. Salmonellosis in dogs. *J. Infect. Dis.* **91:**1–5.

37. **Georgi, J. R.** 1987. Tapeworms. *Vet. Clin. N. Am. Small Anim. Pract.* **17:**1285–1305.

38. **Glaser, C. A., F. J. Angulo, and J. A. Rooney.** 1994. Animal-associated opportunistic infections among persons infected with the human immunodeficiency virus. *Clin. Infect. Dis.* **18:**14–24.

39. **Glickman, L. T., and F. S. Shofer.** 1987. Zoonotic visceral and ocular larva migrans. *Vet. Clin. N. Am. Small Anim. Pract.* **17:**39–53.

40. **Glickman, L. T., P. M. Schantz, and R. H. Cypress.** 1979. Canine and human toxocariasis: review of transmission, pathogenesis and clinical disease. *J. Am. Vet. Med. Assoc.* **175:**1265–1269.

41. **Glickman, L. T., and P. M. Schantz.** 1981. Epidemiology and pathogenesis of zoonotic toxocariasis. *Epidemiol. Rev.* **3:**230–250.

42. **Gnann, J. W., G. S. Bressler, C. A. Bodet, and C. K. Avent.** 1983. Human blastomycosis after a dog bite. *Ann. Intern. Med.* **98:**48–49.

43. **Goldstein, E. J. C., D. M. Citron, B. Wield, V. Blachman, V. L. Sutter, T. A. Miller, and S. M. Finegold.** 1978. Bacteriology of human and animal bite wounds. *J. Clin. Microbiol.* **8:**667–672.

44. **Goldstein, E. J. C.** 1991. Household pets and human infections. *Infect. Dis. Clin. N. Am.* **5:**117–130.

45. **Goldstein, E. J. C.** 1999. Current concepts on animal bites: bacteriology and therapy. *Curr. Clin. Top. Infect. Dis.* **19:**99–111.

46. **Grove, D. I., K. S. Warren, and A. A. F. Mahmoud.** 1976. Algorithms in the diagnosis and management of exotic diseases. X. Echinococcosis. *J. Infect. Dis.* **133:**354–358.

47. **Hald, B., and M. Madsen.** 1997. Healthy puppies and kittens as carriers of *Campylobacter* spp., with special reference to *Campylobacter upsaliensis. J. Clin. Microbiol.* **35:**3351–3352.

48. **Hall, W. H.** 1990. Modern chemotherapy for brucellosis in humans. *Rev. Infect. Dis.* **12:**1060–1099.

49. **Harrison, E. G., Jr., and J. H. Thompson.** 1965. Dirofilariasis of human lung. *Am. J. Clin. Path.* **43:**224–234.

50. **Hasi, D. K., J. A. Collins, and S. C. Flick.** 1978. Canine parasitism. *Canine Pract.* **2:**42–47.

51. **Havin, T. R., and D. D. Juranek.** 1984. Cryptosporidiosis: clinical, epidemiologic and parasitologic review. *Rev. Infect. Dis.* **6:**313–327.

52. **Hewitt, M., G. S. Walton, and M. Waterhouse.** 1971. Pet animal infestations and human skin lesions. *Br. J. Dermatol.* **85:**215–225.

53. **Hicklin, H., A. Verghese, and S. Alvarez.** 1987. Dysgonic fermenter-2 septicemia. *Rev. Infect. Dis.* **9:**884–890.

54. **Humbert, P., S. Buchet, and T. Barde.** 1995. Toxocariasis: a cosmopolitan parasitic zoonosis. *Allerg. Immunol.* (Paris) **27:**284–291.

55. **Huntley, C. C., M. C. Costos, A. Lyerly.** 1965. Visceral larva migrans syndrome: clinical characteristics and immunologic studies in 51 patients. *Pediatrics* **36:**523–536.

56. **Jacquier, P., B. Gottstein, Y. Stingelin, and J. Eckert.** 1991. Immunodiagnosis of toxocariasis in humans: evolution of a new enzyme-linked immunosorbent assay kit. *J. Clin. Microbiol.* **29:**1831–1835.

57. **Juckett, G.** 1997. Pets and parasites. *Am. Fam. Physician* **56:**1763–1774.

58. **Kaldor, J., and B. R. Speed.** 1984. Guillain-Barré syndrome and *Campylobacter jejuni:* a serologic study. *Br. Med. J.* **288:**1867–1870.

59. **Katz, R., J. Ziegler, and H. Blank.** 1965. The natural course of creeping eruption and treatment with thiabendazole. *Arch. Dermatol.* **91:**420.

60. **Khuroo, M. S., N. A. Wani, G. Javid, B. A. Khan, G. N. Yattoo, A. H. Shah, and S. G. Jeelani.** 1997. Percutaneous drainage compared with surgery for hepatic hydatid cysts. *N. Engl. J. Med.* **337:**881–887.

61. **Khuroo, M. S., S. A. Zargar, and R. Mahajan.** 1991. Echinococcus granulosus cyst in the liver: management with percutaneous drainage. *Radiology* **180:**141–145.

62. **Khuroo, M. S., M. Y. Dar, G. N. Yattoo, S. A. Zargar, G. Javaid, B. A. Khan, and M. I. Boda.** 1993. Percutaneous drainage versus albendazole therapy in hepatic hydatidosis: a prospective, randomized study. *Gastroenterology* **104:**1452–1459.

63. **Kosunen, T. U., O. Kauranen, J. Martio, T. P. Aponka, L. Hortling, S. Aittoniemi, O. Penttila, and S. Koskimies.** 1980. Reactive arthritis after *Campylobacter jejuni* enteritis in patients with HLA-B27. *Lancet* i:1312–1313.

64. **Lauer, E. A., W. C. White, and B. A. Lauer.** 1982. Dog bites: a neglected problem in accident prevention. *Am. J. Dis. Child.* **136:**202–204.

65. **Liu, L. X., and P. F. Weller.** 1998. Trichinosis and infections with other tissue nematodes, p. 1206–1208. *In* A. S. Fauci, E. Braunwald, K. J. Isselbacher, J. D. Wilson, J. B. Martin, D. L. Kasper, S. L. Hauser, and D. L. Longo (ed.), *Harrison's Principles of Internal Medicine.* McGraw-Hill, New York, N.Y.

66. **Margolis, B.** 1983. Dog tapeworm infestation in an infant. *Am. J. Dis. Child.* **137:**702.

67. **Marty, P.** 1997. Human dirofilariasis due to *Dirofilaria repens* in France. A review of reported cases. *Parasitologia* **39:**383–386.

68. **Mayer, G., and S. VanOre.** 1983. Recurrent pharyngitis in family of four. *Postgrad. Med.* **74:**277–279.

69. **McClain, J. B., W. R. Ballou, S. M. Harrison, and D. L. Steinweg.** 1984. Doxycycline for leptospirosis. *Ann. Intern. Med.* **100:**696–698.

70. **McDade, J. E.** 1990. Ehrlichiosis—a disease of animals and humans. *J. Infect. Dis.* **161:**609–617.

71. **Merrill, J. R., J. Otis, W. D. Logan, Jr., and B. Davis.** 1980. The dog heartworm (*Dirofilaria immitis*) in man: an epidemic pending or in progress? *JAMA* **243:**1066–1068.

72. **Mohamed, A. E., M. I. Yasawy, and M. A. Al Karawi.** 1998. Combined albendazole and praziquantel versus albendazole alone in the treatment of hydatid disease. *Hepato-Gastroenterology* **45:**1690–1694.

73. **Molina, C. P., J. Ogburn, and P. Adegboyega.** 2003. Infection by *Dipylidium caninum* in an infant. *Arch. Pathol. Lab. Med.* **127:**e157–e159.

74. **Mulder, A. H., P. G. Gerlag, L. H. Verhoef, and A. W. van den Wall Bake.** 2001. Hemolytic uremic syndrome after Capnocytophaga canimorsus (DF-2) septicemia. *Clin. Nephrol.* **55:**167–170.

75. **Nerad, J. L., M. T. Seville, and D. R. Snydman.** 1998. Miscellaneous gram-negative bacilli: Acinetobacter, Cardiobacterium, Actinobacillus, Chromobacterium, Capnocytophaga, and others, p. 1871–1887. *In* S. L. Gorbach, J. G. Bartlett, and N. R. Blacklow (ed.), *Infectious Diseases*, 2nd ed. W. B. Saunders Company, Philadelphia, Pa.

76. **Newton, N. L., and B. Sharma.** 1986. Case report: acute myocardial infarction associated with DF-2 bacteremia after a dog bite. *Am. J. Med. Sci.* **291:**352–354.

77. **Nutman, T. B., and P. F. Weller.** 1998. Cestodes, p. 1224–1227. *In* A. S. Fauci, E. Braunwald, K. J. Isselbacher, J. D. Wilson, J. B. Martin, D. L. Kasper, S. L. Hauser, and D. L. Longo (ed.), *Harrison's Principles of Internal Medicine.* McGraw-Hill, New York, N.Y.

78. **Olsen, S. J., E. E. DeBess, T. E. McGivern, N. Marano, T. Eby, S. Mauvais, V. K. Balan, G. Zirnstein, P. R. Cieslak, and F. J. Angulo.** 2001. A nosocomial outbreak of fluoroquinolone-resistant Salmonella infection. *N. Engl. J. Med.* **344:**1572–1579.

79. **Ortiz, J. J., A. Ayoub, and N. L. Gargala.** 2001. Randomized clinical study of nitazoxanide compared to metronidazole in the treatment of symptomatic giardiasis in children from northern Peru. *Aliment. Pharmacol. Ther.* **15:**1409–1415.

80. **Paderes, C., C. Zanartu, and G. Castillo.** 2001. Environmental contamination with Toxocara sp. eggs in public squares and parks from Santiago, Chile, 1999. *Bol. Chil. Parasitol.* **55:**86–91.

81. **Perez, M., Y. Rikihisa, and B. Wen.** 1996. *Ehrlichia canis*-like agent isolated from a man in Venezuela: antigenic and genetic characterization. *J. Clin. Microbiol.* **34:**2133–2139.

82. **Piampiano, P., M. McLeary, L. W. Young, and D. Janner.** 2000. Brucellosis: unusual presentations in two adolescent boys. *Pediatr. Radiol.* **30:**355–357.

83. Polt, S. S., W. E. Dismukes, A. Flint, and J. Schaefer. 1982. Human brucellosis caused by *Brucella canis*: clinical features and immune response. *Ann. Intern. Med.* **97:**717–719.

84. Puylaert, J. B., R. J. Vermeijden, S. D. van der Werf, L. Doornbos, and R. K. Koumans. 1989. Incidence and sonographic diagnosis of bacterial ileocaecitis masquerading as appendicitis. *Lancet* ii:84–86.

85. Rossignol, J. F., A. Ayoub, and M. S. Ayers. 2001. Treatment of diarrhea caused by *Cryptosporidium parvum*: a prospective randomized, double-blind, placebo-controlled study of nitazoxanide. *J. Infect. Dis.* **184:**103–106.

86. Rubel, D., A. Seijo, B. Cernigoi, A. Viale, and C. Wisnivesky-Colli. 1997. Leptospira interrogans in a canine population of Greater Buenos Aires: variables associated with seropositivity. *Pan Am. J. Public Health* **2:**102–105.

87. Salfield, N. J., and E. J. Pugh. 1987. Campylobacter enteritis in young children living in households with puppies. *Br. Med. J.* **294:**21–22.

88. Sauret, J. M., and N. Vilissova. 2002. Human brucellosis. *J. Am. Board Fam. Pract.* **15:**401–406.

89. Sawyer, L. A., D. B. Fishbein, and J. E. McDade. 1987. Q fever: current concepts. *Rev. Infect. Dis.* **9:**935–946.

90. Schaefer, J. W., and Y. M. Khan. 1991. Echinococcus (hydatid disease): lessons from experience with 59 patients. *Rev. Infect. Dis.* **13:**243–247.

91. Schantz, P. M., and L. T. Glickman. 1978. Toxocaral visceral larva migrans. *N. Engl. J. Med.* **298:**436–439.

92. Schieven, B. C., M. Brennan, and Z. Hussain. 1991. *Echinococcus granulosus* hydatid disease. *ASM News* **57:**407–410.

93. Schmidt, D. R., R. E. Winn, and T. J. Keefe. 1989. Leptospirosis: epidemiologic features of a sporadic case. *Arch. Intern. Med.* **149:**1878–1880.

94. Scott, D. W., and R. T. Horn, Jr. 1987. Zoonotic dermatoses of dogs and cats. *Vet. Clin. N. Am. Small Anim. Pract.* **17:**117–144.

95. Scully, R., E. J. Mark, W. F. McNeely, and B. U. McNeely. 1987. Case records of the Massachusetts General Hospital, case 45-1987. *N. Engl. J. Med.* **317:**1209–1218.

96. Senneville, E., F. Ajana, P. Lecocq, C. Chidiac, and Y. Mouton. 1991. *Rickettsia conorii* isolated from ticks introduced to northern France by a dog. *Lancet* **337:**676.

97. Smith, E. B., and T. F. Claypoole. 1967. Canine scabies in dogs and in humans. *JAMA* **199:**95–100.

98. Spielman, A., and M. Wachtel. 1998. Arthropods, p. 2499–2513. *In* S. L. Gorbach, J. G. Bartlett, and N. R. Blacklow (ed.), *Infectious Diseases*, 2nd ed. W. B. Saunders Company, Philadelphia, Pa.

99. Stehr-Green, J. K., G. Murray, P. M. Schantz, and S. P. Wahlquist. 1987. Intestinal parasites in pet store puppies in Atlanta. *Am. J. Public Health* **77:**345–346.

100. Takafuji, E. T., J. W. Kirkpatrick, R. N. Miller, J. J. Karwacki, P. W. Kelley, M. R. Gray, K. M. McNeil, H. L. Timboe, R. E. Kane, and J. L. Sanchez. 1984. An efficacy trial of doxycycline chemoprophylaxis against leptospirosis. *N. Engl. J. Med.* **310:**497–500.

101. Takeda, N., K. Kikuchi, R. Asano, T. Harada, K. Totsuka, T. Sumiyoshi, T. Uchiyama, and S. Hosoda. 2001. Recurrent septicemia caused by Streptococcus canis after a dog bite. *Scand. J. Infect. Dis.* **33:**927–928.

102. Talan, D. A., D. M. Citron, F. M. Abrahamian, G. J. Moran, E. J. C. Goldstein, and the Emergency Medicine Animal Bite Study Group. 1999. Bacteriologic analysis of infected dog and cat bites. *N. Engl. J. Med.* **34:**85–92.

103. Tan, J. S. 1997. Human zoonotic infections transmitted by dogs and cats. *Arch. Intern. Med.* **157:**1933–1943.

104. Taylor, D. H., and D. L. Morris. 1989. Combination chemotherapy is more effective in post spillage prophylaxis for hydatid disease than either albendazole or praziquantel alone. *Br. J. Surg.* **76:**954.

105. Thomsett, L. R. 1968. Mite infestations of man contracted from dogs and cats. *Br. Med. J.* **3:**93–95.

106. Todorov, T., K. Vutoa, D. Petkov, G. Mechkov, and K. Kolev. 1988. Albendazole treatment of human cystic echinococcosis. *Trans. R. Soc. Trop. Med. Hyg.* **82:**453–459.

107. Tsung, S. H., J. I. Lin, and D. Han. 1982. Pulmonary dirofilariasis in man. *Am. J. Med. Sci.* **283:**106–110.

108. **Turner, J. A.** 1962. Human dipylidiasis (dog tapeworm infection) in the United States. *J. Pediatr.* **61:**763–768.
109. **Tzipori, S., and I. Campbell.** 1981. Prevalence of *Cryptosporidium* antibodies in 10 animal species. *J. Clin. Microbiol.* **14:**455–456.
110. **Weber, D. J., and A. R. Hansen.** 1991. Infections resulting from animal bites. *Infect. Dis. Clin. N. Am.* **5:**663–680.
111. **Weiss, H. B., D. I. Friedman, and J. H. Coben.** 1998. Incidence of dog bite injuries treated in emergency departments. *JAMA* **279:**51–53.
112. **Whiting, D. A.** 1976. The successful treatment of creeping eruption with topical thiabendazole. *S. Afr. Med. J.* **50:**253–255.
113. **WHO Informal Working Group on Echinococcosis.** 1996. Guidelines for treatment of cystic and alveolar echinococcosis in humans. *Bull. W. H. O.* **74:**231–242.
114. **Willard, M. D., B. Sugarman, and R. D. Walker.** 1987. Gastrointestinal zoonoses. *Vet. Clin. N. Am. Small Anim. Pract.* **17:**145–178.
115. **Wilson, J. F., A. C. Diddams, and R. L. Rausch.** 1968. Cystic hydatid disease in Alaska. *Am. Rev. Respir. Dis.* **98:**1–15.
116. **Wilson, K. S., S. Antone, and R. M. Gander.** 1995. The family pet as an unlikely source of group A beta-hemolytic streptococcal infection in humans. *Pediatr. Infect. Dis. J.* **14:**372–375.

Infections of Leisure, Third Edition
Edited by David Schlossberg
© 2004 ASM Press, Washington, D.C.

Chapter 6

Around Cats

Ellie J. C. Goldstein and Craig E. Greene

The origins of the domestic cat are unknown. However, mummified cats have been found in the treasure rooms of the Egyptian pyramids, and their images are inscribed in the royal hieroglyphics. The genus *Felis* includes the modern domestic house cat as well as the puma (cougar), golden cats, jaguarundi, ocelot, serval, lynx, and bobcat. Today it is estimated that more than 56 million cats are kept as household pets in the United States and that 31% of households own cats (43). There are numerous diseases which may be transmitted from cats to humans or that cats and people acquire from common sources, some of which are described in this chapter (5, 16, 26). However, it is likely that the domestic cat can act as a reservoir for many other zoonoses that are as yet unrecognized. The diseases discussed are arranged by the general method of transmission from cat to person, although more than one route is possible for certain infections.

INHALATION

Bordetellosis

Bordetella bronchiseptica is a gram-negative coccobacillus that causes a pertussis-like illness (whooping cough) in humans, especially children. It can be found in the respiratory tract of clinically healthy or ill animals, including laboratory and domestic cats. While a cough is common in dogs infected with *B. bronchiseptica* (kennel cough), it is usually much less prominent in infected cats, which manifest disease by fever, nasal discharge, sneezing, submandibular lymphadenomegaly, and lethargy. If a cat exhibits cough, it may be associated with pneumonia. Vaccines are available for protection of cats against this pathogen; an attenuated intranasal product has only recently been licensed in the United States, and one genetically engineered product was once, but is no longer, available in Europe.

Ellie J. C. Goldstein • R. M. Alden Research Laboratory, Santa Monica, CA 90404, and UCLA School of Medicine, Los Angeles, CA 90024. *Craig E. Greene* • Department of Small Animal Medicine, College of Veterinary Medicine, University of Georgia, Athens, GA 30602.

Humans, especially immunocompromised hosts such as those with human immunodeficiency virus (HIV) infection (AIDS), may infrequently acquire disease from cats and may manifest illness from mild upper respiratory symptoms to frank pneumonia (12). The organism is difficult to cultivate on routine media and may be misidentified by human clinical laboratories. By the time humans become adults, the possible cross-immunity that can be developed because of pertussis vaccination in childhood is most likely to have waned to nonprotective levels.

Plague

Plague is caused by *Yersinia pestis*, a gram-negative coccobacillus. While cat fleas are considered poor vectors for transmission, domestic and wild cats may contract this disease, usually in the summer months (9). Cats are exposed via ingestion of an infected rodent or by their fleas. Cats manifest plague in the same way as humans, with either the bubonic, septicemic, or pneumonic form. In 1996, there were five human cases of plague reported in the United States, two of which were fatal and one in which there was exposure to an infected pet cat (5). Between 1970 and 1995, five persons infected by inhalation were known to be exposed to infected domestic cats (5). This illness is covered further in chapter 9.

Q Fever

Cats may be infected with *Coxiella burnetii*, the rickettsia which causes Q fever. Cat infection may ensue from a tick bite, ingestion of infected body tissues, or inhalation of organisms in a contaminated environment. Most cats are asymptomatic, although in pregnant queens, abortion or birth of stillborn or weak kittens has been observed. Experimentally infected cats maintained *C. burnetii* in their blood for 1 month and excreted it in their urine for 2 months (16). *C. burnetii* has also been isolated from infected cat uteri postpartum. Seroprevalence studies in various parts of the world have shown exposure to *C. burnetii* in 15 to 20% of cats. Humans may occasionally become infected from cats by direct exposure to or inhalation of infected material from parturient or aborted tissue from infected cats.

VECTOR-BORNE SPREAD

Ehrlichiosis

Ehrlichiae are obligate intracellular, rickettsial organisms causing tick-borne disease in many animals and in humans. At least three species of *Ehrlichia* (especially *Ehrlichia chaffeensis* and *Ehrlichia ewingii*) and *Anaplasma phagocytophilum* cause diseases in humans, and these diseases are collectively referred to as "human ehrlichiosis." Some *Ehrlichia* species cross infect mammalian hosts, so cats may serve as reservoirs or sentinels for human infection. Cats can be experimentally infected by intravenous, but not subcutaneous, inoculation with *Ehrlichia equi* and *Ehrlichia risticii;* however, another species observed in feline leukocytes has not yet been identified. Experimental and natural *A. phagocytophilum* infection in cats has been described (4a, 13). This organism can cause a febrile illness. Routes of transmission between cats are unknown, and transmission from cats to humans has not (as yet) been documented.

CSD

Cat scratch disease (CSD) is worldwide in distribution, and in temperate climates there is a fall and winter prevalence (1, 38). A prospective population-based study in Connecticut in 1992 to 1993 found a statewide annual incidence of 3.7/100,000 persons (18). It often affects children (median age, 14 years) and persons <21 years old (80% of cases). In the Connecticut study, the age-specific attack rate was highest for persons <10 years old (9.3/100,000) and decreased with increasing age (18). Exposure was usually associated with a young, newly acquired or stray cat and not usually with longtime pets. Injury has occurred as a bite, scratch, or licks. Approximately 1 week after injury (range, 3 to 10 days), a primary inoculation papule or pustule (0.5 to 1 cm), which often goes unnoticed, may appear at the site of injury in 25 to 60% of patients. The papule may become vesicular and may crust. Subsequent to the inoculation papule, 5 to 120 days later (average, 2 weeks), tender, regional adenopathy may develop. Adenopathy, which often lasts >3 weeks, may be the only symptom in half the cases and suppurates in approximately 15% of cases. Since this is usually a benign and usually self-limiting disease (6 to 12 weeks) in immunocompetent individuals, it often goes unnoticed or unreported. Some healthy patients experience a "flu-like" illness. Most patients who seek medical attention will present because of the adenopathy, especially if it involves the head and neck area and/or fever (low grade, 50% of patients). Consequently, the differential diagnosis often centers on these problems. Depending on the area of the adenopathy, various diseases should be excluded, including streptococcal pharyngitis, infectious mononucleosis, toxoplasmosis, cytomegalovirus infection, syphilis, lymphogranuloma venereum, cellulitis, Hodgkin's disease, dental abscess, etc.

Accompanying symptoms include fatigue and malaise (28%), fever (101 to 106°F) (31%), splenomegaly (12%), exanthema (4%), parotid swelling (2%), and seizures (1 to 2%). Other syndromes include ocular granuloma (Perinaud's oculoglandular syndrome—conjunctival granuloma, periauricular adenopathy, and nonsuppurative conjunctivitis), erythema nodosum, thrombocytopenic purpura, figurate erythema, osteomyelitis, pneumonia, and liver abscesses. The most serious complication is the development of acute encephalopathy and altered consciousness. Spontaneous recovery is usual with encephalopathy as well, usually within 2 weeks. Endocarditis due to *Bartonella quintana* has been reported for homeless men and those exposed to cats and their fleas; *Bartonella henselae* has also been reported as an unusual cause of endocarditis in humans (7, 8, 36). In human bartonellosis, atypical cases can occur, and immunocompromised patients may have diverse and unusual manifestations (2) (see "Bacillary [Epithelioid] Angiomatosis" below).

Cats are the natural reservoir host for *B. henselae*, and it produces an intra-erythrocytic subclinical bacteremia. The organism was isolated from the blood of

~40% of a covenant of cats in San Francisco, Calif. (6). Naturally infected cats can maintain bacteremia for several months, although the organism can cause endocarditis (8). Impounded or formerly stray cats were more likely to be bactermic than long-term domestic pet cats. Other factors associated with bacteremia are the presence of fleas (which can readily transmit *Bartonella* from one cat to another) and cat age of <1 year. Cats develop increasing immunity to infection with age, which may occur from natural exposure to the organism. Limited trials have shown that cats can be treated for *Bartonella* infection, as are humans, with a similar variety of antimicrobials (tetracyclines, quinolones, etc.) (17).

Diagnosis is often made on clinical grounds. A history of feline contact (usually an immature cat) and, if possible, the identification of an inoculation site should be sought. Other diagnostic possibilities should be excluded. If there is an unusual reason to pursue the diagnosis, then a lymph node biopsy sample showing granulomatous formation, preferably with stellate microabscesses, is supportive. The modified Warthin-Starry stain of the node may show organisms but is difficult to interpret in many pathology laboratories due to the infrequency of its use, the unavailability of positive controls, and a variety of other technical factors. Isolation of the organism from human specimens is ideal but is also technically difficult for most laboratories even with the correct media. In contrast, isolation from infected cats is quite rewarding due to the high numbers of organisms. The organism is a slow-growing (2 to 3 weeks), fastidious gram-negative bacterium. It grows on chocolate agar as well as CDC agar. The colonies are small, nonhemolytic, rough, dry, and yellow to gray. Growth on human blood agar is superior to that on horse or sheep blood agar. It is oxidase and catalase negative and is X factor dependent.

Serologic evidence of recent infection with *B. henselae* is also helpful, but the tests are often either unavailable or not standardized. A new, modified immuno-fluorescent-antibody assay has been noted (32) to have a sensitivity of 85% and a specificity of ~98% for both immunoglobulin G (IgG) and IgM components. The IgM remained positive for less than 3 months and the IgG decreased over time, with 25% of patients remaining seropositive for >1 year; no association was found between titers and clinical manifestations or duration of disease.

Therapy at this time is supportive (38a). Aspiration of a necrotic node is preferable to excision and may be necessary in some cases. Chronic draining sinus tracts can develop. The role of antimicrobial therapy remains undetermined (31, 33). Recent data suggest that bacillary angiomatosis and hepatosplenic disease respond more favorably (rapidly and consistently) than typical CSD to antimicrobial therapy for unclear reasons. Organisms in granulomas may be "walled off" from penetration by antibacterials. Rifampin has been used successfully, and with rapid rate of response, in hepatosplenic cases (2). The combination of doxycycline and rifampin has been used successfully to treat CSD-associated retinitis (37). *Bartonella* organisms are noted to be macrolide susceptible, and reports have noted the clinical success of azithromycin in treating typical CSD (3). Susceptibility studies have suggested that isolates may be variably susceptible to other antibiotics, with much strain-to-strain variation (31). Clinical success and failure have been attributed to the same antimicrobial agents, including gentamicin, tetracyclines, ciprofloxacin, and sulfamethoxazole-trimethoprim (21, 33, 45). In vitro resistance of *B. henselae* to broad-spectrum cephalosporins correlated with clinical therapeutic failure.

Prevention is accomplished by control of fleas in pets and discussion with a veterinarian about pet health, especially for immunocompromised prospective pet owners. No vaccine exists for cats. Blood culture of a prospective pet cat and, if indicated, subsequent antimicrobial therapy may be prudent for certain household situations.

Bacillary (Epithelioid) Angiomatosis

Patients with HIV infection may develop Kaposi's sarcoma-like papular lesions after cat scratch or contact (24, 25, 41, 44). Lesions may also be found in immunocompetent patients as well. Lesions may be nodular, subcutaneous, or even polypoid and may be pigmented or nonpigmented. Lesions contain a distinctive pattern of vascular proliferation on histopathological sections. CSD and bacillary angiomatosis have organisms that appear similar on Warthin-Starry stain. Lesions are often multiple and appear on a variety of body surfaces. Lesions may also be osseous and appear in the fibula, radius, femur, and tibia, as well as present as hepatic abscesses, splenic involvement, colonic mucosal lesions, and even as extensive bone marrow infiltration. Systemic symptoms, including fever, night sweats, and weight loss, may also be associated with disease. This disease was originally thought to be a variant of CSD in an immunocompromised patient population and is difficult to differentiate from it on clinical grounds. *B. henselae* and *B. quintana* have been isolated from patients with bacillary angiomatosis and bacillary peliosis and have been shown to be the etiologic agents of these diseases. Host immunoincompetency, as opposed to lymphatic containment of the organisms, is likely responsible for the systemic spread.

Rickettsia felis ("Flea-Borne Spotted Fever")

A newly described rickettsial organism, *R. felis*, is transmitted to humans, who are incidental hosts, by the cat flea (*Ctenocephalides felis*), which can become infected transovarially and transstadially. Opossums and cats are reservoirs. Human cases have been reported in Texas, California, Oklahoma, and Europe (23a). It has been found in cats in Yucatan, England, and South America (23a, 46). The human illness, manifested as a febrile exanthema, is probably more widespread than generally appreciated.

FECAL-ORAL

Campylobacteriosis

Campylobacter jejuni has emerged as one of the most frequent bacterial causes of diarrheal diseases in the United States. The organism is a motile, curved, microaerophilic gram-negative rod that inhabits the gastrointestinal tract of clinically healthy and diarrheic animals and has been isolated from cat feces. Newly acquired, young cats are more likely to be carriers. Those cats with diarrhea pose a greater zoonotic risk. Most cases of human infection are acquired from contaminated food, especially undercooked poultry, and water.

In humans, a flu-like illness with fever, malaise, etc., will precede the development of cramping diarrhea. Infection is usually self-limiting; however, colitis, bacteremia, and metastatic infections may result. A reactive arthritis or Guillain-Barré syndrome may also occur after resolution of the diarrheal illness.

Prevention of infection by hand washing after cat contact and prior to eating should be common sense. Cats should also not be fed raw or poorly cooked meat. Therapy consists of symptomatic treatment. Antimicrobial agents such as erythromycin or the fluoroquinolones (norfloxacin, ciprofloxacin, levofloxacin, moxifloxacin, etc.) have proven effective. While resistance remains rare in the United States, some strains from Europe and Southeast Asia have been reported to be resistant to quinolones and/or to macrolides. The use of antimicrobials in animal food as a growth promoter is suspected of being responsible for this resistance. Some companies and countries have encouraged the use of these agents in animals only for therapeutic purposes and not for prophylaxis or growth enhancement.

Helicobacteriosis

Helicobacter bizzozeronii (*Helicobacter heilmannii*) has been isolated from a few people with gastritis, and in some reports cats have been associated (28). In addition, it was reported that a researcher exposed to cat stomachs developed gastritis, which was attributed to infection with *Helicobacter felis* (16). *Helicobacter pylori* has also been demonstrated in the gastric mucosa of cats in research colonies; the presumed source of infection was animal caretakers. Further genetic comparisons of human and feline isolates will be needed to determine the direct relationship of these findings.

Cryptosporidiosis

Human cryptosporidiosis was first reported in 1976 and has become recognized as an important cause of gastrointestinal illness (23). National reporting began in the United States in 1995, with 2,972 human cases (5). Recent outbreaks linked to the water supplies of urban cities (>400,000 cases in Milwaukee, Wis.) have generated public concern and awareness as well as "made-for-TV" movies. The disease is particularly problematic in AIDS patients, in whom it causes not only diarrhea but also cholecystitis. The diarrhea is often profuse and watery and is associated with cramping abdominal pain, fever, and emesis. Immunocompetent patients sometimes have a mild and self-limiting form of illness, while immunocompromised patients have prolonged and severe courses that warrant attempts at therapeutic intervention. Weight loss and volume depletion with electrolyte imbalance may even require hospitalization. Infection is often in the small intestine (ileum) and may be focal in nature. Cryptosporidial cholecystitis may be manifested by right upper quadrant pain, emesis, and a thickened gallbladder wall and dilated ducts on ultrasound. In AIDS patients it must also be differentiated from cytomegalovirus acalculous cholecystitis. Cryptosporidia have also been isolated from sputum and lung tissue from immunocompromised hosts, although its role in pulmonary disease is less well defined.

Cats and many other species of mammals, birds, and reptiles may act as definitive hosts for cryptosporidia. Experimental infection in healthy cats and young kittens resulted in nonsymptomatic infections and colonization. In naturally infected cats, watery diarrhea may be self-limiting. Immunocompromised cats have more symptoms, including chronic, large-volume, watery diarrhea; anorexia; and weight loss. In cats, infection with feline leukemia or immunodeficiency virus or the presence of other intestinal pathogens is associated with more severe disease and increased shedding.

Infection has been transmitted between species, such as from animals to humans, as well as from human to human. *Cryptosporidium parvum* genospecies subtype 1 infects only people, while subtype 2 is adapted to cows but infects a wide variety of mammalian hosts, including cats and people. Cats have their own genospecies, which also infects people. Cat-to-human transmission has been reported; however, cattle are thought to be the main source of animal-related human infections. After ingestion, the sporozoite excysts and enters the villous intestinal border. Several asexual developmental forms ensue. Ultimately, thin-walled oocysts may invade other cells, while thick-walled oocysts are excreted into the feces. These oocysts are quite hardy and difficult to destroy. Crowding of either animals or humans (e.g., as occurs in day care centers or underdeveloped countries) and unsanitary practices are associated with an increased risk of acquiring cryptosporidiosis.

Diagnosis is made by demonstrating the organism in stool specimens or tissue biopsy samples. Routine ova and parasite examination of stool specimens will fail to identify this pathogen, as special stains or immunodiagnostic tests are required for identification. Consequently, cryptosporidium exam must be specifically ordered; cryptosporidiosis is probably underdiagnosed and underreported. For cats, a positive test may not be associated with active infection. Definitive therapy remains imperfect. Many drugs, such as spiramycin and paromomycin (Humatin), have met with limited success. Patients often turn to alternative nonallopathic treatment modalities, which also meet with limited success.

Toxoplasmosis

Toxoplasma gondii, the causative agent of toxoplasmosis, is a ubiquitous, obligate intracellular protozoan that can affect almost all warm-blooded animals, including humans. Domestic cats and their relatives are definitive hosts of *T. gondii*. Millions of oocysts are excreted in the feces daily, and ingestion of infested food or water may cause disease in cats. Cat excretion of oocysts is self-limiting and occurs for only 1 to 3 weeks after initial infection. However, approximately 1% (~560,000) of cats in the United States are thought to be infected and excreting oocysts on any given day. Congenital or lactational transmission in cats (tachyzoites) and ingestion of tissue cysts (bradyzoites) in contaminated meats (most common) can also lead to feline disease.

Following ingestion, bradyzoites are released from the infected muscle and penetrate the epithelium of the cat small intestine. Subsequently, the parasite develops within the intestinal epithelium and disseminates into tissues while also going through a variety of stages until it forms unsporulated and uninfective oocysts which are passed in the feces. This process may take between 3 days and 3 weeks to be completed. As soon as 2 to 3 days after being shed, uninfective oocysts begin to sporulate, depending on climate and temperature factors, and they may remain infective and viable for 1 year in the soil. They do not sporulate at <4 or >37°C. Consequently, the disease is less prevalent in cold and arid climates.

Human infection may occur after ingestion of uncooked or undercooked meat of livestock (especially pork or goat) that contains tissue cysts; ingestion is probably the most usual method of zoonotic transmission. Single tissue cysts, which may contain thousands of organisms, are common in skeletal muscle, heart muscle, and brain tissue. However, infection may develop from exposure to fecal oocysts when changing cat litter boxes or gardening in areas where cat feces have been deposited.

The clinical spectrum of human disease is variable and includes asymptomatic forms (common) and acute or chronic symptomatic forms. Human congenital transmission occurs when a woman becomes acutely infected, usually asymptomatically, during pregnancy. This may result in spontaneous abortion or stillbirth. While congenital toxoplasmosis is currently rare in the United States, no statistical correlation between disease and cat ownership has been proven (34). A variable percentage of infants born after such exposure may develop a wide variety of sequelae, including mental and psychomotor retardation, cerebral calcifications, chorioretinitis, jaundice, hepatosplenomegaly, anemia, and pneumonia. "The incidence of transplacental transmission and severity of congenital disease depend on gestational age at which maternal seroconversion occurs" (34). Each presentation must be differentiated from other causes of similar problems, such as the other etiologic agents of the TORCH syndrome complex (toxoplasmosis, other [syphilis, sepsis, listeriosis, etc.], rubella, cytomegalovirus, herpes).

Approximately 10 to 20% of immunocompetent individuals manifest symptomatic toxoplasmosis, usually with cervical adenopathy that does not require therapy. This regional adenopathy needs to be differentiated from that due to streptococcal pharyngitis, infectious mononucleosis, Hodgkin's disease, CSD, sarcoidosis, and cytomegalovirus infection. The disease manifestations are both protean and nonspecific. Other symptoms may include fever, malaise, fatigue, myalgias, sore throat, and rash. While most cases of disease are self-limiting, rarely lasting more than 3 to 6 months, some patients have prolonged symptoms, including depression, and some infections disseminate, with development of myocarditis, pneumonia, retinal disease, or encephalitis. A disseminated form of acute cutaneous toxoplasmosis may occur. Patients with disseminated disease often benefit from therapy. Immunocompromised hosts, including AIDS patients, HIV-infected patients, and cancer patients (especially those on chemotherapy), may develop more serious disease manifestations, including brain abscess, retinitis, encephalopathy, pneumonia, and hepatitis. Immunocompromised patients always require therapy for acute toxoplasmosis or any complication of recurrent (reactivated) disease.

Diagnosis is made by serologic studies or by isolation or cytologic demonstration of the organism from blood or body fluids or by histologic demonstration of the trophozoite. Most cases are diagnosed by serologic means. However, a high prevalence rate of *T. gondii*-specific antibodies, sometimes even at high levels (>1:512), in the general population may make this difficult. Both false-positive and false-negative tests can occur. However, a negative serologic test result virtually excludes the diagnosis in an immunocompetent individual. In cats, a positive serotest result measuring IgG indicates that the cat is not an exposure risk, as the oocyst shedding phase has already occurred during prior exposure.

The need for therapy depends on the immune status of the host, host defenses, and location of infection. The standard therapy has been sulfadiazine and pyrimethamine. The duration of therapy depends on specific host factors and the site of infection. Prevention of disease in AIDS patients may be accomplished with the use of sulfonamide-based compounds used for the prevention of *Pneumocystis carinii* pneumonia. If an AIDS patient does develop cerebral toxoplasmosis, he or she will require prolonged therapy. Trimethoprim-sulfamethoxazole has been used instead of sulfadiazine. Alternative therapy with clindamycin plus pyrimeththamine has been advocated for sulfonamide-allergic patients. Spiramycin has been used in therapy of pregnant women and infants with congenital infection.

Prevention of infection should be advocated for immunocompromised patients at risk for disease. They should be instructed not to change cat litter boxes or to do so daily so that the oocysts do not have a chance to sporulate prior to exposure. In addition, they should not garden in areas where cats may have defecated or beatclean rugs, which may be contaminated by cat feces.

Salmonellosis

There has been a continual increase in the number of cases of human salmonellosis reported in the United States over the past several years (5). A small number of these approximately 50,000 annual cases may come from exposure to household pets, usually reptiles or amphibians. In these instances the victims are usually children who acquire infection from direct fecal-oral exposure. Cats may acquire infection from infected foods, especially offal, live prey, uncooked meat or fish meal, or contaminated water. If one feeds his or her cat any of these potentially contaminated products, good hand washing is in order. Cats may also pick up salmonellosis from staying in a contaminated kennel. The prevalence of infection in cats being exclusively fed commercial rations is very low; however, up to 18% of normal and healthy-appearing cats may be infected or carriers when foodstuffs are not restricted. Cats may acquire infection, often *Salmonella enterica* serovar Typhimurium, from ingestion of birds, which occurs in association with the seasonal songbird migration in the northeastern United States.

Infected cats can shed organisms orally and conjunctivally as well as fecally. Their fur may become contaminated, as may their water dishes. They may manifest illness as a gastroenterologic disease with diarrhea, excessive salivation, or emesis or as a systemic illness with fevers, etc. In utero infection may occur. Kittens less than 7 weeks old may not manifest symptoms even if bacteremic.

The characteristics of human salmonellosis can be divided into asymptomatic (most usual), enterocolitis, enteric fever with bacteremia, metastatic complications, and chronic carrier state. The enterocolitis must be differentiated from other infectious diarrheal illnesses such as campylobacteriosis, shigellosis, and viral disease and noninfectious diarrheal diseases. The incubation period is 6 to 48 h. Cramping abdominal pain, emesis, nausea, and diarrhea are common. Occasionally, salmonellosis must be differentiated from appendicitis and other surgical causes of the acute abdomen.

Diagnosis is made by isolation of the organism from stool cultures or blood cultures. Most infections are asymptomatic or mild and self-limiting and do not require antimicrobial therapy. However, for patients with serious infection, such as enteric fever, bacteremia, or metastatic complications, or for immunocompromised hosts, antimicrobial therapy is advocated. The choice of antimicrobial must be determined by considering local resistance patterns for empirical therapy. Agents used have included ampicillin, chloramphenicol, and trimethoprim-sulfamethoxazole. Recently, the fluoroquinolones (norfloxacin, ciprofloxacin, levofloxacin, and trovafloxacin) have shown efficacy in salmonellosis. They are an attractive choice since they are active against almost all other enteric bacterial pathogens as well. However, resistance has developed, albeit rarely to date, and they are contraindicated for pregnant women and children whose epiphyseal plates have not yet closed. Success has also been achieved using some parenterally administered expanded-spectrum cephalosporins. Prevention by practicing good hand washing after petting cats, changing litter boxes, or feeding raw fish or meat products is prudent.

Anaerobiospirillum Diarrhea

Anaerobiospirillum species are anaerobic spiral bacteria with bipolar tufts of flagella that have been associated with cases of human diarrhea (29). Two species, *Anaerobiospirillum succiniciproducens* and *Anaerobiospirillum thomasii*, have been isolated from cats with diarrhea (30). *A. succiniciproducens* has been implicated as a cause of human bacteremia and sepsis. *A. thomasii* has been implicated as a cause of human diarrhea. Human disease included 3 to 7 days of diarrhea, fever, abdominal pain, and emesis. Malnick et al. (29) developed a selective medium that allowed its detection in the feces of 7 of 10 asymptomatic cats sampled during elective surgery. Consequently, cats may act as a vector in human disease.

Yersinia pseudotuberculosis Gastroenteritis

Y. pseudotuberculosis is a well-established cause of human diarrheal disease, diffuse abdominal illness sometimes mimicking acute appendicitis, and sepsis. Serotyping and endonuclease restriction analysis proved that two young children had become infected and symptomatic after having drunk water from puddles in a garden that was contaminated by feces from cats. Cats may be asymptomatic carriers but may also exhibit clinical infection with anorexia, vomiting, and severe diarrhea, which are most likely to occur in the winter and spring (14).

Toxocariasis

Toxocara cati is a helminthic parasite that affects cats and may incidentally infect humans. Cats may be infected transplacentally or may become infected via oral intake of infected feces (11). After ingestion, the ova hatch in the small intestine and migrate to other body organs, including the liver and lungs. Organisms that are coughed up or subsequently swallowed will then mature in the small intestinal lumen. Excreted ova subsequently develop in the soil, taking weeks to mature. Human infection results from ingestion of infected soil or animal feces and is most usual in toddlers with pica and playing in areas where cats defecate.

Most human infection is asymptomatic. Some patients develop a cough or wheezing or an asthmatic presentation from the parasites' pulmonary migration. Some patients present with hepatomegaly, abdominal pain, and eosinophilia. This must be differentiated from other parasitic diseases such as strongyloidiasis, trichinosis, ascariasis, anisakiasis, schistosomiasis, and echinococcosis. The organism may migrate to any part of the body and may localize in the retina, causing blindness.

Diagnosis is usually made by clinical grounds. Serologic studies are available but are not specific. The organism is occasionally found incidentally in tissue biopsy. Therapy for this form of disease is usually symptomatic, as the disease is usually self-limiting.

Occasionally, *T. cati* can cause cutaneous larva migrans, or the creeping eruption. More commonly, cats are infected with *Ancylostoma braziliense* and subsequently shed ova. This is also a disease of children who play in areas where cats defecate. It is more common in the southeastern United States and in areas with a temperate climate and sandy or shady soil. Larvae come into contact with human skin and burrow under it, causing itching and paresthesias. The lesion can become erythematous along a serpiginous tract. Eosinophilia may be present. Disease is usually self-limiting but may be treated with thiabendazole, orally or topically.

Opisthorchiasis

Opisthorchis felineus is a common liver fluke of cats that can occasionally be transmitted to humans. It is a disease of fish-eating mammals, such as cats, and is endemic in Southeast Asia and Eastern Europe but not the United States. Embryonated eggs are excreted in the feces by the definitive host. The eggs are ingested by specific snail species and develop until they are released as cercariae into freshwater, where they penetrate into the intermediate fish host. Human infection comes from ingestion of rare or raw infected fish. The parasites mature into adults in the bile ducts. Most patients are asymptomatic; however, signs of cholangitis and hepatitis may develop. Diagnosis is made by finding eggs in a fecal sample. Praziquantel is used for therapy.

Dipylidiasis

Dipylidium caninum is a common cat tapeworm that may infect humans, usually children. Fleas ingest eggs which then develop into the cysticercus stage. When fleas are ingested, the tapeworm subsequently develops in the intestinal tract; humans become infected when they ingest fleas. The patient may develop eosinophilia and mild gastrointestinal discomfort. Diagnosis is made by demonstration of proglottids in a stool sample. Niclosamide is used for therapy. This disease needs to be distinguished from other parasitic causes of eosinophilia.

BITE, SCRATCH, OR PUNCTURE

Rabies

Approximately 7,000 animals per year are proven positive for rabies in the United States. While domestic animals account for less than 10% of all rabid animals, over the past 10 years rabid cats have been more common than rabid dogs. Vaccination of cats is not legally mandated in all areas as it is for dogs, making them more susceptible to infection. Cats acquire rabies from exposure to infected wildlife and a "spillover effect." Rabid cats may develop frenzied rabies but more often become reclusive. Rabies is covered in chapter 10.

Erysipelothrix Infection

Erysipelothrix rhusiopathiae is a geographically widespread, facultative, gram-positive rod that may be isolated from soil, water, and animals. Human disease is usually associated with cellulitis acquired by animal contact and occurs usually in slaughterhouse workers. A recent report (40) notes *E. rhusiopathiae* isolation from two infected wounds secondary to cat bites. Human disease may be manifested by a painful, ulcerating, and progressive papular skin lesion that is associated with pain or stiffness in the local joint. Disease may be self-limiting and disappear in approximately 3 weeks. A human disseminated form which may include a vasculitic rash and endocarditis can also occur. The source animals are often not clinically ill. A new species, *Erysipelothrix tonsillarum*, has been shown to cause septicemia and endocarditis in dogs but has not yet been associated with human illness. Therapy with penicillin or a cephalosporin may be useful in localized cases as well as for disseminated disease.

Anthrax

Anthrax is caused by *Bacillus anthracis*, a large gram-positive spore-forming rod. Infections in humans are almost always the result of contact with infected animals or their by-products (especially goat hair). The alkaline soil of many tropical and subtropical regions allows vegetative spore growth, resulting in a soilborne systemic disease of domestic animals. Domestic herbivores have the highest prevalence of infection, and cats are uncommonly affected. Soil may remain contaminated for many years. In cats, anthrax is manifested by inflammation, edema, and necrosis of the upper gastrointestinal tract. Spread to regional lymph nodes, liver, and spleen is frequent. Human infection usually results from handling infected tissues, carcasses, or animal skin. Inhalation anthrax is a rare phenomenon in humans in the United States but has recently gained attention because of potential threats of bioterrorism. Before the autumn of 2001, the last case of inhalation anthrax reported in the United

States was in 1992; in the 1960s and 1970s, there were an average of one or two cases (range, zero to six) reported annually in the United States (5).

In humans, cutaneous lesions account for >95% of cases. One to five days after exposure, a small and often pruritic papule may form at the inoculation site. The area, although painless, develops a brawny edema; the lesion enlarges and the center becomes necrotic. Regional adenopathy and lymphangitis may be associated with the skin lesion. The lesion of anthrax should be covered. The differential diagnosis includes brown recluse spider bite, orf, CSD, erythema gangrenosum, tularemia, and plague.

Diagnosis is achieved by Gram staining of the exudate and isolation of the organism. The laboratory should be warned if the diagnosis is suspected. Several serologic tests are available but will not be of help in rapidly progressive cases. Therapy with intravenous penicillin G and subsequent oral penicillin for 7 to 10 days is generally effective for cutaneous disease. There are rare reports of penicillin-resistant *B. anthracis*. Inhalation anthrax is difficult to diagnose and is therefore usually fatal.

Pasteurella multocida Infection

Most people associate *P. multocida* with infected dog and cat bite wounds (15); indeed, almost all feline species commonly carry this organism in their oropharynx as part of the normal flora. Additionally, when cats lick their paws, they are in effect inoculating *P. multocida* onto their claws.

It is estimated that 400,000 persons are bitten or severely scratched by cats annually in the United States. Many of these wounds never become infected and are trivial in severity. However, infection resulting from cat bites and scratches is an important and frequent medical problem. Most people are bitten or scratched by cats they know, and these injuries occur while handling the cat. Cat bites become infected more frequently than do dog bites. Cats teeth are small but sharp, and when the bite is to the hand, it can easily penetrate the joints, bones, and tendons. Infections following cat bites are usually cellulitis, often with a gray malodorous discharge but without lymphangitis or regional adenopathy, but also include septic arthritis, tenosynovitis, and osteomyelitis. Consequently, the use of antimicrobial therapy as prophylactic therapy in cases of moderate to severe wounds, wounds to the hands (especially those that have come near a joint), or those causing pain is warranted to reduce the incidence of infection. Other organisms, both aerobic and anaerobic feline oral flora, can be cultured from many wounds.

Pasteurella infection in humans has also been associated both with general animal contact and, in approximately 15 to 20% of cases, such as respiratory infection, without known animal contact. The possibility of more remote contact and persistence of the isolate on the skin or mucous membranes has been entertained.

In 1992, Holst et al. (22) characterized 159 strains of *Pasteurella* recovered from human infections and studied their distribution, which was as follows: *Pasteurella multocida* subsp. *multocida*, 60%; *Pasteurella multocida* subsp. *septica*, 13%; *Pasteurella canis*, 18%; *Pasteurella stomatis*, 6%; and *Pasteurella dagmatis*, 3%. They did not fully differentiate the distribution of species in the 87 of 159 cases associated with cat bites and contact. However, they did note different ecological niches for the different species and subspecies and slightly different pathogenic potentials. *P. multocida* subsp. *multocida* and *P. multocida* subsp. *septica* were usually associated with more severe infections; the former was associated with almost all bacteremic cases, and the latter was associated with several cases of central nervous system infection.

The bacteriology of 57 infected cat bite wounds has been recently studied in a prospective, multicenter project which shows the great diversity of isolates (40). Women accounted for 72% of cat bite victims, compared to 38% for dog bites. Cat bites presented as abscesses 19% of the time, while purulent wounds accounted for 39% and nonpurulent cellulitis accounted for 42%. Cat bites had a median of six bacterial isolates per wound and were mixed cultures (both aerobes and anaerobes) 63% of the time. The prevalence and distribution of *Pasteurella* species are different for dog and cat bites. Surprisingly, *Pasteurella* species were present in 75% of wounds in the following distribution: *P. multocida* subsp. *multocida*, 54%; *P. multocida* subsp. *septica*, 28%; *P. dagmatis*, 7%; *P. stomatis*, 4%; and *P. canis*, 2%.

Most wounds can be treated with outpatient management. If there is any edema, then the affected body part should be elevated. Failure to adequately elevate the injured part is one of the most common causes of therapeutic failure. The location of punctures, especially in relation to the bones and joints of the hand, should be noted. Prophylactic therapy with an antimicrobial agent such as penicillin or amoxicillin-clavulanic acid is inexpensive and prudent. Alternative agents could include trimethoprim-sulfamethoxazole, doxycycline, fluoroquinolones (ciprofloxacin, levofloxacin, trovafloxacin, etc.), and possibly cefuroxime axetil. The duration of therapy for prophylaxis is 3 to 5 days, while therapy for established infection such as cellulitis often requires 10 to 14 days. More serious complications such as septic arthritis and osteomyelitis require prolonged courses of antimicrobials. Occasionally, anti-inflammatory agents reduce the posttraumatic arthritis that subsequently develops in a minority of cases. In some areas, rabies prophylaxis may be considered (see chapter 10). Tetanus toxoid should be administered if the patient is not current on his or her immunizations.

Mixed Aerobic and Anaerobic Bacterial Infections

There are approximately 400,000 infected cat bites annually in the United States and an even greater number of cat scratches that get infected. Cat claws become infected when cats are grooming and inoculate normal flora onto their claws. Cat bites are most often to the hand (63%) and upper extremity (23%) and a few (9%) are to the lower extremities. Most victims are women (72%) with a median age of 39 years (40). Presentation to the emergency department for medical help is usually associated with a nonpurulent but infected wound (42%), while 39% have purulent wounds and 19% have abscesses. The wounds will grow 2 to 13 isolates, with 63% having both aerobic and anaerobic bacteria cultured from the wounds. A plethora of different bacteria may be cultured from these wounds, as noted by Talan et al. (40), and include not only *P. multocida* and other *Pasteurella* species (75%) but also numerous other bacteria, including streptococci (46%), staphylococci (35%), *Neisseria* spp. (19%), *Corynebacterium* spp. (28%), *Moraxella* spp. (35%), *Bacteroides* spp. (especially *Bacteroides tectus*) (28%), *Fusobacterium* spp. (33%), and *Porphyromonas* spp. (30%). Conrads et al. recently reported a new species of fusobacterium, *Fusobacterium canifelinum*, that is associated with cat and dog bites and is resistant to fluoroquinolones (8a). Almost all isolates come from the normal flora of the biting cat.

Sporotrichosis

Sporothrix schenckii is an endemic, dimorphic fungus that can cause ulcerated, verrucous, or erythematous and nodular skin infection after direct inoculation by cat bite or scratch (10). On cats, lesions are seen on the head, limbs, or tail base and are often draining puncture wounds similar to fight wound abscesses. Cats may further spread disease by licking and grooming. In humans, sporotrichosis may also cause nodular pulmonary lesions after inhalation of infected soil. Cutaneous sporotrichosis is more common in the cooler, distal extremities, with painless, smooth or verrucous lesions that may ulcerate and have raised erythematous borders. Lesions may have a deep red or purplish coloration. Secondary lesions may occur along lymphatic channels and in lymph nodes. Osteoarticular disease also occurs and may affect the hands, elbows, ankles, and knees. AIDS patients may develop disseminated disease, including meningitis and parenchymal brain lesions. Cats have been reported to be bacteremic from naturally acquired infection (39).

Diagnosis is made by culture of tissue or blood. Biopsy samples will reveal granulomatous changes, but the organism is often difficult to identify in specimens. Therapy with a saturated solution of potassium iodine has been previously employed. Patients started off with 5 to 10 drops of solution thrice daily, increasing to up to 40 to 50 drops thrice daily or until side effects such as nausea, diarrhea, anorexia, and parotid enlargement limited therapy. de Lima Barros et al. (10) described 24 human cases related to transmission by domestic cats; all patients responded to itraconazole therapy.

Feline Orthopox

Infection with cowpox virus (an orthopoxvirus) is the most common poxvirus infection in cats. Infection is more common in Europe, and cats, usually rural cats that hunt rodents, are usually incidental hosts. Cats often start with a single lesion on the head, neck, or forelimb that occurs from a bite or skin wound inoculation. Dissemination occurs, with the cats manifesting coryza and diarrhea; secondary bacterial infections also occur. Both cat-to-cat transmission and cat-to-human transmission have been reported (4, 19). Cat-to-human transmission is unlikely when basic hygiene is followed after contact.

Tularemia

Tularemia is caused by a small, gram-negative coccobacillus, *Francisella tularensis*, that grows poorly on routine culture media. It is ubiquitous and most often found in wild mammals, such as rabbits, but may affect cats. Four subspecies are recognized; the different subspecies are associated with different geographic locations worldwide. *Francisella tularensis* subsp. *tularensis* is found predominantly in the United States; *Francisella tularensis* subsp. holarcita is found in Europe, the former Soviet Union, and Japan; *Francisella tularensis* subsp. *mediasiatica* is found in Kazakhstan and Uzbekistan; and *Francisella tularensis* subsp. *novicida* is found in North America (42). *F. tularensis* survives in amoebae and is therefore associated with waterways (42). Cat infection usually results from a bite by an infected tick, which may serve as both reservoir and vector, or by hunting or ingestion of infected rabbits. Young cats may die from disseminated infection. Older cats may develop draining abscesses as well as fever and adenopathy. Cat-associated human tularemia has occurred in conjunction with bite wounds. The organism is highly virulent and has an infectious dose of 10 to 50 CFU. Consequently, the local endemicity of infected animals and appropriate vectors should alert the physician to this possibility. A study of the epidemiology of tularemia in the southwestern and central United States showed that 17 of 1,041 (1.6%) human cases diagnosed between 1981 and 1987 were associated with cat scratches or bites (5).

The ulceroglandular form of tularemia is most common and causes regional adenopathy and ulcerative skin lesions. This manifestation must be differentiated from other skin infections, including staphylococcal or streptococcal infection, bite wound infection due to *P. multocida*, and CSD. Pneumonia, without sputum production, may develop in ~15% of patients with ulceroglandular disease. Most cases are diagnosed by a compatible clinical picture and antibody titers, since isolation of the organism is difficult and, if accomplished, may pose health risks to the laboratory technologists.

Standard therapy consists of streptomycin (10 to 20 mg/kg of body weight/ day intramuscularly for 7 to 14 days). Tetracyclines and chloramphenicol have been used successfully but may be associated with increased rates of relapse. Fluoroquinolones and some cephalosporins, such as ceftriaxone, have in vitro activity against *F. tularensis*, but studies documenting clinical proof of efficacy are lacking.

SOILBORNE

Histoplasmosis

Histoplasma capsulatum is an imperfect dimorphic fungus that is endemic in the central United States and may be found in other temperate and tropical climates. The free-living mycelial stage of *H. capsulatum* grows in the soil and produces both micro- and macroconidia. Inhalation of microconidia leads to conversion to the yeast phase in the body and subsequent pulmonary infection, which in turn may lead to dissemination. Soil, organically enriched by bird droppings, is the most frequent source of human exposure. Cats are also susceptible to histoplasmosis, and common-source outbreaks involving animals and people have occurred. As with most systemic fungal infections, direct animal-to-animal or animal-to-human spread is unlikely. Cats <4 years old and female cats seem to be more prone to developing histoplasmosis. There is no breed predilection. Infected cats that develop disseminated disease usually die but may also develop ulcerated skin lesions.

Direct cat-to-human transmission has not been reported. Histoplasmosis in cats can be treated with itraconazole (20). Human disease may be treated with itraconazole or amphotericin B.

DIRECT CONTACT

Dermatophilosis

Cats may become infected with *Dermatophilus congolensis,* an actinomycete that causes abscesses in muscles and lymph nodes and fistulous tracts. Humans handling infected cats may become accidentally infected. Human infection is manifested by an exudative, pustular dermatitis at the site of contact. The lesions spontaneously resolve within 2 weeks and do not usually require antimicrobial therapy. In cats, the hair should be clipped around the lesion and kept dry. Repeated bathing, application of iodine solutions, and in some cases the use of penicillin-related compounds are therapeutic.

Scabies

Sarcoptes scabiei, which causes a condition known as the "seven-year itch," can infect cats and be transmitted to humans. Scabies mites cause hypersensitivity in human hosts often manifested by pruritic, papular lesions at areas where they burrow into the skin. The itching increases at night. Cat scabies mites are unable to burrow into human skin to complete their life cycle, and so a cutaneous scraping test will not be diagnostic. Rather, diagnosis is made by clinical presentation. Therapy consists of ridding the affected pet of mites and laundering clothes and bedding.

Cheyletiella Mite Infestation

Cheyletiella species are animal mites, some of which can infest cats and may occasionally cause human infestation.

Dermatophytosis

Domestic cats can harbor a wide variety of molds and yeasts in the hair of their coats and on their skin. Both symptomatic disease and asymptomatic carriage may occur. These organisms include *Epidermophyton floccosum, Microsporum* species, and *Trichophyton* species. These dermatophytes spread between animals and potentially from animals to humans and also from humans to animals. Infections often involve the hair shaft and follicle, from which infectious arthrospores are disseminated to the local environment and remain viable for months. Up to 89% of cats may harbor dermatophytes, of which *Microsporum canis* is the most common. Fomites contaminated by cat hair can also act as a vector. The incubation period is often 1 to 3 weeks.

In cats, the most common manifestation is a patchy alopecia but may include a scaling or granulomatous dermatitis. A variety of lesions have been observed that mimic other skin conditions. Since transmission is possible, and cats can be subclinical carriers, they are often treated with clipping of the hair, with topical antifungal bathing over their entire body, and some may require oral antifungal agents as well. Additionally, the environment must be cleaned of hairs and dander to stop transmission. Approximately 50% of humans exposed to cat dermatophytes develop symptomatic infection, including ringworm and tinea capitis. In humans the infection can manifest as alopecia, scaling or crusting lesions and ulcers and nodules. Secondary bacterial infection may also occur.

Diagnosis is made by culture of skin scrapings and examination of scrapings using potassium hydroxide digestion or by using a Wood's lamp. As for cats, human therapy usually consists of topical antifungals such as clotrimazole, miconazole, etc., or in severe cases oral agents such as fluconazole or itraconazole. Again, cleaning the environment of cat hairs and dander from carpets, bedding, clothing, etc., is essential for control. Air conditioning and heating filters must also be changed regularly. Pets may need to be restricted from bedrooms. Cats may be treated with topical agents such as lime sulfur dip or miconazole shampoo with or without chlorhexidine. The same products in lotions are less effective in penetrating cat hair. Oral agents such as itraconazole are of most benefit with the least side effects.

Uncertain Associations

Hepatitis E

Hepatitis E virus is present in Southeast and Central Asia and the Middle East but rare in the United States; it is thought to be enterically transmitted. Transmission from humans to nonhuman primates has been reported as well as infection in swine and rodents (35). Kuno et al. (27) reported a case of hepatitis E virus infection in a 47-year-old Japanese man whose pet cat had antibody to hepatitis E virus.

REFERENCES

1. **Adal, K. A., C. J. Cockerell, and W. A. Petri, Jr.** 1994. Cat scratch disease, bacillary angiomatosis, and other infections due to *Rochalimaea. N. Engl. J. Med.* **330:**1509–1515.
2. **Arisoy, E. S., A. G. Correa, M. L. Wagner, and S. L. Kaplan.** 1999. Hepatosplenic cat-scratch disease in children: selected clinical features and treatment. *Clin. Infect. Dis.* **28:**778–784.
3. **Bass, J. W., B. C. Freitas, A. D. Freitas, C. L. Sisler, D. S. Chan, J. M. Vincent, D. A. Person, J. R. Claybaugh, R. R. Whitter, M. E. Weisse, R. L. Regnery, and L. N. Slater.** 1998. Prospective randomized double blind placebo-controlled evaluation of azithromycin for treatment of cat-scratch disease. *Pediatr. Infect. Dis. J.* **17:**447–452.
4. **Baxby, D., M. Bennett, and B. Getty.** 1994. Human cowpox: a review based on 54 cases, 1969–1993. *Br. J. Dermatol.* **131:**598–607.
4a. **Bjoersdorff, A., L. Svendenius, J. H. Owens, and R. F. Massung.** 1999. Feline granulocytic ehrlichiosis—a report of a new clinical entity and characterisation of the infectious agent. *J. Small Anim. Pract.* **40:**20–24.
5. **Centers for Disease Control and Prevention.** 1997. Summary of notifiable diseases, United States, 1996. *Morb. Mortal. Wkly. Rep.* **45(53):**1–103.
6. **Chomel, B. B., R. C. Abbott, R. W. Kasten, K. A. Floyd-Hawkins, P. H. Kass, C. A. Glaser, N. C. Pedersen, and J. E. Koehler.** 1995. *Bartonella henselae* prevalence in domestic cats in California: risk factors and association between bacteremia and antibody titers. *J. Clin. Microbiol.* **33:**2445–2450.
7. **Chomel, B. B., R. W. Kasten, J. E. Sykes, H. J. Boulouis, and E. B. Breitschwerdt.** 2003. Clinical impact of persistent *Bartonella* bacteremia in humans and animals. *Ann. N. Y. Acad. Sci.* **990:**267–278.

8. **Chomel, B. B., A. C. Wey, R. W. Kasten, B. A. Stacy, and P. Labelle.** 2003. Fatal case of endo-carditis associated with *Bartonella henselae* I infection in a domestic cat. *J. Clin. Microbiol.* **41:**5337–5339.

8a.**Conrads, G., D. M. Citron, S. Jang, and E. J. C. Goldstein.** *Fusobacterium canifelinum* sp. novum from the oral cavity of cats and dogs. *Syst. Appl. Microbiol.,* in press.

9. **Craven, R. B., and A. M. Barnes.** 1991. Plague and tularemia. *Infect. Dis. Clin. N. Am.* **5:**165–175.

10. **de Lima Barros, M. B., A. de Oliveira Schubach, M. C. Galhardo, T. M. Schubach, R. S. dos Reis, M. J. Conceicao, and A. C. do Valle.** 2003. Sporotrichosis with widespread cutaneous lesions: re-port of 24 cases related to transmission by domestic cats in Rio de Janeiro, Brazil. *Int. J. Dermatol.* **42:**677–681.

11. **Despommier, D.** 2003. Toxocariasis: clinical aspects, epidemiology, medical ecology, and molecu-lar aspects. *Clin. Microbiol. Rev.* **16:**265–272.

12. **Dworkin, M. S., P. S. Sullivan, S. E. Buskin, R. D. Harrington, J. Olliffe, R. D. MacArthur, and C. E. Lopez.** 1999. *Bordetella bronchiseptica* infection in human immunodeficiency virus-infected patients. *Clin. Infect. Dis.* **28:**1095–1099.

13. **Foley, J. E., C. M. Leutenegger, J. S. Dumler, N. C. Pedersen, and J. E. Madigan.** 2003. Evidence for modulated immune response to *Anaplasma phagocytophila* sensu lato in cats with FIV-induced im-munosuppression. *Comp. Immunol. Microbiol. Infect. Dis.* **26:**103–113.

14. **Fukushima, H., M. Gomyoda, S. Ishikura, T. Nishio, S. Moriki, J. Endo, S. Kaneko, and M. Tsubokura.** 1989. Cat-contaminated environmental substances lead to *Yersinia pseudotuberculo-sis* infection in children. *J. Clin. Microbiol.* **27:**2706–2709.

15. **Goldstein, E. J. C., D. M. Citron, B. Wield, U. Blachman, V. L. Sutter, T. A. Miller, and S. M. Finegold.** 1978. Bacteriology of human and animal bite wounds. *J. Clin. Microbiol.* **8:**667–672.

16. **Greene, C. E. (ed.).** 1998. *Infectious Diseases of the Dog and Cat,* 2nd ed. The W. B. Saunders Co., Philadelphia, Pa.

17. **Greene, C. E., R. McDermott, P. H. Jameson, and A. M. Marks.** 1996. *Bartonella henselae* infection in cats: evaluation during primary infection, treatment, and rechallenge infection. *J. Clin. Microbiol.* **34:**1682–1685.

18. **Hamilton, D. H., K. M. Zangwill, J. L. Hadler, and M. L. Cartter.** 1995. Cat-scratch disease—Connecticut, 1992–1993. *J. Infect. Dis.* **172:**570–573.

19. **Hawranek, T., M. Tritscher, W. H. Muss, J. Jecel, N. Nowotny, J. Kolodziejek, M. Emberger, H. Schaeppi, and H. Hintner.** 2003. Feline orthopoxvirus infection transmitted from cat to human. *J. Am. Acad. Dermatol.* **49:**513–518.

20. **Hodges, R. D., A. M. Legendre, L. G. Adams, M. D. Willard, R. P. Pitts, K. Monce, C. C. Needles, and H. Ward.** 1994. Itraconazole for the treatment of histoplasmosis in cats. *J. Vet. Intern. Med.* **8:**409–413.

21. **Holley, H. P., Jr.** 1991. Successful treatment of cat-scratch disease with ciprofloxacin. *JAMA* **265:**1563–1565.

22. **Holst, E., J. Rolof, L. Larsson, and J. P. Nielsen.** 1992. Characterization and distribution of *Pas-teurella* species recovered from infected humans. *J. Clin. Microbiol.* **30:**2984–2987.

23. **Juranek, D. D.** 1995. Cryptosporidiosis: sources of infection and guidelines for prevention. *Clin. Infect. Dis.* **21**(Suppl. 1):57–61.

23a.**Kenny, M. J., R. J. Birtles, M. J. Day, and S. E. Shaw.** 2003. Rickettsia felis in the United Kingdom. *Emerg. Infect. Dis.* **9:**1023–1024.

24. **Koehler, J. E., and J. W. Tappero.** 1993. Bacillary angiomatosis and bacillary peliosis in patients in-fected with human immunodeficiency virus. *Clin. Infect. Dis.* **17:**612–624.

25. **Koehler, J. E., F. D. Quinn, T. G. Berger, P. E. LeBoit, and J. W. Tappero.** 1992. Isolation of *Rochali-maea* species from cutaneous and osseous lesions of bacillary angiomatosis. *N. Engl. J. Med.* **327:**1625–1631.

26. **Kravetz, J. D., and D. G. Federman.** 2002. Cat-associated zoonoses. *Arch. Intern. Med.* **162:**1945–1952.

27. **Kuno, A., K. Ido, N. Isoda, Y. Satoh, K. Ono, S. Satoh, H. Inamori, K. Sugano, N. Kanai, T. Nishizawa, and H. Okamoto.** 2003. Sporadic acute hepatitis E of a 47-year-old man whose pet cat was positive for antibody to hepatitis E virus. *Hepatol. Res.* **26:**237–242.

28. **Lee, A.** 1992. *Helicobacter pylori* and *Helicobacter*-like organisms in animals: overview of mucus-colonizing organisms, p. 259–275. *In* B. J. Rathbone and R. U. Heatley (ed.), *Helicobacter pylori and Gastroduodenal Disease*, 2nd ed. Blackwell Scientific, London, England.

29. **Malnick, H., K. Williams, J. Phil-Ebosie, and A. S. Levy.** 1990. Description of a medium for isolating *Anaerobiospirillum* spp., a possible cause of zoonotic disease, from diarrheal feces and blood of humans and use of the medium in a survey of human, canine, and feline feces. *J. Clin. Microbiol.* **28:**1380–1384.

30. **Malnick, H.** 1997. *Anaerobiospirillum thomasii* sp. nov., an anaerobic spiral bacterium isolated from the feces of cats and dogs and from diarrheal feces of humans, and emendation of the genus *Anaerobiospirillum*. *Int. J. Syst. Bacteriol.* **47:**381–384.

31. **Maurin, M., S. Gasquet, C. Ducco, and D. Raoult.** 1995. MICs of 28 antibiotic compounds for 14 *Bartonella* (formerly *Rochalimaea*) isolates. *Antimicrob. Agents Chemother.* **39:**2387–2391.

32. **Metzkor-Cotter, E., Y. Kletter, B. Avidor, M. Varon, Y. Golan, M. Ephros, and M. Giladi.** 2003. Long-term serological analysis and clinical follow-up of patients with cat scratch disease. *Clin. Infect. Dis.* **37:**1149–1154.

33. **Mui, B. S. K., M. E. Mulligan, and W. L. George.** 1990. Response of HIV-associated disseminated cat scratch disease to treatment with doxycycline. *Am. J. Med.* **89:**229–231.

34. **Pinard, J. A., N. S. Leslie, and P. J. Irvine.** 2003. Maternal serologic screening for toxoplasmosis. *J. Midwifery Womens Health* **48:**308–316.

35. **Purcell, R. H., and S. U. Emerson.** 2000. Hepatitis E virus, p. 1958–1970. *In* G. L. Mandell, J. E. Bennett, and R. Dolin (ed.), *Principles and Practice of Infectious Diseases*, 5th ed. Churchill Livingstone, Philadelphia, Pa.

36. **Raoult, D., P. E. Fournier, M. Drancourt, T. J. Marrie, J. Etienne, J. Cosserat, P. Cacoub, Y. Poinsignon, P. Leclerq, and A. M. Sefton.** 1996. Diagnosis of 22 new cases of *Bartonella* endocarditis. *Ann. Intern. Med.* **125:**646–652.

37. **Reed, J. B., D. K. Scales, M. T. Wong, and C. P. Lattuada, Jr.** 1998. Cat scratch disease retinitis, therapy. *Ophthalmology* **105:**459–466.

38. **Regnery, R., and J. Tappero.** 1997. Unraveling mysteries associated with cat-scratch disease, bacillary angiomatosis, and related syndromes. *Emerg. Infect. Dis.* **1:**16–21.

38a. **Rolain, J. M., P. Brouqui, J. E. Koehler, C. Maguina, M. J. Dolan, and D. Raoult.** 2004. Recommendations for treatment of human infections caused by *Bartonella* species. *Antimicrob. Agents Chemother.* **48:**1921–1933.

39. **Schubach, T. M., A. Schubach, T. Okamoto, I. V. Pellon, P. C. Fialho-Monteiro, R. S. Reis, M. B. Barros, M. Andrade-Perez, and B. Wanke.** 2003. Haematogenous spread of Sporothrix schenckii in cats with naturally acquired sporotrichosis. *J. Small Anim. Pract.* **44:**395–398.

40. **Talan, D. A., D. M. Citron, F. A. Abrahamian, G. J. Moran, E. J. C. Goldstein, and the Emergency Medicine Animal Bite Infection Study Group.** 1999. The bacteriology and management of dog and cat bite wound infections presenting to emergency departments. *N. Engl. J. Med.* **340:**85–92.

41. **Tappero, J. W., J. Mohle-Boetani, J. E. Koehler, B. Swaminathan, T. G. Berger, P. E. LeBoit, L. L. Smith, J. D. Wenger, R. W. Pinner, C. A. Kemper, and A. L. Reingold.** 1993. The epidemiology of bacillary angiomatosis and bacillary peliosis. *JAMA* **269:**770–775.

42. **Titball, R. W., and A. Sjostedt.** 2003. *Francisella tularensis:* an overview. *ASM News* **69:**558–563.

43. **U.S. Department of Commerce.** 1990. *Statistical Abstracts of the United States, 1990*, p. 234. U.S. Department of Commerce, Washington, D.C.

44. **Welch, D. F., D. A. Pickett, L. N. Slater, A. G. Steigerwalt, and D. J. Brenner.** 1992. *Rochalimaea henselae* sp. nov., a cause of septicemia, bacillary angiomatosis, and parenchymal bacillary peliosis. *J. Clin. Microbiol.* **30:**275–280.

45. **Wolfson, C., J. Branley, and T. Gottlieb.** 1996. The Etest for antimicrobial susceptibility testing of *Bartonella henselae*. *J. Antimicrob. Chemother.* **38:**963–968.

46. **Zavala-Velazquez, J. E., J. A. Ruiz-Sosa, R. A. Sanchez-Elias, G. Becerra-Carmona, and D. H. Walker.** 2000. *Rickettsia felis* rickettsiosis in Yucatan. *Lancet* **356:**1079–1080.

Infections of Leisure, Third Edition
Edited by David Schlossberg
© 2004 ASM Press, Washington, D.C.

Chapter 7

Feathered Friends

Matthew E. Levison

Although many people these days work at leisure time activities, diseases are most commonly acquired from birds during the course of work in the usual sense of the term, not leisure. However, travel for pleasure to areas where the diseases are highly endemic puts people at risk of acquiring some of these bird-related diseases (histoplasmosis and togavirus infections), as does ownership of birds as pets (psittacosis).

Infectious diseases can be transmitted to humans from birds by one of several mechanisms (Table 1). In group 1 infections, birds are the natural reservoirs for the infectious agent, which causes illness among them. The diseased birds then disseminate the infectious agent into the environment, and humans become infected as accidental hosts. Examples of such infections include psittacosis, Newcastle disease, avian influenza, and yersiniosis. In group 2 and 3 infections, birds are the natural reservoirs for the infectious agent but do not become ill themselves. The infectious agents disseminate from the colonized birds into the environment directly (for example, salmonellosis and mites) in group 2 infections or by means of insect vectors (for example, eastern equine, St. Louis, western equine, and Japanese B encephalitis) in group 3 infections, involving humans as accidental hosts. In group 4 infections, birds are not the natural reservoirs, but they facilitate growth of the organisms in the environment by means of their fecal matter. Examples of the last category include the fungal diseases histoplasmosis and cryptococcosis (1).

PSITTACOSIS

Pathogen

Chlamydia psittaci is an obligate intracellular bacterial parasite.

Matthew E. Levison • Drexel University College of Medicine, 3300 Henry Ave., Philadelphia, PA 19129.

Table 1. Bird-related diseases

Natural reservoir(s)	Disease	Illness(es) in:		Mode(s) of spread
		Birds	Humans	
Group 1				
Birds	Psittacosis	Intestinal, respiratory	Respiratory	Aerosolized bird feces
Domestic and wild fowl	Newcastle disease	Respiratory, neurological	Conjunctivitis	Aerosols, contaminated hands
	Influenza	Respiratory, intestinal, neurological	Respiratory	Aerosols
Domestic and wild turkeys	Yersiniosis	Intestinal	Intestinal	Contaminated food
Group 2				
Domestic and wild birds	Mite infestation	None	Pruritic rash	Indirect and direct contact
Domestic fowl	Salmonellosis	None	Diarrhea	Contaminated food
Group 3 (domestic and wild birds)	Arbovirus infections	None	Encephalitis, polyarthritis, rash	Insect vector
	Histoplasmosis	None	Respiratory	Aerosols
Group 4 (soil fertilized by bird droppings)	Cryptococcosis	None	Respiratory, neurological	Aerosols

Source of Infection

The natural reservoirs of *C. psittaci* are wild and domestic birds. Infection in birds is usually latent but may become apparent when resistance is compromised by conditions such as crowding, prolonged transport, or nutritional deficiencies. In birds the infection is primarily gastrointestinal and respiratory and results in diarrhea, fever, conjunctival congestion, and respiratory distress. The agent is shed in the liquid feces, contaminating the environment and the bird's feathers. As the fecal matter dries, the chlamydiae become airborne, which is facilitated by the motion of the feathers. In addition to coprophagy and cannibalism, birds acquire the disease by inhalation of infectious aerosols, i.e., airborne particles less than 5 μm in diameter. Airborne particles of this size do not settle out by gravity but remain suspended for prolonged periods; only ventilation and filtration by the lungs remove these particles from the atmosphere. Humans acquire the disease by inhalation of infectious aerosols.

Human Activity

Psittacosis is mainly an occupational disease among workers in turkey processing plants (8, 9), duck or goose pluckers, pigeon breeders, and pet store employees.

Human Disease

C. psittaci causes atypical pneumonia, that is, pneumonia usually characterized by an insidious onset, a predominance of constitutional symptoms (such as fever, headache, and myalgias), shortness of breath, and a nonproductive hacking cough. Chest X rays show focal infiltrates, usually at the lung bases. More severe illness may be accompanied by nausea, vomiting, diarrhea, delirium, and hepatosplenomegaly. The illness is usually self-limiting and lasts 1 to 2 weeks, but the course can be shortened by the use of antibiotic therapy, e.g., doxycycline. The case/fatality ratio is less than 1% with appropriate therapy, except for the rare cases acquired from other people, where the disease has been noted to be more severe, with high mortality. The organisms can be recovered in culture from sputum and blood. Isolation of the organism should only be attempted in laboratories that use strict isolation techniques. Diagnosis is usually confirmed by a fourfold rise in serum complement-fixing antibody titers between onset and convalescence.

Treatment for adults consists of 2 weeks of doxycycline at 100 mg orally every 12 h. The macrolide azithromycin achieves high intracellular concentrations, is bactericidal, has a long half-life that allows single daily dosing, is well tolerated after oral administration, and may prove equally or more efficacious.

Control

Chemoprophylaxis of psittacine birds with 0.5% chlortetracycline for 3 to 4 weeks prior to shipment or after arrival or mass treatment and quarantine of flocks that are identified by serologic screening as being infected have been used successfully to control the disease (3).

NEWCASTLE DISEASE

Pathogen

The Newcastle disease agent is an RNA virus that is related to the mumps virus. In birds, the severity of clinical picture produced by Newcastle virus varies depending on the strain of virus and the species of bird and usually involves respiratory and neurological findings. More-virulent strains produce hemorrhagic lesions in the digestive tract, associated with high mortality. More-susceptible species of birds include chickens. A carrier state may exist in psittacines and some other wild birds.

Source of Infection

Domestic fowl, especially poultry, and wildfowl are the natural reservoirs of the virus. Sources of the virus include respiratory secretions, carcasses, and feces of infected birds. Transmission among birds occurs by aerosol inhalation; the ingestion of secretions, especially feces, of an infected bird; or contact with contaminated water, feed, implements, premises, or human clothing.

Human Activity

The disease occurs primarily in poultry slaughterhouse workers, laboratory personnel, and vaccinators of the live Newcastle disease virus vaccines. It is transmitted by rubbing the eyes with contaminated hands or by inhalation of infectious aerosols (6).

Human Disease

After an incubation period of several days, patients usually develop conjunctivitis with minimal constitutional symptoms; some patients develop an influenza-like illness, thought to be the consequence of aerosol exposure.

Control

The disease has been controlled by the routine use of Newcastle disease virus vaccines in the poultry industry.

AVIAN INFLUENZA (5, 19)

Pathogen

Influenza is caused by either influenza A or B virus; the more important of the two, and the cause of pandemics in humans, is influenza A virus. A third genus, influenza C virus, is also recognized. The influenza virus genome is divided into eight separate segments of RNA. The antigenic specificity of the viral nucleoprotein determines group specificity, while the antigenic specificities of the two surface proteins (hemagglutinin [H] and neuraminidase [N]) determine type specificity. Influenza A viruses of 15 H and 9 N types are known to circulate in humans and other animals, whereas influenza B virus infects only humans. H is the main determinant of the host range of influenza A viruses. Types H1, H2, and H3 are known most commonly to cause human infection. Swine can be infected by H1 and H2; horses can be infected by H3 and H7; seals can be infected by H1, H4, and H7; and ducks and other aquatic birds can be infected by all 15 H types of influenza A viruses. The influenza virus produces a respiratory infection in swine and horses that is similar to that in humans. Influenza in avian species varies from inapparent infection to a lethal infection involving the gastrointestinal tract, central nervous system, and respiratory tract.

Before 1997, strains infecting domestic birds were not known to produce disease by direct transfer to humans, although seroprevalence studies in southern China revealed that inapparent infection with avian strains had occurred in up to 38% of the local human population. However, transmission of influenza has been demonstrated between pigs and humans and possibly between pigs and birds. Within a cell of an intermediate nonhuman host, such as the pig, coinfected by strains with different host specificities, reassortment of the eight segments of the genome of each strain may result in a new strain with a novel combination of surface proteins. Thus, the numerous H and N types of nonhuman origin create a reservoir of influenza viruses available for genetic reassortment with circulating human strains. Reassortment results in a so-called antigenic shift.

If the recombinant strain is capable of infecting humans and being efficiently spread from person to person, it may produce a pandemic in the human population, which is highly susceptible because the prevalent antibody does not recognize this novel strain of influenza virus. Pandemics have occurred every 10 to 40 years (e.g., 1889, 1918, 1957, 1968, and 1977). Each of these pandemics was characterized by its sudden appearance; the first occurrence of cases in China during the more recent pandemics; restriction to H1, H2, and H3; and an antigenic specificity of the pandemic strain distinctly different from those of influenza viruses then circulating in humans. The H1N1 strain that caused the 1918 pandemic is thought to be of avian origin and to have undergone reassortment with a human strain in pigs; it persists in swine to this day as swine influenza virus.

The probability of reassortment between human and domestic-animal influenza viruses increases in proportion to the contact between humans and the domestic animals. Such close contact, for example, through the presence of numerous live-bird markets, occurs in communities in Southeast Asia, where most influenza epidemics have first arisen. Pandemics spread along routes of travel at any season from one country to another. They involve people of all ages, with high attack and mortality rates, especially in young adults. The 1918 pandemic occurred in three waves associated in part with troop movements in World War I; 21 million people died worldwide, and 549,000 people died in the United States.

Mutations of the influenza virus genome result in changes in the H and N proteins on the outer surface of the virus. These surface proteins function in binding the virus to and releasing it from the host cell. Viral mutations arise continuously in the infected host and may become predominant by circumventing the preexisting host immune response that suppresses the wild-type organism but allows the mutant to propagate. The result of this so-called antigenic drift is not sufficient to compromise immunity completely, as would occur with infection by a pandemic strain. Antigenic drift results in the regional epidemics that occur, usually in the late fall and winter, every few years. Attack rates in these seasonal epidemics tend to be lower than those during a pandemic, and mortality is variable. Because attack rates approach 20 to 30%, outbreaks of influenza disrupt community and business life and cause dramatic increases in the use of health care services.

Source of Infection

Influenza is spread in crowded, enclosed, poorly ventilated spaces by means of infectious aerosol particles, less than 5 μm in diameter, that are generated by infected persons. Because of their light weight, the particles remain suspended in the air for prolonged periods unless dissipated by ventilation. Particles the size of aerosols effectively bypass defenses in the upper respiratory tract (i.e., the mucociliary barrier). Because influenza is highly contagious and has a short incubation period (about 2 days), the infection spreads through a susceptible population quickly, usually infecting most of those susceptible within several weeks.

Human Activity

The identification of an influenza virus that is new to the human population is a cause of great concern for public health, because a pandemic can occur from the emergence and sustained person-to-person transmission of a novel strain to which humans have no immunity. As a result of ongoing influenza surveillance in

Hong Kong, an outbreak of influenza was recently found to be caused by a strain of influenza A (H5N1) virus (18a, 19). This strain had previously been noted to infect only shorebirds and domestic birds. In May 1997, however, a strain of influenza virus was isolated from a 3-year-old boy who died of complications of influenza (respiratory, renal, and liver failure and disseminated intravascular coagulopathy). It took 3 months to identify the strain as influenza A (H5N1) virus in a Dutch laboratory that is one of the World Health Organization Influenza Reference Centers. No further isolates were found during the next 5 months, despite continued surveillance. However, 17 additional cases were identified in November and December 1997. The 18 patients ranged from 1 to 60 years of age, and 10 were female. Eight required mechanical ventilation, and six died. Like that described for influenza pandemics, disease was seen primarily in children and young adults, and the mortality was high and was concentrated in young adults. The cases were not geographically clustered within Hong Kong, and no cases occurred outside of Hong Kong. No cases have occurred since the last week in December 1997, when large-scale killing of flocks of chickens and ducks was initiated in Hong Kong.

DNA analysis of the virus genome revealed all gene segments of the isolate to be of avian origin, with no evidence of genetic reassortment with recent human influenza A virus genes. The isolate retained pathogenicity for avian species, and laboratory contamination was found to be unlikely. There were outbreaks of avian influenza on farms in Hong Kong from March to May 1997 due to H5N1 viruses, and a case control study suggested that contact with poultry was the strongest risk factor for developing disease. There were sick chicks at the initial patient's preschool, although there was no evidence of direct contact or that the chicks were infected with influenza virus.

The H protein cleavage site that is characteristic of highly pathogenic avian viruses, and that is believed to enable the virus to spread systemically in birds from the respiratory tract to other sites in the infected host, such as the heart and brain, was found in the H5N1 strain. The H5N1 strain was closely related to avian strains isolated from wild shorebirds in Asia. The strain is likely to have spread from these shorebirds to domestic birds and then among flocks of the domestic birds. Although wild birds have not been proven to be the source of the Hong Kong outbreak, shared use of water sources, such as ponds that become contaminated with feces of wild ducks and other waterfowl, presumably introduces low-pathogenicity influenza virus into domestic flocks; if allowed to circulate, the virus can evolve into a highly pathogenic form. However, because the strain apparently lacks the genes encoding the ability for efficient person-to-person transmission, the disease spread no further than to the few humans who had contact with infected domestic birds.

An H5N1 outbreak recurred in the Far East in 2004. From January to March, 22 confirmed human cases of influenza A (H5N1) were reported in Vietnam, with 15 deaths, and 12 cases were reported in Thailand, with 8 deaths. All patients with confirmed cases were hospitalized with severe pneumonia; most were children or young adults who tended poultry on farms or kept poultry as pets. There was no evidence of person-to-person spread. Infection in humans coincided with a widespread epidemic caused by the same highly pathogenic H5N1 strain among poultry in Vietnam and Thailand. Concurrent H5N1 outbreaks occurred in poultry populations in South Korea, Japan, China, Indonesia, Laos, and Cambodia without confirmed human cases. Outbreaks of highly pathogenic avian influenza virus can be extremely difficult to control. Control efforts in the recent Asian outbreaks required culling millions of infected and exposed birds in the poultry stock in the affected countries.

Human Disease

Influenza is a dramatic respiratory tract infection that strikes suddenly with shaking chills, fever, headache, myalgias, and a nonproductive persistent cough. In most patients the disease lasts several days and the outcome is benign. Some patients, usually those with underlying chronic heart or lung disease, develop overwhelming viral pneumonia. Others may develop secondary bacterial pneumonia during or shortly after the attack. These complications result in mortality in excess of a given norm for the time and place in which the epidemic occurs. This mortality may result not only from influenza itself but also from the underlying conditions, especially heart and lung disease. Generally, 80 to 90% of influenza-associated excess mortality occurs among persons ≥65 years old.

Control

Control of influenza is best achieved by means of an effective vaccine. The influenza vaccine is made from egg-grown viruses that are highly purified and inactivated and cannot cause infection. Since 1976, the vaccines have contained two type A strains (H1N1 and H3N2) and one type B strain. The vaccines are available in both whole and split (subvirion) preparations. Both preparations are well tolerated and they are equally immunogenic in adults, but the split preparation is better tolerated in children. Because the antigenic specificity of the circulating strain usually varies annually and infection or vaccination with one strain provides little protection against infection by a subsequent, more distantly related strain of the same type, vaccines must be kept current. High-risk members of the population must be revaccinated annually with vaccine appropriate for the strain that is anticipated to be in circulation during the subsequent winter. The appearance of a new strain that is anticipated to be implicated in the next winter's outbreak in North America must be detected by means of a worldwide surveillance program, especially in Southeast Asia, early enough to allow sufficient lead time for vaccine production. The implicated strain must be adapted to egg culture, and a high-yield clone suitable for mass production must be selected.

Influenza vaccines are efficacious in 70 to 90% of young adults for reduction of clinical illness caused by the same strain or closely related strains. In older persons the efficacy may be only 30 to 40% in preventing clinical illness, although vaccines are more effective in preventing pneumonia, hospitalization, and death and in preventing institutional outbreaks in nursing homes. Development of a vaccine for the H5N1 strain that caused the 1997 outbreak in Hong Kong has been problematic because of difficulty in adapting the strain to egg culture.

Amantadine (200 mg/day in most adults and 100 mg/day in persons over 65 years of age) or rimantadine is effective for prevention of influenza A virus infection in unimmunized patients during an influenza A outbreak and for therapy (for 5 to 7 days) of early influenza A infection. An in vitro assay revealed that the H5N1 strain involved in the 1997 Hong Kong outbreak was sensitive to amantadine. Drugs that selectively block viral neuraminidase activity are also available for prophylaxis and treatment of influenza A and B infections.

Vaccines are also available for immunization against the bacterial pathogens, *Streptococcus pneumoniae* and *Haemophilus influenzae* type b, that may cause secondary bacterial pneumonia. Influenza and pneumococcal vaccines are strongly recommended for health care workers, persons over 65 years of age, and persons of any age who are at risk for adverse consequences of influenza or bacterial pneumonia because of underlying conditions, such as human immunodeficiency virus infection, diabetes mellitus, hemoglobinopathies, immunosuppression, or chronic renal, pulmonary, cardiac, or liver disease. Revaccination with pneumococcal vaccine in 5 years is now recommended by the Centers for Disease Control and Prevention for certain high-risk persons who have relatively rapid falls in antibody titers after initial vaccination. The currently available 23-valent pneumococcal vaccine covers 88% of the serotypes causing systemic disease as well as 8% of related serotypes. The increasing prevalence of multiantibiotic resistance in pneumococci makes immunization of high-risk individuals with the pneumococcal vaccine of utmost importance. The use of aspirin in children and young adults with influenza is risky because of the possible development of Reye's syndrome as a complication.

YERSINIOSIS

Pathogen

Yersinia pseudotuberculosis is an enteric facultatively anaerobic gram-negative bacillus in the family *Enterobacteriaceae*, like *Escherichia coli, Proteus mirabilis, Klebsiella pneumoniae*, etc. *Yersinia* grows well at refrigerator temperatures, unlike other enteric pathogens, and also at 37°C on routine media. So-called cold enrichment is used to differentially isolate *Yersinia* from clinical material.

Source of Infection

The natural reservoirs for *Y. pseudotuberculosis* are believed to be domestic and wild animals, including turkeys, guinea pigs, sheep, cats, and rabbits (22, 23).

Human Activity

The mechanisms by which the disease is transmitted to humans are unknown, but contamination of food from the animal reservoir is thought to be an important factor. Humans acquire the disease by the fecal-oral route.

Human Disease

Yersiniosis presents as an acute abdominal infection that simulates acute appendicitis, with fever, right lower quadrant pain, and vomiting. The course is usually benign and lasts for about 1 week unless interrupted by surgery for suspected acute appendicitis; however, symptoms may persist for months (20).

Although it has not been subjected to critical analysis, effective treatment is thought to consist of a 2-week course of either doxycycline or a fluoroquinolone, e.g., ciprofloxacin (750 mg every 12 h).

Control

In view of the obscure modes of transmission to humans, control of yersiniosis is problematic, but it should involve protection of food and water against fecal contamination by fowl and other animals.

MITES

Pathogen

Mites that infest wild and domestic birds have four stages (i.e., egg, larva, nymph, and adult) in their life cycles, which can be completed within 1 week under favorable circumstances.

Source of Infection

The natural reservoirs for these mites are birds. Humans are accidental hosts. The adults of the species *Dermanyssus gallinae* feed on birds at night and during the day infest the buildings that house the birds; there, the female mites lay eggs after feeding on the host's blood. Other species of mites, e.g., *Ornithonyssus bursa* and *Ornithonyssus sylviarum*, complete their entire life cycles on birds.

Human Activity

People who work during the day in buildings that house infested birds can become accidental hosts of *D. gallinae*, whereas human infestation by *Ornithonyssus* occurs mainly from handling birds.

Human Disease

Intensely pruritic papular urticaria develops at sites on the skin where the mites have bitten.

Control

The most effective method to control mite bites is spraying clothing with insect repellent, such as products that contain dimethylphthalate.

SALMONELLOSIS

Pathogen

Non-*Salmonella enterica* serovar Typhi salmonellae are enteric facultatively anaerobic gram-negative bacilli in the family *Enterobacteriaceae*. Identification is based on serotyping. Over 1,000 serotypes are known to infect humans. The majority of these strains can be grouped with polyvalent antisera into groups A to E. Definitive identification of a serotype depends on reactivity to antisera directed against somatic O and flagellar H antigens. The relative frequencies at which specific serotypes are isolated vary among different geographic areas. *Salmonella enterica* serovar Typhimurium is the most frequent salmonella serotype isolated in the United States.

Source of Infection

Whereas serovar Typhi is specific for humans, the natural reservoirs of non-serovar Typhi salmonellae are a large variety of both wild and domestic animals (7). Animal-to-animal transmission can be facilitated by contamination of animal feed whose main ingredients are meal made from bone and meat. The most common source of human disease is poultry products, such as eggs, chicken, turkey, and ducks, but meat from other animals is also involved. Salmonellae on raw meat can contaminate utensils and surfaces where food is prepared and then be transferred to previously uncontaminated food. Cooking temperatures may not be high enough to lower the bacterial count sufficiently, and in fact, the cooking temperatures, for example, in the center of a stuffed turkey or a soft-boiled or quick-scrambled egg, may actually foster bacterial growth.

Human Activity

Salmonellosis is acquired by ingestion of food or water contaminated by large numbers of organisms, e.g., $>10^5$ CFU/ml, when eating out or at home. Traveler's diarrhea is usually caused by any one of a variety of enteric pathogens but is most commonly caused by enteropathogenic *E. coli* rather than non-serovar Typhi *Salmonella*. Direct transmission from person to person without food or water as the intervening vehicle does occur, usually by means of the fecal-oral route during male homosexual activity. Person-to-person spread has also been implicated in nursery and hospital outbreaks, which involve patients in whom host defenses in the gastrointestinal tract, such as gastric acidity, small intestinal motility, and colonic bacterial flora, are compromised so that lower inoculum concentrations, i.e., $<10^5$ CFU/ml, are able to colonize the bowel and subsequently induce disease. Gastrointestinal defenses may be compromised by antacids, gastrectomy, agents that slow intestinal motility, and antibiotics. Some diseases, such as cirrhosis, lymphoma, and human immunodeficiency virus infection, which impair systemic host defenses, also increase susceptibility to salmonellosis. *Salmonella* colonizes and invades the intestinal mucosa and then may gain access to the bloodstream to produce transient bacteremia. Metastatic infection, usually in tissues that are previously diseased, such as in hematomas, neoplasms, bone infarcts, degenerative arthritis, or even atherosclerotic abdominal aneurysms, may follow episodes of transient bacteremia. Control of *Salmonella* bacteremia is impaired in patients with an underlying hemolytic condition, such as sickle cell anemia. In fact, in patients with sickle cell anemia, *Salmonella* rather than *Staphylococcus aureus* is the most common cause of osteomyelitis in areas of bone compromised by ischemia or necrosis.

Human Disease

Non-serovar Typhi *Salmonella* causes an acute, self-limiting, febrile, diarrheal disease of about 1 week's duration. Patients can carry *Salmonella* in the intestinal tract for several weeks or, more rarely, for up to several months during convalescence. Transient bacteremia is unusually detected in adult patients but is more frequently detected in infants (up to 50% in patients during the first week of life) and in elderly patients, and it is more common with some *Salmonella* species, such as *Salmonella enterica* serovar Choleraesuis.

Control

Control is currently based on the education of cooks at home and in commercial establishments about appropriate methods to reduce contamination of food. Antibiotic therapy of infected patients, even with new potent agents, such as the fluoroquinolones, does not shorten the course of the illness or ameliorate the symptoms and fails to shorten the duration of the convalescent carrier state (16). The methods recommended for prevention of traveler's diarrhea apply to salmonellosis: use no ice in drinks; drink only bottled, carbonated beverages, hot tea or coffee, or beer; brush the teeth with any of the aforementioned liquids; eat only cooked, hot food; and eat no raw vegetables (e.g., salads), undercooked meats or fish, or unpeeled fruits (see chapter 13 for more on travel-related illnesses).

ARTHROPOD-BORNE VIRUSES

Pathogens

Arthropod-borne viruses (also called arboviruses) are a heterogeneous group of RNA viruses that share a mode of vector-borne transmission. These species belong to either the alphaviruses (*Togaviridae*) or flaviviruses. Eastern equine encephalitis (EEE), western equine encephalitis (WEE), Ross River, and Sindbis viruses are alphaviruses, and St. Louis encephalitis (SLE) (10, 15), Japanese encephalitis (11, 17), Murray Valley encephalitis, West Nile, Central Europe encephalitis, and Russian spring-summer encephalitis viruses are flaviviruses.

Source of Infection

The distributions of EEE, WEE, and SLE viruses overlap extensively. For example, EEE virus has been isolated from eastern Canada, the Gulf and Atlantic coasts of the United States, the Caribbean islands, and Central and South America. WEE and SLE viruses also are distributed from Canada to Argentina. Japanese encephalitis virus is found in most countries of the Far East and in India. Sindbis virus is found in Africa, Scandinavia, countries of the former Soviet Union, and Asia; Ross River virus is found in northern and eastern Australia and Oceania; and Murray Valley virus is found in southern Australia and New Guinea. The natural reservoirs of these viruses are native wild birds, among which arthropod vectors spread the viruses. Mosquitoes transmit most arboviruses, but ticks (arachnids) transmit a few (Central Europe encephalitis and Russian spring-summer viruses). Viral amplification in other vertebrate species may lead to epidemic outbreaks that involve domestic animals and humans, who are accidental hosts.

Human Activity

Habitation or travel in an area where arboviruses are endemic places a person at risk.

Human Disease

All of these viruses, except Sindbis and Ross River viruses, produce an acute illness, with sudden onset of fever, headache, decreased sensorium, and stiff neck. More severe cases are complicated by progressive delirium, convulsions, coma, death, or residual neurological deficits in those who recover. Although EEE occurs less frequently than SLE or WEE, it has greater morbidity and mortality. Most SLE cases occur in those >60 years of age, in whom the disease is particularly severe, whereas Murray Valley virus infection is more frequent and especially severe in children. Sindbis and Ross River viruses produce a mild illness characterized by fever, polyarthritis, jaundice, and a maculopapular or vesicular rash.

Control

Effective vaccines are available against Japanese encephalitis, WEE, and EEE. However, only the vaccine for Japanese encephalitis has been extensively used in humans. Mass vaccination programs have been carried out in several countries in the Far East, including Japan, Korea, and China, with good results in Japan. The vaccine is now available in the United States for prolonged travel to regions where the disease is endemic. Prevention of these infections is usually limited to avoidance of mosquito bites through the use of protective clothing, insect repellents on the body and clothing, and mosquito netting in dwellings in areas where the disease is endemic. Eradication of the insect vectors has been effective, but it is costly.

WNV

Of special note is West Nile virus (WNV). WNV was first isolated in Uganda in 1937 and first isolated in the United States in 1999. WNV is now seen throughout the United States, in Canada, and in the Caribbean basin. The 2002 WNV epidemic in the United States was the largest arboviral meningoencephalitis outbreak ever documented in the western hemisphere and the largest reported meningoencephalitis epidemic. As a newly introduced species, WNV is having a major effect on the North American ecosystem. WNV and SLE virus are closely related; both are transmitted by *Culex* mosquitoes and amplified in birds, but unlike SLE, WNV is an avian neuropathogen and causes high mortality in many avian species, including crows (which have the highest rate of WNV infection), blue jays, ravens, and raptors, such as eagles, hawks, and owls. In addition, WNV is a neuropathogen in other vertebrate species, such as horses, rabbits, squirrels, chipmunks, goats, and reptiles. A major die-off due to WNV infection is reported for many species of birds, mammals, and reptiles, although over time species are expected to adapt. The usual sentinel event that signals WNV activity in a region is sighting dead crows. WNV infection in birds is characterized by high-level viremia of sufficient magnitude to maintain a reservoir of infected mosquitoes. WNV can also pass transovarially from adult mosquitoes to their eggs, so that larvae are hatched already infected, and probably can also winter over in other unknown hosts. Although many species of mosquito are vectors of WNV, *Culex* species are the most common. WNV can also be found in bird feces and saliva, and perhaps birds of prey can acquire the infection by eating infected prey, or through their droppings, or pass the virus to their chicks transovarially.

Most human WNV infections are acquired by a bite of an infected mosquito, but a few patients have become infected by accidental percutaneous inoculation in the laboratory, by administration of blood and blood products and by transplantation of organs from infected donors, possibly by breast-feeding, and by transplacental transmission with evidence of congenital severe central nervous system damage in the child. WNV causes illness in humans from June to November in southern states and July to October in northern states, with peak activity in late August. The incubation period is 2 to 14 days. Infected patients are usually asymptomatic, but a few will have a nonspecific acute febrile illness, with headache, myalgias, swollen lymph nodes, and back pain, that resolves rapidly. Less than 1% develop meningitis, encephalitis, or acute flaccid paralysis after an initial mild febrile illness. Severe neurological illness and neurological residua, e.g., oculomotor palsies, muscle weakness, and movement disorders, which may mimic stroke, Parkinsonism, or poliomyelitis, are seen most frequently in older or immunocompromised patients, and relative higher mortality rates occur in these groups. The overall mortality rate for WNV infection is 6 to 7%.

Infection is thought to confer immunity against subsequent exposure. No antiviral drugs are known to be effective in prevention or treatment of WNV infection. Control of WNV includes spraying with insecticide for control of adult mosquitoes and larvae in the summertime, draining or treating stagnant water in urban and suburban areas during the mosquito season (mosquitoes lay their eggs in standing water, e.g., in fountains, bird baths, wading pools), and using personal protective measures to reduce mosquito exposure (e.g., DEET [*N,N*-diethyl-*m*-toluamide] on exposed skin, permethrin or DEET on clothing, clothing that minimizes exposed skin, sleeping under mosquito nets impregnated with permethrin, and limiting outdoor exposure at dawn and dusk, when mosquito biting is most intense). Bird-based surveillance is used to monitor regional WNV activity in an area before the recognition of human cases.

Although mosquito-borne transmission is the major mode of WNV transmission, transfusion-associated transmission has also been identified. In June 2003, the blood supply of the United States was screened for circulation of WNV RNA by testing pooled samples from 6 to 16 donors, using investigational nucleic acid amplification tests (NATs). Compared with screening each donor's plasma individually, such pooling dilutes viremic plasma by 6- to 16-fold and potentially reduces the assay's sensitivity. About 4.5 million people receive blood or blood products annually. Between June and December 2003, 818 WNV-positive donations in the United States that could have potentially transmitted WNV to recipients if transfused were interdicted by the NATs. However, six cases of WNV infection have been attributed to transfusion of blood that had been screened by testing pooled samples and had been found to be negative for WNV RNA, presumably because of very low levels of WNV. Individual donor testing for WNV RNA is being considered for 2004 in regions with high WNV infection rates.

Diagnosis of WNV infection is based on serologic tests and detection of WNV RNA by nucleic acid amplification. The viremia is typically low level and of short duration during the incubation period. Viremia has usually resolved by the time of onset of symptoms. WNV can be detected in the cerebrospinal fluid, and immunoglobulin M antibody specific for WNV can be detected in cerebrospinal fluid within 3 to 5 days of onset of clinical disease and in serum by day 6. Immunoglobulin G antibody appears several days later, and acute- and convalescent-phase serum samples, collected at least 2 weeks apart, can be run simultaneously to assess for a fourfold or greater rise in antibody titer. Antibodies against other flaviviruses can cross-react in serologic tests for WNV.

HISTOPLASMOSIS

Pathogen

Histoplasma capsulatum is a dimorphic fungus: the yeast form grows in vitro at 37°C and in tissues; the mycelial form grows in vitro at room temperature. One variety of the organism (*Histoplasma capsulatum* var. *duboisii*) has been isolated only in central Africa. The other variety is distributed worldwide, usually in major river valleys. In the United States, infection is concentrated in the Mississippi, Missouri, and Ohio river valleys (2, 12). Histoplasmosis is endemic in most of Latin America.

Source of Infection

The natural reservoir is soil, especially soils fertilized by bird or bat guano. Birds themselves are not infected, although some bats are infected and eliminate the fungus in their droppings. When contaminated soil is disturbed, for example, by bulldozing or razing old buildings, infectious aerosols of microconidia may be created, and in poorly ventilated caves, tunnels, and mines inhabited by bats, the air may become heavily laden with infectious aerosols when the ground is disturbed by human activity (14, 18).

Human Activity

Infection occurs in humans by inhalation of infectious aerosols when working at construction sites or when visiting caves, tunnels, and abandoned mines in which bat droppings have accumulated.

Human Disease

In areas where the disease is endemic, infection is common, although the precise prevalence may vary from area to area. From 20 to over 80% of the population in areas of endemicity have positive reactions to the histoplasmin skin test, which indicates past or current infection with *H. capsulatum*.

The pathogenesis of histoplasmosis is thought to be identical to that of tuberculosis. The inhaled aerosols, particles less than 3 µm in diameter, which may consist of only one or two infectious microconidia, easily bypass defense mechanisms in the upper respiratory tract and airways to lodge in the alveoli. In the lung, the microconidia may begin to grow and divide. Some particles may be engulfed by macrophages, which are eventually carried to regional lymph nodes. From there the intracellular pathogens are disseminated via the lymphatics into the bloodstream and then throughout the body to lodge in other reticuloendothelial organs, such as the bone marrow, liver, and spleen (primary lymphohematogenous dissemination).

Clinical disease presents in a variety of ways. Acute pulmonary histoplasmosis resembles atypical pneumonia, the severity of which depends on the number of infectious particles inhaled. Fever, headache, myalgias, and a dry, hacking cough develop initially. Several weeks after exposure to the infectious aerosol, some patients develop erythema nodosum and arthralgias, probably when the immune response first develops. With the onset of the immune response, further growth of the organisms is curtailed and the balance between the patient and the fungus then temporarily shifts in favor of the patient. Not all the organisms are killed, however; residual foci of latent infection remain, which can reactivate at any time in the future if host defenses should fail. In most patients, acute pulmonary histoplasmosis is a self-limiting process and the only residual signs of this initial encounter with histoplasma microconidia are diffusely scattered foci of fine pulmonary or splenic calcifications.

Progressive pulmonary disease develops in a few patients. The initial pulmonary infiltrates develop into a fibronodular pattern and cavities that enlarge over months to years but may become quiescent in some patients. Progressive pulmonary histoplasmosis is seen in older men with prior pulmonary disease.

Progressive dissemination with involvement primarily of the lung, liver, and bone marrow occurs rarely. Most of these patients have defects in cell-mediated immunity, e.g., patients with AIDS or severe debility, the very young, or the very old. The tempo of the illness may be acute or chronic, and it is invariably fatal if untreated. It is manifested by hepatosplenomegaly, fever, night sweats, and mucosal ulcerations. Involvement of the bone marrow may produce anemia, leukopenia, and thrombocytopenia.

H. capsulatum var. *duboisii* produces granulomatous lesions in skin, subcutaneous soft tissue, and bone in the form of abscesses and ulcerations.

A positive histoplasmin skin test indicates the presence of cellular immunity, but the test may be negative early in the course of disease or for patients with disseminated disease. It is used only for epidemiological purposes, not to diagnose a specific individual's illness. Indeed, the skin test may itself elicit an antibody response and confound the results of subsequent serologic testing. Testing of serologic response, sputum culture, and culture and histology of biopsied tissues, e.g., bone marrow, liver, and mucosal lesions, are the main diagnostic methods.

Treatment is reserved for those patients with severe acute pulmonary, chronic progressive, or disseminated disease. Amphotericin B (0.5 to 0.7 mg/kg of body weight intravenously daily for a total dose of 2 to 2.5 g) has been the standard therapy. Ketoconazole in doses of 400 mg orally daily for 6 or more months has proven equally effective (13).

Control

Control of the organism in the environment is difficult. Spraying the ground with 3% Formalin has been recommended, as has the use of face masks when disturbing dirt or buildings where birds have roosted.

CRYPTOCOCCOSIS

Pathogen

Cryptococcus neoformans is a urease-positive yeast that has worldwide distribution. The organism exists in tissues in an encapsulated form and in soil in an unencapsulated form. It reproduces both asexually as a yeast and sexually as a basidiomycete. *Cryptococcus* is identified in clinical specimens by detection of its polysaccharide capsule by means of the India ink preparation, by use of mucicarmine staining of the polysaccharide capsule around the organism in tissue sections, or by means of an antibody to the capsular polysaccharide antigen in serum and other body fluids.

Source of Infection

Birds carry the organism in their intestinal tracts without becoming ill. The organism is isolated from bird feces and soil contaminated with bird feces. The creatinine in the feces serves as a source of nitrogen for the organisms. Inhalation of an infectious aerosol, which is generated from contaminated dust or soil, is thought to be the mode of infection for humans. However, the exact form of the infectious agent is unknown. The size of the encapsulated yeast (4 to 7 μm in diameter) may be too large for it to be an efficient aerosol. However, the unencapsulated yeast or the basidiospore, which measures 2 μm in diameter, may be a more appropriate size for the infectious particle.

Human Activity

Work in areas where pigeons roost or where soil is contaminated with pigeon feces poses a danger.

Human Disease

The portal of infection is thought to be the respiratory tract, although only a minority of patients develop a respiratory illness. At the time most patients present with clinical cryptococcosis, they have extrapulmonary involvement, usually of the central nervous system; the asymptomatic primary pulmonary infection has either resolved spontaneously or left a residual pulmonary nodule (cryptococcoma). For the few patients with symptomatic pulmonary infection, the patient complains of fever, chest pain, cough, and hemoptysis, and unless the patient is immunocompromised, the disease has not disseminated to extrapulmonary sites. Dissemination is likely in patients with AIDS, lymphoma, diabetes mellitus, and cirrhosis and those being treated with corticosteroids. Involvement of the central nervous system presents insidiously over weeks, with severe headache and progressive deterioration in mental status. The patient may have a stiff neck and focal cranial nerve signs. The cerebrospinal fluid has a lymphocytic pleocytosis (5 to 500 leukocytes/mm^3), low glucose concentration (<45 mg/100 ml), and high protein concentration (>45 mg/100 ml). In patients with AIDS, but less so in others, the organisms are so numerous in the cerebrospinal fluid that they are readily visible in the India ink preparation. In any case, the antibody test for capsular polysaccharide in the cerebrospinal fluid and serum is positive for over 95% of patients and is rarely falsely positive. In fact, the test in serum is more sensitive than that in cerebrospinal fluid for patients with AIDS. Patients may have focal neurological involvement as a consequence of cerebral cryptococcomas. Other sites for the development of disseminated disease include bone, skin, and the prostate. The prostate has been implicated as a frequent site for relapsing infection after a course of antibiotic therapy.

Effective treatment for cryptococcal meningitis in patients without AIDS has been shown to be amphotericin B at 0.3 mg/kg intravenously daily combined with 5-flucytosine at 150 mg/kg in four divided oral doses daily for 6 weeks (4). In patients with AIDS, 5-flucytosine has been associated with an excessive bone marrow-suppressive effect and amphotericin B alone fails to eradicate the disease. After an initial course of 0.4 to 0.6 mg of amphotericin B per kg for at least 6 weeks, relapse of cryptococcal meningitis can be prevented in most patients with AIDS by giving 0.6 mg/kg intravenously weekly. Almost equally effective is fluconazole at 200 to 400 mg daily for 10 to 12 weeks after the last positive cerebrospinal fluid culture. However, because of a slower initial response in clearance of cryptococci from the cerebrospinal fluid and excessive early mortality with fluconazole compared to that with amphotericin B therapy, initial treatment with amphotericin B at 0.6 mg/kg intravenously daily for 2 weeks followed by fluconazole at 200 mg daily for the rest of the patient's life is recommended for patients with AIDS.

Control

Control of pigeon populations in areas of human habitation has been attempted for aesthetic and health reasons, with varying success.

REFERENCES

1. **Acha, P. N., and B. Szyfres.** 1987. *Zoonoses and Communicable Diseases Common to Man and Animals*, 2nd ed. Pan American Health Organization, Washington, D.C.
2. **Ajello, L.** 1967. Comparative ecology of respiratory mycotic disease agents. *Bacteriol. Rev.* **31:**6–24.
3. **Armstein, P., B. Eddie, and K. F. Meyer.** 1968. Control of psittacosis by group chemotherapy of infected parrots. *Am. J. Vet. Res.* **29:**2213–2227.
4. **Bennett, J. E., W. E. Dismukes, R. J. Duma, G. Medoff, M. A. Sande, H. Gallis, J. Leonard, B. T. Fields, M. Bradshaw, H. Haywood, Z. A. McGee, T. R. Cate, C. G. Cobbs, J. F. Warner, and D. W.**

Alling. 1979. A comparison of amphotericin B alone and combined with flucytosine in the treatment of cryptococcal meningitis. *N. Engl. J. Med.* **301**:126–131.

5. Reference deleted.

6. **Brandly, C. A.** 1964. The occupational hazard of Newcastle disease to man. *Lab. Anim. Care* **14**:433–440.

7. **Bryan, F. L.** 1981. Current trends in food-borne salmonellosis in the United States and Canada. *J. Food Prot.* **44**:394–402.

8. **Center for Disease Control.** 1974. Follow-up on turkey-associated psittacosis. *Morb. Mortal. Wkly. Rep.* **23**:309–310.

9. **Centers for Disease Control.** 1982. Psittacosis associated with turkey processing—Ohio. *Morb. Mortal. Wkly. Rep.* **30**:638–640.

10. **Centers for Disease Control.** 1987. Arboviral infections of the central nervous system—United States, 1986. *Morb. Mortal. Wkly. Rep.* **36**:450–455.

11. **Gatus, B. J., and M. R. Rose.** 1983. Japanese B encephalitis; epidemiology, clinical and pathologic aspects. *J. Infect.* **6**:213–218.

12. **Goodwin, R. A., and R. M. DesPrez.** 1978. State of the art. Histoplasmosis. *Am. Rev. Respir. Dis.* **117**:929–956.

13. **Graybill, J. R., and D. J. Drutz.** 1980. Ketoconazole: a major innovation for treatment of fungal disease. *Ann. Intern. Med.* **93**:921–923.

14. **Hoff, G. L., and W. J. Bigler.** 1981. The role of bats in the propagation and spread of histoplasmosis: a review. *J.Wildl. Dis.* **17**:191–196.

15. **Luby, J. P., S. E. Sulkin, and J. P. Sanford.** 1969. The epidemiology of St. Louis encephalitis: a review. *Annu. Rev. Med.* **20**:329–350.

16. **Neill, M. A., S. M. Opal, J. Heelan, R. Giusti, J. E. Cassidy, R. White, and K. H. Mayer.** 1991. Failure of ciprofloxacin to eradicate convalescent fecal excretion after acute salmonellosis: experience during an outbreak in healthcare workers. *Ann. Intern. Med.* **114**:195–199.

17. **Rosen, L.** 1986. The natural history of Japanese encephalitis virus. *Annu. Rev. Microbiol.* **40**:395–414.

18. **Schech, W. F., L. J. Wheat, J. L. Ho, M. L. French, R. J. Weeks, R. B. Kohler, C. E. Deane, H. E. Eitzen, and J. D. Band.** 1983. Recurrent urban histoplasmosis, Indianapolis, Indiana, 1980–1981. *Am. J. Epidemiol.* **118**:301–312.

18a.**Snacken, R., A. P. Kendal, L. R. Haaheim, and J. M. Wood.** 1999. The next influenza pandemic: lessons from Hong Kong, 1997. *Emerg. Infect. Dis.* **5**:195–203.

19. **Subbarao, K., A. Klimov, J. Katz, H. Regnery, W. Lim, H. Hall, M. Perdue, D. Swayne, C. Bender, J. Huang, M. Hemphill, T. Rowe, M. Shaw, X. Xu, K. Fukuda, and N. Cox.** 1998. Characterization of an avian influenza (H5N1) virus isolated from a child with a fatal respiratory illness. *Science* **279**:393–396.

20. **Tertti, R., K. Granfors, O.-P. Lehtonen, J. Mertsola, A. L. Makela, I. Valimaki, P. Hanninen, and A. Toivanen.** 1984. An outbreak of *Yersinia pseudotuberculosis* infection. *J. Infect. Dis.* **149**:245–250.

21. **Tesh, R. B.** 1982. Arthritides caused by mosquito-borne viruses. *Annu. Rev. Med.* **33**:31–40.

21a.**Treanor, J. J.** 2000. Influenza virus, p. 1823–1848. *In* G. L. Mandell, J. E. Bennett, and R. Dolin (ed.), *Principles and Practice of Infectious Diseases,* 5th ed. Churchill Livingstone, New York, N.Y.

22. **Wallner-Pendleton, E., and G. Cooper.** 1983. Several outbreaks of *Yersinia pseudotuberculosis* in California turkey flocks. *Avian Dis.* **27**:524–526.

23. **World Health Organization Scientific Working Group.** 1980. Enteric infections due to *Campylobacter, Yersinia, Salmonella* and *Shigella. Bull. W. H. O.* **58**:519–537.

Infections of Leisure, Third Edition
Edited by David Schlossberg
© 2004 ASM Press, Washington, D.C.

Chapter 8

Less Common House Pets

Bruno B. Chomel

Many infectious diseases in humans can be acquired through contact with pets. Dogs and cats may be the most common pets around the world, but there are also many other vertebrates that share our household environment. Almost 60% of all households in the United States have at least one pet, and 15 to 20% have pet birds, but the pet population also includes several million rodents (estimated population, 16.8 million), reptiles (8.8 million), and aquarium fish (185 million), not to mention less common species (e.g., the miniature pig) and exotic species, including wild carnivores, wild rodents, and pet monkeys (129, 139). It is estimated that 20 million American homes have aquariums at any given time (62). Pet rabbits are among the most common specialty and exotic pets, accounting for almost 5 million animals present in approximately 2% of the households (139). Specialty or exotic pet ownership increased from 6.7% of all households in 1991 to 10.7% in 1996 (52) but somehow decreased between 1996 and 2001 (139). It is estimated that between 1996 and 2001 the number of pet ferrets increased by 25.3%, with an estimated 1 million ferrets present in 0.5% of all households (139). A 12.6% increase in pet turtle ownership was also reported for the same period (139). Similarly, the estimated number of households with reptiles doubled from approximately 850,000 to 1.7 million during the period from 1991 to 2001 (33).

The objective of this chapter is not to cover every species that can be kept as pets and every disease, especially the rare and exotic ones, that they can transmit to us but rather to focus on the most common "other house pets" and the major health threat that they can represent. Only a brief discussion at the end of this chapter is devoted to more uncommon pets, especially ferrets and primates. However, because of the recent outbreak of monkeypox in prairie dogs and humans, which occurred in the spring of 2003 in the United States, a few words are devoted to the risk of ownership of exotic pets.

Bruno B. Chomel • Department of Population Health and Reproduction, School of Veterinary Medicine, University of California, Davis, Davis, CA 95616.

PET RABBITS AND RODENTS

Zoonoses transmitted by pet rabbits and pet rodents are quite rare (Table 1). Most of the health problems encountered with these animals are related to allergies or bites. A major distinction should be made between the domestic pets (rabbits, guinea pigs, hamsters, mice, or rats) and wild or exotic rodents kept as pets. If the first group is rarely involved in transmitting zoonoses, a special warn-

Table 1. Zoonoses potentially transmitted by pet rabbits and rodents

Animal	Zoonosis (pathogen)[a]			
	Viral	Bacterial	Parasitic	Mycotic
Rabbit	[Rabies] [Monkeypox]	**Pasteurellosis** **Salmonellosis** Yersiniosis [Listeriosis] [Tuberculosis] [Tularemia]	**Cheyletiellosis** [*Baylisascaris* infection]	**Dermatophytosis** (*T. mentagrophytes, Microsporum*)
Mouse	**LCM** [HFRS]	**Salmonellosis** Pasteurellosis Yersiniosis Mycoplasmosis [RBF] [Leptospirosis]	**Taeniasis** (*H. nana, H. diminuta*)	**Dermatophytosis** (*T. mentagrophytes*)
Rat, Gambian rat	**HFRS** **Monkeypox** **Encephalomyocarditis** [Rabies] [Cowpox] **Hepatitis E?**	**Salmonellosis** **Pasteurellosis** Yersiniosis **RBF** [Leptospirosis] [Tularemia?] [Plague?]	**Taeniasis** (*H. nana, H. diminuta*) Acariasis (*Trixacarus diversus*)	**Dermatophytosis** (*T. mentagrophytes* var. *quinckeanum*) [Sporotrichosis]
Guinea pig	LCM?	**Salmonellosis** **Yersiniosis** Campylobacteriosis **Pasteurellosis** Plague	**Acariasis** (*T. caviae*)	**Dermatophytosis** (*T. mentagrophytes*)
Hamster	**LCM**	**Campylobacteriosis** **Salmonellosis** Yersiniosis **Pasteurellosis**	**Acariasis** **Taeniasis** (*H. nana*)	**Dermatophytosis**
Gerbil	None	**Salmonellosis**	**Taeniasis** (*H. nana*)	None
Prarie dog	**Monkeypox**	**Plague**	None	None
Squirrel	**Monkeypox**	**Pasteurellosis** **RBF** **Tularemia** [Relapsing fever] [Rocky Mountain spotted fever] [Epidemic typhus]	None	None

[a]Boldface indicates the most common zoonoses; brackets indicate rare zoonoses.

ing should be given for wild animals and exotic pets. As a general rule, wildlife and exotic animals should not be sold or kept as pets. As examples of potential zoonotic risks, woodchucks could transmit rabies, as 49 wild woodchucks (*Marmota monax*) were diagnosed as rabid in 2001 and 2002 in the United States (82), and squirrels could transmit tularemia, rat-bite fever (RBF), or leptospirosis. However, a recent trend in pet ownership has emerged, especially in developed countries, which is the purchase of exotic pets imported from various parts of the world, where many zoonoses are endemic, or ownership of unconventional pets. This danger is well illustrated by an outbreak of tularemia which was identified among commercially distributed prairie dogs (*Cynomys ludovicianus*) at a commercial exotic-animal distributor in Texas (30); approximately 250 of an estimated 3,600 prairie dogs caught in South Dakota and that had transited by this facility died. Potentially infected rodents were distributed to wholesalers, retailers, and persons in several states or exported to Belgium, the Czech Republic, Japan, The Netherlands, and Thailand. An unusually high number of sick or dead prairie dogs were reported from Texas and the Czech Republic (30). Prairie dogs have been documented to also be infected with other human pathogens (e.g., *Yersinia pestis*, the agent of plague). In May 1998, a heavy die-off among prairie dogs at a Texan exotic-animal retailer led to a positive diagnosis of plague in that colony (8). Any wild animal should be handled with caution and referred to wildlife specialists. The recent outbreak (May 2003) of monkeypox in the midwestern United States is also a reminder that exotic pets can be a source of infection of native species that are highly susceptible to infections that they have never encountered before and can be a very effective source of human infection.

Rabbits

The domestic or European rabbit (*Oryctolagus cuniculus*), which can be housed indoors or outdoors and fed a readily available pelleted feed, makes a good pet that can be house-trained. The rabbit is certainly an excellent pet for children, as diseases of major public health importance are rarely encountered in domestic rabbits. Biting is uncommon, but rabbits can inflict painful scratches with their rear limbs if improperly restrained (67).

Infectious Zoonoses

Among the organisms causing infectious diseases in rabbits, *Pasteurella multocida* may cause cutaneous infection in susceptible persons (66). Other diseases to which rabbits are susceptible, e.g., salmonellosis and tularemia, are extremely rare and are more commonly transmitted to humans by wild animals. Cases of listeriosis have been reported to occur in farm rabbitries but do not seem to be of concern from pet rabbits. On the contrary, direct zoonotic transmission of *Yersinia pseudotuberculosis* infection from domestic rabbits has been documented (57). Cerebral larva migrans caused by *Baylisascaris procyonis* was reported to occur in pet rabbits infected by bedding straw contaminated with raccoon feces, but human contamination from these pets is very unlikely (44). Very rare cases of rabies and tuberculosis have been diagnosed in rabbits. More commonly, some external parasites of the rabbit may be transmitted to humans and cause infections, which include fur mite (*Cheyletiella parasitivorax*) acariasis and dermatophytosis (*Trichophyton menta-grophytes*).

Cheyletiella (rabbit fur mite) infestation. The rabbit fur mite, *C. parasitivorax*, is uncommon in the domestic rabbit. It is an external parasite of the skin and hair that does not excavate tunnels or furrows in the skin. The life cycle is completed in about 35 days. Adult females and eggs can survive for 10 days off the animal's body, but the larvae, nymphs, and adult males are not very resistant and die in about 2 days in the environment (1). Lesions in rabbits involve hair loss and a mild, scaly, oily dermatitis. In humans, the disease consists of a papular and pruritic eruption on the arms, thorax, waist, and thighs. Human infestation is transitory, as the mites do not reproduce on human skin. In a recent human case, treatment with benzyl benzoate (Ascabiol) resolved all the patient's symptoms (134). To prevent human infestation, infested rabbits should be treated with insecticides (e.g., methyl carbamate) once a week for 3 to 4 weeks.

Dermatophytosis. Fungal skin infections (ringworm) due to *T. mentagrophytes* are relatively rare. A few recent cases related to rabbit exposure have been reported in the scientific literature. Two human cases of tinea corporis due to *Arthroderma benhamiae* (teleomorph of *T. mentagrophytes*) were described for the first time in Japan (102). The two persons acquired the infection from their crossbred rabbit. Similarly, two cases of tinea gladiatorum due to *T. mentagrophytes* var. *quinckeanum* were described. A pet rabbit was probably the primary source of infection, which was then spread further by human-to-human contact to four other members of the same wrestling team, who were affected by tinea corporis (126).

In rabbits, irritation and inflammation of skin areas occur, with crusts, scabs, and hair loss. Some rabbits (about 4%) are asymptomatic carriers (18). Affected animals should be isolated. Antifungal treatment with topical or systemic griseofulvin (25 mg/kg of body weight) for 4 weeks is effective. The spectrum of ringworm in humans varies from subclinical colonization to an inflammatory scaly eruption that spreads peripherally and causes localized alopecia. Diagnosis is made by identifying hyphae in skin scrapings on a potassium hydroxide slide or by isolation in fungal culture media, the only method that allows identification of the species. In humans, topical treatment with clotrimazole (Lotrimin or Mycelex) or miconazole (Monistat-derm) twice a day for 2 to 4 weeks is usually sufficient. Application of ketoconazole cream twice daily for 2 months was used for the two Japanese patients (102). When extensive lesions are observed, oral griseofulvin (Fulvicin, Grifulvin V, or Grisactin) should be used. For adults, the dosage is 500 mg twice a day for at least 4 weeks (38). For children, the usual dose of oral microcrystalline griseofulvin is 10 to 15 mg/kg (up to 500 mg) given in one or two doses, preferably with fatty food, such as ice cream or whole milk. Treatment should be continued for 4 to 8 weeks.

Rodents

Although rodents, especially mice and rats, are definitively associated with transmission to humans of major fatal diseases, such as plague, typhus, and leptospirosis, they can be very good pets. The albino rat, the domestic variety of the brown rat (*Rattus norvegicus*), and the albino domestic mouse (*Mus musculus*) are kept by many people. However, guinea pigs, hamsters, and gerbils are the most common house pets among the rodents. It should be noted that introduction and ownership of gerbils are illegal in California. Furthermore, following the monkey-pox outbreak in prairie dogs, restrictions on African rodents, prairie dogs, and certain other animals were recently set by the U.S. government (34). New World flying squirrels (mainly *Glaucomys volans* and *Glaucomys sabrinus*) have also gained some popularity as household pets, with an estimated 5,000 to 8,000 owners in the United States (115).

As mentioned by Wagner and Farrar (136), the most important concerns about rodents for pet owners are bites and allergies. Human allergies to rodent dander are common. Symptoms are characterized by cutaneous (reddening, itching, and hives) and respiratory problems.

Zoonotic diseases from pet rodents are relatively rare. Among these, salmonellosis, lymphocytic choriomeningitis (LCM), and, more recently, monkeypox virus infection are of major concern. Rodent-borne zoonotic diseases are presented below in the following order: viral zoonoses, bacterial zoonoses, parasitic zoonoses, and fungal zoonoses.

Viral Zoonoses

LCM. LCM virus (LCMV) is found in many rodent species and spreads to humans through contact with infected aerosols, direct animal contact, or rodent bites. The natural reservoir of the disease is the domestic mouse (*M. musculus*), which usually does not present any symptoms (1, 38, 61, 67).

Epidemiology. LCMV (an RNA virus of the family *Arenaviridae*) is transmitted horizontally among rodents through secretions (urine, saliva, and feces) and vertically to the embryos, especially in mice. Infected offspring develop a persistent infection and shed the virus during most of their life spans. Outbreaks have been reported to occur in laboratory mice, and cases have occurred in humans in houses where infected mice were caught. In humans, the disease is sporadic, but outbreaks may occasionally occur. Such outbreaks of LCM, related to the use of hamsters as pets, occurred in the late 1960s and early 1970s in Germany and the United States. In Germany, 47 cases in humans associated with pet hamsters were reported within a 2-year period (2). In the United States, a nationwide epidemic occurred in late 1973 and early 1974, totaling at least 181 cases in 12 states, with 57 cases in New York State (14) and California. All were associated with pet hamsters from a single breeder in Birmingham, Ala. This breeder was an employee of a biological-product firm whose tumor cell lines were found to be positive for LCM. The same cell source was also incriminated in a prior outbreak at the University of Rochester Medical Center, Rochester, N.Y. (64). Since the suspension of the sale of pet hamsters by the Birmingham breeder and of the distribution of positive tumor cell lines by the biological-product firm, no further outbreaks have been reported in the United States. More recently, four cases in humans of acute meningitis due to LCM occurred in southern France in 1993 after close contact with pet Syrian hamsters (116).

Symptoms. In hamsters, LCMV infection is usually not associated with signs of illness (46) and can be detected only by laboratory tests. In humans, the course of infection varies from clinically unapparent to a flu-like infection, with fever, headache, and severe myalgia, occurring 5 to 10 days after infection. A small number of patients progress to aseptic meningitis, which is characterized by a very high lymphocyte count in the cerebrospinal fluid. On rare occasions, there may be meningoencephalitis. Chronic sequelae are not common, and fatal cases are rare.

Diagnosis. Diagnosis of infection in humans is based on isolation of the virus from the blood or from nasopharyngeal or cerebrospinal fluid samples taken early in the attack and inoculated onto tissue cultures or injected intracerebrally into LCM-free adult mice. Serodiagnostic tests include indirect immunofluorescence assay, enzyme-linked immunosorbent assay (ELISA), and immunoglobulin G (IgG) Western blotting. Serum screening is performed by indirect immunofluorescence assay and titration of IgM and IgG antibodies by ELISA (116).

Treatment. Since the disease is self-limiting, treatment is for symptomatic relief only.

Monkeypox. The first outbreak of human monkeypox infection in the western hemisphere began in May 2003 in the midwestern United States and was attributed to contact with infected exotic pets. Seventy-one suspected cases of monkeypox were investigated, primarily in Wisconsin, Indiana, and Illinois (32). Most of the affected people reported close contact with ill prairie dogs, although at least one case is thought to be related to an ill rabbit (which had contact with a sick prairie dog). No patients have been confirmed to have had exposure to persons with monkeypox as their only possible exposure. Prairie dogs appear to have been infected through contact with Gambian giant rats and dormice that originated in Ghana. Traceback investigations to identify the source of introduction of monkeypox into the United States identified a Texas animal distributor that had imported a shipment of approximately 800 small mammals from Ghana on 9 April 2003 that contained 762 African rodents, including rope squirrels (*Funisciurus* spp.), tree squirrels (*Heliosciurus* spp.), Gambian giant rats (*Cricetomys* spp.), brushtail porcupines (*Atherurus* spp.), dormice (*Graphiurus* spp.), and striped mice (*Hybomys* spp.) (32). The U.S. Department of Health and Human Services issued an embargo order on the import of rodents from Africa, effective 11 June 2003. In addition, the U.S. Department of Health and Human Services has also prohibited the distribution, sale, transport, or intentional release into the wild of prairie dogs and six African rodent species (34).

In humans, the signs and symptoms of monkeypox are characterized, after an incubation period of approximately 12 days, by fever, headache, muscle aches, backache, swollen lymph nodes, a general feeling of discomfort, and exhaustion. Within 1 to 3 days after onset of fever, the patient develops a papular rash, often first on the face but sometimes initially on other parts of the body. The lesions usually develop through several stages before crusting and falling off. The illness typically lasts for 2 to 4 weeks. No specific treatment is available, but smallpox vaccination has been used in people in contact with infected humans and people exposed to infected rodents (32).

Cowpox. Human cowpox is a relatively rare zoonosis which occurs sporadically in the United Kingdom and across Europe and in some western states of the former Soviet Union. The virus circulates in wild rodents, mainly field and bank voles and wood mice in the United Kingdom (11). A young boy was bitten by a rodent when swimming in a Dutch canal and developed cowpox (109). More recently, a cowpox virus was isolated from the ulcerative eyelid lesions of a young Dutch girl who owned many pets (turtles, hamsters, guinea pigs, birds, ducks, cats, and a dog) and had cared for a clinically ill wild rat that later died (140).

Rabies. Because bites from pet rodents are frequent events, one must be concerned with rabies. No case of rabies has ever been reported from bites by pet rodents. However, one should be very careful any time a wild rodent kept as a pet has bitten a person. Cases of rabies have been reported to occur in woodchucks, squirrels, and even a rat (82, 100).

HFRS, or Korean hemorrhagic fever, and hantavirus pulmonary syndrome (HPS). Hemorrhagic fever with renal syndrome (HFRS) describes a group of rodent-borne viral diseases (hantaviruses) that are endemic or occur as focal epidemics on the Eurasian continent and in Japan. In general, hantavirus isolates from Asia or eastern Europe (Hantaan, Dobrava, and Seoul viruses) are considered more pathogenic to humans than the northern European strains (Puumala virus). Wild rodents in rural areas or wild rats in cities (36) are the reservoirs of the virus, which they can shed for several weeks. Several outbreaks involving laboratory personnel (86) infected by laboratory rats have been reported in Japan and Europe. Hantaviruses cause chronic, apparently asymptomatic infections of their rodent hosts, but associated cases in humans may reveal the animal infection. The disease in laboratory personnel has been characterized by fever and a flu-like syndrome, with fever and myalgia and, a few days later, oliguria, proteinuria, and hematuria. Usually, patients recover without sequelae. The infection is contracted by handling infected animals or from contaminated aerosols. Most laboratory rat suppliers employ a screening test and destroy infected colonies. The diagnosis of infection is based on viral isolation and, more often, on serodiagnosis by indirect immunofluorescence or ELISA.

In the United States, HPS was first reported in the spring of 1993, caused by a virus called Sin Nombre virus. There were 353 reported human cases by early November 2003 (http://www.cdc.gov/ncidod/diseases/hanta/hps/noframes/caseinfo.htm), with a fatality rate of 38%. Most of the cases have been reported in the western states, especially New Mexico, Arizona, and Colorado. The reservoir of Sin Nombre virus is *Peromyscus maniculatus*, the deer mouse. Other hantaviruses have been identified in humans and various rodent species in North America, such as Black Creek Canal virus, which has been identified in Florida, with the cotton rat (*Sigmodon hispidus*) as the reservoir (77). Other viruses, such as Monongahela, New York, and Bayou viruses, also cause HPS and are found in eastern Canada and the eastern and southeastern United States. In South and Central America, several hantaviruses have been identified as causing HPS, including Andes virus in Argentina and Chile; Andes-like viruses, including Oran, Lechiguanas, and Hu39694 viruses in Argentina; Laguna Negra virus in Bolivia and Paraguay; Bermejo virus in Argentina; Juquitiba virus in Brazil; and Choclo virus in Panama (77, 130). No cases in humans acquired by contact with pet rodents have been reported.

Encephalomyocarditis. Encephalomyocarditis is a rare disease in humans caused by an RNA virus of the family *Picornaviridae*. Sporadic cases have been reported, and the virus has been isolated from children in Germany and The Netherlands; in the United States, epizootics have occurred in pigs (1). Rodents, especially of the genus *Rattus*, have been considered the main reservoirs of the virus, and they transmit the virus to rats and other species through bites. However, no case from a rodent source has been identified in humans.

Hepatitis E. Hepatitis E virus (HEV) is an important cause of enterically transmitted human hepatitis in developing countries. However, autochthonous cases of hepatitis E have been reported in the United States and other industrialized countries. The source of HEV infection in these cases is unknown, but zoonotic transmission has been suggested. Recent cases from consumption of raw deer or wild boar meat have been reported from Japan (94, 132). Antibodies to HEV have been detected in many animals in areas where HEV is endemic and in domestic swine and rats in the United States (53, 70). In the United States, an antibody prevalence of almost 60% was reported for rats, with higher prevalence in rodents from urban habitats than in animals captured from rural areas (53). A 12% seroprevalence of HEV antibodies was reported for rats trapped in a valley in Nepal where HEV was hyperendemic, and HEV RNA was detected in four animals (70). Phylogenetic analysis of the four genome sequences showed that they were identical and closely related to two human isolates from Nepal and distinct from the sequences of HEV isolated elsewhere (70). Similarly, in Japan, 114 of 362 (31.5%) Norway rats (*R. norvegicus*) and 12 of 90 (13.3%) black rats (*Rattus rattus*) were positive for anti-HEV IgG (72). Rats could play a role as a potential reservoir of HEV, but no cases of human infection from a pet rat have been reported yet.

Bacterial Zoonoses

Pasteurellosis. Among bite-transmitted zoonoses, infection by *P. multocida* is certainly the most common in domestic pets. Although most of the cases occur from cat and dog bites, rodents nevertheless harbor *P. multocida* in their oral cavities and can at times transmit the organism through a bite wound. *P. multocida* is likely to be the pathogen if cellulitis develops within a few hours after the bite (1). Swelling, reddening, and intense pain in the region are the main signs and symptoms. If the incubation period is longer, staphylococcal or streptococcal infection is more likely. A recent case of *P. pneumotropica* peritonitis was reported to occur in a child maintained on peritoneal dialysis following contamination of the dialysis tube by a pet hamster (17). *P. pneumotropica* has been isolated primarily from rodents. The patient responded well to intraperitoneal tobramycin and vancomycin. Cultures of samples from infected bite wounds should always be performed in order to administer the appropriate antibiotics. Treatment should be carried out with amoxicillin-clavulanate potassium (Augmentin), 500 mg three times daily for 5 to 7 days, or doxycycline, 100 mg orally twice a day.

RBF. RBF is a rare disease that can be transmitted by rats, which are healthy carriers of *Streptobacillus moniliformis* or *Spirillum minus* in the nasopharynx. Streptobacillary RBF is a rare disease in the United States. Of 14 cases on record since 1958, 7 originated from the bites of laboratory rats (6, 21). Bites by wild rodents (rats and squirrels) can also transmit the infectious agent (21). Infection has also followed consumption of contaminated raw milk (6). According to a case report from New Mexico, a 15-year-old boy was infected after he drank water from an open irrigation ditch next to a baseball field (28). In Europe, a case of septic arthritis of the hip due to *S. moniliformis* after a bite on the finger of a 14-year-old boy from a rat for sale in a pet shop was also reported (49). The case was successfully treated by arthrotomy, drainage, and joint lavage followed by administration of penicillin. In The Netherlands, a 43-year-old woman presented, after being bitten by a pet rat, with a generalized febrile illness; an exanthema with mixed maculopapulous and pustulous eruptions on the lower halves of the extremities, elbows, knees, palms, and soles; and severe arthralgia and asymmetric arthritis (122). These cases highlight a possible danger of keeping rats as pets. Streptobacillary RBF has an incubation period of 2 to 10 days, a rapidly healing point of inoculation, and abrupt onset of irregularly relapsing fever, asymmetric polyarthritis, shaking chills, vomiting, headache, arthralgia, myalgia, and regional lymphadenopathy. Two to four days after onset, a maculopapular rash appears on the extremities. Endocarditis is a possible complication. Diagnosis of RBF is made by culture of the organism from the blood or joint fluid (38). Recommended therapy for RBF is penicillin G or tetracycline (21). Clindamycin can also be effective.

Spirillary RBF is an even less common disease, with an incubation period of 1 to 6 weeks (5). Clinically, *S. minus* infection differs from streptobacillary fever in the rarity of arthritic symptoms, a distinctive rash, and a common reactivation of the healed wound when symptoms appear.

Tularemia. Tularemia, also known as "rabbit fever," is an acute febrile illness caused by *Francisella tularensis*. Rodents are very susceptible to the disease, which usually culminates in a fatal septicemia. Because the disease is mainly transmitted from rodent to rodent by ticks and fleas, pet rabbits or rodents should not be a major risk for the transmission of tularemia. There have been documented cases of transmission from domestic cats and, more recently, from the bite of a squirrel kept as a household pet, which died minutes after biting a child (91). Recent cases among commercially distributed prairie dogs from Texas raised concerns about human risk of contamination in the United States and abroad (30).

Plague. Plague is endemic in many wild rodents in the western United States. Although several cases in humans have been associated with pets, especially cats (51), there are no reports in the literature of transmission to humans from pet rodents. The potential commercial distribution of plague-infected prairie dogs in Texas in 1998 should remind people of the danger of using wild animals as pets (8). Recurrent outbreaks of plague in Peru were also associated with the presence indoors of infected guinea pigs, used as both pets and sources of food by the natives (P. Arambulo, personal communication).

Epidemic typhus. Epidemic typhus is caused by *Rickettsia prowazekii* and is usually transmitted from person to person by the human body louse. Sporadic cases have been reported in the United States for people living in rural areas after contacts with flying squirrels (50, 113, 115). From 1976 to 2001, approximately one-third of the 39 *R. prowazekii* infections documented in the United States occurred after contact with flying squirrels or their nests (113).

Leptospirosis. Although rodents, especially rats, are known to harbor and shed various *Leptospira interrogans* serovars for long periods, very few cases of human infection from pet rodents have been reported. In one instance, *L. interrogans* serovar Ballum was contracted from a pet mouse (59). Outbreaks in personnel working with laboratory rats and mice have been documented in Europe and the United States (57).

Salmonellosis. Guinea pigs are highly susceptible to salmonella infection and develop severe clinical disease (septicemia). In guinea pigs, high mortality is the rule. Fish et al. (54) reported a family outbreak of salmonellosis due to contact with guinea pigs raised on a commercial ranch in Canada. Mice and rats are also very susceptible and may carry subclinical infections for long periods. These infections are usually caused by *Salmonella enterica* serovar Typhimurium or *S. enterica* serovar Enteritidis. If salmonellosis occurs in a child who has a pet rodent, the pet's feces should be cultured for *Salmonella*. However, shedding may be only intermittent.

Yersiniosis. Infections with *Y. pseudotuberculosis* and *Yersinia enterocolitica* may be contracted from pet rodents. Guinea pigs are very commonly infected with *Y. pseudotuberculosis* (5). The course of the disease in these animals is usually subacute. Loss of weight and diarrhea are often the only clinical signs. Healthy carriers are common. In rats and mice, the infection is common, but usually without any symptoms. Children can be infected by fecal-oral contamination. In humans, the disease is mainly observed in children, adolescents, and young adults. The most common clinical form, after 1 to 3 weeks of incubation, is mesenteric adenitis, or pseudoappendicitis, with acute abdominal pain in the right iliac fossa, fever, and vomiting. The disease is usually more common in young males. Diagnosis requires the isolation and identification of the etiologic agent. Serologic tests by ELISA are also available. When the disease is mild (uncomplicated pseudoappendicular syndrome), antimicrobial chemotherapy is not useful (19). *Y. pseudotuberculosis* is usually sensitive to ampicillin, aminoglycosides, or tetracycline (12). *Y. enterocolitica* is also found in rodents, which are usually healthy carriers (123). Chinchillas are very susceptible to the infection, and several epizootics have occurred in Europe and the United States (1). Guinea pigs also are commonly infected by *Y. enterocolitica*, but serotypes found in rodents usually do not affect humans. *Y. enterocolitica* affects mainly young children. The major symptoms are an acute enteritis with watery diarrhea, sometimes bloody, lasting 3 to 14 days, and abdominal pain. Diagnosis is based on isolation of the agent from the feces of patients. An ELISA on paired sera is also useful to determine infection. Aminoglycosides and trimethoprim-sulfamethoxazole are the most appropriate antibiotics (12).

Campylobacteriosis. Campylobacter infection can occur in some rodent species. Proliferative ileitis, a specific enteric syndrome of hamsters, is probably caused by a strain of *Campylobacter*. Hamsters certainly represent a potential source of human infection, but no hamster-associated cases have been reported (61). In humans, campylobacter infection is characterized by diarrhea, abdominal pain, cramps, fever, and vomiting. The diarrhea is frequently bloody. The incubation period is 2 to 5 days, and the disease usually does not last more than a week. Usually treatment is limited to fluid replacement therapy.

Parasitic Zoonoses

Cestodiasis or taeniasis (tapeworm). Cestodes, or tapeworms, infect a wide range of species, including rabbits and rodents (1). *Hymenolepis nana*, the dwarf tapeworm, is found in rodents, especially hamsters. *Hymenolepis diminuta* is the rat tapeworm, but it may also be found in other rodents. Hymenolepiasis occurs primarily in children. The prepatent period is 15 to 30 days. Usually, the infestation is asymptomatic in humans, but if parasites are present in large numbers, gastrointestinal disorders, such as abdominal pain, nausea, vomiting, and diarrhea, may occur. Eggs of some *Hymenolepis* spp. are infective to the definitive host when passed in the feces. Humans may acquire the infection from infected rodents either by ingestion of eggs from fecally contaminated fingers or from contaminated food or water. When eggs of the directly transmitted *Hymenolepis* spp. are ingested, they hatch in the intestine, liberating an oncosphere that enters a mucosal villus and develops into a cysticercoid larva within 5 days. The cysticercoid ruptures the villus, travels into the lumen, and attaches to the lower small intestine. It reaches the adult phase in 2 weeks and starts to release eggs. Diagnosis of infection is made by microscopic identification of the eggs in the feces. Praziquantel (Biltricide) and niclosamide (Yomesan or Niclocide) are effective for treatment of hymenolepis infection (1, 12, 66, 67). Treatment of infected rodents can be done with 1 mg of niclosamide per 10 g of body weight given at 7-day intervals or 0.3% active ingredient in the feed for 7 days (136).

Acariasis (*Trixacarus caviae*). Several external parasites can infest rodents. Among these, *T. caviae*, a parasite mainly found in guinea pigs, can be transmitted to humans. In guinea pigs, the infection is usually asymptomatic. Stress and/or poor care can lead to severe alopecia, dermatitis, and pruritus on the body and legs. The skin is thickened, dry, and scaly. Treatment is based on a solution of 1:40 lime sulfur in water applied to the skin and repeated weekly for 6 weeks or once-a-week application of 10% lindane for 3 weeks. Ivermectin injected subcutaneously at 200 mg/kg is a useful treatment for ectoparasitism (5). In humans, pruritic skin lesions on the hands, arms, or neck can be observed in children. Diagnosis may be established by recovering the mite from its burrow and identifying it microscopically. For infected children, crotamiton (Eurax) in one application per day for 2 to 5 days is the most common treatment; lindane (1% γ-benzene hexachloride) (Kwell) may also be used (12, 67).

Fungal Zoonoses

Dermatophytosis. Tinea favus of rats and mice, caused by *T. mentagrophytes* var. *quinckeanum*, is widespread (67). Mice and guinea pigs are the important sources of human infection with *T. mentagrophytes* var. *mentagrophytes* or *Microsporum gypseum* (108). The rat, chinchilla, and hamster are much less common sources of ringworm in humans (108). The lesion, localized on the head or trunk, is white and scabby, but rodents often have no noticeable lesions. The infection is transmitted to humans and dogs. (For diagnosis and treatment, see "Dermatophytosis" under "Rabbits" above.) In rodents, oral griseofulvin at 15 to 25 mg/kg orally once daily for 3 to 5 weeks is the recommended treatment (108).

Sporotrichosis. A few human cases of lymphocutaneous sporotrichosis caused by *Sporothrix schenckii* have been associated with rodent bite accidents (108).

HEDGEHOGS

Salmonellosis has been diagnosed in patients who own hedgehogs as pets (26). The African pygmy hedgehog (*Atelerix albiventris*) has been associated with cases of *S. enterica* serovar Tilene infection in children in the United States and Canada (89, 141). It is estimated that 40,000 households own such a pet in the United States (115). Ringworm cases (inflammatory tinea corporis) caused by *T. mentagrophytes* var. *erinacei* have been reported from owners of pet African pygmy hedgehogs (114). Human cases are easily treated with oral itraconazole (200 mg daily for 7 days). The hedgehog can be treated by application of a miconazole-containing veterinary lotion. The African pygmy hedgehog has not yet been documented to carry any mycobacterial diseases; however, infection by various *Mycobacterium* species (*Mycobacterium marinum* and *Mycobacterium avium*) has been reported for the European hedgehog (115). Therefore, hedgehogs are not recommended pets for patients with human immunodeficiency virus infection.

REPTILES AND AMPHIBIANS

Reptiles are once again popular pets in the United States. In 2001, an estimated 8.8 million pet reptiles were owned by approximately 3% of households (25, 139). There is a large international trade in live reptiles, with the United States accounting for 80% of this trade. In 1995, 2.5 million reptiles were imported in the United States. Meanwhile, over 10,000 green iguanas were imported annually in the United Kingdom during the 1990s (111). Table 2 lists the major zoonoses transmitted by reptiles and amphibians.

Bacterial Zoonoses

Salmonellosis
Salmonellosis is certainly the most frequent and major zoonosis transmitted by reptiles, especially turtles (22, 84) and iguanas (25). Recently, the Centers for Disease Control and Prevention emphasized the risk associated with ownership of amphibians (33). Reptile and amphibian contacts are estimated to account for 74,000 (6%) of the approximately 1.2 million sporadic *Salmonella* infections that occur each year in the United States (33). Of all zoonoses, *Salmonella* infections present the most significant hazard to children, who are at greater risk of disease than adults because they are frequently in close contact with animals and their hand washing practices are often not well developed (4). For instance, in 1994, 413 (81%) of 513 *S. enterica* serovar Marina cases occurred in children aged <1 year (29).

Pet turtles have been recognized as a major source of human salmonellosis since Hershey and Mason isolated *S. enterica* serovar Hartford from the pet turtle of a 7-month-old infant with serovar Hartford gastroenteritis (20). Subsequent investigations established that 14% of the estimated 2 million cases of human salmonellosis in the United States in 1970 and 1971 were linked to pet turtles, mainly

Table 2. Major zoonoses potentially transmitted by reptiles and aquarium fishes

Animal	Zoonosis (pathogen)[a]			
	Viral	Bacterial	Parasitic	Mycotic
Turtle	None	**Salmonellosis** Yersiniosis Campylobacteriosis [*Aeromonas* infection]	None	[Dermatophytosis]
Lizard, snake	None	**Salmonellosis** **Yersiniosis** [*E. tarda* infection] [*Plesiomonas* infection] [*S. marcescens* infection]	Pentastomiasis [*Mesocestoides* infection]	[Dermatophytosis]
Frog	None	**Salmonellosis**	None	[Dermatophytosis]
Fish	None	**Mycobacteriosis** [*Erysipelothrix* infection] [*A. hydrophila* infection] [*E. tarda* infection] [Melioidosis] [*S. iniae* infection] [*Vibrio* infection] [*Y. enterocolitica* infection]	None	None

[a]Boldface indicates the most common zoonoses; brackets indicate rare zoonoses.

the red-eared turtle (*Pseudemys scripta elegans*) (37). With annual sales of 15 million turtles, zoonotic salmonellosis was a growing problem. By 1975, commercial distribution of turtles less than 4 in. long was banned within the United States by the Food and Drug Administration. A 77% decrease in turtle-associated salmonellosis was noted following enactment of the ban (39, 42). Nonetheless, an estimated 3 million to 4 million turtles are shipped annually from the United States and sold around the world. Consequently, several outbreaks of salmonellosis have been reported in Japan (60), the United Kingdom (7, 15), Puerto Rico (131), Israel (35), and France (118). For instance, an outbreak caused by *S. enterica* serovar Tel-el-kebir was reported in Ireland among owners of terrapin turtles (89). In a study of salmonellosis in people from southwestern Germany, owners of puppies, kittens, or turtles were almost seven times (odds ratio = 6.8; $P = 0.002$) more likely to have *Salmonella* infection than were healthy controls (80). Turtles are usually healthy carriers of salmonellae, and shedding is very irregular, but they may shed salmonellae for up to 11 months. The problem of salmonella infection in turtles arises from the widespread contamination and persistence of the microorganism in turtle breeding ponds and nesting areas. Turtles can acquire the organism in ovo or after hatching (78). The pattern of *Salmonella* excretion in amphibians and reptiles was studied in a vivarium over a 3-year period (107). *Salmonella* could be isolated about twice as often from animals kept under arid or mesic conditions than from animals living in humid or aquatic environments. Animals feeding on mice ($P = 0.04$) and reptiles in general ($P = 0.04$) more commonly excreted *Salmonella*. Use of antibiotics for attempted control of salmonellae in pet turtle husbandry has been widely practiced. In their attempt to eradicate salmonellae with gentamicin sulfate, turtle farmers have created an even greater health hazard through selection of antibiotic-resistant strains (41). Treatment of pet turtles is not recommended, and infected reptiles should be destroyed. However, knowledge of the potential health hazards, along with proper sanitation, is usually sufficient to prevent human infection. Pet turtles should not be displayed in classrooms where children can handle them or have contact with their containers. Identification of the microorganism from stool culture and an antibiogram should be performed any time salmonellosis is suspected. Similarly, culture should be performed from the pet reptile or from its aquarium. In humans, primary treatment of salmonellosis consists of fluid and electrolyte replacement. Antibiotics are not recommended, except in severe forms, as they not only fail to shorten the duration of the illness but also may prolong the carrier state.

Salmonella infection can be acquired not only from pet turtles but also from other reptiles and amphibians, such as lizards or snakes (55), chameleons (138), and frogs (10, 33), or from aquarium fish (99). The 1990s were characterized by an explosion in pet reptile ownership in the United States. Because the most popular reptile species (iguanas, for example) do not breed if closely confined, most reptiles are captured in the wild and imported. From 1989 through 1993, reptile imports to the United States increased by 82%, from 1.1 million to 2.1 million. During the same period, iguana imports increased by 431%, from 143,000 to 760,000 animals (3). Pet iguana-associated salmonellosis cases in two infants residing in Indiana were reported in 1990 (23), and more recently many other cases were reported from several states (23, 24, 33, 40, 97), underscoring the important role played by reptiles, particularly pet lizards, in the transmission of zoonoses. In several cases, a rare *S. enterica* serotype, Marina, was involved, and there was no direct contact between the pet iguana and the infant (23, 24). These cases demonstrate that direct contact between the reptile and the infant is not necessary for transmission to occur. Similarly, a human case of salmonellosis acquired through a platelet transfusion from a donor with a boa constrictor was reported (75). Isolation of rare serotypes of *Salmonella* spp. often alerts public health staff about possible transmission of infection from reptiles to humans. For instance, isolations of serovar Marina and *Salmonella enterica* serovar Poona from humans increased, respectively, from 2 and 199 in 1989 to 47 and 341 in 1998 (29). Similarly, cases associated with savanna monitor lizards (*Varanus exanthemapicus*) imported as pets from Ghana and Togo were caused by a rare serotype, Poona (97). An outbreak of salmonellosis among children attending a Komodo dragon exhibit at a zoo was the cause of at least 65 cases of serovar Enteritidis infection (58). It was estimated that in 1995 there were as many as 6,700 reptile-caused salmonella infections in the United States, but the incidence may be closer to 80,000 cases per year, 80% of them in children. In Canada, an estimated 3 to 5% of all cases of salmonellosis in humans are associated with exposure to exotic pets (141).

A high proportion of reptiles (more than 90%) are asymptomatic carriers of *Salmonella*. Reptiles can become infected through transovarial transmission or direct contact with other infected reptiles or contaminated reptile feces. High rates of fecal carriage of *Salmonella* can be related to the eating of feces by hatchlings, a typical behavior for iguanas and other lizards. In a cohort study of 12 captive iguanas, fecal shedding of *Salmonella* was monitored for 10 weeks (16). All 12 iguanas were found to shed *Salmonella* at least once, and multiple serotypes were isolated from 7 of the 12 animals. Salmonellae were isolated from 83% of the fecal samples tested. In a limited survey in a green-iguana farm in El Salvador to identify sources of *Salmonella* in green iguanas and their environment, *Salmonella* spp. were isolated from the intestine of both adult (3 of 20) and hatchling (8 of 20) iguanas and from the surfaces of 40% (7 of 16) of the egg surfaces tested (98). Soil samples from a breeding pen and a nest in that farm were both positive for *Salmonella* spp.

Edwardsiella Infection

Human infection with *Edwardsiella tarda* is uncommon. This organism can be found in cold-blooded animals, reptiles, and fish (goldfish, catfish, and bass). In humans, the organism may cause gastroenteritis resembling *Salmonella* infections. Wound infections, such as cellulitis or gas gangrene associated with trauma to mucosal surfaces, and systemic disease, such as septicemia, meningitis, cholecystitis, and osteomyelitis, have been reported. At least one case associated with a pet turtle was reported in the United States (101). This bacterium is susceptible to most commonly prescribed antibiotics, but fatal gastrointestinal and extraintestinal infections have been described (76).

Plesiomonas Infection

Plesiomonas (*Aeromonas*) *shigelloides* is a gram-negative rod that causes progressive ulcerative stomatitis in snakes ("mouth rot disease"). It may cause gastroenteritis in humans. A case of acute gastroenteritis in a zoo animal keeper infected by handling a sick boa constrictor has been reported (43). Diagnosis is made by stool culture. Treatment with trimethoprim-sulfamethoxazole (Bactrim or Septra) for 5 days is usually effective.

Yersinia Infection

Y. enterocolitica has been found in water and on cold-blooded animals, such as frogs and fish (69, 142). However, the serotypes involved are not usually found in humans.

Campylobacter fetus

During the course of a *Salmonella enterica* serovar Agona case investigation, *C. fetus* was isolated for the first time from a pet turtle (68). This suggests that turtles, in addition to being reservoirs for *Salmonella* species, may also be reservoirs for *C. fetus*.

Serratia marcescens Cellulitis

A case of cellulitis caused by *S. marcescens* was reported to have occurred in an 8-year-old boy who was bitten by a pet iguana on his left index finger (74). The *Serratia* isolate was resistant to ampicillin and cefazolin but was susceptible to ampicillin-sulbactam and gentamicin.

Parasitic Zoonoses of Reptiles

Pentastomiasis

Pentastomes (*Armillifer* spp.) are annulate metazoa that are almost exclusively parasites of the reptilian respiratory system. Snakes are the definitive hosts, and many wild rodents, on which snakes feed, are the intermediate hosts. The female parasite deposits eggs in the respiratory cavities of the reptiles. The eggs are expectorated or swallowed and then eliminated with the feces. Humans can become accidental hosts by handling infected reptiles and placing contaminated hands to the mouth. In humans, the infection is usually asymptomatic. The encapsulated larvae may be found during laparotomies or can be diagnosed by radiographic examination (1, 71).

Mesocestoides (Cestoda) Infection

Infections with *Mesocestoides* spp., cestodes of mammals and birds, occur infrequently in humans (120). One case occurred in California in 1990 in a child who was exposed to a large variety of animals in a day care center. That case was unique in that the day care facility housed all the animals necessary for the complete life cycle of this cestode. Niclosamide was used to treat this child, with apparent success.

Fungal Zoonoses of Reptiles and Amphibians

Very limited information is available on fungal diseases of reptiles and amphibians. It does not appear that reptiles and amphibians are a major source of fungal zoonoses. Dermatophytosis caused by *Trichophyton* and *Microsporum* species in reptilian species has rarely been reported (121). Treatment of these infections in reptiles is mainly based on the use of itraconazole and ketoconazole (15 to 30 mg/kg orally once daily for at least 2 weeks) or amphotericin B and nystatin.

ORNAMENTAL (AQUARIUM) FISH

In the United States, about 20 million household aquariums are maintained, accommodating an annual sale of approximately 600 million pet fish (124), mostly from foreign countries (in Southeast Asia and South America) and from Florida. In Australia, it is estimated that 12 to 14% of the population keep ornamental fish as pets (87). However, very few cases of zoonosis are reported (Table 2), and no major outbreaks of human disease for which diseased fish were directly responsible have been reported recently (124). The main pathogens acquired topically from fish (through spine puncture or open wounds) are *Aeromonas hydrophila*, *Edwardsiella tarda*, *Erysipelothrix rhusiopathiae*, *M. marinum*, *Streptococcus iniae*, *Vibrio vulnificus*, and *Vibrio damselae* (87). *S. iniae* has recently emerged as a public health hazard associated with aquaculture, and *M. marinum* often infects home aquarium hobbyists. With the expansion of aquaculture and popularity of recreational fishing, medical practitioners can expect to see more infections of this nature. Among these bacterial diseases of fish, mycobacteriosis is certainly of major concern.

Mycobacteriosis

Mycobacterial infections are certainly among the major zoonoses that can be transmitted by aquarium fish (45, 87, 133). Mycobacterial infections are increasingly reported for fish fanciers who keep an aquarium (79). *M. marinum, Mycobacterium fortuitum*, and *M. platypoecilus* have been associated with both fish and human disease for many years. Skin ulcers due to *M. marinum*, contracted from fish tanks, have been reported. In two cases, a cut on the hand had preceded the cleaning of a home fish aquarium (81). Infection by *M. marinum*, also known as "swimming pool granuloma," is characterized, after inoculation on an abraded skin and an incubation period of 2 to 3 weeks, by papulonodules, ulcers, or verrucous plaques. These may progress into sporotrichoid lesions or into deeper infections involving tendons and bone. In infected fish, granulomatous lesions are usually observed. A diagnosis can be made by isolating and identifying the organism. Histopathological examination shows a nonspecific inflammatory infiltrate in the acute phase. In chronic lesions the histopathological pattern is a tuberculoidlike granuloma. Infected fish should be destroyed, and the aquarium should be disinfected (with 5% calcium hypochlorite solution) before other fish are added (88). In humans, infection resolves following treatment with minocycline (Minocin), 100 mg twice daily orally for 6 to 8 weeks (38). Use of rifampin (Rifadin or Rimactane) has also been very successful (48), although indications for therapy are controversial.

Melioidosis and Exotic Fish

Melioidosis is an uncommon disease in humans, with a wide range of clinical manifestations from inapparent infection to a rapid fatal septicemia. *Burkholderia* (previously *Pseudomonas*) *pseudomallei*, the infectious agent, is endemic in Southeast Asia, where it is saprophytic in certain soils and waters. Recent studies have shown that the water of tanks in which exotic aquarium fishes were imported was contaminated with this bacillus. Disinfection of aquariums with bleach between water changes should be recommended in pet stores to prevent the spread of infection (47).

Erysipelothrix Infection

Erysipelothrix insidiosa infection has been reported to occur in humans contaminated by handling fish (87, 110). It is mainly an occupational disease affecting fishermen. The organism can be found on the surface of the fish and produces skin lesions known as "fish roses" in humans. *Erysipelothrix* infection is almost invariably introduced through minor skin wounds. Local erysipeloid most commonly occurs on the hands, with the occasional complication of local lymphangitis and lymphadenitis. As reported by Lehane and Rawlin (87), 11 of 49 recorded cases of *E. insidiosa* septicemia in the United States between 1912 and 1988 were associated with fish contact. Despite the potential of this organism to infect aquarium owners, no cases have been reported to occur in humans as a result of aquarium fish contamination. Penicillin is the appropriate treatment for erysipeloid (125), as well as cephalosporins (87).

S. iniae Infection

S. iniae is a pathogen of fish capable of causing invasive disease and outbreaks in aquaculture farms (137). It can also produce invasive infection, characterized mainly by cellulitis but also by sepsis, endocarditis, meningitis, and arthritis, after skin injuries during handling of whole fresh fish. In 1995 and 1996, nine Asian patients in Toronto, Canada, had invasive S. iniae infections (27). Eight of the nine patients had bacteremic cellulitis (137). No cases associated with aquarium fish owners have been reported. More recently, two cases (one case of cellulitis and one case of osteomyelitis) were reported for two Chinese patients after handling fresh fish for cooking (85). Most of the human cases have been reported in Asia and were related to fish preparation. Older age and underlying conditions were also identified as risk factors for developing invasive infection (85).

E. tarda and Ornamental Fish

Protracted diarrhea in a 2-month-old Belgian infant was associated with E. tarda, and the same organism was isolated from a tropical aquarium fish in the home of the patient (135). Similarly, fibrinopurulent arthritis in a young man who had his knee punctured by a silver cobbler (Arius midgleyi) was reported in Australia (87). He recovered after treatment, which included intravenous gentamicin.

Aeromonas and Comamonas Bacteremia

A case of Comamonas bacteremia that could be related to tropical fish exposure was described. The patient was treated successfully with levofloxacin. Comamonas species are environmental gram-negative rods that rarely cause human infection (127). A. hydrophila infection in a wound can lead to cellulitis, muscle necrosis, or septicemia (87).

Vibrio vulnificus and Vibrio damselae

Vibriosis is a common infection of fish. Wound infection by these bacteria may be mild or self-limiting or lead to severe cellulitis and myositis, sometimes mimicking gas gangrene (87). In Australia, V. vulnificus infection occurred in a 68-year-old man who was spiked in the buttock by the dorsal spine of a flathead. He had acute septicemia associated with cellulitis, skin necrosis, necrotizing fasciitis, and myositis, which resolved after administration of doxycycline (95). Similarly, a few cases of wound infections caused by V. damselae were reported in Australia, with one fatal case in a 61-year-old man who received a puncture wound by a catfish spine (87).

WILD CARNIVORES: FERRETS

Among the large variety of house pets, wild carnivores, especially ferrets, have experienced increasing popularity; an estimated 6,000 ferrets are sold annually (13). There are approximately 12 million to 17 million pet ferrets in about 4 million households (3 to 4 ferrets per owner) in the United States (104). Despite the fact that

Table 3. Major zoonoses transmitted by ferrets[a]

Viral	Bacterial	Parasitic	Mycotic
Influenza	**Campylobacteriosis**	Cryptosporidiosis	Dermatophytosis
Rabies	**Salmonellosis**	Toxocariasis	
SARS CoV	Tuberculosis	Giardiasis	
	Leptospirosis		
	Listeriosis		

[a]Boldface indicates the most common zoonoses.

ferrets are enjoyable pets, much concern has been raised following severe injuries to children by ferrets kept as house pets. The state of California does not allow ferrets or several other exotic animals as house pets (117). As pets, ferrets can also represent a health hazard by transmitting several zoonoses to humans (Table 3).

Rabies

Like other carnivores, ferrets are susceptible to rabies. In the United States, fewer than 30 cases of rabies in domestic ferrets have been reported since 1958, most often from pet ferrets, some of which were acquired from pet shops (104, 117). Rabies immunization of ferrets with an inactivated vaccine has been shown to be effective for at least a year (117). The U.S. Department of Agriculture granted approval on 8 February 1990 for the use of this vaccine in ferrets 3 months of age or older. Annual booster vaccinations are required. Since 1998, the National Association of State Public Health Veterinarians has recommended in its compendium of animal rabies control that ferrets be treated like dogs and cats for postexposure management. Therefore, the previous requirement that all ferrets that have bitten human beings be killed and their brains examined for rabies is no longer applicable (103).

Influenza

Ferrets are very susceptible to influenza viruses and have served for years as animal models in the laboratory (13, 92). In ferrets, influenza is characterized by sneezing, fever, lethargy, mucoserous nasal discharge, conjunctivitis, and photophobia. The course of the influenza infection usually lasts less than a week. The disease can be severe in young ferrets. Cases of influenza in humans have occurred from contamination by aerosols from infected ferrets (92). Similarly, ferrets can be infected by humans shedding the virus.

SARS

An acute and often severe respiratory illness emerged in the southern part of the People's Republic of China in late 2002 and rapidly spread to different areas of Asia as well as several countries around the world. When the outbreak of this apparently novel infectious disease, termed severe acute respiratory syndrome (SARS), came to an end in July 2003, it had caused over 8,000 probable cases worldwide and more than 700 deaths. A novel coronavirus (CoV) was identified as the cause of the 2003 global outbreak of SARS (83). Genetic analysis and epidemiological studies suggest that the SARS CoV was introduced into humans not long ago, and SARS CoV-like viruses were isolated in Himalayan palm civets (*Paguma larvata*) and raccoon dogs (*Nyctereutes procyonoides*) in a retail live-animal market in Guangdong Province, southern China (65). Furthermore, a higher seroprevalence (13%) of SARS CoV IgG antibody in workers in live-animal markets in Guangzhou, Guangdong Province, than in persons in control groups (1 to 3%) was reported, suggesting indirect support for the hypothesis of an animal origin for SARS (31). Finally, ferrets and domestic cats were shown to be experimentally susceptible to the SARS CoV, and it was also shown that they could efficiently transmit the virus to previously uninfected animals that were housed with them (93). It is noteworthy that only the ferrets developed clinical signs (lethargy, conjunctivitis) after infection and some of them died of their infection. Therefore, owners of pet ferrets should be concerned about the risk of infection of their pets by a SARS or SARS-related virus and the possible transmission to humans.

Other Potential Zoonotic Pathogens

Ferrets can harbor several pathogenic microorganisms in their digestive tracts, especially *Salmonella* and *Campylobacter*. In a 9-month survey of ferrets used in biomedical research, 4% had *Salmonella* and 18% had *Campylobacter jejuni* or *Campylobacter coli* isolated from their feces (56). Although no cases have been reported to occur in humans from ferret contamination, ferrets must be considered possible reservoirs for *Campylobacter* and *Salmonella* organisms. Ferrets should not be allowed to roam freely, and their feces should be discarded in a hygienic manner (92). Ferrets can harbor many other zoonoses, such as cryptosporidiosis (*Cryptosporidium* causes ill thrift and mucoid diarrhea), tuberculosis, and listeriosis. Ferrets share many parasites with dogs and cats (e.g., *Toxocara* and *Ancylostoma* spp.) as well as dermatophytes (*Microsporum canis* and *T. mentagrophytes*). However, fungal diseases are uncommon in the domestic ferret. A few cases of disseminated coccidioidomycosis have been reported for ferrets from the southwestern United States, and all cases of dermatophytosis reported for ferrets occurred in animals that had been exposed to cats (63). Ferrets respond poorly to treatment compared with dogs and cats (63). A complete description of these infections has been published by Marini et al. (92).

PET BATS

Among the uncommon exotic pet species, bats may represent a major public health issue, as bats can be infected with various lethal viruses, such as rabies, Hendra, and Nipah viruses (73, 90). A case of rabies was diagnosed in France in 1999 in a pet African bat (*Rousettus* sp.), imported from either Togo or Egypt and sold by a Belgian exotic-pet dealer to another pet dealer in Bordeaux, where the owner, who was from Nîmes, bought it (9). The virus was identified to be a Lagos bat lyssavirus (lyssavirus genotype 2). Cases of rabies have also been reported to occur in bats belonging to the same species kept in a zoological garden collection in Denmark (9). The incriminated virus was a European bat lyssavirus (EBL1a). Similarly, rabies is of major concern for people working in animal rehabilitation centers. The first human case of Australian bat lyssavirus was reported to occur in a 39-year-old female animal handler from Queensland, in November 1996, within 5 weeks after she was scratched and possibly bitten by a yellow-bellied sheath-tailed bat (*Saccolaimus flaviventris*) (96).

NONHUMAN PRIMATES

During the last 25 years, laws restricting importation of nonhuman primates into the United States have considerably reduced the number of primates appearing in the pet trade. However, nonhuman primates sometimes find their way into the hands of pet owners. Until the 1974 prohibition, New World primates, especially the squirrel monkey, were used extensively in the pet trade (112). Because of close phylogenetic ties between humans and nonhuman primates, zoonoses transmitted by monkeys are numerous, some of them being particularly severe in humans. For public health reasons, as well as for animal welfare and environmental protection, I strongly support the policy that monkeys should not be kept as pets. It is not my purpose to present all the zoonoses that can be transmitted by primates, as excellent reviews have been published (106, 112, 119, 128). A short table of the major and most severe zoonoses is included for information (Table 4).

Among the major zoonoses, salmonellosis and shigellosis are certainly the most frequent in monkeys, as gastrointestinal illnesses are very common. Nonhuman primates are also very susceptible to respiratory infections, and tuberculosis must be considered a major risk for monkeys and their owners or caretakers. Monkeys are very susceptible to *Mycobacterium tuberculosis*, *Mycobacterium bovis*, and *M. avium*, and suspect animals should not be treated. Monkeys are also very susceptible to some viral diseases, such as measles. Infected children can easily transmit the virus to pet monkeys. Some viral diseases of the nonhuman primates may be deadly to humans who are infected. An example is herpes B virus, which may be shed by healthy monkeys (mainly macaques) in their saliva. In a recent study of nonoccupational exposure incidents involving macaques in the United States, children were more than three times as likely to be bitten as adults. Herpes B virus must be as-

Table 4. Major zoonoses transmitted by nonhuman primates[a]

Viral	Bacterial	Parasitic	Mycotic
Hepatitis A	**Salmonellosis**	**Amoebiasis**	Dermatophytosis
Measles	**Shigellosis**	**Balantidosis**	(*T. mentagrophytes*,
Herpes B	**Tuberculosis**	*Hymenolepis* infection	*Microsporum* spp.)
[Rabies]	Campylobacteriosis	*Strongyloides* infection	
[Ebola and Marburg	Yersiniosis	Giardiasis	
virus infections]	Klebsiellosis		
[Monkeypox]	[Tularemia]		

[a]Boldface indicates the most common zoonoses; brackets indicate rare zoonoses.

sumed to be a potential health hazard in macaque bite wounds; this risk makes macaques unsuitable as pets (105). In monkeys, rabies is a rare disease, but cases have been reported to occur in pet monkeys vaccinated with live modified strains; thus, only inactivated rabies vaccines should be used to immunize monkeys.

CONCLUSION

Zoonotic diseases transmitted by domestic pets are quite uncommon events but should be systematically considered when disease occurs in both animals and humans or in the pet's household. In order to reduce such a risk, acquisition of exotic pets or wild animals as pets should not be encouraged. Regular veterinary care is strongly suggested to keep pets healthy and prevent any human infection.

REFERENCES

1. **Acha, P., and B. Szyfres.** 1987. *Zoonoses and Communicable Diseases Common to Man and Animals*, 2nd ed., p. 963. Pan American Health Organization, Washington, D.C.
2. **Ackermann, R., W. Stille, W. Blumenthal, E. B. Helm, K. Keller, and O. Baldus.** 1972. Syrische goldhamster als Ubertrager von Lymphozytarer Choriomeningitis. *Dtsch. Med. Wochenschr.* **97:** 1725–1731.
3. **Ackman, D. M., P. Drabkin, G. Birkhead, and P. Cieslak.** 1995. Reptile-associated salmonellosis in New York State. *Pediatr. Infect. Dis. J.* **14:**955–959.
4. **Altman, R., J. C. Gorman, L. L. Bernhardt, and M. Goldfield.** 1972. Turtle-associated salmonellosis. II. The relationship of pet turtles to salmonellosis in children in New Jersey. *Am. J. Epidemiol.* **95:**518–520.
5. **Anderson, L. C.** 1987. Guinea pig husbandry and medicine. *Vet. Clin. N. Am. Small Anim. Pract.* **17:**1045–1060.
6. **Anderson, L. C., S. L. Leary, and P. J. Manning.** 1983. Rat bite fever in animal research laboratory personnel. *Lab. Anim. Sci.* **33:**292–294.
7. **Anonymous.** 1981. Reptilian salmonellosis. *Lancet* **ii:**130–131.
8. **Anonymous.** *Promed* (Internet/e-mail service), 19981007.
9. **Aubert, M., O. Lemarignier, C. Gibon, M. B. Alvado-Brette, P. Brie, and F. Rosenthal.** 1999. Un cas de rage dans le Gard sur une rousette d'Egypte considérée comme animal familier. *Bull. Epidemiol. Mens. Rage Anim. France* **29(4–6):**1–4.
10. **Bartlett, K. H., T. J. Trust, and H. Lior.** 1977. Small pet aquarium frogs as a source of *Salmonella*. *Appl. Environ. Microbiol.* **33:**1026–1029.
11. **Baxby, D., and M. Bennett.** 1997. Poxvirus zoonoses. *J. Med. Microbiol.* **46:**17–20.
12. **Benenson, A.** 1990. *Control of Communicable Diseases in Man*, 15th ed., p. 532. American Public Health Association, Washington, D.C.
13. **Besch-Williford, C. L.** 1987. Biology and medicine of the ferret. *Vet. Clin. N. Am. Small Anim. Pract.* **17:**1155–1183.
14. **Biggar, R. J., J. P. Woodall, P. D. Walter, and G. E. Haughie.** 1975. Lymphocytic choriomeningitis outbreak associated with pet hamsters. Fifty-seven cases from New York State. *JAMA* **232:**494–500.
15. **Borland, E. D.** 1975. *Salmonella* infection in dogs, cats, tortoises and terrapins. *Vet. Rec.* **96:**401–402.
16. **Burnham, B. R., D. H. Atchley, R. P. DeFusco, K. E. Ferris, J. C. Zicarelli, J. H. Lee, and F. J. Angulo.** 1998. Prevalence of fecal shedding of *Salmonella* organisms among captive green iguanas and potential public health implications. *J. Am. Vet. Med. Assoc.* **213:**48–50.
17. **Campos, A., J. H. Taylor, and M. Campbell.** 2000. Hamster bite peritonitis: *Pasteurella pneumotropica* peritonitis in a dialysis patient. *Pediatr. Nephrol.* **15:**31–32.
18. **Canny, C. J., and C. S. Gamble.** 2003. Fungal diseases of rabbits. *Vet. Clin. Exot. Anim.* **6:**429–433.
19. **Carniel, E., and H. H. Mollaret.** 1990. Yersiniosis. *Comp. Immunol. Microbiol. Infect. Dis.* **13:**51–58.

20. **Center for Disease Control.** 1963. *Salmonella Surveillance Report No. 10*, p. 22–24. Center for Disease Control, Atlanta, Ga.

21. **Centers for Disease Control.** 1984. Rat bite fever in a college student, California. *Morb. Mortal. Wkly. Rep.* **33**:318–320.

22. **Centers for Disease Control.** 1986. Turtle-associated salmonellosis—Ohio. *Morb. Mortal. Wkly. Rep.* **35**:733–734, 739.

23. **Centers for Disease Control.** 1992. Iguana-associated salmonellosis—Indiana, 1990. *Morb. Mortal. Wkly. Rep.* **41**:38–39.

24. **Centers for Disease Control.** 1992. Lizard-associated salmonellosis—Utah. *Morb. Mortal. Wkly. Rep.* **41**:610–611.

25. **Centers for Disease Control and Prevention.** 1995. Reptile-associated salmonellosis—selected states, 1994–1995. *Morb. Mortal. Wkly. Rep.* **44**:347–350.

26. **Centers for Disease Control and Prevention.** 1995. African pigmy hedgehog-associated salmonellosis—Washington, 1994. *Morb. Mortal. Wkly. Rep.* **44**:462–463.

27. **Centers for Disease Control and Prevention.** 1996. Invasive infection due to *Streptococcus iniae*—Ontario, 1995–1996. *Morb. Mortal. Wkly. Rep.* **45**:650–653.

28. **Centers for Disease Control and Prevention.** 1998. Rat-bite fever—New Mexico, 1996. *Morb. Mortal. Wkly. Rep.* **47**:89–91.

29. **Centers for Disease Control and Prevention.** 1999. Reptile-associated salmonellosis—selected states, 1996–1998. *Morb. Mortal. Wkly. Rep.* **48**:1009–1013.

30. **Centers for Disease Control and Prevention.** 2002. Outbreak of tularemia among commercially distributed prairie dogs, 2002. *Morb. Mortal. Wkly. Rep.* **51**:688, 699.

31. **Centers for Disease Control and Prevention.** 2003. Prevalence of IgG antibody to SARS-associated coronavirus in animal traders—Guangdong Province, China, 2003. *Morb. Mortal. Wkly. Rep.* **52**:986–987.

32. **Centers for Disease Control and Prevention.** 2003. Update: multistate outbreak of monkeypox—Illinois, Indiana, Kansas, Missouri, Ohio, and Wisconsin, 2003. *Morb. Mortal. Wkly. Rep.* **52**:642–646.

33. **Centers for Disease Control and Prevention.** 2003. Reptile-associated salmonellosis—selected states, 1998–2002. *Morb. Mortal. Wkly. Rep.* **52**:1206–1209.

34. **Centers for Disease Control and Prevention, Food and Drug Administration, Department of Health and Human Services.** 2003. Control of communicable diseases; restrictions on African rodents, prairie dogs, and certain other animals. Interim final rule; opportunity for public comment. *Fed. Regist.* **68**:62353–62369.

35. **Chassis, G., E. M. Gross, Z. Greenberg, M. Tokar, N. Platzner, R. Mizrachi, and A. Wolff.** 1986. Salmonella in turtles imported to Israel from Louisiana. *JAMA* **256**:1003.

36. **Childs, J. E., G. E. Glass, T. G. Ksiazek, C. A. Rossi, J. G. Oro, and J. W. Leduc.** 1991. Human-rodent contact and infection with lymphocytic choriomeningitis and Seoul viruses in an inner-city population. *Am. J. Trop. Med. Hyg.* **44**:117–121.

37. **Chiodini, R. J., and J. P. Sundberg.** 1981. Salmonellosis in reptiles: a review. *Am. J. Epidemiol.* **113**:494–499.

38. **Chretien, J. H., and V. F. Garagusi.** 1990. Infections associated with pets. *Am. Fam. Pract.* **41**:831–845.

39. **Cohen, M. L., M. Potter, R. Pollard, and R. A. Feldman.** 1980. Turtle-associated salmonellosis in the United States. Effect of public health action, 1970–1976. *JAMA* **243**:1247–1249.

40. **Dalton, C., R. Hoffman, and J. Pape.** 1995. Iguana-associated salmonellosis in children. *Pediatr. Infect. Dis. J.* **14**:319–320.

41. **D'Aoust, J. Y., E. Daley, M. Crozier, and A. M. Sewell.** 1990. Pet turtles: a continuing international threat to public health. *Am. J. Epidemiol.* **132**:233–238.

42. **D'Aoust, J. Y., and H. Lior.** 1978. Pet turtle regulations and abatement of human salmonellosis. *Can. J. Public Health* **69**:107–108.

43. **Davis, W. A., II, J. H. Chretien, V. F. Garagusi, and M. A. Goldstein.** 1978. Snake-to-human transmission of *Aeromonas (Pl) shigelloides* resulting in gastroenteritis. *South. Med. J.* **71**:474–476.

44. **Deeb, B. J., and R. F. DiGiacomo.** 1994. Cerebral larva migrans caused by *Baylisascaris* sp. in pet rabbits. *J. Am. Vet. Med. Assoc.* **205**:1744–1747.

45. **De Guzman, E., and E. B. Shotts.** 1988. Bacterial culture and evaluation of diseases of fish. *Vet. Clin. N. Am. Small Anim. Pract.* **18:**365–374.
46. **Deibel, R., J. P. Woodall, W. J. Decher, and G. D. Schryver.** 1975. Lymphocytic choriomeningitis virus in man. Serologic evidence of association with pet hamsters. *JAMA* **232:**501–504.
47. **Dodin, A., and M. Galimand.** 1981. La mélioidose: maladie de pathologie comparée. *Bull. Soc. Sci. Vet. Med. Comp.* **83:**255–258.
48. **Donta, S. T., P. W. Smith, R. E. Levitz, and R. Quintiliani.** 1986. Therapy of *Mycobacterium marinum* infections. Use of tetracyclines vs. rifampin. *Arch. Intern. Med.* **146:**902–904.
49. **Downing, N. D., G. D. Dewnany, and P. J. Radford.** 2001. A rare and serious consequence of a rat bite. *Ann. R. Coll. Surg. Engl.* **83:**279–280.
50. **Duma, R. J., D. E. Sonenshine, F. M. Bozeman, J. M. Veazey, Jr., B. L. Elisberg, D. P. Chadwick, N. I. Stocks, T. M. McGill, G. B. Miller, Jr., and J. N. MacCormack.** 1981. Epidemic typhus in the United States associated with flying squirrels. *JAMA* **245:**2318–2323.
51. **Eidson, M., J. P. Thilsted, and O. J. Rollag.** 1991. Clinical, clinicopathologic, and pathologic features of plague in cats: 119 cases (1977–1988). *J. Am. Vet. Med. Assoc.* **199:**1191–1197.
52. **Enriquez, C., N. Nwachuku, and C. P. Gerba.** 2001. Direct exposure to animal enteric pathogens. *Rev. Environ. Health* **16:**117–131.
53. **Favorov, M. O., M. Y. Kosoy, S. A. Tsarev, J. E. Childs, and H. S. Margolis.** 2000. Prevalence of antibody to hepatitis E virus among rodents in the United States. *J. Infect. Dis.* **181:**449–455.
54. **Fish, N. A., A. L. Fletch, and W. E. Butler.** 1968. Family outbreak of salmonellosis due to contact with guinea pigs. *Can. Med. Assoc. J.* **99:**418–420.
55. **Fonseca, R. J., and L. M. Dubey.** 1994. *Salmonella montevideo* sepsis from a pet snake. *Pediatr. Infect. Dis. J.* **13:**550.
56. **Fox, J. G., J. A. Adkins, and K. O. Maxwell.** 1988. Zoonoses in ferrets. *Lab. Anim. Sci.* **38:**500–501.
57. **Fox, J. G., C. E. Newcomer, and H. Rozmiarek.** 1984. Selected zoonoses and other health hazards, p. 613–648. *In* J. G. Fox, B. J. Cohen, and F. M. Loew (ed.), *Laboratory Animal Medicine.* Academic Press, New York, N.Y.
58. **Friedman, C. R., C. Torigian, P. J. Shillam, R. E. Hoffman, D. Heltzel, J. L. Beebe, G. Malcolm, W. de Witt, L. Hutwagner, and P. M. Griffin.** 1998. An outbreak of salmonellosis among children attending a reptile exhibit at a zoo. *J. Pediatr.* **132:**802–807.
59. **Friedmann, C. T. H., E. L. Spiegel, E. Aaron, and R. McIntyre.** 1973. *Leptospira ballum* contracted from pet mice. *Calif. Med.* **118:**51–52.
60. **Fujita, K., K. I. Murono, and H. Yoshioka.** 1981. Pet-linked salmonellosis. *Lancet* **ii:**525.
61. **Goscienski, P. J.** 1983. Zoonoses. *Pediatr. Infect. Dis. J.* **2:**69–81.
62. **Gratzeck, J. B.** 1984. Tropical fish: keeping a giant industry healthy, p. 347–357. *In Animal Health, 1984 Yearbook of Agriculture.* U.S. Department of Agriculture, Washington, D.C.
63. **Greenacre, C. B.** 2003. Fungal diseases of ferrets. *Vet. Clin. Exot. Anim.* **6:**435–448.
64. **Gregg, M. B.** 1975. Recent outbreaks of lymphocytic choriomeningitis in the United States of America. *Bull. W. H. O.* **52:**549–553.
65. **Guan, Y., B. J. Zheng, Y. Q. He, X. L. Liu, Z. X. Zhuang, C. L. Cheung, S. W. Luo, P. H. Li, L. J. Zhang, Y. J. Guan, K. M. Butt, K. L. Wong, K. W. Chan, W. Lim, K. F. Shortridge, K. Y. Yuen, J. S. Peiris, and L. L. Poon.** 2003. Isolation and characterization of viruses related to the SARS coronavirus from animals in southern China. *Science* **302:**276–278.
66. **Harkness, J. E.** 1987. Rabbit husbandry and medicine. *Vet. Clin. N. Am. Small Anim. Pract.* **17:**1019–1044.
67. **Harkness, J. E., and J. E. Wagner.** 1983. *The Biology and Medicine of Rabbits and Rodents,* 2nd ed., p. 2104. Lea & Febiger, Philadelphia, Pa.
68. **Harvey, S., and J. R. Greenwood.** 1985. Isolation of *Campylobacter fetus* from a pet turtle. *J. Clin. Microbiol.* **21:**260–261.
69. **Harvey, S., R. Greenwood, M. J. Pickett, and R. H. Mah.** 1976. Recovery of *Yersinia enterocolitica* from streams and lakes of California. *Appl. Environ. Microbiol.* **32:**352–354.
70. **He, J., B. L. Innis, M. P. Shrestha, E. T. Clayson, R. M. Scott, K. J. Linthicum, G. G. Musser, S. C. Gigliotti, L. N. Binn, R. A. Kuschner, and D. W. Vaughn.** 2002. Evidence that rodents are a reservoir of hepatitis E virus for humans in Nepal. *J. Clin. Microbiol.* **40:**4493–4498.

71. Hendrix, C. M., and B. L. Blagburn. 1988. Reptilian pentastomiasis: a possible emerging zoonosis. *Compend. Small Anim.* **10:**46–51.

72. Hirano, M., X. Ding, T. C. Li, N. Takeda, H. Kawabata, N. Koizumi, T. Kadosaka, I. Goto, T. Masuzawa, M. Nakamura, K. Taira, T. Kuroki, T. Tanikawa, H. Watanabe, and K. Abe. 2003. Evidence for widespread infection of hepatitis E virus among wild rats in Japan. *Hepatol. Res.* **27:**1–5.

73. Hoar, B. R., B. B. Chomel, F. J. Argaz Rodriguez, and P. A. Colley. 1998. Zoonoses and potential zoonoses transmitted by bats. *J. Am. Vet. Med. Assoc.* **212:**1714–1720.

74. Hsieh, S., and F. E. Balb. 1999. *Serratia marcescens* cellulitis following an iguana bite. *Clin. Infect. Dis.* **28:**1181–1182.

75. Jafari, M., J. Forsberg, R. O. Gilcher, J. W. Smith, J. M. Crutcher, M. McDermott, B. R. Brown, and J. N. George. 2002. *Salmonella* sepsis caused by a platelet transfusion from a donor with a pet snake. *N. Engl. J. Med.* **347:**1075–1078.

76. Janda, J. M., and S. L. Abbott. 1993. Infections associated with the genus *Edwardsiella:* the role of *Edwardsiella tarda* in human disease. *Clin. Infect. Dis.* **17:**742–748.

77. Jay, M., M. S. Ascher, B. B. Chomel, M. Madon, D. Sesline, B. A. Enge, B. Hjelle, T. G. Ksiazek, P. E. Rollin, P. H. Kass, and K. Reilly. 1997. Seroepidemiologic studies of hantavirus infection among wild rodents in California. *Emerg. Infect. Dis.* **3:**183–190.

78. Kaufmann, A. F., M. D. Fox, G. K. Morris, B. T. Wood, J. C. Feeley, and M. K. Frix. 1972. Turtle-associated salmonellosis. III. The effects of environmental salmonellae in commercial turtle breeding ponds. *Am. J. Epidemiol.* **95:**521–528.

79. Kiesch, N. 2000. Aquariums and mycobacterioses. *Rev. Med. Brux.* **21:**A255–A256. (In French.)

80. Kist, M. J., and S. Freitag. 2000. Serovar specific risk factors and clinical features of *Salmonella enterica* ssp. *enterica* serovar Enteritidis: a study in South-West Germany. *Epidemiol. Infect.* **124:**383–392.

81. Kleeburg, H. H. 1975. Tuberculosis and other mycobacterioses, p. 303–360. *In* W. T. Hubbert, W. F. McCulloch, and P. R. Schnurrenberger (ed.), *Diseases Transmitted from Animals to Man,* 6th ed. Charles C Thomas, Publisher, Springfield, Ill.

82. Krebs, J. W., J. T. Wheeling, and J. E. Childs. 2003. Rabies surveillance in the United States during 2002. *J. Am. Vet. Med. Assoc.* **223:**1736–1748.

83. Ksiazek, T. G., D. Erdman, C. Goldsmith, S. R. Zaki, T. Peret, S. Emery, et al. 2003. A novel coronavirus associated with severe acute respiratory syndrome. *N. Engl. J. Med.* **348:**1953–1966.

84. Lamm, S. H., A. Taylor, Jr., E. J. Gangarosa, H. W. Anderson, W. Young, M. H. Clark, and A. R. Bruce. 1972. Turtle associated salmonellosis. I. An estimation of the magnitude of the problem in the United States, 1970–1971. *Am. J. Epidemiol.* **95:**511–517.

85. Lau, S. K., P. C. Woo, H. Tse, K. W. Leung, S. S. Wong, and K. Y. Yuen. 2003. Invasive *Streptococcus iniae* infections outside North America. *J. Clin. Microbiol.* **41:**1004–1009.

86. LeDuc, J. W. 1987. Epidemiology of Hantaan and related viruses. *Lab. Anim. Sci.* **37:**413–418.

87. Lehane, L., and G. T. Rawlin. 2000. Topically acquired bacterial zoonoses from fish: a review. *Med. J. Aust.* **173:**256–259.

88. Leibovitz, L. 1980. Fish tuberculosis (mycobacteriosis). *J. Am. Vet. Med. Assoc.* **176:**415.

89. Lynch, M., M. Daly, B. O'Brien, F. Morrison, B. Cryan, and S. Fanning. 1999. *Salmonella tel-el-kebir* and terrapins. *J. Infect.* **38:**182–184.

90. Mackenzie, J. S., H. E. Field, and K. J. Guyatt. 2003. Managing emerging diseases borne by fruit bats (flying foxes), with particular reference to henipaviruses and Australian bat lyssavirus. *J. Appl. Microbiol.* **94**(Suppl.):59S–69S.

91. Magee, J. S., R. W. Steele, N. R. Kelly, and R. F. Jacobs. 1989. Tularemia transmitted by a squirrel bite. *Pediatr. Infect. Dis. J.* **8:**123–125.

92. Marini, R. P., J. A. Adkins, and J. G. Fox. 1989. Proven or potential zoonotic diseases of ferrets. *J. Am. Vet. Med. Assoc.* **195:**990–994.

93. Martina, B. E., B. L. Haagmans, T. Kuiken, R. A. Fouchier, G. F. Rimmelzwaan, G. Van Amerongen, J. S. Peiris, W. Lim, and A. D. Osterhaus. 2003. SARS virus infection of cats and ferrets. *Nature* **425:**915.

94. Matsuda, H., K. Okada, K. Takahashi, and S. Mishiro. 2003. Severe hepatitis E virus infection after ingestion of uncooked liver from a wild boar. *J. Infect. Dis.* **188:**944.

95. **Maxwell, E. L., B. C. Mayall, S. R. Pearson, and P. A. Stanley.** 1991. A case of *Vibrio vulnificus* septicaemia acquired in Victoria. *Med. J. Aust.* **154:**214–215.

96. **McCall, B. J., J. H. Epstein, A. S. Neill, K. Heel, H. Field, J. Barrett, G. A. Smith, L. A. Selvey, B. Rodwell, and R. Lunt.** 2000. Potential human exposure to Australian bat lyssavirus, Queensland, 1996–1999. *Emerg. Infect. Dis.* **6:**259–264.

97. **Mermin, J., B. Hoar, and F. J. Angulo.** 1997. Iguanas and *Salmonella marina* infection in children: a reflection of the increasing incidence of reptile-associated salmonellosis in the United States. *Pediatrics* **99:**399–402.

98. **Mitchell, M. A., and S. M. Shane.** 2000. Preliminary findings of *Salmonella* spp. in captive green iguanas (*Iguana iguana*) and their environment. *Prev. Vet. Med.* **45:**297–304.

99. **Mokhayer, B., and H. Tadjbakhche.** 1978. Isolement de *Salmonella havana* d'une épizootie sévissant sur les poissons rouges (queue de voile et comète). *Bull. Soc. Sci. Vet. Med. Comp.* **80:**147–150.

100. **Moro, M. H., J. T. Horman, H. R. Fischman, J. K. Grigor, and E. Israel.** 1991. The epidemiology of rodent and lagomorph rabies in Maryland, 1981 to 1986. *J. Wildl. Dis.* **27:**452–456.

101. **Nagel, P., A. Serritella, and T. J. Layden.** 1982. *Edwardsiella tarda* gastroenteritis associated with a pet turtle. *Gastroenterology* **82:**1436–1437.

102. **Nakamura, Y., R. Kano, E. Nakamura, K. Saito, S. Watanabe, and A. Hasegawa.** 2002. Case report. First report on human ringworm caused by *Arthroderma benhamiae* in Japan transmitted from a rabbit. *Mycoses* **45:**129–131.

103. **National Association of State Public Health Veterinarians.** 2003. Compendium of animal rabies prevention and control, 2003. *Morb. Mortal. Wkly. Rep.* **52**(RR-5):1–6.

104. **Niezgoda, M., D. J. Briggs, J. Shaddock, D. W. Dreesen, and C. E. Rupprecht.** 1997. Pathogenesis of experimentally induced rabies in domestic ferrets. *Am. J. Vet. Res.* **58:**1327–1331.

105. **Ostrowski, S. R., M. J. Leslie, T. Parrott, S. Abelt, and P. E. Piercy.** 1998. B-virus from pet macaque monkeys: an emerging threat in the United States? *Emerg. Infect. Dis.* **4:**117–121.

106. **Parrott, T. Y.** 1986. An introduction to diseases of nonhuman primates. *Compend. Small Anim.* **8:**733–738.

107. **Pfleger, S., G. Benyr, R. Sommer, and A. Hassl.** 2003. Pattern of *Salmonella* excretion in amphibians and reptiles in a vivarium. *Int. J. Hyg. Environ. Health* **206:**53–59.

108. **Pollock, C.** 2003. Fungal diseases of laboratory rodents. *Vet. Clin. Exot. Anim.* **6:**401–413.

109. **Postma, B. H., R. J. A. Dierpersloot, G. J. C. M. Niessen, and R. P. Droog.** 1991. Cowpox-virus-like infection associated with rat bite. *Lancet* **337:**733–734.

110. **Reboli, A., and E. Farrar.** 1989. *Erysipelothrix rhusiopathiae*: an occupational pathogen. *Clin. Microbiol. Rev.* **2:**354–359.

111. **Redrobe, S.** 2002. Reptiles and disease—keeping the risks to a minimum. *J. Small Anim. Pract.* **43:**471–472.

112. **Renquist, D. M., and R. A. Whitney.** 1987. Zoonoses acquired from pet primates. *Vet. Clin. N. Am. Small Anim. Pract.* **17:**219–240.

113. **Reynolds, M. G., J. S. Krebs, J. A. Comer, J. W. Sumner, T. C. Rushton, C. E. Lopez, W. L. Nicholson, J. A. Rooney, S. E. Lance-Parker, J. H. McQuiston, C. D. Paddock, and J. E. Childs.** 2003. Flying squirrel-associated typhus, United States. *Emerg. Infect. Dis.* **9:**1341–1343.

114. **Rosen, T.** 2000. Hazardous hedgehogs. *South. Med. J.* **93:**936–938.

115. **Rosen, T., and J. Jablon.** 2003. Infectious threats from exotic pets: dermatological implications. *Dermatol. Clin.* **21:**229–236.

116. **Rousseau, M. C., M. F. Saron, P. Brouqui, and A. Bourgeade.** 1997. Lymphocytic choriomeningitis virus in southern France: four case reports and review of the literature. *Eur. J. Epidemiol.* **13:**817–823.

117. **Rupprecht, C. E., J. Gilbert, R. Pitts, K. R. Marshall, and H. Koprowski.** 1990. Evaluation of an inactivated rabies virus vaccine in domestic ferrets. *J. Am. Vet. Med. Assoc.* **196:**1614–1616.

118. **Sanchez, R., A. Martin, A. Bailly, and M. F. Dirat.** 1988. Salmonellose digestive associée à une tortue domestique. A propos d'un cas. *Med. Mal. Infect.* **18:**458–459.

119. **Satterfield, W. C., and W. R. Voss.** 1987. Nonhuman primates and the practitioner. *Vet. Clin. N. Am. Small Anim. Pract.* **17:**1185–1202.

120. **Schultz, L. J., R. R. Roberto, G. W. Rutherford, B. Hummert, and I. Lubell.** 1992. *Mesocestoides* (Cestoda) infection in a California child. *Pediatr. Infect. Dis. J.* **11:**332–334.

121. **Schumacher, J.** 2003. Fungal diseases of reptiles. *Vet. Clin. Exot. Anim.* **6:**327–335.
122. **Schuurman, B., A. J. van Griethuysen, J. H. Marcelis, and A. M. Nijs.** 1998. Rat bite fever after a bite from a tame pet rat. *Ned. Tijdschr. Geneeskd.* **142:**2006–2009.
123. **Seguin, B., Y. Boucaud-Maitre, P. Quenin, and G. Lorgue.** 1986. Recherche de *Yersinia enterocolitica* et des espèces apparentées chez le rat d'égout: présence d'une souche pathogène humaine. *Med. Mal. Infect.* **16:**28–30.
124. **Shotts, E. B.** 1980. Bacteria associated with fish and their relative importance, p. 517–525. *In* J. H. Steele (ed.), *CRC Handbook Series in Zoonoses, Section A,* vol. II. CRC Press, Boca Raton, Fla.
125. **Shotts, E. B.** 1987. Bacterial diseases of fish associated with human health. *Vet. Clin. N. Am. Small Anim. Pract.* **17:**241–247.
126. **Skorepova, M., J. Stork, and J. Hrabakova.** 2002. Case reports. Tinea gladiatorum due to *Trichophyton mentagrophytes. Mycoses* **45:**431–433.
127. **Smith, M. D., and J. D. Gradon.** Bacteremia due to *Comamonas* species possibly associated with exposure to tropical fish. *South. Med. J.* **96:**815–817.
128. **Soave, O.** 1981. Viral infections common to human and nonhuman primates. *J. Am. Vet. Med. Assoc.* **179:**1385–1388.
129. **Stehr-Green, J. K., and P. Schantz.** 1987. The impact of zoonotic diseases transmitted by pets on human health and the economy. *Vet. Clin. N. Am. Small Anim. Pract.* **17:**1–15.
130. **Tager Frey, M., P. C. Vial, C. H. Castillo, P. M. Godoy, B. Hjelle, and M. G. Ferres.** 2003. Hantavirus prevalence in the IX Region of Chile. *Emerg. Infect. Dis.* **9:**827–832.
131. **Tauxe, R. V., J. G. Rigau-Pérez, J. G. Wells, and P. A. Blake.** 1985. Turtle-associated salmonellosis in Puerto Rico. *JAMA* **254:**237–239.
132. **Tei, S., N. Kitajima, K. Takahashi, and S. Mishiro.** 2003. Zoonotic transmission of hepatitis E virus from deer to human beings. *Lancet* **362:**371–373.
133. **Thoen, C. O., A. G. Karlson, and E. M. Himes.** 1981. Mycobacterial infections in animals. *Rev. Infect. Dis.* **3:**960–972.
134. **Tsianakas, P., B. Polack, L. Pinquier, B. Levy Klotz, and C. Prost-Squarcioni.** 2000. *Cheyletiella* dermatitis: an uncommon cause of vesiculobullous eruption. *Ann. Dermatol. Venereol.* **127:**826–829.
135. **Vandepitte, J., P. Lemmens, and L. de Swert.** 1983. Human edwardsiellosis traced to ornamental fish. *J. Clin. Microbiol.* **17:**165–167.
136. **Wagner, J. E., and P. L. Farrar.** 1987. Husbandry and medicine of small rodents. *Vet. Clin. N. Am. Small Anim. Pract.* **17:**1061–1087.
137. **Weinstein, M. R., M. Litt, D. A. Kertesz, P. Wyper, D. Rose, M. Coulter, A. McGeer, R. Facklam, C. Ostach, B. M. Willey, A. Borczyk, and D. E. Low.** 1997. Invasive infections due to a fish pathogen, *Streptococcus iniae. N. Engl. J. Med.* **337:**589–594.
138. **Willis, C., T. Wilson, M. Greenwood, and L. Ward.** 2002. Pet reptiles associated with a case of salmonellosis in an infant were carrying multiple strains of *Salmonella. J. Clin. Microbiol.* **40:**4802–4803.
139. **Wise, J. K., B. L. Heathcott, and M. L. Gonzales.** 2002. Results of the AVMA survey on companion animal ownership in US pet-owning households. *J. Am. Vet. Med. Assoc.* **221:**1572–1573.
140. **Wolfs, T. F., J. A. Wagenaar, H. G. Niesters, and A. D. Osterhaus.** 2002. Rat-to-human transmission of cowpox infection. *Emerg. Infect. Dis.* **8:**1495–1496.
141. **Woodward, D. L., R. Khakhria, and W. M. Johnson.** 1997. Human salmonellosis associated with exotic pets. *J. Clin. Microbiol.* **35:**2786–2790.
142. **Zamora, J., and R. Enriquez.** 1987. *Yersinia enterocolitica, Y. frederiksenii* and *Y. intermedia* in *Cyprinus carpio* (Linneo 1758). *Zentbl. Vetmed. Reihe B* **34:**155–159.

Infections of Leisure, Third Edition
Edited by David Schlossberg
© 2004 ASM Press, Washington, D.C.

Chapter 9

Man's Worst Friend (the Rat)

James G. Fox

Historically, the rat has been considered a scourge to humankind. For example, the rat is a reservoir for plague called the Black Death, which accounted for millions of deaths in Europe during the Middle Ages. At least three pandemics (in the 5th and 6th, 8th through 14th, and 19th through 21st centuries) of plague ravaged civilizations, and pandemics undoubtedly have "plagued" humankind prior to recorded history. Also, numerous other diseases are spread to humans by the rat; thus, Hans Zinsser's quote from his text *Rats, Lice and History*, "Man and rat will always be pitted against each other as implacable enemies," conveys the general revulsion that society holds for the wild rat (162).

Numerous methods have been used by countless countries attempting to eradicate the rat, but it continues to successfully colonize both urban and rural settings on a global level. One novel approach introduced first in Asia and Europe and then the United States was the use of domestic ferrets for rodent control.

With the life cycle and transmission of *Yersinia pestis* closely linked to rats and their fleas, tremendous efforts were mounted to eradicate the rat host and its flea, *Xenopsylla cheopis*. For example, in the Philippines, rat catcher groups of 300 men were assigned the formidable task of eliminating the omnipresent pest (63). When rats were encountered, they were killed immediately. Some of these work forces had fox terriers imported specially from Australia, because of their agility and quickness. Others utilized trained ferrets which responded to their masters' calls, like dogs. The ferrets were even more effective than dogs in killing rats. A ferret would grasp the rats in its jaws, and the ferret's teeth would then sever the rat's spinal column (63). Undoubtedly, ferrets performed a similar role in locales throughout the world to control rat infestations and hence reduce the likelihood of further spread of the dreaded pestilence.

One author recommended that, when rats are hunted in plague-infested areas, the rats and the sack containing the dead rats be submerged in a germicidal solution as soon as they are killed (71). It was strongly urged that rats in plague areas as well

James G. Fox • Division of Comparative Medicine, Massachusetts Institute of Technology, 77 Massachusetts Ave., Cambridge, MA 02139.

as the bag containing the rats be incinerated. Even though attention was given to treating rat bite wound infection in ferrets, discussions on ferrets hunting plague-infected rats and becoming infected with the plague bacillus were not found.

The practice of using ferrets to control wild rodents also became popular in the United States during the early part of the 20th century, and tens of thousands of ferrets were raised and sold for this purpose. The Department of Agriculture distributed bulletins announcing the use of ferrets for rodent abatement (47). Because rodents are extremely fearful of ferrets and flee even their scent, only a few ferrets were needed to disperse literally hundreds of rodents from granaries, barns, and warehouses. A ferret handler would deploy his ferrets on an infested farm or granary, and the animal would then "ferret out" the rodents from their hiding places and nests. Men and terrier dogs, strategically located, would eradicate the rodents as they emerged from hiding. Alternatively, small farms or granaries would maintain ferrets and allow the territorial imperative for up to about 650 ft (200 m)—considered to be the ranging domain of a ferret—with an adequate food source. The introduction of commercially available rodenticides, however, has dramatically reduced the popularity of ferrets as rodent exterminators (47).

During the early 1900s, rodenticides containing live cultures of *Salmonella enteritidis* were distributed on a large-scale basis by commercial and public health organizations in an attempt to eliminate feral rats. These cultures were known as "rat viruses" and were widely used in Europe, England, and the United States as "rat poisons" (153). However, the enthusiasm for their use waned when it was discovered that the spread of the organisms could not be limited; predictably, the baiting program was implicated in several epidemics among exposed human populations (153). Surprisingly, as late as the 1950s in England, *S. enteritidis* (serovar Danzy) was isolated from adults living 4 mi apart. The source of infection was traced to contaminated cakes from a local bakery. Mice which had acquired the infection from living serovar Danzy cultures in rodenticide baits had infected food in the bakery (19).

On a global scale, there has been a dramatic increase in the number of feral cats. During the last decade, it has been estimated that 50 million to 60 million feral cats inhabit the United States. This tremendous number raises the question of whether they play a role in controlling the wild rat population in both rural and urban settings. Though the predatory habits of feral cats have a profound effect on reducing the number of wild birds and small rodents and reptiles, feral cats supposedly do not kill rats weighing over 200 g.

The black roof rat (*Rattus rattus*), which coexisted with humans in the crowded, unsanitary environs of the medieval era, has been largely displaced by the more aggressive, larger brown Norway rat (*Rattus norvegicus*) (30, 109, 128). This species of rat lives more distant from contemporary, better-constructed urban domiciles by taking up residence in backyards, sewers, industrial buildings, dumps, or granaries. In this environment, the rat often competes for food and territory with other wild rodents and therefore can share zoonotically transmitted diseases. Fortunately, human fleas, which accounted for widespread human-to-human transmission of plague, have almost been eliminated from cities in the United States, and thus the likelihood of epidemics initiated by rat zoonoses has been reduced. Nevertheless, zoonotic transmission of rat diseases still occurs, and as major cities suffer from overcrowding, structural decay, and inadequate waste removal, the rat population will increase and the probability of transmission of these diseases to the homeless or underprivileged will correspondingly increase.

Contrary to the image of the rat depicted by Zinsser, the laboratory rat, used extensively for decades in biomedical research, has provided immeasurable benefit to humankind's understanding of disease processes, their control, and their elimination. However, the use of rats in research and the current popularity of rats as "pocket pets" also afford the opportunity for those in contact with these rats to become infected with rat-borne diseases. The purpose of this chapter, therefore, is to highlight those zoonotic diseases of the rat, and in certain cases the same diseases in other rodents, which have clinical relevance in the United States and its territories (50).

RAT BITES

Relapsing fevers following rat bites have been noted clinically for more than 2,000 years, being first recognized in India. Early recorded descriptions of the disease are found in the Yale University medical archives of the 19th century. The Japanese were the first to use the term *Rattenbisskrankheit*, or rat-bite fever (85).

Approximately 40,000 rat bites are reported annually according to one carefully researched report (30). Several studies indicate that over two-thirds of the rat bites occur in children under 10 years of age. Adults attacked are usually debilitated or otherwise helpless. Most bites occur on the hands and feet, but bites may also be present on the head and face of infants, sometimes with disfiguring consequences. Occasionally, deaths due to rat bites have been recorded for infants or debilitated adults (109). It has been estimated in one study that 2% of rodent bites in humans become infected (101). Several bacterial pathogens have been isolated from rat bites, including *Leptospira interrogans*, *Pasteurella multocida*, and *Staphylococcus* species; however, the most commonly isolated microorganisms are *Streptobacillus moniliformis* and *Spirillum minus* (150, 151).

BACTERIAL DISEASES

Rat-Bite Fever

Rat-bite fever can be caused by either of two microorganisms, *Streptobacillus moniliformis* or *Spirillum minus*. *Streptobacillus moniliformis* causes the diseases designated streptobacillary fever, streptobacillary rat-bite fever, and streptobacillosis. Haverhill fever and epidemic arthritic erythema are diseases associated with ingestion of water, food, or raw milk contaminated with *Streptobacillus moniliformis*. Sodoku, derived from Japanese (rat [so] and poison [doku]), spirillosis, and spirillary rat-bite fever are caused by *Spirillum minus*. The bite of an infected rat is the usual source of infection. In some cases, other animal bites, including those of mice, gerbils, squirrels, weasels, ferrets, dogs, and cats, or rare traumatic injuries unassociated with animal contact cause the infection. Exposure to cats and dogs that prey on wild rodents may also be the source of the organisms.

These organisms are present in the oral cavity and upper respiratory passages of asymptomatic rodents, usually rats (155). In one study, *Streptobacillus moniliformis* was isolated as the predominant microorganism from the upper trachea of laboratory rats (103). Other small surveys indicate isolation of the organism in 0 of 15, 7 of 10, 2 of 20, and 7 of 14 laboratory rats and in 4 of 6 wild rats (56). Presumably the incidence of *Streptobacillus moniliformis* is now lower in high-quality, commercially reared specific-pathogen-free (SPF) rats. Surveys of wild rats indicate 0 to 25% rates of infection with *Spirillum minus* (72). *Spirillum minus* does not grow in vitro and requires inoculation of culture specimens into laboratory animals, with subsequent identification of the bacteria by dark-field microscopy. *Streptobacillus moniliformis* grows slowly on artificial media, but only in the presence of 15% blood and serum, usually 10 to 20% rabbit or horse serum incubated at reduced partial pressures of oxygen (46). Sodium polyanethol sulfonate, sometimes found in blood-based media because of its properties as a bacterial growth promoter, should not be used due to its inhibitory effects on *Streptobacillus moniliformis*. Growth on agar consists of 1- to 2-mm gray, glistening colonies. The API ZYM diagnostic system can be used for rapid biochemical analysis and diagnosis. In a recent survey of 45 *S. moniliformis* isolates, 91% were from humans; the most frequent source was blood (78%), followed by aspirates (12%) and wounds (10%) (59a).

Rat-bite fever is not a reportable disease, which makes its prevalence, geographic location, racial data, and source of infection in humans difficult to assess. The disease, though uncommon in humans, has nonetheless appeared among researchers or students working with laboratory rodents, particularly rats (6). Historically, wild-rat bites and subsequent illness (usually in small children) relate to poor sanitation and overcrowding (72). One survey of rat bites in Baltimore, Md., tabulated rat-bite fever in 11 of 87 cases (18). The disease can also occur in individuals who have no history of rat bites but reside or work in rat-infested areas. Acute febrile diseases, especially if associated with animal bites, are routinely treated with penicillin or other antibiotics. Therefore, accurate data regarding prevalence are usually not provided.

Streptobacillus moniliformis incubation varies from a few hours to 2 to 10 days, whereas *Spirillum minus* incubation ranges from 1 to 6 weeks (Table 1). Fever is present in either form. Inflammation associated with the bite and lymphadenopathy are frequently accompanied by headache, general malaise, myalgia, and chills (7, 29, 57, 94). The discrete macular rash that often appears on the extremities may generalize into pustular or petechial sequelae. Arthritis occurs in 50% of all cases of *Streptobacillus moniliformis* infection but is less common in *Spirillum minus* infection. *Streptobacillus moniliformis* may be cultured from serous to purulent effusion which is recovered from affected larger joints.

If antibiotic treatment, usually penicillin at doses of 400,000 to 600,000 U daily for 7 days, is not instituted early, complications such as pneumonia, hepatitis, pyelonephritis, enteritis, and endocarditis may develop (6, 7, 29, 57, 94, 113, 116, 123, 139). If endocarditis is present, the penicillin should be given parenterally at doses of 15×10^6 to 20×10^6 U daily for 4 to 6 weeks. Streptomycin and tetracyclines are also effective antibiotics for those individuals with penicillin associated allergies. Death has occurred in cases of *Streptobacillus moniliformis* infection involving preexisting valvular disease.

Table 1. Clinical signs of rat-bite fever[a]

Clinical features	Streptobacillary fever (*Streptobacillus moniliformis*)	Spirillosis (*Spirillum minus*)
Incubation period	2–10 days	1–6 wk
Fever	+++	+++
Chills	+++	+++
Myalgia	+++	+++
Rash	++; morbilliform, petechial	++; maculopapular
Lymphadenitis	+	++
Arthralgia, arthritis	++	+−
Indurated bite wound	−	+++
Recurrent fever/constitutional signs (untreated)	Irregular periodicity	Regular periodicity

[a]Modified from reference 85. Symbols: + indicates positive clinical signs, with increasing numbers of plus signs indicating increasing severity; − indicates that clinical signs are not present.

Plague

"The houses were filled with dead bodies and the streets with funerals; neither age or sex was exempt; slaves and plebians were suddenly taken off amidst the lamentations of their wives and children, who, while they assisted the sick and mourned the dead, were seized with disease and, perishing, were burned on the same funeral pyre. To the knights and senators, the disease was less mortal though these also suffered in the common calamity" (63). This graphic account of the dreaded disease the bubonic plague was recorded in imperial Rome in the second century A.D. This pestilence occurred again and again during the ensuing centuries. By the 14th century, the disease appeared in the Far East, spread to Asia Minor, and followed trade routes to Europe. It did not make its arrival in the United States until the early 1900s, when the disease appeared in California, where it still exists endemically in ground squirrels and chipmunks.

Human infections due to *Y. pestis*, a gram-negative coccobacillus, in the United States are sporadic and limited, usually resulting from contact with infected fleas or rodents. Since 1924 and 1925, when a plague epidemic ravaged Los Angeles, Calif., neither urban plague nor rat-borne plague has been diagnosed in the United States (32). All reported cases since then have occurred in states located west of the 101st meridian.

Although wild rat populations still serve as the primary reservoir of plague, with transmission of *Y. pestis* to humans via fleas (particularly *X. cheopis*) in many parts of the world, and remain a continued threat in the United States, sciurid rodents (rock squirrels, California ground squirrels, chipmunks, and prairie dogs) are the primary plague reservoirs in the western part of the United States (77, 91, 122). Cricetid rodents, such as the wood rat, are occasionally cited as reservoir hosts. The oriental rat flea, *X. cheopis*, the common vector of plague, is well established throughout the United States, particularly in the southern states and southern California. It is important to remember that more than 1,500 species of fleas and 230 species of rodents are infected with *Y. pestis*. Only 30 to 40 rodent species, however, are permanent reservoirs of the infection (90). Plague is infrequently reported in the United States, with annual incidences in recent decades ranging between a low of 1 case in 1972 and a high of 40 cases in 1983 (32). Ninety percent of the cases have been diagnosed in New Mexico, Colorado, and California. Urban development (particularly in New Mexico) encroached into rodent habitats where plague was enzootic, placing the human populations at increased risk of contracting the disease. In addition to rodent epidemics, dogs and, increasingly, cats either have served as passive transporters of the disease or have been actively infected (90, 119, 122). From 1977 to 1991, the Centers for Disease Control confirmed 16 human plague cases (50% mortality) acquired through inhalation of *Y. pestis*-infected droplets expelled from cats with secondary plague pneumonia (90). The disease occurs seasonally, with the highest proportion of cases occurring from May through September.

Transmission of *Y. pestis* via the flea to the human involves a complex interaction of the bacterium with the flea. Fleas become infected with *Y. pestis* after engorging blood from a bacteremic animal or human. Some fleas clear the bacteria even though they have ingested large numbers of yersiniae. However, *Y. pestis* most often replicates to large numbers in the midgut of the flea, which is normally sterile (105). Interestingly, the organisms do not invade cells or tissues of the flea, but after 72 h they aggregate into clumps in the midgut or attach to the proventriculus of the flea. The proventriculus, a valve-like chamber between the flea's esophagus and midgut, is lined with spinelike structures which mechanically disrupt cells, allowing the blood to enter the midgut. After a week the yersiniae grow to large numbers and block the proventriculus. Once the proventriculus is blocked, the flea cannot ingest further blood into the midgut and starves to death (105). In an attempt to feed more often because of the blockage, the flea draws hosts blood into its esophagus, where the blood mixes with yersiniae growing in this location and proventriculus. The blood, now infected with yersiniae, flows back into the wound inflicted by the flea and the mammal becomes infected with *Y. pestis*. Experiments have shown that only blocked fleas can transmit *Y. pestis* to susceptible hosts. Interestingly, *Y. pestis* has evolved bacterial factors that allow it to invade the host by downregulating immune responses (e.g., the Yops and the LerV effector proteins) as well as growth factors that allow Yersinia to colonize and replicate in the flea. The hemin storage protein (Hms) is required by Yersinia for colonization and blockage of the proventriculus by *Y. pestis* (66). A second virulence factor is *Yersinia* murine toxin (Ymt), so named because it is lethal when injected into mice. Its presence is essential to the survival of *Y. pestis* in fleas. Apparently Ymt acts from the intracellular level in *Y. pestis* and protects the bacterium from antibacterial activity normally present in the midgut of fleas (67). Clearly, these examples among many illustrate how the organism has evolved a genetic repertoire that has allowed it to survive not only in the mammalian host but also in the flea.

Human infection is usually the result of a bite from an infected flea but can also occur via cuts or abrasions in the skin or via infected aerosols coming in contact with the oropharyngeal mucous membrane. Although today the association between plague and rats seems obvious, not until the bacillus *Y. pestis* was isolated and cultured could this association be definitively proven. After the discovery of the infectious nature of the disease, it was soon established that epidemics among human populations closely coincided with epizootics of the disease in rats, particularly *R. rattus*. It still was not apparent how the two diseases in the two hosts were linked. The hypothesis, first conceived by P. L. Simond of Spain, that the plague bacillus was transmitted by the rat flea was first discounted but later was proven to be correct (63).

Bubonic plague in humans is usually characterized by fever (2 to 7 days postexposure) and buboes (large, tender, swollen lymph nodes). If untreated, the disease may progress to severe pneumonic or systemic plague. Inhaled infective particles, particularly from animals with plague pneumonia, may also result in the pneumonic form of the disease.

Primary pneumonic plague historically occurred by inhalation of infectious droplets from a pneumonic plague patient. However, in the last several decades this form of the disease has occurred from exposure to infected animals (usually cats) which have developed secondary pneumonia due to septicemic spread of the organism (32, 90, 119, 122). Owners or veterinarians attending these sick animals are then infected by inhaling infected aerosols generated by the plague bacteria.

A presumptive diagnosis can be made by visualizing bipolar-staining, ovoid, gram-negative rods on microscopic examination of fluid from buboes, blood, sputum, or spinal fluid; confirmation can be made by culture. Complement fixation, passive hemagglutination, and immunofluorescence staining of specimens can be used for serologic confirmation.

Mortality without antibiotic therapy, particularly in cases of pneumonic plague, exceeds 50%. Although *Y. pestis* is susceptible to a wide variety of antibiotics, multiple-antibiotic-resistant strains are being isolated with increasing frequency (36). Aminoglycosides such as streptomycin and gentamicin are the most effective antibiotics in vivo against *Y. pestis*. Chloramphenicol is the drug of choice for treating plague meningitis and endophthalmitis (32, 98). For individuals exposed to *Y. pestis*, prophylactic therapy with tetracycline for a 7-day period is often prescribed.

An inactivated plague vaccine is available for laboratory personnel working with the organism and for high-risk individuals (e.g., wildlife management employees, Peace Corps volunteers) exposed to plague reservoirs in areas of endemicity.

Rodent and flea control, particularly in areas of high endemicity, is an indispensable part of containing exposure to plague, as is restricting certain locales for recreational use.

Yersiniosis

Yersinia enterocolitica is now recognized as a cause of enteritis in humans. Cultural identification of the organism takes advantage of the fact that the bacterium replicates in culture media at refrigeration temperatures, which allows selective growth conditions to be utilized. Pigs and dogs are considered natural reservoirs for *Y. enterocolitica* serovar 3. Biovar 4 is a common cause of the disease in humans. This strain has also been isolated from *R. norvegicus* and *R. rattus* in Japan (76). It has been suggested that rats may play a role in the ecology of *Y. enterocolitica* in swine herds. Control of wild rat populations in swine farms may reduce the potential transmission of this organism by pork products. More recently, another pathogenic strain, serovar O8, was isolated from wild rodents: wood mice, geisha mice, and a vole (74). This strain, however, was not evident in random samples of brown or black rats taken from selected locales in Japan (74). Further epidemiological studies are needed in the United States to determine the importance of wild rats as reservoirs for *Y. enterocolitica*.

Leptospirosis

Leptospirosis is solely a zoonotic disease of livestock, pet and stray dogs, and wildlife, including wild rats. Reservoir hosts of leptospirosis, in addition to rats, include mice, field moles, hedgehogs, gerbils, squirrels, rabbits, and hamsters (53, 144). Human-to-human transmission is extremely rare. *Leptospira interrogans* (comprising >200 serovars) has been isolated worldwide. Although particular serotypes usually have distinct host species, most serotypes can be carried by several hosts. *Leptospira* is well adapted to a variety of mammals, particularly wild animals and rodents.

In the chronic form, the organism is carried and shed in the urine inconspicuously for long periods. Rodents are the only major group of animals that can shed leptospires throughout their life span without clinical manifestations (53, 144). Active shedding of leptospires by rodents can go unrecognized until personnel handling the animals become clinically infected or are infected by exposure to water or food contaminated by urine.

Leptospira interrogans serotype Icterohaemorrhagiae was first recovered in 1918 in the United States from wild rats sampled in New York, N.Y. In one study in Detroit, Mich., more than 90% of adult brown Norway rats were infected with serovar Icterohaemorrhagiae (141). In an earlier study conducted in Baltimore, 45.5% of 1,643 rats were infected with *Leptospira*; higher prevalence rates were found for older rats (~60%) (84). Other studies confirm the high prevalence of this organism in wild rats inhabiting cities in the United States (3, 124). Rats and mice are also common animal hosts for another serotype, *L. interrogans* serotype Ballum, although it has been found in other wildlife as well. Water can often be contaminated with infected rat urine. The infection can persist unnoticed in laboratory rodents; the carrier rates for laboratory-maintained rodents in the United States are unknown but are probably low (56). However, there was a report of leptospirosis in a research colony of mice in the United States that was housed in a large research institution (3).

Because leptospirosis in humans is often difficult to diagnose, the low incidence of reported infection in humans may be misleading. From 1974 to 1979 only 498 cases were reported, for an incidence of 0.05 per 100,000 people per year (124). Outbreaks in personnel working with laboratory mice have been documented in the United States (8, 133). In one study, 8 of 58 employees handling infected laboratory mice (80% of breeding females were excreting serotype Ballum in their urine) contracted leptospirosis (133). In several European laboratories, personnel have been infected with leptospires from laboratory rats (56).

Infection with *Leptospira* most frequently results from handling infected animals (contaminating the hands with urine) or from aerosol exposure during cage cleaning (8, 54, 133). Skin abrasions or mucous membranes may serve as the portal of entry. All secretions and excretions from infected animals should be considered infective. In one instance, a man apparently was infected after his daughter used his toothbrush to clean a contaminated pet mouse cage (14). Handling infected wild rats also increases the risk of contracting leptospires (88). A young man died of acute leptospirosis acquired by falling into a heavily polluted river contaminated with serotype Icterohaemorrhagiae (124). Rodent bites can also transmit the disease (87). In the Detroit area, children from the inner city had a significantly higher level of serotype Icterohaemorrhagiae antibody than children living in the suburbs. Therefore, children living in rat-infested tenements may be at increased risk of infection (35).

The disease may vary from inapparent infection to severe infection and death. Infected individuals experience a biphasic disease (42, 124, 133). They become suddenly ill with weakness, headache, myalgia, malaise, chills, and fever and usually exhibit leukocytosis. During the second phase of the disease, conjunctival suffusion and a rash may occur. Upon examination of the patient, renal, hepatic, pulmonary, and gastrointestinal findings may be abnormal. Penicillin is the drug of choice in treating early onset of leptospirosis infection (42, 138). Ampicillin and doxycycline also have been effective in treating people with leptospirosis. Tetracycline has been used successfully to eradicate serotype Ballum in a mouse colony (132).

Because of the variability in clinical symptoms and lack of pathognomonic pathological findings in humans and animals, serologic diagnosis or actual isolation of leptospires is imperative (42). As an aid to diagnosis, leptospires can sometimes be observed by examination or direct staining of body fluids or fresh tissue suspensions (137). The definitive diagnosis in humans or animals is made by culturing the organisms from tissue or fluid samples or by animal inoculation (particularly in 3- to 4-week-old hamsters) and subsequent culture and isolation. Culture media with long-chain fatty acids with 1% bovine serum albumin are routinely used as a detoxicant (42). Serologic assessment is accomplished by indirect hemagglutination, agglutination analysis, complement fixation, microscopic agglutination, and fluorescent-antibody techniques (42). The serologic test most frequently used is the modified microtiter agglutination test. Titers of 1:100 or greater are considered significant.

Borrelia Species (Tick-Borne Relapsing Fever)

Tick-borne relapsing fever occurs primarily in foci in the western part of the United States but also occurs in other parts of the world. The disease is caused by at least 15 *Borrelia* species and is transmitted to humans from a variety of rodents (chipmunks, squirrels, rats, mice, and prairie dogs) and hedgehogs via soft ticks of the genus *Ornithodoros*. The rat has also been used experimentally to study the pathogenesis of the disease (137).

Salmonellosis

The genus *Salmonella* consists of gram-negative bacteria with approximately 2,000 serotypes. Nontyphoidal salmonellosis is caused by any of these serotypes.

Other than *Salmonella typhi*, the causative agent of typhoid fever, salmonellosis occurs worldwide and is important in humans and animals. Although there is some debate about the taxonomy of the genus *Salmonella*, according to one view *S. typhi* and *Salmonella choleraesuis* have only one serotype each, whereas the remaining 2,000 serotypes are within the species *S. enterica*. References to the *S. enterica* serotypes are abbreviated such that "enterica" is dropped, e.g., *Salmonella enterica* serotype Typhimurium is called *Salmonella typhimurium*. *S. typhimurium* is the serotype most commonly associated with disease in both animals and humans. Other serotypes most commonly reported from humans and animals are *Salmonella heidelberg*, *Salmonella agona*, *Salmonella montevideo*, and *Salmonella newport*. Salmonellae are pathogenic to a variety of animals.

Rats are extremely susceptible to infection with *Salmonella* spp. In studies performed in the 1920s through 1940s, the prevalence of *Salmonella* in wild rats surveyed in the United States varied from 1 to 18%, compared to 19% in wild rats in Europe (3, 9, 56, 153). In experimental studies, when rats were dosed orally with *Salmonella*, 10% shed the organism in the two months after inoculation, and a few were found to remain carriers when examined 5 months after experimental challenge. These rats, when placed with other naive rats, were capable of initiating new epizootics (110). Fortunately, the disease in laboratory rats, though common before 1939, has been found to occur rarely in U.S. commercially reared rats since that time. However, because rats are used experimentally to study *Salmonella* pathogenesis, personnel working with these animals must take appropriate precautions to prevent zoonotic transmission.

Salmonellae are ubiquitous in nature and are routinely found in water or food contaminated with animal or human excreta. Fecal-oral transmission is the primary mode for spread of infection from animal to animal or to human. Rat feces can remain infective for 148 days when maintained at room temperature (154). Transmission is enhanced by crowding and poor sanitation.

As with other diseases transmitted by the fecal-oral route, control depends on eliminating contact with contaminated feces, food, or water or animal reservoirs excreting the organism. *Salmonella* survives for months in feces and is readily cultured from sediments in ponds and streams previously contaminated with sewage or animal feces. Fat and moisture in food promote survival of *Salmonella*. Pasteurization of milk and proper cooking of food (56°C for 10 to 20 min) effectively destroy *Salmonella*. Municipal water supplies should be routinely monitored for coliform contamination (104).

Clinical signs of salmonellosis in humans include acute sudden gastroenteritis, abdominal pain, diarrhea, nausea, and fever. Diarrhea and anorexia may persist for several days. Organisms invading the intestine may create septicemia without severe intestinal involvement; most clinical signs are attributed to hematogenous spread of the organisms. As with other microbial infections, the disease's severity relates to the organism's serotype, the number of bacteria ingested, and the host's susceptibility. In experimental studies with volunteers, several serovars induced a spectrum of clinical disease from brief enteritis to serious debilitation. Incubation varied from 7 to 72 h. Cases of asymptomatic carriage, persisting for several weeks were common (72).

Salmonellae are flagellated, nonsporulating, aerobic gram-negative bacilli that can be readily isolated from feces on selective media designed to suppress bacterial growth of other enteric bacteria. *Salmonella* serotyping requires antigenic analysis (28).

Salmonella gastroenteritis is usually mild and self-limiting. With careful management of fluid and electrolyte balance, antimicrobial therapy is not necessary. In humans, antimicrobial therapy may prolong rather than shorten the period during which *Salmonella* is shed in the feces (99, 104). In one double-blind placebo study of infants, oral antibiotics did not significantly affect the duration of *Salmonella* carriage. Bacteriological relapse after antibiotic treatment occurred in 53% of the patients, and 33% of these suffered a recurrence of diarrhea, whereas none of the placebo group relapsed (99).

Other Possible Bacterial Infections

Campylobacteriosis, a common diarrheal disease in humans caused by *Campylobacter jejuni* and *Campylobacter coli*, affects a variety of animals, including rats. Animals can be responsible for zoonotic spread of this organism; however, to date, rats have not been incriminated (48, 160).

Helicobacter cinaedi (formerly *Campylobacter cinaedi*) is a fastidious microaerophile which was first isolated from the lower bowel of homosexuals with proctitis and colitis. It has also been isolated from the blood of homosexual patients with human immunodeficiency virus as well as from children and adult women (27, 100, 102, 111, 112, 148). In a recent retrospective study of 23 patients with *H. cinaedi*-associated illness, 22 of the patients had the organism isolated from blood by using an automated blood culture system in which a slightly elevated growth index was noted (79). This study also described a new *H. cinaedi*-associated syndrome consisting of bacteremia and fever accompanied by leukocytosis and thrombocytopenia. Recurrent cellulitis and/or arthritis is also noted in a high percentage of infected immunocompromised patients (20, 79). Although *H. cinaedi* is primarily recovered from immunocompromised individuals, the organism is also recovered from chronic alcoholics as well as immunocompetent men and women. It should be stressed that many hospital and veterinary laboratories have difficulty isolating this organism. Because of the slow growth of *H. cinaedi*, laboratory diagnosis is unlikely if blood culture procedures that rely on visual detection in culture media are used (20, 78, 79). Dark-field microscopy or use of acridine orange staining of blood culture media, rather than Gram staining, increases the likelihood of seeing the organism. Likewise, fecal isolation is difficult; selective antibiotic media are required, and recovery is facilitated by passing fecal homogenates through a 0.45-μm-pore-size filter (55). Also, in a recent study, several strains of both *H. cinaedi* and *Helicobacter fennelliae* were inhibited by concentrations of cephalothin and cefazolin used frequently in selective media for isolation of enteric microaerophilic bacteria. These organisms also require an environment rich in hydrogen for optimum in vitro growth.

H. cinaedi has also been recovered from blood and fecal specimens from children and a neonate with septicemia and meningitis. The mother of the neonate had cared for pet hamsters during the first two trimesters of her pregnancy (102). Because *H. cinaedi* has been isolated from normal intestinal flora of hamsters, it was suggested that the pet hamsters served as a reservoir for transmission to the mother (55). The mother had a diarrheal illness during the third trimester of pregnancy; the newborn was likely to have been infected during the birthing process, although this was not proven (102). Further studies are needed to confirm the zoonotic risk of handling *H. cinaedi*-infected hamsters (55). Also of interest is the isolation, based on cellular fatty acid identification analysis, of *H. cinaedi* from the feces of dogs and a cat (78). More recently it has been isolated from a macaque monkey with idiopathic colitis and hepatitis (52) as well as from asymptomatic macaques (44a). Until diagnostic laboratories embark on routine attempts to isolate *Helicobacter* spp. from feces, the extent of their presence in companion and pocket pets and their zoonotic potential will remain unknown.

Tetracycline and various aminoglycosides appear to be effective in treating infections with *H. cinaedi*. Apparent relapses of *H. cinaedi* bacteremia in patients treated with ciprofloxacin, despite its previous use to successfully treat *H. cinaedi* infection, and the occurrence of in vitro resistance of *H. cinaedi* isolates to ciprofloxacin suggest that this antibiotic should be used with caution (45, 78, 79).

Of recent interest are the increasingly recognized enterohepatic *Helicobacter* spp. which cause both hepatic and intestinal disease in mice and rats (49). One of these, *Helicobacter bilis*, has been found in Chilean patients with chronic cholecystitis and in patients with hepatocellular carcinoma and hepatobiliary carcinoma (51, 92). Given that these bacteria persist in the lower bowel of rodents and are shed in the feces of infected animals, it will be interesting to note, after further studies are conducted, whether these new helicobacters will be linked to zoonotic transmission from wild rodents.

Of the gastric helicobacters, *Helicobacter pylori* is the best known and the most important in terms of global impact on human disease. However, two other gastric helicobacters, "*Helicobacter heilmannii*" and *Helicobacter felis*, are associated with gastric disease in humans and are worthy of discussion (62, 83).

A diagnosis of infection with "*H. heilmannii*," first observed and reported for three humans in 1987, has been made on morphological grounds by a variety of authors assessing human gastric biopsy samples (62, 65, 96, 97, 130, 135, 142). The frequency of occurrence is between 0.25 and 0.60% depending on the study. However, as many as 6% of patients in Thailand and China have been reported to be infected with "*H. heilmannii*" (157, 159). "*H. heilmannii*"-infected patients have a chronic, active gastritis or chronic gastritis consisting of a lymphoplasmacytic inflammation. "*H. heilmannii*" is located in the deep part of the gastric pit of human patients, whereas *H. pylori* colonizes more frequently the mucous layer of surface epithelia. The gastric *Helicobacter*-like organisms can also invade parietal cells in a manner similar to that of these organisms in other mammals. Stolte et al. systematically compared the histologies of "*H. heilmannii*" and *H. pylori* in a large group of patients (134). Two hundred two patients with "*H. heilmannii*" infection were compared with an equal number of *H. pylori*-infected individuals. "*H. heilmannii*"-associated gastritis was more mild than *H. pylori* gastritis (134). "*H. heilmannii*" also has been associated with primary gastric low-grade lymphoma in humans (96, 115). Similar to *H. pylori*-associated lymphoma, clinical remission of the lymphoma in five patients was noted after antibiotic eradication of the gastric helicobacter (73, 96, 118). These helicobacters can persist in humans for years, and presumably the same is true for other mammals.

Eradication of "*H. heilmannii*" by antimicrobial therapy also has resulted in the resolution of gastritis and peptic ulcer disease (59, 62, 65). "*H. heilmannii*" infections have been successfully treated with bismuth alone and with combination therapies that included metronidazole or amoxicillin (5, 62, 65).

In addition to dogs and cats as potential zoonotic hosts of these gastric helicobacters, swine and wild rats may be sources of infections for humans (58, 95).

Beta-hemolytic group G streptococci have been isolated from rats with cervical lymphadenitis, as well as from the pharynx of normal laboratory rats (31). *Streptococcus* species of group G cause a wide variety of clinical diseases in humans, including septicemia, pharyngitis, endocarditis, pneumonia, and meningitis. Asymptomatic carriage of group G streptococci also is common in humans. At present, however, there is no documented evidence that streptococci from rats are transmitted to, or acquired by, humans (121).

Pathogenic *Staphylococcus aureus* of human phage type can cause clinical disease in mice and rats. This organism has been introduced into SPF barrier-maintained mouse colonies and SPF rats and guinea pigs; the same phage type was isolated from their animal caretakers (13, 33, 129). Colonization by normal *S. aureus* strains in the nasopharyngeal area of humans presumably minimizes the zoonotic potential of animal-originated *S. aureus*.

VIRAL DISEASES

HFRS and Nephropathia Epidemica (Hantaan Virus)

Hemorrhagic fever with renal syndrome (HFRS) and nephropathia epidemica are terms used to describe a group of rodent-borne diseases caused by several hantaviruses (family *Bunyaviridae*) (82, 158). In southeast Asia the disease is endemic, whereas focal epidemics throughout the Eurasian continent and Japan have been recorded. American soldiers became infected with the disease during the Korean War. The severity of the disease depends on the particular immunotype of the virus as well as the respective natural reservoir host.

Korean hemorrhagic fever occurs seasonally in agricultural workers, with bimodal peaks in the populations of the reservoir host (the striped field mouse, *Apodemus agrarius*) and its ectoparasites. HFRS is characterized by fever, headache, myalgia, and hemorrhagic manifestations that may lead to shock from massive capillary leakage of plasma protein. Though mortality previously occurred at a significant rate, it has now been reduced to 6% with hospitalization and dialysis (145).

Nephropathia epidemica, a less severe form, is encountered in Scandinavia, the western Soviet Union, and several countries of Europe. The etiologic virus has been isolated and named Puumala virus by Finnish researchers (25a). The natural reservoir is the bank vole, *Clethrionomys glareolus*. Infected persons, usually adult men with vole contact, exhibit sudden onset of fever, abdominal or lower back pain, elevated serum creatinine levels, and polyuria; fatalities are rare.

In the late 1970s, a disease resembling HFRS was reported among laboratory workers in Japan, Belgium, and Korea. Retrospective epidemiological evaluation of the first laboratory-associated outbreak and additional urban outbreaks in Japan revealed that the reservoir of the disease was laboratory and wild rats. Over 100 cases of HFRS in humans have been linked to exposure to laboratory rats infected with the virus (146, 147). Infected persons exhibited a range of illness, from a nonspecific influenza-like episode to acute renal insufficiency and hemorrhagic diathesis. Because the worldwide distribution of infected laboratory rats or their tissues has occurred, testing of potentially contaminated colonies and transplantable rat tumor banks was undertaken. Transmission of hantavirus infection was reported in Belgium and the United Kingdom as well as Japan (37, 86). One individual in the United States had serologic evidence of infection, and in Great Britain a mild clinical case was diagnosed. Caesarian rederivation procedures employed for imported animals probably prevented or eliminated the spread of infection at most institutions.

Hantaan-related virus infection in wild rats, both *R. rattus* and *R. norvegicus*, raised concern regarding the potential spread of disease by international shipping. Sea ports throughout the world, including many in the United States, harbor rats infected with Hantaan or a related virus. To date, serologic evidence of disease in the United States has been noted, but no human clinical cases have been associated with this type of exposure (25).

Prospect Hill virus, another hantavirus, has been isolated from meadow voles (*Microtus pennsylvanicus*) in Maryland; it has not been associated with human disease, although serologic surveys indicate inapparent infection throughout the United States, with a distribution of virus limited to the geographic distribution of the animal host.

HPS

In 1993, an outbreak of acute respiratory illness with significant mortality was linked to a newly recognized hantavirus (21). This zoonotic disease, now known as hantavirus pulmonary syndrome (HPS), was discovered in the southwestern part of the United States. This disease provided the first example of what is now recognized as being caused by a complex of New World hantaviruses, each associated with a particular rodent species belonging to the subfamily Sigmondontinae, family Muridae. The prototype virus, Sin Nombre (SN) virus, which replicates in its natural host, the deer mouse (*Peromyscus maniculatus*) (131), causes more than 95% of the cases of HPS in North America, which are primarily seen in the southwestern United States (68, 125).

Three other hantaviruses distinct from SN virus are also recognized as etiologic agents of HPS in North America; their rodent reservoir hosts are the white-footed mouse, *Peromyscus leucopus*, which serves as the host for the New York hantavirus (131); the cotton rat, *Sigmodon hispidus*, the reservoir host for Black Creek Canal virus (120); and the rice rat, *Oryzomys palustris,* which is the host for the newly recognized Bayou virus (143). The last two viruses have been isolated in Florida, Louisiana, and eastern Texas.

A newly recognized hantavirus found in the pygmy rice rat (*Oligoryzomys microtis*) in Bolivia and Argentina has been linked to zoonotic HPS in humans residing in these countries (12). Serologic tests to detect antibodies to hantavirus as well as confirmatory Western immunoblotting are used to presumptively diagnose the disease in humans exposed to these various rodents (68). Reverse transcription-PCR with specific primers is used to definitely diagnose the virus in infected human or rodent biological and tissue samples (69).

Humans at risk are those who reside or work in areas heavily infested with reservoir hosts of hantaviruses. Patients with HPS often present to an emergency room with persistent and worsening dyspnea. Prodromal signs include fatigue and somnolence, with increasing shortness of breath and low-grade fever. Chest radiographs show interstitial and increasing bilateral interstitial alveolar infiltrates and pleural effusion. Patients often require 100% oxygen endotracheal intubation and positive and expiratory pressure support.

Elevation in creatine kinase and serum creatinine and proteinuria can indicate renal insufficiency and myositis associated with HPS; these later clinical manifestations are more commonly observed in HPS caused by viruses of the oryzomine and *Sigmodon* clade and much less frequently with SN virus infection (69, 125).

Hantaviruses do not cause disease in their respective rodent hosts, although virus can be detected in the salivary glands and numerous visceral organs of chronically infected animals. The virus is shed in the saliva, feces, and urine; transmission to humans is generally believed to occur via aerosols generated from contaminated rodent excreta (145). There is also the potential for transmission to occur via ectoparasites. Identification of infected rodents or infected rodent tissue prior to entry into the laboratory is crucial in preventing zoonotic disease. Enzyme-linked immunosorbent assay, indirect immunofluorescence assay, and immunoblotting are available for serodiagnosis, in addition to PCR-based assays.

Monkeypox

Human monkeypox, caused by an orthopoxvirus, was first diagnosed in the Democratic Republic of the Congo in 1970, shortly after eradication of smallpox in that country in 1968. It is now recognized as a zoonotic disease that occurs primarily in the rain forest located in west and central Africa.

Besides zoonotic transmission, limited person-to-person transmission can also occur, especially where monkeypox is endemic. The first documented evidence of community-acquired monkeypox was obtained in the United States in 2003 (22). The source of the two outbreaks was identified as a common Illinois distributor where prairie dogs and Gambian giant pouched rats were being housed together. The Gambian giant rats had been imported from Ghana in April 2003 by a Texas importer who subsequently sold them to the Illinois distributor. The diseased prairie dogs were then sold to pet stores in the region and were further disseminated at pet swaps. The shipment from Ghana contained approximately 800 small mammals of nine different species. The actual source(s) could therefore have been multiple, which highlights the serious public health hazard posed by introduction of exotic species such as rodents from Africa. Because of this hazard and pursuant to 42 CFR 70.2 and 21 CFR 1240.30, the Centers for Disease Control and Prevention and the Food and Drug Administration have prohibited their transportation or importation into the United States.

Although clinically similar in some ways to smallpox, monkeypox differs from smallpox both biologically and epidemiologically (16). The disease has an incubation period of 7 to 17 days. The prodrome consists of a fever, backache, fatigue, and headache (114). In the large U.S. outbreak with 72 confirmed or suspected cases as of 30 July 2003, patients had a prodrome consisting of headaches, myalgias, chills, and drenching sweats. Over one-third of the patients had nonproductive coughs. The monkeypox rash occurring on the head, trunk, or extremities includes papules, vesicles, macules, and pustules that become encrusted over a 14- to 21-day period (75, 114). The major clinical difference between monkeypox and smallpox is the pronounced lymphadenopathy noted in the majority of patients infected with monkeypox (75) (Fig. 1). Mortality rates in areas where monkeypox is endemic vary from 1 to 10%, with higher death rates among children. The outbreak in the United States which occurred in Illinois, Indiana, and Wisconsin (median age, 26 years [range, 4 to 53 years]) affected over 50 humans, 14 of whom required hospitalization.

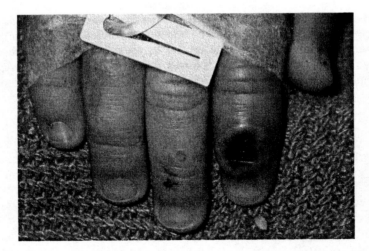

Figure 1. Infected finger of a child with monkeypox (Marshfield, Wis., index case). The patient was bitten by a prairie dog on 27 May 2003; the primary inoculation site was the right index finger. The photo was taken 14 days after the prairie dog bites (11 days after the onset of febrile illness, hospital day 5). Courtesy of Kurt Reed, Marshfield Clinic, Marshfield, Wis.

Infected monkeypox patients or those suspected of having the disease should follow standard contact and airborne transmission precautions. Appropriate diagnosis and management of exposed and ill pets should also be instituted to minimize spread of the disease. Pet owners who suspect their animal of having a disease compatible with monkeypox should isolate the animal from humans and other animals and contact their state and local health department. They are also advised to wear a mask and gloves when handling the animal. In most instances, it is advisable for a veterinarian to examine the suspect animal. Illness noted in affected rodents includes fever, cough, blepharoconjunctivitis, and lymphadenopathy, followed by a nodular rash. Mortality is variable. If animals are suspected to be infected with monkeypox virus, whole blood in EDTA or sera can be collected and refrigerated at 4°C before being shipped to a laboratory. If ill animals are euthanized, necropsy of these animals should be performed only in biosafety level 3 laboratories by personnel recently immunized with smallpox vaccine. Entire carcasses can be preserved for later viral isolation by freezing at −70°C. Diagnosis of the disease in infected humans or animals is made by viral isolation in tissue culture, electron microscopic observation of the poxvirus in infected tissues, and PCR-based assays. Sera also can be evaluated for antibodies to the virus.

Treatment for the disease consists of supportive therapy if needed. No specific treatment has been recommended. In areas of endemicity, smallpox vaccine has been reported to reduce the risk of monkeypox among those individuals previously vaccinated. It is not known whether postexposure use of smallpox vaccine or antiviral therapy would be beneficial in treating monkeypox infection in humans.

Rabies

Rabies virus, a rhabdovirus, has been recognized as a clinical disease for centuries in both Europe and Asia. When the virus is inoculated into animals (usually via a bite), it almost always produces a fatal disease in all warm-blooded species; rats should therefore be listed as a susceptible host.

Rabies occurs on all continents except Australia. Some islands, such as the Hawaiian Islands, New Zealand, and Great Britain, are also fortunate in not having rabies in their domestic or wild animal population. Rabies occurs infrequently in humans, but its presence in natural reservoirs, such as wild carnivores, bats, and, rarely, certain rodents such as squirrels, is endemic in certain parts of the United States as well as other parts of the world. Rabies in skunks, raccoons, and bats has increased markedly in the last several decades and now accounts for more than 85% of all reported cases in the United States (93). From 1971 through 1989, woodchucks accounted for 68% of the 200 rodent cases reported in the United States (93). Other rodents, including rats, are almost never infected with rabies, and no human cases of rabies of rodent origin have been reported in the last 50 years. However, in the Federal Republic of Germany, from 1961 to 1967, nine Norway rats and eight muskrats were reportedly infected with rabies and had supposedly bitten humans (56).

RICKETTSIAL DISEASES

Murine Typhus (Endemic Typhus)

Murine typhus is caused by *Rickettsia typhi*. Although this disease has been recognized for centuries, it was not distinguished from epidemic typhus until the 1920s. The absence of louse infestation in humans, its seasonal occurrence, and its sporadic nature help differentiate murine typhus from louse-borne typhus (i.e., epidemic typhus). Epidemic typhus is seen in the eastern United States only in association with flying squirrels (41).

Murine typhus is primarily a disease of rats, with its principal vectors being the oriental rat flea, *X. cheopis*, and another flea, *Nasopsyllus fasciatus*. These fleas also naturally colonize the house mouse, *Mus musculus*. The cat flea, *Ctenocephalides felis* (as well as seven other species of fleas), has also been implicated in the spread of the disease. Rickettsiae are ingested by fleas via a blood meal; they multiply in the gut and are subsequently passed out in the dejecta of the flea. Infection in rats and humans is the result of contamination of the puncture wound by flea feces (43). Recent experimental evidence indicates that a flea bite also can directly transmit the infection (43). *R. typhi* is resistant to drying and remains infectious for up to 100 days in rat feces.

Murine typhus is distributed worldwide, and in the United States, it is usually diagnosed in southeastern states, including those on the Gulf of Mexico, as well as areas along the northern portion of the Mississippi River (17). It also is associated with human populations subjected to areas of high-density wild rat colonies, such as ports, granaries, farms, or rat-infested inner-city buildings. Laboratory personnel have been infected with this agent when inoculating rodents and handling infected animals (17).

Since the 1970s there has been a shift in the distribution of human cases of murine typhus to a more rural locale in southern California and central and southern Texas (2). In southern California, Orange County was considered an unusual locale for murine typhus because it is a wealthy suburb where rat infestation was uncommon. Epidemiological studies indicated that opossums had a high rate of seropositivity for murine typhus and the cat fleas infesting the opossums were infected with either *R. typhi* or a newly recognized rickettsia first called the ELB agent and later named *Rickettsia felis* (1, 156). Findings extended to a survey of fleas on dogs, cats, and opossums in California, Texas, and Georgia also confirmed that fleas were infected with *R. typhi* or *R. felis*, helping explain the spread of murine typhus into rural areas of the United States. Also, human cases of typhus caused by *R. felis* as determined by PCR have been recorded (126). Exact taxonomic specification of *R. felis* has not been possible because no isolates have been obtained for detailed comparative analysis.

After infection with the rickettsia, the incubation period is 7 to 14 days. Because murine typhus is difficult to differentiate either clinically or anatomically from other rickettsial diseases, specific serologic tests are extremely important in making the correct diagnosis (43). The acute febrile disease is usually characterized by general malaise, headache, rash, and chills, with signs ranging from mild to severe. An encephalitic syndrome can also occur (98). In one report, 25% of 180 patients with the disease were described as having delirium, stupor, or coma (136). Fortunately, these findings resolve with lowering of the febrile response. The fatality rate for all ages is about 2% but increases with age. In a recent study of 22 patients residing in the Canary Islands, murine typhus was diagnosed based on a titer of immunoglobulin M antibody against *R. typhi* of ≥1:40, or at least a fourfold increase in immunoglobulin G titers against *R. typhi* by direct immunofluorescence within 8 weeks after symptoms appeared (63a). These patients had, in addition to fevers of intermediate duration, a distinct clinical presentation characterized by a higher incidence of complications, especially renal damage (including acute kidney failure and abnormal urinalysis). Interestingly, all had contact with animals, most frequently dogs (63a).

Recovery of rickettsial organisms or antigens from biological specimens is inconsistent and is not routinely done except in labs equipped to process and identify these samples. It must be remembered that rickettsiae are hazardous and have accounted for numerous infections of laboratory personnel. Currently, serologic diagnosis is accomplished by enzyme-linked immunosorbent assay and radioimmunoassay; however, the indirect immunofluorescence assay technique remains the most commonly used. Unfortunately, this test cannot distinguish epidemic from endemic typhus. The Centers for Disease Control and Prevention considers a fourfold rise in titer detected by any technique (except Weil-Felix) as evidence of rickettsial infection. A complement fixation titer of 1:16 or higher in a single serum sample from a patient with clinically compatible signs is also considered diagnostic (93).

Proper antibiotic therapy is the most effective measure to prevent morbidity or mortality due to rickettsial infections. Tetracycline and chloramphenicol have proven to be effective in hastening recovery and preventing neurological sequelae, such as deafness due to involvement of cranial nerve VIII (98).

Fleas can be controlled by applying insecticides (organochlorines, as well as others) as residual powders or sprays in areas where rats nest or traverse. It is imperative that insecticides be applied prior to using rodenticides; this will prevent fleas from leaving the dead rodents and feeding on human hosts (10).

Rickettsialpox

A variety of rodents are infected with other rickettsial diseases. *M. musculus* is the natural host for the causative agent of rickettsialpox, *Rickettsia akari*, a member of the spotted fever group of rickettsiae (11, 17). This organism is also isolated from *R. rattus* and *R. norvegicus*, and the rat under certain circumstances may transmit the disease to humans. The disease is transmitted by the mite *Liponyssoides* (*Allodermanyssus*) *sanguineus*. The disease is diagnosed in New York City and other eastern cities, as well as Russia, Egypt, and South Africa (11). The incubation period is approximately 10 to 24 days, and the clinical disease is similar to that noted in murine typhus. The rash of rickettsialpox commences as a discrete maculopapular rash, which then becomes vesicular. The palms and soles are usually not involved. About 90% of affected persons develop an eschar, with a shallow ulcer covered by a brown scab (11, 43). Although headaches are common and may be accompanied by stiff necks, lumbar cerebrospinal fluid (CSF) samples are normal. Pulmonary and gastrointestinal involvement also is almost never encountered. Diagnosis, treatment, and control are similar to those described for murine typhus and *Y. pestis* infection.

MYCOSES

Dermatophytes

In almost all rat- and mouse-associated ringworm infections in humans, *Trichophyton mentagrophytes* has been isolated as the etiologic agent (Table 2) (4, 15, 23, 34, 38, 136). Classical murine ringworm, reportedly caused by *Trichophyton quinckeanum*, is usually restricted to feral rodents, but successful crossing of cultures of this strain with tester strains of perfect-state *T. mentagrophytes* (*Arthroderma benhamiae*) proves that *T. quinckeanum* is not a distinct species and is indistinguishable from *T. mentagrophytes* (108).

Dermatophytes are distributed worldwide, with some species reportedly more common in certain geographic locations. From a study of 1,288 animals from 15 different species of small mammals in their natural habitats, 57 *T. mentagrophytes* strains were isolated most commonly from the bank vole (*C. glareolus*), followed by the common shrew (*Sorex araneus*) and house mouse (*M. musculus*) (26). Agricultural workers exposed to these mammals in granaries and barns risked contracting *T. mentagrophytes* infections; indeed, 77% of 137 agricultural workers were infected with ringworm. Only 23% of the workers showed signs of infection (26).

Table 2. *T. mentagrophytes* infection associated with laboratory mice or rats or pet mice

Probable source of infection	No. of persons infected	Lesions appearing on infected mice or rats	Reference
Pet white mice, inbred albino laboratory mice (VSBS, A2G)	7 children, 2 lab technicians	2 of 104; diffuse alopecia	89
Laboratory mice	6 lab technicians		4
Laboratory mice	2 lab technicians	0 of 96 (222 cultured); survey of commercial stock	38
BALB/c C3H/BI mice	6 lab technicians	<1% of all mice; carrier rate, 90%	34
White mice	1 lab worker	% not determined, alopecia, increased scaling on head and back; 10 mice	15
White mice	1 bacteriologist	40 of 600; crusted or crustless plaques, circular with prominent periphery; general alopecia; mortality in some mice	23
Wistar rats	1 technician	20% of colony with alopecia and scaly skin	38
Rats	1 technician	Alopecia with crusting and erythema	108

In laboratory mice and rats, ringworm infection is often asymptomatic, going unrecognized until laboratory personnel become infected (Table 2) (38). In one study, for the 8-month period before dermatophyte-infected mice were treated, almost half the people handling the mice developed ringworm, although less than 1% of the mice showed any signs of disease (34).

Transmission occurs via direct or indirect contact with asymptomatic carrier animals, skin lesions of infected rodents, contaminated grain, or animal bedding. Causal fungi present in air or dust or on surfaces of animal holding rooms are also transmittal sources (136).

Ringworm is considered a nonfatal, usually self-limiting infection, and, because it is sometimes asymptomatic, it is often ignored by the affected person. The dermatophytes cause scaling, erythema, and occasionally vesicles and fissures; the fungi cause thickening and discoloration of the nails. On the skin of the trunk and extremities, lesions may be circular with a central clearing. The location of the fungus signifies the clinical category, for example, tinea capitis or tinea unguium. When humans are infected by one of the dermatophytes recovered from mice, the fungus appears on the body and/or extremities, most commonly on the arms and hands.

Zoophilic *T. mentagrophytes* produces an acute inflammatory response which often undergoes rapid resolution; the infection may produce furunculosis, widespread tinea corporis, and deep involvement of the hair follicles.

Topical fungicides or griseofulvin per os is effective in eradicating dermatophytes from animals and humans. Strict environmental and personal hygiene helps lower the incidence of ringworm. Personnel should wear rubber gloves when touching infected rodents.

HELMINTH DISEASES

Roundworms

Angiostrongylus (Parastrongylus) cantonensis (Rat Lungworm)

A clinical syndrome known as eosinophilic meningitis is caused in humans by accidental ingestion of raw aquatic animals, e.g., prawns (transport hosts) and snails or slugs (intermediate hosts), harboring infective larvae of the lungworm or by eating larvae which have contaminated vegetables. In humans, the infective larvae migrate to the central nervous system (CNS) and may undergo one or two molts, but they do not develop into adult worms; thus, the human is a dead-end host. The rat serves as the reservoir host where the adult worms develop and pass infective eggs in their feces, which are then ingested by the intermediate host. Spread of the organism to rats has been linked to dispersal of the African land snail (*Achatina fulica*) (10, 81).

Historically, this disease was restricted to the Far East and the Pacific Rim, including Hawaii and Tahiti. More recently, the disease has been reported in Cuba and the lungworm has been recovered from rats in Puerto Rico and New Orleans, La. (10, 81). It is therefore likely that the disease will be more commonly diagnosed in the Americas in the future.

The disease may often be subclinical or have an indistinct 2- to 4-month prepatent period. The distinguishing clinical feature of the disease is the presence of elevated eosinophils (>10%) of the leukocytes found in abnormal CSF. Other CNS signs can also be present, such as severe headache, meningeal irritation (nuchal rigidity), and increased intracranial pressure. Visual impairment may occur if there is ocular involvement. A febrile response is usually mild to absent. Only the most severe infections result in permanent impairment or, in some cases, death (80).

Occasionally (in <10% of cases), larval or young adult worms can be recovered from the CSF. The infection must be distinguished from other helminth CNS infections, such as paragonimiasis, fascioliasis, trichinosis, strongyloidiasis, cysticercosis, echinococcosis, and ascariasis. A microenzyme-linked immunosorbent assay for antibodies directed against the antigens of the parasite in either serum or CSF has been recently developed and is helpful in confirming the diagnosis (81).

Effective anthelmintic regimens have not been developed (although ivermectin shows promise in animal trials), and potential therapeutic intervention designed to kill the parasite may actually exacerbate the inflammatory response and clinical signs. Clinical treatment is usually supportive to relieve headache and nausea. In some cases corticosteroids have been used. Thiabendazole has been used with some success during the first week of infection (80). Prevention of the infection is obviously preferred. This is accomplished by avoidance of eating raw vegetables and underwashed or unfrozen snails and aquatic crustaceans in areas of endemicity.

Tapeworms

Hymenolepis nana, the Dwarf Tapeworm of Humans

The dwarf tapeworm is a common parasite of both rats and mice. The infection in humans occurs most frequently in children who live in warm climates. The presence of *H. nana* in humans is noted worldwide, and it is the most frequently detected tapeworm in the United States (17). *H. nana* is unique among tapeworms because it does not require an intermediate host to complete its life cycle. The adult tapeworm develops after the egg is ingested; the hooked oncosphere invades the intestinal mucosa and develops into a cysticercoid larva, and 2 weeks later the larva matures into an adult worm. The *H. nana* eggs can contaminate hands, eating utensils, food, or aerosolized dust and then be accidentally ingested. Internal autoinfection may also occur. The tapeworm can also use fleas and beetles to proceed through its life cycle; these in turn are then ingested by humans. Personal hygiene, sanitation, and rodent control are important in preventing transmission. Humans with mild infection and in a good nutritional state usually have no symptoms, or the infection may cause diarrhea, anorexia, vomiting, pruritus of the nose and anus, or urticaria. In severe infections, signs are consistently present and include diarrhea, abdominal pain, anorexia, and CNS signs (17). Niclosamide for 5 to 7 days is the treatment of choice after demonstration of the characteristic eggs in the feces.

Hymenolepis diminuta, the Rat Tapeworm

H. diminuta is especially common in the Norway rat and the black rat; however, it is rarely found in humans (44), though it has been seen in patients from several parts of the United States (17).

The rat tapeworm requires an intermediate host for larval development. This is usually the larval stage of rat fleas, but other arthropods, such as many beetle species, earwigs, and meal moths, can serve as intermediate hosts.

Symptoms of the infection are usually not noted, and diagnosis is made by recovery of the eggs in feces. The eggs are distinguished from *H. nana* by the lack of polar filaments.

Treatment with niclosamide, similar to the regimen used to treat *H. nana,* is recommended. Control is dependent on elimination of rodents from the premises.

ARTHROPOD INFESTATIONS

Several arthropods found on rats, mice, and other wild rodents are vectors of human disease, and some cause allergic dermatitis as well (Table 3) (161). Fleas are seldom found in laboratory rodents but are common parasites of feral rodents. The oriental rat flea, *X. cheopis,* and another flea, *N. fasciatus,* naturally infest both mice and rats; they are vectors for murine typhus and *Y. pestis.* That *X. cheopis* easily establishes itself in animal facilities can be demonstrated by the flea bites which two students received while working in animal rooms housing mice (161).

Ornithonyssus bacoti, the Tropical Rat Mite

O. bacoti can be found on many rodents; the brown Norway rat and the black roof rat are probably the primary host species (10). Since the time of the first report of human *O. bacoti*-associated dermatitis in Australia in 1913 and a 1923 report of a case in a man in the United States, many other cases have been described throughout the world (Table 4) (24, 39, 40, 50, 60, 64, 117, 140, 149, 152).

O. bacoti is an obligate blood-sucking parasite, usually tan but red when engorged with blood. Both the male and female feed on a rodent as their preferred host. The female is 700 μm to 1 mm in length; the male is smaller. Eggs are laid in bedding or wall crevices by the female, which survives for about 70 days and feeds about every 2 days during this period. The mite has five developmental stages: adult, egg, nonfeeding larva, blood-sucking protonymph, and nonfeeding deutonymph. After feeding, the adults and protonymphs leave their host and seek refuge in cracks and crevices. The life cycle from adult to egg requires 7 to 16 days at room temperature. Unfed protonymphs have survived for 43 days (17).

The mite often gains access to the premises on wild rodents and lives in crevices. If wild rodents are not readily available or are captured, the mite will seek blood elsewhere, either from laboratory rodents (if in an animal research facility) or from humans. In some infestations, the rodent shows no clinical signs. However, in more chronic cases, dermatitis and anemia may develop. In the past, this mite has been a troublesome parasite for certain laboratory animals, especially rats, mice, and hamsters (106).

Table 3. Selected ectoparasites of rodents with zoonotic potential[a]

Species	Disease(s) in humans	Host(s)	Agent(s) transmitted
Mites			
Obligate skin mites (*Sarcoptes scabiei* subspecies)	Scabies	Mammals	
Trixacarus caviae	Dermatitis	Guinea pigs	
Nest-inhabiting parasites			
Ornithonyssus bacoti	Dermatitis, murine typhus, rickettsialpox	Rodents and other vertebrates	Coxsackievirus, WEE[b] virus, SLE[c] virus, *Rickettsia typhi*, *Rickettsia akari*, *Francisella tularensis*
Liponyssoides sanguineus	Dermatitis, rickettsialpox	Rodents, particularly *Mus musculus*	*R. akari*
Haemogamasus pontiger	Dermatitis	Rodents, insectivores, straw bedding	
Haemolaelaps casalis	Dermatitis	Birds, mammals, straw, hay	
Eulaelaps stabularis	Dermatitis, tularemia	Small mammals, straw bedding	*F. tularensis*
Ixodids (ticks)			
Dermacentor variabilis	Irritation, RMSF,[d] tularemia, tick paralysis, other diseases	Wild rodents, cottontail rabbits, dogs from areas of endemicity	*Rickettsia rickettsii*, *F. tularensis*
Amblyomma americanum	Irritation, RMSF, tularemia	Wild rodents, dogs	
Ixodes scapularis	Irritation, possible tularemia	Dogs, wild rodents	
Ixodes dammini	Human babesiosis, Lyme disease	Wild rodents, especially *Peromyscus*	*Borrelia burgdorferi*, *Babesia microti*
Fleas			
Xenopsylla cheopis	Dermatitis, plague, murine typhus, *Hymenolepis nana* infection, *Hymenolepis diminuta* infection	Rat, mouse, wild rodents	Rodent tapeworms, *Yersinia pestis*, *R. typhi*
Nasopsyllus fasciatus	Dermatitis, plague, *H. nana* infection, *H. diminuta* infection, murine typhus	Rat, mouse, wild rodents	Rodent tapeworms, *Y. pestis*, *R. typhi*
Leptopsylla segnis	*H. diminuta* infection, *H. nana* infection, murine typhus	Rat	Rodent tapeworms, harbors *Salmonella*, *R. typhi*

[a]Found in laboratory animals and causes allergic dermatitis or from which zoonotic agents have been recovered in nature (see reference 161).
[b]WEE, western equine encephalitis.
[c]SLE, St. Louis equine encephalitis.
[d]RMSF, Rocky Mountain spotted fever.

Table 4. Reports of *O. bacoti*-induced dermatitis in humans: United States, 1931 through 1982

Host	Person(s) afflicted	Environment	Lesions	Anatomical location	Reference
Rat	200 adults and children	Residence, theater	Adults: urticarial wheals, papules; children: papules, urticarial wheals, vesicles	Adults: ankles, trunk, back, neck; children: beltline, upper part of shoulders	39
Rat	4 women, 1 man	Department store	Wheals, papules, few wheals with central puncture	Women: arms, forearms; man: hands, ankles, legs, beltline, shoulders, neck	152
Rat	Employees	Department store	Macular skin eruptions		117
Rat	Infants, adult occupants	Foundling home	Papular urticaria, grouping of bites		60
Rat	8-yr-old boy; 5 siblings and both parents affected with milder symptoms	Residence	Excoriated urticarial papules	Trunk, upper part of arms, buttocks	40
Norway rat	60-yr-old woman	Residence	1- to 4-mm papules, excoriated macules	Neck, shoulders, back, scalp, forearm, arms, abdomen	64
Rat	56-yr-old father and 2 sons; 73-yr-old woman	Residence (apartment over food store)	"Insect bites," papular excoriated dermatitis	Thorax, extremities, buttocks, genitalia, entire body	149
Rat	69-yr-old woman	Residence	Papules with erythema	Breast, shoulders, arm	24
Rat	3 female adults, 3 children	Residence	Papular urticaria, erythematous	Neck, shoulders, arms, legs, abdomen, back	140
Mouse	5 research personnel, 2 animal care technicians	Animal research laboratory	Several millimeters to >1-cm raised erythematous papules and nodules	Wrists, arm, abdomen, chest	50

Tropical rat mites produce painful, pruritic lesions on humans. Examination of patients often discloses papular lesions on the wrists, arms, abdomen, and chest. Raised erythematous papules and nodules several millimeters to more than 1 cm in size occur singly or in linear configuration. Epidemiologically, cases usually occur in clusters that involve a common source of exposure to the mite. Experimentally, cases have been shown to be a vector of pathogens. In the laboratory, mite transmission of various rickettsial species, *Pasteurella tularensis*, and coxsackievirus between different laboratory animals has been shown (70, 106, 107, 127).

Affected individuals are treated with topical lindane. Papular dermatitis regresses 7 to 10 days posttherapy. Recurrence of *Ornithonyssus* infestations is common unless the premises and laboratory animals have been treated with an appropriate insecticide and any feral rodents have been eradicated. Lindane can also be used to eradicate the mites from research rodent colonies (61).

REFERENCES

1. **Adams, J. R., E. T. Schmidtmann, and A. F. Azad.** 1990. Infection of colonized cat fleas, *Ctenocephalides felis* (Bouche), with a rickettsia-like microorganism. *Am. J. Trop. Med. Hyg.* **43**:400–409.
2. **Adams, W. H., R. W. Emmons, and J. E. Brooks.** 1970. The changing ecology of murine (endemic) typhus in Southern California. *Am. J. Trop. Med. Hyg.* **19**:311–318.
3. **Alexander, A. D.** 1984. Leptospirosis in laboratory mice. *Science* **224**:1158.
4. **Alteras, I.** 1965. Human infection from laboratory animals. *Sabouraudia* **3**:143–145.
5. **Andersen, L. P., A. Norgaard, S. Holck, J. Blom, and L. Elsborg.** 1996. Isolation of a "*Helicobacter heilmannii*"-like organism from the human stomach. *Eur. J. Clin. Microbiol. Infect. Dis.* **15**:95–96.
6. **Anderson, L. C., S. L. Leary, and P. J. Manning.** 1983. Rat-bite fever in animal research laboratory personnel. *Lab. Anim. Sci.* **33**:292–294.
7. **Arkless, H. A.** 1970. Rat-bite fever at Albert Einstein Medical Center. *Pa. Med.* **73**:49.
8. **Barkin, R. M., J. C. Guckian, and J. W. Glosser.** 1974. Infection by *Leptospira ballum*: a laboratory-associated case. *South. Med. J.* **67**:155 passim.
9. **Bartram, J. T., H. Welsh, and M. Ostroleur.** 1940. Incidence of members of the Salmonella group in rats. *J. Infect. Dis.* **67**:222–226.
10. **Beaver, P. C., and R. C. Jung.** 1985. *Animal Agents and Vectors of Human Disease*, 5th ed. Lea & Febiger, Philadelphia, Pa.
11. **Benenson, A. S. (ed.).** 1985. *Control of Communicable Disease in Man*, 14th ed. American Public Health Association, Washington, D.C.
12. **Bharadwaj, M., J. Botten, N. Torrez-Martinez, and B. Hjelle.** 1997. Rio Mamore virus: genetic characterization of a newly recognized hantavirus of the pygmy rice rat, *Oligoryzomys microtis*, from Bolivia. *Am. J. Trop. Med. Hyg.* **57**:368–374.
13. **Blackmore, D. K., and R. A. Francis.** 1970. The apparent transmission of staphylococci of human origin to laboratory animals. *J. Comp. Pathol.* **80**:645–651.
14. **Boak, R. A., W. D. Linscott, and R. E. Bodfish.** 1960. A case of *Leptospirosis ballum* in California. *Calif. Med.* **93**:163–165.
15. **Booth, B. H.** 1952. Mouse ringworm. *Arch. Dermatol. Syphilol.* **66**:65–69.
16. **Breman, J.** 2000. Monkeypox: an emerging infection for humans?, p. 45–67. *In* W. M. Scheld, W. A. Craig, and J. M. Hughes (ed.), *Emerging Infections 4*. ASM Press, Washington, D.C.
17. **Brettman, L. R., S. Lewin, R. S. Holzman, W. D. Goldman, J. S. Marr, P. Kechijian, and R. Schinella.** 1981. Rickettsialpox: report of an outbreak and a contemporary review. *Medicine* (Baltimore) **60**:363–372.
18. **Brooks, J. E.** 1973. A review of commensal rodents and their control. *Rev. Environ. Control* **3**:405–453.
19. **Brown, C. M., and M. T. Parker.** 1957. Salmonella infection in rodents in Manchester. *Lancet* **273**:1277–1279.

20. **Burman, W. J., D. L. Cohn, R. R. Reves, and M. L. Wilson.** 1995. Multifocal cellulitis and mono-articular arthritis as manifestations of *Helicobacter cinaedi* bacteremia. *Clin. Infect. Dis.* **20:**564–570.

21. **Centers for Disease Control and Prevention.** 1993. Update: hantavirus disease—southwestern United States, 1993. *Morb. Mortal. Wkly. Rep.* **42:**570–572.

22. **Centers for Disease Control and Prevention.** 2003. Multistate outbreak of monkeypox—Illinois, Indiana, and Wisconsin, 2003. *Morb. Mortal. Wkly. Rep.* **52:**537–540.

23. **Cetin, E. T., M. Tahsinoglu, and S. Volkan.** 1965. Epizootic of Trichophyton mentagrophytes (interdigitale) in white mice. *Pathol. Microbiol.* **28:**839–846.

24. **Charlesworth, E. N., and R. W. Clegern.** 1977. Tropical rat mite dermatitis. *Arch. Dermatol.* **113:**937–938.

25. **Childs, J. E., G. E. Glass, G. W. Korch, R. R. Arthur, K. V. Shah, D. Glasser, C. Rossi, and J. W. Leduc.** 1988. Evidence of human infection with a rat-associated Hantavirus in Baltimore, Maryland. *Am. J. Epidemiol.* **127:**875–878.

25a.**Chin, J. (ed.).** 2000. *Control of Communicable Diseass Manual,* 17th ed. American Public Health Association, Washington, D.C.

26. **Chmel, L., L. Buchvald, and M. Valentova.** 1975. Spread of *Trichophyton mentagrophytes* var. Gran. infection to man. *Int. J. Dermatol.* **14:**269–272.

27. **Cimolai, N., M. J. Gill, A. Jones, B. Flores, W. E. Stamm, W. Laurie, B. Madden, and M. S. Shahrabadi.** 1987. "*Campylobacter cinaedi*" bacteremia: case report and laboratory findings. *J. Clin. Microbiol.* **25:**942–943.

28. **Coffey, E. M., and W. C. Eveland.** 1967. Experimental relapsing fever initiated by *Borrelia hermsi*. I. Identification of major serotypes by immunofluorescence. *J. Infect. Dis.* **117:**23–28.

29. **Cole, J. S., R. W. Stoll, and R. J. Bulger.** 1969. Rat-bite fever. Report of three cases. *Ann. Intern. Med.* **71:**979–981.

30. **Committee on Urban Pest Management.** 1980. *Urban Pest Management.* National Academy Press, Washington, D.C.

31. **Corning, B. F., J. C. Murphy, and J. G. Fox.** 1991. Group G streptococcal lymphadenitis in rats. *J. Clin. Microbiol.* **29:**2720–2723.

32. **Craven, R. B., and A. M. Barnes.** 1991. Plague and tularemia in animal associated human infections. *Infect. Dis. Clin. N. Am.* **5:**165–175.

33. **Davey, D. G.** 1962. The use of pathogen free animals. *Proc. R. Soc. Med.* **55:**256–262.

34. **Davies, R. R., and J. Shewell.** 1964. Control of mouse ringworm. *Nature* **202:**406–407.

35. **Demers, R. Y., A. Thiermann, P. Demers, and R. Frank.** 1983. Exposure to Leptospira icterohaemorrhagiae in inner-city and suburban children: a serologic comparison. *J. Fam. Pract.* **17:**1007–1011.

36. **Dennis, D. T., and J. M. Hughes.** 1997. Multidrug resistance in plague. *N. Engl. J. Med.* **337:**702–704.

37. **Desmyter, J., C. van Ypersele de Strihou, and G. van der Groen.** 1984. Hantavirus disease. *Lancet* **ii:**158.

38. **Dolan, M. M., A. Kligman, P. G. Kobylinski, and M. A. Motsavage.** 1958. Ringworm epizootics in laboratory mice and rats: experimental and accidental transmission of infection. *J. Investig. Dermatol.* **30:**23–25.

39. **Dove, W. E., and B. Shelmire.** 1931. The tropical rat mite, *Liponyssus bacoti* Hirst 1914: the cause of a skin eruption of man, and a possible vector of endemic typhus fever. *JAMA* **96:**579–584.

40. **Dowlati, Y., and H. C. Maguire, Jr.** 1970. Rat mite dermatitis: a family affair. *Arch. Dermatol.* **101:**617–618.

41. **Duma, R. J., D. E. Sonenshine, F. M. Bozeman, J. M. Veazey, Jr., B. L. Elisberg, D. P. Chadwick, N. I. Stocks, T. M. McGill, G. B. Miller, Jr., and J. N. MacCormack.** 1981. Epidemic typhus in the United States associated with flying squirrels. *JAMA* **245:**2318–2323.

42. **Faine, S.** 1991. Leptospirosis, p. 367–393. *In* A. Evans and P. S. Brachman (ed.), *Bacterial Infections in Humans.* Plenum Medical Book Co., New York, N.Y.

43. **Farhang-Azad, A., R. Traub, and S. Baqar.** 1985. Transovarial transmission of murine typhus rickettsiae in *Xenopsylla cheopis* fleas. *Science* **227:**543–545.

44. **Faust, E. L., and P. F. Russel.** 1970. *Craig & Faust Clinical Parasitology,* 8th ed. Lea & Febiger, Philadelphia, Pa.

44a. **Fernandez, K. R., L. M. Hansen, P. Vandamme, B. L. Beaman, and J. V. Solnick.** 2002. Captive rhesus monkeys (*Macaca mulatta*) are commonly infected with *Helicobacter cinaedi. J. Clin. Microbiol.* **40:**1908–1912.

45. **Flores, B. M., C. L. Fennell, K. K. Holmes, and W. E. Stamm.** 1985. In vitro susceptibilities of *Campylobacter*-like organisms to twenty antimicrobial agents. *Antimicrob. Agents Chemother.* **28:** 188–191.

46. **Fox, J., C. Newcomer, and H. Rozmiarek.** 2002. Selected zoonoses, p. 1060–1128. *In* J. Fox, L. Anderson, F. Loew, and F. Quimby (ed.), *Laboratory Animal Medicine,* 2nd ed. Academic Press, Boston, Mass.

47. **Fox, J. G.** 1998. *Biology and Diseases of the Ferret,* 2nd ed. Williams and Wilkins, Baltimore, Md.

48. **Fox, J. G.** 1991. Campylobacter infections and salmonellosis. *Semin. Vet. Med. Surg. (Small Anim.)* **6:**212–218.

49. **Fox, J. G.** 2002. The non-*H. pylori* helicobacters: their expanding role in gastrointestinal and systemic diseases. *Gut* **50:**273–283.

50. **Fox, J. G., and J. B. Brayton.** 1982. Zoonoses and other human health hazards, p. 403–423. *In* H. L. Foster, J. D. Small, and J. G. Fox (ed.), *Biology of the Laboratory Mouse,* vol. II. Academic Press, New York, N.Y.

51. **Fox, J. G., F. E. Dewhirst, Z. Shen, Y. Feng, N. S. Taylor, B. J. Paster, R. L. Ericson, C. N. Lau, P. Correa, J. C. Araya, and I. Roa.** 1998. Hepatic *Helicobacter* species identified in bile and gallbladder tissue from Chileans with chronic cholecystitis. *Gastroenterology* **114:**755–763.

52. **Fox, J. G., L. Handt, B. J. Sheppard, S. Xu, F. E. Dewhirst, S. Motzel, and H. Klein.** 2001. Isolation of *Helicobacter cinaedi* from the colon, liver, and mesenteric lymph node of a rhesus monkey with chronic colitis and hepatitis. *J. Clin. Microbiol.* **39:**1580–1585.

53. **Fox, J. G., and N. S. Lipman.** 1991. Infections transmitted by large and small laboratory animals. *Infect. Dis. Clin. N. Am.* **5:**131–163.

54. **Friedmann, C. T., E. L. Spiegel, E. Aaron, and R. McIntyre.** 1973. *Leptospirosis ballum* contracted from pet mice. *Calif. Med.* **118:**51–52.

55. **Gebhart, C. J., C. L. Fennell, M. P. Murtaugh, and W. E. Stamm.** 1989. *Campylobacter cinaedi* is normal intestinal flora in hamsters. *J. Clin. Microbiol.* **27:**1692–1694.

56. **Geller, E. H.** 1979. Health hazards for man, p. 402. *In* H. J. Baker, J. R. Lindsey, and S. H. Weisbroth (ed.), *The Laboratory Rat,* vol. I. Academic Press, New York, N.Y.

57. **Gilbert, G. L., J. F. Cassidy, and N. M. Bennett.** 1971. Rat-bite fever. *Med. J. Aust.* **2:**1131–1134.

58. **Giusti, A. M., L. Crippa, O. Bellini, M. Luini, and E. Scanziani.** 1998. Gastric spiral bacteria in wild rats from Italy. *J. Wildl. Dis.* **34:**168–172.

59. **Goddard, A. F., R. P. Logan, J. C. Atherton, D. Jenkins, and R. C. Spiller.** 1997. Healing of duodenal ulcer after eradication of *Helicobacter heilmannii. Lancet* **349:**1815–1816.

59a. **Graves, M. H., and J. M. Janda.** 2001. Rat-bite fever (Streptobacillus moniliformis): a potential emerging disease. *Int. J. Infect. Dis.* **5:**151–155.

60. **Haggard, C. N.** 1955. Rat mite dermatitis in children. *Pediatrics* **15:**322–324.

61. **Harris, J. M., and J. J. Stockton.** 1960. Eradication of the tropical rat mite *Ornithonyssus bacoti* (Hirst 1913) from a colony of mice. *Am. J. Vet. Res.* **21:**316–318.

62. **Heilmann, K. L., and F. Borchard.** 1991. Gastritis due to spiral shaped bacteria other than *Helicobacter pylori*: clinical, histological, and ultrastructural findings. *Gut* **32:**137–140.

63. **Heiser, V.** 1936. *An American Doctor's Odyssey.* W. W. Norton Publishers, New York, N.Y.

63a. **Hernandez-Cabrera, M., A. Angel-Moreno, E. Santana, M. Bolanos, A. Frances, A. Martin-Sanchez, and J. Perez-Arellano.** 2004. Murine typhus with renal involvement in Canary Islands, Spain. *Emerg. Infect. Dis.* **10:**740–743.

64. **Hetherington, G. W., W. R. Holder, and D. B. Smith.** 1971. Rat mite dermatitis. *JAMA* **215:**1499–1500.

65. **Hilzenrat, N., E. Lamoureux, I. Weintrub, E. Alpert, M. Lichter, and L. Alpert.** 1995. *Helicobacter heilmannii*-like spiral bacteria in gastric mucosal biopsies. Prevalence and clinical significance. *Arch. Pathol. Lab. Med.* **119:**1149–1153.

66. **Hinnebusch, B. J., R. D. Perry, and T. G. Schwan.** 1996. Role of the *Yersinia pestis* hemin storage (hms) locus in the transmission of plague by fleas. *Science* **273:**367–370.

67. **Hinnebusch, B. J., A. E. Rudolph, P. Cherepanov, J. E. Dixon, T. G. Schwan, and A. Forsberg.** 2002. Role of *Yersinia* murine toxin in survival of *Yersinia pestis* in the midgut of the flea vector. *Science* **296:**733–735.

68. **Hjelle, B., S. Jenison, N. Torrez-Martinez, B. Herring, S. Quan, A. Polito, S. Pichuantes, T. Yamada, C. Morris, F. Elgh, H. W. Lee, H. Artsob, and R. Dinello.** 1997. Rapid and specific detection of Sin Nombre virus antibodies in patients with hantavirus pulmonary syndrome by a strip immunoblot assay suitable for field diagnosis. *J. Clin. Microbiol.* **35:**600–608.

69. **Hjelle, B., N. Torrez-Martinez, F. T. Koster, M. Jay, M. S. Ascher, T. Brown, P. Reynolds, P. Ettestad, R. E. Voorhees, J. Sarisky, R. E. Enscore, L. Sands, D. G. Mosley, C. Kioski, R. T. Bryan, and C. M. Sewell.** 1996. Epidemiologic linkage of rodent and human hantavirus genomic sequences in case investigations of hantavirus pulmonary syndrome. *J. Infect. Dis.* **173:**781–786.

70. **Hopla, C. E.** 1951. Experimental transmission of tularemia by the tropical rat mite. *Am. J. Trop. Hyg.* **31:**768–782.

71. **Hovell, M.** 1924. *Rats and How to Destroy Them.* John Bale, Sons & Danielson Ltd., London, England.

72. **Hull, T. G.** 1955. *Diseases Transmitted from Animals to Man,* 4th ed. Charles C Thomas, Springfield, Ill.

73. **Hussell, T., P. G. Isaacson, J. E. Crabtree, and J. Spencer.** 1996. *Helicobacter pylori*-specific tumour-infiltrating T cells provide contact dependent help for the growth of malignant B cells in low-grade gastric lymphoma of mucosa-associated lymphoid tissue. *J. Pathol.* **178:**122–127.

74. **Iinuma, Y., H. Hayashidani, K. Kaneko, M. Ogawa, and S. Hamasaki.** 1992. Isolation of *Yersinia enterocolitica* serovar O8 from free-living small rodents in Japan. *J. Clin. Microbiol.* **30:**240–242.

75. **Jezek, Z., M. Szczeniowski, K. M. Paluku, and M. Mutombo.** 1987. Human monkeypox: clinical features of 282 patients. *J. Infect. Dis.* **156:**293–298.

76. **Kaneko, K. I., S. Hamada, Y. Kasai, and E. Kato.** 1978. Occurrence of *Yersinia enterocolitica* in house rats. *Appl. Environ. Microbiol.* **36:**314–318.

77. **Kaufman, A. F., J. M. Boyce, and W. J. Martone.** 1980. Trends in human plague in the United States. *J. Infect. Dis.* **141:**522.

78. **Kiehlbauch, J. A., D. J. Brenner, D. N. Cameron, A. G. Steigerwalt, J. M. Makowski, C. N. Baker, C. M. Patton, and I. K. Wachsmuth.** 1995. Genotypic and phenotypic characterization of *Helicobacter cinaedi* and *Helicobacter fennelliae* strains isolated from humans and animals. *J. Clin. Microbiol.* **33:**2940–2947.

79. **Kiehlbauch, J. A., R. V. Tauxe, C. N. Baker, and I. K. Wachsmuth.** 1994. *Helicobacter cinaedi*-associated bacteremia and cellulitis in immunocompromised patients. *Ann. Intern. Med.* **121:**90–93.

80. **Kliks, M. M., K. Kroenke, and J. M. Hardman.** 1982. Eosinophilic radiculomyeloencephalitis: an angiostrongyliasis outbreak in American Samoa related to ingestion of *Achatina fulica* snails. *Am. J. Trop. Med. Hyg.* **31:**1114–1122.

81. **Kliks, M. M., W. K. Lau, and N. E. Palumbo.** 1988. Neurologic angiostronglyiasis: parasitic eosinophilic meningoencephalitis, p. 754–767. *In* A. Balows (ed.), *Laboratory Diagnosis of Infectious Diseases: Principles and Practice,* vol. I. Springer-Verlag, New York, N.Y.

82. **LeDuc, J. W.** 1987. Epidemiology of Hantaan and related viruses. *Lab. Anim. Sci.* **37:**413–418.

83. **Lee, A., S. L. Hazell, J. O'Rourke, and S. Kouprach.** 1988. Isolation of a spiral-shaped bacterium from the cat stomach. *Infect. Immun.* **56:**2843–2850.

84. **Li, H., and D. E. Davis.** 1952. The prevalence of carriers of leptospira and salmonella in Norway rats of Baltimore. *Am. J. Hyg.* **56:**90–100.

85. **Lipman, N. S.** 1996. Rat bite fevers, p. 451–455. *In* D. Schlossberg (ed.), *Current Therapy of Infectious Diseases.* Mosby Yearbook, Inc., Philadelphia, Pa.

86. **Lloyd, G., E. T. Bowen, N. Jones, and A. Pendry.** 1984. HFRS outbreak associated with laboratory rats in UK. *Lancet* **i:**1175–1176.

87. **Looke, D. F.** 1986. Weil's syndrome in a zoologist. *Med. J. Aust.* **144:**597, 600–601.

88. **Luzzi, G. A., L. M. Milne, and S. A. Waitkins.** 1987. Rat-bite acquired leptospirosis. *J. Infect.* **15:**57–60.

89. **Mackenzie, D.** 1961. *Trichophyton mentagrophytes* in mice: infections of humans and incidence amongst laboratory animals. *Sabouraudia* **1:**178–182.

90. **Macy, D. W.** 1998. Plague, p. 295–300. *In* C. E. Greene (ed.), *Infectious Disease of the Dog and Cat,* 2nd ed. W. B. Saunders Co., Philadelphia, Pa.

91. **Mann, J. M., W. J. Martone, J. M. Boyce, A. F. Kaufmann, A. M. Barnes, and N. S. Weber.** 1979. Endemic human plague in New Mexico: risk factors associated with infection. *J. Infect. Dis.* **140:**397–401.

92. **Matsukura, N., S. Yokomuro, S. Yamada, T. Tajiri, T. Sundo, T. Hadama, S. Kamiya, Z. Naito, and J. G. Fox.** 2002. Association between *Helicobacter bilis* in bile and biliary tract malignancies: *H. bilis* in bile from Japanese and Thai patients with benign and malignant diseases in the biliary tract. *Jpn. J. Cancer Res.* **93:**842–847.

93. **McDade, J. E., and D. B. Fishbein.** 1988. Rickettsiaceae: the rickettsiae, p. 864–890. *In* E. H. Lennette, P. Halonen, and F. A. Murphy (ed.), *Laboratory Diagnosis of Infectious Disease: Principles and Practice,* vol. II. Springer-Verlag, New York, N.Y.

94. **McGill, R. C., A. M. Martin, and P. N. Edmunds.** 1966. Rat-bite fever due to *Streptobacillus moniliformis. Br. Med. J.* **i:**1213–1214.

95. **Mendes, E., et al.** 1994. Are pigs a reservoir host for human Helicobacter infection? *Am. J. Gastroenterol.* **89:**1296. (Abstract 45.)

96. **Morgner, A., N. Lehn, L. P. Andersen, C. Thiede, M. Bennedsen, K. Trebesius, B. Neubauer, A. Neubauer, M. Stolte, and E. Bayerdorffer.** 2000. *Helicobacter heilmannii*-associated primary gastric low-grade MALT lymphoma: complete remission after curing the infection. *Gastroenterology* **118:**821–828.

97. **Morris, A., M. R. Ali, L. Thomsen, and B. Hollis.** 1990. Tightly spiral shaped bacteria in the human stomach: another cause of active chronic gastritis? *Gut* **31:**139–143.

98. **Mushatt, D. M., and N. E. Hyslop, Jr.** 1991. Neurologic aspects of North American zoonoses. *Infect. Dis. Clin. N. Am.* **5:**703–731.

99. **Nelson, J. D., H. Kusmiesz, L. H. Jackson, and E. Woodman.** 1980. Treatment of Salmonella gastroenteritis with ampicillin, amoxicillin, or placebo. *Pediatrics* **65:**1125–1130.

100. **Ng, V. L., W. K. Hadley, C. L. Fennell, B. M. Flores, and W. E. Stamm.** 1987. Successive bacteremias with "*Campylobacter cinaedi*" and "*Campylobacter fennelliae*" in a bisexual male. *J. Clin. Microbiol.* **25:**2008–2009.

101. **Ordog, G. J., S. Balasubramanium, and J. Wasserberger.** 1985. Rat bites: fifty cases. *Ann. Emerg. Med.* **14:**126–130.

102. **Orlicek, S. L., D. F. Welch, and T. L. Kuhls.** 1993. Septicemia and meningitis caused by *Helicobacter cinaedi* in a neonate. *J. Clin. Microbiol.* **31:**569–571.

103. **Paegle, R. D., R. P. Tewari, W. N. Bernhard, and E. Peters.** 1976. Microbial flora of the larynx, trachea, and large intestine of the rat after long-term inhalation of 100 per cent oxygen. *Anesthesiology* **44:**287–290.

104. **Pavia, A. T., and R. V. Tauxe.** 1991. Salmonellosis: nontyphoidal, p. 573–592. *In* A. S. Evans and P. S. Brachman (ed.), *Bacterial Infections of Humans. Epidemiology and Control.* Plenum, New York, N.Y.

105. **Perry, R.** 2003. A plague of fleas—survival and transmission of *Yersinia pestis. ASM News* **69:**336–338.

106. **Petrov, V. G.** 1971. On the role of the mite *Ornithonyssus bacoti* Hirst as a reservoir and vector of the agent of tularemia. *Parazitologiia* **1:**7–14.

107. **Philip, C. B., and L. E. Hughes.** 1948. The tropical rat mite, *Liponyssus bacoti,* as an experimental vector of rickettsial pox. *Am. J. Trop. Hyg.* **28:**697–705.

108. **Povar, M. L.** 1965. Ringworm (*Trichophyton mentagrophytes*) infection in a colony of albino Norway rats. *Lab. Anim. Care* **15:**264–265.

109. **Pratt, H. D., B. F. Bjornson, and K. S. Littig.** 1976. Control of domestic rats and mice. Publication no. (CDC) 76-8141. U.S. Department of Health, Education, and Welfare, Atlanta, Ga.

110. **Price-Jones, C.** 1927. Infection of rats by Gartner's bacillus. *J. Pathol. Bacteriol.* **30:**45.

111. **Quinn, T. C., S. E. Goodell, C. Fennell, S. P. Wang, M. D. Schuffler, K. K. Holmes, and W. E. Stamm.** 1984. Infections with *Campylobacter jejuni* and *Campylobacter*-like organisms in homosexual men. *Ann. Intern. Med.* **101:**187–192.

112. **Quinn, T. C., W. E. Stamm, S. E. Goodell, E. Mkrtichian, J. Benedetti, L. Corey, M. D. Schuffler, and K. K. Holmes.** 1983. The polymicrobial origin of intestinal infections in homosexual men. *N. Engl. J. Med.* **309:**576–582.

113. **Raffin, B. J., and M. Freemark.** 1979. Streptobacillary rat-bite fever: a pediatric problem. *Pediatrics* **64:**214–217.

114. **Reed, K. D., J. W. Melski, M. B. Graham, R. L. Regnery, M. J. Sotir, M. V. Wegner, J. J. Kazmier-czak, E. J. Stratman, Y. Li, J. A. Fairley, G. R. Swain, V. A. Olson, E. K. Sargent, S. C. Kehl, M. A. Frace, R. Kline, S. L. Foldy, J. P. Davis, and I. K. Damon.** 2004. The detection of monkeypox in humans in the Western Hemisphere. *N. Engl. J. Med.* **350:**342–350.

115. **Regimbeau, C., D. Karsenti, V. Durand, L. D'Alteroche, C. Copie-Bergman, E. H. Metman, and M. C. Machet.** 1998. Low-grade gastric MALT lymphoma and *Helicobacter heilmannii* (*Gastrospirillum hominis*). *Gastroenterol. Clin. Biol.* **22:**720–723.

116. **Richter, C. P.** 1954. Incidence of rat bites and rat bite fever in Baltimore. *JAMA* **128:**324.

117. **Riley, W. A.** 1940. Rat mite dermatitis in Minnesota. *Minn. Med.* **23:**423–424.

118. **Roggero, E., E. Zucca, G. Pinotti, A. Pascarella, C. Capella, A. Savio, E. Pedrinis, A. Paterlini, A. Venco, and F. Cavalli.** 1995. Eradication of *Helicobacter pylori* infection in primary low-grade gastric lymphoma of mucosa-associated lymphoid tissue. *Ann. Intern. Med.* **122:**767–769.

119. **Rollag, O. J., M. R. Skeels, L. J. Nims, J. P. Thilsted, and J. M. Mann.** 1981. Feline plague in New Mexico: report of five cases. *J. Am. Vet. Med. Assoc.* **179:**1381–1383.

120. **Rollin, P. E., T. G. Ksiazek, L. H. Elliott, E. V. Ravkov, M. L. Martin, S. Morzunov, W. Livingstone, M. Monroe, G. Glass, S. Ruo, et al.** 1995. Isolation of Black Creek Canal virus, a new hantavirus from *Sigmodon hispidus* in Florida. *J. Med. Virol.* **46:**35–39.

121. **Rolston, K. V.** 1986. Group G streptococcal infections. *Arch. Intern. Med.* **146:**857–858.

122. **Rosner, W. W.** 1987. Bubonic plague. *J. Am. Vet. Med. Assoc.* **191:**406–409.

123. **Roughgarden, J. W.** 1965. Antimicrobial therapy of rat bite fever. *Arch. Intern. Med.* **116:**39.

124. **Sanger, J. G., and A. B. Thiermann.** 1988. Leptospirosis. *J. Am. Vet. Med. Assoc.* **193:**1250–1254.

125. **Schmaljohn, C., and B. Hjelle.** 1997. Hantaviruses: a global disease problem. *Emerg. Infect. Dis.* **3:**95–104.

126. **Schriefer, M. E., J. B. Sacci, Jr., J. S. Dumler, M. G. Bullen, and A. F. Azad.** 1994. Identification of a novel rickettsial infection in a patient diagnosed with murine typhus. *J. Clin. Microbiol.* **32:**949–954.

127. **Schwab, M. R., R. Allen, and S. E. Sulkin.** 1952. The tropical rat mite (*Liponyssus bacoti*) as an experimental vector of coxsackie virus. *Am. J. Trop. Hyg.* **1:**982–986.

128. **Schwartz, E.** 1942. Notes on commensal rats. *Am. J. Trop. Med.* **22:**577–579.

129. **Shults, F. S., P. C. Estes, J. A. Franklin, and C. B. Richter.** 1973. Staphylococcal botryomycosis in a specific-pathogen-free mouse colony. *Lab. Anim. Sci.* **23:**36–42.

130. **Solnick, J. V., J. O'Rourke, A. Lee, B. J. Paster, F. E. Dewhirst, and L. S. Tompkins.** 1993. An uncultured gastric spiral organism is a newly identified Helicobacter in humans. *J. Infect. Dis.* **168:**379–385.

131. **Song, J. W., L. J. Baek, D. C. Gajdusek, R. Yanagihara, I. Gavrilovskaya, B. J. Luft, E. R. Mackow, and B. Hjelle.** 1994. Isolation of pathogenic hantavirus from white-footed mouse (*Peromyscus leucopus*). *Lancet* **344:**1637.

132. **Stoenner, H. G., E. F. Grimes, F. B. Thraikill, and E. Davis.** 1958. Elimination of *Leptospira ballum* from a colony of Swiss albino mice by use of chlortetracycline hydrochloride. *Am. J. Trop. Med. Hyg.* **7:**423–426.

133. **Stoenner, H. G., and D. Maclean.** 1958. Leptospirosis (ballum) contracted from Swiss albino mice. *Arch. Intern. Med.* **101:**706–710.

134. **Stolte, M., G. Kroher, A. Meining, A. Morgner, E. Bayerdorffer, and B. Bethke.** 1997. A comparison of *Helicobacter pylori* and *H. heilmannii* gastritis. A matched control study involving 404 patients. *Scand. J. Gastroenterol.* **32:**28–33.

135. **Stolte, M., E. Wellens, B. Bethke, M. Ritter, and H. Eidt.** 1994. *Helicobacter heilmannii* (formerly *Gastrospirillum hominis*) gastritis: an infection transmitted by animals? *Scand. J. Gastroenterol.* **29:**1061–1064.

136. **Stuart, B. M., and R. L. Pullen.** 1945. Endemic (murine) typhus fever: clinical observations of 180 cases. *Ann. Intern. Med.* **23:**520–525.

137. **Sulzer, C. R., T. W. Harvey, and M. M. Galton.** 1968. Comparison of diagnostic techniques for the detection of leptospirosis in rats. *Health Lab. Sci.* **5:**171–173.

138. **Taber, E., and R. D. Feigin.** 1979. Spirochetal infections. *Pediatr. Clin. N. Am.* **26:**377.

139. **Taylor, A. F., T. G. Stephenson, and H. A. Giese.** 1984. Rat bite fever in a college student. *Morb. Mortal. Wkly. Rep.* **33:**318.

140. Theis, J., M. M. Lavoipierre, R. LaPerriere, and H. Kroese. 1981. Tropical rat mite dermatitis. Report of six cases and review of mite infestations. *Arch. Dermatol.* **117:**341–343.

141. Thiermann, A. B. 1977. Incidence of leptospirosis in the Detroit rat population. *Am. J. Trop. Med. Hyg.* **26:**970–974.

142. Thomson, M. A., P. Storey, R. Greer, and G. J. Cleghorn. 1994. Canine-human transmission of *Gastrospirillum hominis. Lancet* **343:**1605–1607.

143. Torrez-Martinez, N., M. Bharadwaj, D. Goade, J. Delury, P. Moran, B. Hicks, B. Nix, J. L. Davis, and B. Hjelle. 1998. Bayou virus-associated hantavirus pulmonary syndrome in Eastern Texas: identification of the rice rat, *Oryzomys palustris,* as reservoir host. *Emerg. Infect. Dis.* **4:**105–111.

144. Torten, M. 1979. Leptospirosis, p. 363–421. *In* J. H. Steele (ed.), *CRC Handbook Series in Zoonoses,* vol. 1. CRC Press, Cleveland, Ohio.

145. Tsai, T. F. 1987. Hemorrhagic fever with renal syndrome: clinical aspects. *Lab. Anim. Sci.* **37:**419–427.

146. Tsai, T. F. 1987. Hemorrhagic fever with renal syndrome: mode of transmission to humans. *Lab. Anim. Sci.* **37:**428–430.

147. Umenai, T., H. W. Lee, P. W. Lee, T. Saito, T. Toyoda, M. Hongo, K. Yoshinaga, T. Nobunaga, T. Horiuchi, and N. Ishida. 1979. Korean haemorrhagic fever in staff in an animal laboratory. *Lancet* **i:**1314–1316.

148. Vandamme, P., E. Falsen, B. Pot, K. Kersters, and J. De Ley. 1990. Identification of *Campylobacter cinaedi* isolated from blood and feces of children and adult females. *J. Clin. Microbiol.* **28:**1016–1020.

149. Wainschel, J. 1971. Rat mite bite. *JAMA* **216:**1964.

150. Weber, D. J., and A. R. Hansen. 1991. Infections resulting from animal bites. *Infect. Dis. Clin. N. Am.* **5:**663–677.

151. Weber, D. J., J. S. Wolfson, M. N. Swartz, and D. C. Hooper. 1984. Pasteurella multocida infections. Report of 34 cases and review of the literature. *Medicine* (Baltimore) **63:**133–154.

152. Weber, L. F. 1940. Rat mite dermatitis. *JAMA* **114:**1442.

153. Weisbroth, S. 1979. Bacterial and mycotic diseases, p. 194–230. *In* H. Baker (ed.), *The Laboratory Rat,* vol. I. Academic Press, New York, N.Y.

154. Welch, H., M. Ostrolenk, and M. T. Bartram. 1941. Role of rats in the spread of food poisoning bacteria in Salmonella group. *Am. J. Public Health* **31:**332–340.

155. Wilkins, E. G., J. G. Millar, P. M. Cockcroft, and O. A. Okubadejo. 1988. Rat-bite fever in a gerbil breeder. *J. Infect.* **16:**177–180.

156. Williams, S. G., J. B. Sacci, Jr., M. E. Schriefer, E. M. Andersen, K. K. Fujioka, F. J. Sorvillo, A. R. Barr, and A. F. Azad. 1992. Typhus and typhuslike rickettsiae associated with opossums and their fleas in Los Angeles County, California. *J. Clin. Microbiol.* **30:**1758–1762.

157. Yali, Z., N. Yamada, M. Wen, T. Matsuhisa, and M. Miki. 1998. Gastrospirillum hominis and Helicobacter pylori infection in Thai individuals: comparison of histopathological changes of gastric mucosa. *Pathol. Int.* **48:**507–511.

158. Yanagihara, R. 1990. Hantavirus infection in the United States: epizootiology and epidemiology. *Rev. Infect. Dis.* **12:**449–457.

159. Yang, H., J. A. Goliger, M. Song, and D. Zhou. 1998. High prevalence of *Helicobacter heilmannii* infection in China. *Dig. Dis. Sci.* **43:**1493.

160. Young, V., D. Schauer, and J. Fox. 2000. Animal models of *Campylobacter* infection, p. 287–301. *In* I. Nachamkin and M. Blaser (ed.), Campylobacter, 2nd ed. ASM Press, Washington, D.C.

161. Yunker, C. E. 1964. Infections of laboratory animals potentially dangerous to man: ectoparasites and other arthropods, with emphasis on mites. *Lab. Anim. Care* **14:**455–465.

162. Zinsser, H. 1935. *Rats, Lice and History.* Little, Brown and Company, Boston, Mass.

Infections of Leisure, Third Edition
Edited by David Schlossberg
© 2004 ASM Press, Washington, D.C.

Chapter 10

Rabies: Ancient Malady, New Twists

John W. Krebs

Rabies is one of the oldest recognized zoonotic diseases. Its antiquity is illustrated by the ancient origins of terms describing this disease. The Latin word *rabies* is believed to derive from the Sanskrit *rabhas*, meaning "to do violence." Early recognition of the infectivity of the saliva of rabid dogs led Roman writers to describe the infectious material as a poison for which the Latin word was *virus* (80). *Lyssavirus*, the genus to which rabies and rabies-related viruses belong, owes its name to the Greek *lyssa* or *lytta*, meaning "madness." The first recorded description of canine rabies was apparently made by Democritus around 500 B.C. Aristotle, writing of rabies in his *Natural History of Animals*, described dogs suffering from a madness causing irritability and noted that other animals became diseased after being bitten by these sick dogs. In most areas of the world where the disease is endemic, dogs and other carnivores remain the common sources of human rabies infection, resulting in little change over time in the epidemiology of the disease. However, in the United States, there is evidence of a new and growing trend during the past 2 decades for human rabies to be the result of infection with variants of the virus associated with bats.

Rabies was enzootic or epizootic in domestic and wild animals in the United States for much of the 19th and 20th centuries; however, the disease has never affected large numbers of people in this country. During the first half of this century, an average of about 50 cases of human rabies (range, 18 [1950] to 105 [1928]), most the result of infection spread by dogs, were reported each year (80) (Centers for Disease Control and Prevention [CDC] records and Office of Vital Statistics). Following the control of canine rabies in the 1940s and 1950s, the number of indigenously acquired human rabies cases fell to an average of about two per year during the 1960s and 1970s (5). In developing nations throughout much of the world, the domestic dog remains the animal most frequently reported as rabid, but in the United States and many other industrialized nations, rabies today is

---

John W. Krebs • Viral and Rickettsial Zoonoses Branch, Division of Viral and Rickettsial Diseases, Centers for Disease Control and Prevention, 1600 Clifton Rd. NE, G-13, Atlanta, GA 30333.

primarily a disease of wildlife. Between 1980 (when potent and safe tissue culture-derived rabies vaccines were introduced in the United States) and 2002, 32 persons in the United States acquired rabies. All but three of these indigenously acquired cases were attributed to insectivorous bats (89, 97). Although the exact circumstances of the exposures were in most instances unknown, some of these infections may have been acquired during the pursuit of leisure activities (18, 22, 23, 32, 33, 35–37, 39–42, 44, 45, 48, 50, 51, 53–55).

Rabies in wildlife is now directly and indirectly responsible for most of the economic and public health burden of the disease in the United States; since 1960, more wild than domestic animals have been reported as rabid in this country. Annual expenditures for rabies prevention and control may exceed $1,000,000 per 100,000 population in some parts of the United States, with the principal component of these expenditures being the routine vaccination of pets against the disease (109). Ongoing analyses of possible savings via wildlife vaccination programs to control rabies have demonstrated the need for further research to determine optimal bait distribution densities and to better define distributions of costs and cost-savings ratios (94).

In contrast to the situation in the United States, canine rabies remains a serious threat for persons traveling to and living in developing countries. Largely because of the ubiquitous presence of dogs in these countries, rates of human rabies sometimes exceed 1 per 100,000 population per year, and more than 1,000 per 100,000 persons each year may receive postexposure rabies treatment (12). U.S. residents are at a much higher risk of exposure to rabies in these developing countries than in the United States and occasionally have developed the disease when they failed to receive proper postexposure treatment (69). Four Americans living outside the United States have contracted the disease since 1980 (19, 20, 86, 97); four other individuals (U.S. citizens or residents) acquired the disease during visits to India, Haiti, Nepal, and the Philippines (34, 38, 46, 89). Nine persons from countries where canine rabies is enzootic developed the disease while in the United States, and with one possible exception, all are believed to have acquired the disease before coming to this country (21, 24–26, 28, 31, 36, 43, 51, 89, 106). The epidemiology and strategies for preventing rabies within the United States are different from those observed and implemented in other areas of the world and are addressed separately.

EPIDEMIOLOGY OF RABIES IN THE UNITED STATES

Demographic changes resulting in ever-expanding suburban sprawl and changes in recreational land use, including increased popularity of hiking, camping, and drive-through wildlife parks, as well as hunting activities and close contact with pets, provide countless situations for human contact with a variety of animal species in the United States. Thus, rabies prevention strategies in this country focus on education and on a working knowledge of the epizootiology of the disease in animals, rather than sole reliance on the treatment of exposed individuals and on vaccination and control of dog populations, as is the case in much of the developing world.

Wildlife

In the United States, rabies is primarily a disease of wildlife. Reported rabies cases among wild animals have increased markedly since 1960, when their total first exceeded those reported among domestic animals. Numbers of reported cases among wild animals have since continued to exceed those among domestic animals, although the relative contributions of those species most frequently reported as rabid have changed markedly. In 1990, reported cases in raccoons first exceeded those in skunks, and in 1991, reported cases of rabies among wildlife exceeded 90% of all reported cases for the first time, due primarily to the increasing reports of rabies in raccoons (86, 110). During 2002, cases in one or more wild species were reported in 49 of the 50 states (Table 1; Fig. 1) (80, 89).

Within broad areas of the United States, rabies infections of terrestrial animals occur in geographically discrete regions where disease transmission is primarily

Table 1. Rabies in animals and humans. United States, 2002 (includes Puerto Rico)

Type of animal	No. of states reporting cases	No. of cases	% Change from 2001
Total	49[a]	7,970	+7.2
Wild animals	49	7,375	+19.1
Raccoons	23	2,891	+4.5
Skunks	38	2,433	+6.6
Bats	47	1,373	+7.8
Foxes	29	508	+16.3
Mongooses[b]	1	67	−4.3
Groundhogs	10	49	+4.3
Bobcats	10	33	+17.9
Deer	4	9	+800.0
Coyotes	3	4	−42.9
Beavers	2	2	−33.0
Javelina	1	2	—[c]
Fisher	1	1	—
Otters	1	1	−80.0
Rabbits	1	1	−66.0
Wolf-dog hybrid	1	1	—
Domestic animals	40	592	+19.1
Cats	33	299	+10.7
Dogs	25	99	+11.2
Cattle	24	116	+41.5
Horses and mules	23	58	+13.7
Goats and sheep	7	15	+400.0
Llama	1	3	—
Ferret	1	1	—
Swine	1	1	−50.0
Humans	3	3	+200.0

[a]Hawaii is rabies free.
[b]Puerto Rico only.
[c]—, no case reported during 2001.

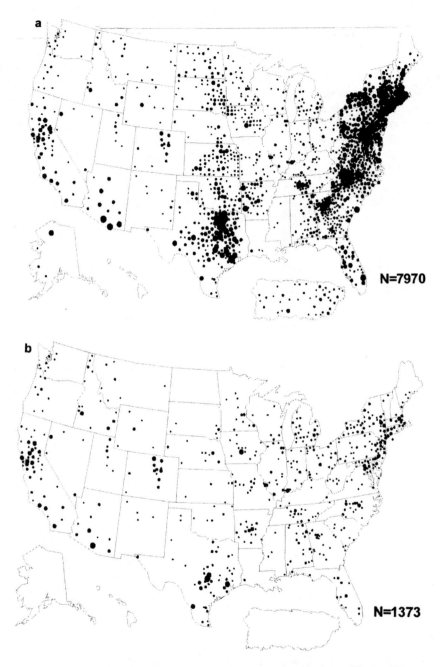

Figure 1. (a) Reported cases of rabies in all animals, United States and Puerto Rico, 2002; (b) reported cases of rabies in bats, United States, 2002. Cases are shown by county; dot size is proportional to the number of cases in a county.

between members of the same species. Spillover infection from these species to other animal species may occur within a region, but such cases are sporadic and rarely initiate sustained intraspecific transmission. Once established, transmission within a species can persist at enzootic levels for decades and perhaps centuries. Compartmentalization of the disease by species and geographic area has led to the evolution of distinctive variants of rabies virus which can be identified by reaction with panels of monoclonal antibodies (105) or by patterns of nucleotide substitution identified by genetic analysis (107). Temporally dynamic boundaries can be identified in a given geographic area both for the principal animal species, or reservoir for rabies, and for the variant of rabies virus associated with the reservoir species (Fig. 2). Affected areas usually expand gradually and are bounded by natural barriers to animal movements, such as mountain ranges or bodies of water; however, unusual animal dispersal patterns or human-mediated translocation of infected animals can result in more rapid and unexpected introduction of rabies into new areas.

Raccoons (*Procyon lotor*) have been recognized as a reservoir for rabies in the southeastern states since the 1950s. An outbreak that began during the late 1970s in the mid-Atlantic states was attributed to the probable translocation by humans of infected raccoons from the long-recognized epizootic in the Southeast (85). Although described as separate epizootics, these two outbreaks have continued to expand and have now merged as one, which includes all of the eastern coastal states as well as Alabama, Pennsylvania, Vermont, West Virginia, eastern Ohio, and most recently, parts of Tennessee (14, 47, 52, 58, 62, 63, 89, 100, 115).

Three different variants of rabies virus are responsible for disease in skunk (primarily *Mephitis mephitis*) reservoirs in the north-central and south-central states and in California. A long-standing reservoir for rabies in red and arctic foxes

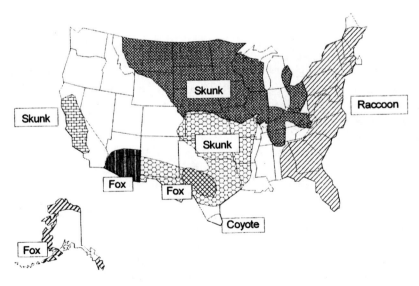

Figure 2. Distribution of major terrestrial reservoirs of rabies in the United States.

(*Vulpes vulpes* and *Alopex lagopus*, respectively) is known in Alaska. The disease spread during the 1950s to include foxes from the Northwest Territories, across Canada, and adjoining areas of the New England states. Rabies remains a persistent problem in foxes in Alaska, while reports of rabid foxes have declined in Canada, and foxes infected with this rabies virus variant have been only intermittently reported in New England. Two different variants of rabies virus are present in small but persistent reservoirs in gray foxes (*Urocyon cinereoargenteus*) in Arizona and Texas. An epizootic of rabies in coyotes (*Canis latrans*) and dogs in southern Texas is the result of long-standing interaction between unvaccinated domestic dogs and coyotes at the Texas-Mexico border (64).

Geographic separation currently allows recognition of eight distinct geographic areas, each with its respective reservoir species (Fig. 2). In each of these areas, other rabid terrestrial animals (including domestic species) appear to acquire the disease as a result of spillover from the wildlife reservoir species (105). Multiple, independent reservoirs for variants of rabies virus circulating in several species of bats overlay the distribution of the disease in terrestrial animals (Fig. 1b). Geographic boundaries for enzootic rabies in bats cannot be defined beyond the known ranges of individual species. Sporadic transmission of rabies from bats to terrestrial mammals (spillover) may occur, but there is no evidence that bats are a source of enzootic rabies in terrestrial mammals. In fact, genetic analyses indicate net differences of 15 to 20% between rabies virus sequences in bats and terrestrial mammals (88).

Raccoons account for the largest proportion of rabies cases in the United States. Since 1990, when reported cases of rabies in raccoons exceeded those in skunks for the first time (110), raccoons have remained the species most frequently reported as rabid. In 2002, 2,891 cases of rabies in raccoons were reported (59% more than the 1,821 raccoon cases reported in 1990).

Raccoon rabies is now established in all of the eastern seaboard states (as well as in Alabama, West Virginia, eastern Ohio, and parts of Tennessee) (89). In response to the expansion of this epizootic into areas previously free of the disease (New Jersey in 1989; New York State in 1990; Connecticut in 1991; Massachusetts in 1992; Rhode Island, New Hampshire, Vermont, and Maine by 1995; and Ohio and Tennessee by 2003), public health officials have been forced to allocate limited resources for public education, vaccination programs for domestic animals, and postexposure prophylaxis for humans (14, 47, 52, 58, 62, 63, 87, 89, 100, 109, 115). Despite the spread of the disease and the marked increase in the number of cases, no raccoon-associated human cases were reported in the United States until the report of a single such case in Virginia in 2003 (56). During the 1980s and 1990s, a new approach to the control of rabies in raccoons was developed, and it is now being field tested in raccoons.

Oral vaccines for wildlife have controlled and apparently nearly eliminated fox rabies in Switzerland and in large areas of Germany and France (111, 112). A recombinant rabies vaccine for raccoons is now being tested in this species in the United States (76, 77, 90, 102). The vaccine vector is the Copenhagen strain of vaccinia virus; the glycoprotein of rabies virus is inserted in the thymidine kinase region of the virus (101).

Enzootic transmission of rabies in skunks has been recognized in three major regions in the United States since the late 1960s (59). One region stretches from Alberta, Canada, south and east to portions of Tennessee and Virginia, and a second region extends from Nebraska and Missouri south to (and presumably across) the Mexican border. The variant of the rabies virus circulating in skunks in a third region in northern California is similar to that found in skunks in the north-central states. Although the number of reported rabid skunks decreased throughout most of the 1980s, subsequent increases have been noted, specifically a 37.1% increase from 1995 to 2002. Most increases are heavily augmented as a result of transmission of rabies from raccoons to skunks in the eastern United States. The last case of human rabies that appears to have been skunk associated occurred in 1981 (18).

Four human rabies cases that occurred between 1964 and 1970 were definitely attributable to exposure during recreational activities. All involved children sleeping (camping) or playing outdoors. Three were bitten by skunks, and the fourth was bitten by an unknown animal (9, 75, 78, 110). No human cases definitely known to be associated with recreational activities in the United States have been reported since 1970.

Bats are the most widely distributed wild animals in the United States. Rabies is present in at least 30 species of bat indigenous to the United States and the temperate parts of Canada, and rabid bats are found in all states except Hawaii. Although the vast majority of animal rabies cases are attributable to the dominant terrestrial species in the area, bats do appear to be responsible for isolated cases of rabies in other animals (104). Of importance in this regard is the fact that 29 of the 32 human rabies infections acquired in the United States between 1980 and 2002 were attributed to variants of the rabies virus associated with bats (22, 23, 32, 33, 35–37, 39–42, 44, 45, 48, 50, 51, 53–55, 89, 97). More remarkable is the fact that genetic analysis revealed that most of these infections (21 of 29) were caused by a single variant of rabies virus that is associated with rabid silver-haired (*Lasionycteris noctivagans*) and eastern pipistrelle (*Pipistrellus subflavus*) bats. Although none of these cases were attributable to specific recreational pursuits, two spelunkers developed rabies in 1960 (65, 83).

It is unclear why exposures from members of this order (Chiroptera [bats]) of mammals appear to pose such a rabies health threat to humans in the United States (Table 2). The number of bats reported as rabid gradually increased from the 1950s, when rabies was recognized in insectivorous bats in the United States, to the 1970s; this increase was likely due to factors associated with surveillance awareness. Following this period, the numbers of reported cases of rabies in bats remained fairly constant, ranging between approximately 600 and 1,000 per year from 1976 through 1997 before increasing to a record 1,373 cases in 2002. While not accurately known, the number of humans bitten by bats is not particularly large, and rabid *L. noctivagans* and *P. subflavus* bats are not common among bats submitted to state health departments for testing (67). While the reason that bats pose such a serious threat to humans is unknown, it is clear that even seemingly insignificant exposures to bats must be carefully evaluated (3, 40, 57). Recommendations regarding evaluation of humans potentially exposed to bats have been

Table 2. Human rabies, United States, 1980 to 2002: location and presumed animal source[a]

Date of death	State of residence	Exposure history[b]	Rabies virus variant[c]
4 July 1981	Oklahoma	Unknown	Skunk, South Central
11 September 1981	Arizona	Dog bite, Mexico	Dog, Mexico
28 January 1983	Massachusetts	Dog bite, Nigeria	Dog, Nigeria
9 March 1983	Michigan	Unknown (interaction?)	Bat (Ln/Ps)
8 August 1984	Texas	Unknown, Laos	Dog, Laos
29 September 1984	Pennsylvania	Unknown	Bat (Msp)
1 October 1984	California	Dog bite, Guatemala	Dog, Guatemala
20 May 1985	Texas	Unknown, Mexico	Dog, Mexico
15 December 1987	California	Unknown, Philippines	Dog, Philippines
3 February 1989	Oregon	Unknown, Mexico	Dog, Mexico
5 June 1990	Texas	Bat bite, Texas	Bat (Tb)
20 August 1991	Texas	Unknown (interaction?)	Dog or coyote
25 August 1991	Arkansas	Unknown (interaction?)	Bat (Ln/Ps)
10 October 1991	Georgia	Unknown (interaction?)	Bat (Ln/Ps)
8 May 1992	California	Dog bite, India	Dog, India
11 July 1993	New York	Unknown (interaction?)	Bat (Ln/Ps)
9 November 1993	Texas	Unknown	Bat (Ln/Ps)
21 November 1993	California	Dog bite, Mexico	Dog, Mexico
18 January 1994	California	Unknown	Bat (Ln/Ps)
21 June 1994	Florida	Unknown, Haiti	Dog, Haiti
11 October 1994	Alabama	Unknown (interaction?)	Bat (Tb)
15 October 1994	West Virginia	Unknown (interaction?)	Bat (Ln/Ps)
23 November 1994	Tennessee	Unknown (interaction?)	Bat (Ln/Ps)
27 November 1994	Texas	Unknown (interaction?)	Dog or coyote
15 March 1995	Washington	Unknown (interaction?)	Bat (Msp)
21 September 1995	California	Unknown (interaction?)	Bat (Tb)
23 October 1995	Connecticut	Unknown (interaction?)	Bat (Ln/Ps)
9 November 1995	California	Unknown (interaction?)	Bat (Ln/Ps)
8 February 1996	Florida	Dog bite, Mexico	Dog, Mexico
20 August 1996	New Hampshire	Dog bite, Nepal	Dog, Southeast Asia
15 November 1996	Kentucky	Unknown	Bat (Ln/Ps)
19 December 1996	Montana	Unknown	Bat (Ln/Ps)
5 January 1997	Montana	Unknown (interaction?)	Bat (Ln/Ps)
18 January 1997	Washington	Unknown (interaction?)	Bat (Ef)
17 October 1997	Texas	Unknown (interaction?)	Bat (Ln/Ps)
23 October 1997	New Jersey	Unknown (interaction?)	Bat (Ln/Ps)
31 December 1998	Virginia	Unknown	Bat (Ln/Ps)
20 September 2000	California	Unknown (interaction?)	Bat (Tb)
9 October 2000	New York	Dog bite, Ghana	Dog, Africa
10 October 2000	Georgia	Unknown (interaction?)	Bat (Tb)
25 October 2000	Minnesota	Bat bite, Minnesota	Bat (Ln/Ps)
1 November 2000	Wisconsin	Unknown (interaction?)	Bat (Ln/Ps)
4 February 2001	California	Unknown	Dog, Philippines
31 March 2002	California	Unknown (interaction?)	Bat (Tb)
31 August 2002	Tennessee	Unknown (interaction?)	Bat (Ln/Ps)
28 September 2002	Iowa	Unknown	Bat (Ln/Ps)

[a]All laboratory-confirmed cases of rabies in human beings who developed the disease in the United States through 2002. Excluded are three persons who were exposed to the disease and died of their infections while outside the United States for whom no rabies virus isolates were available and three persons who died of rabies during 2003, one of whom was infected with the raccoon rabies virus variant, one of whom was infected with a bat variant, and one of whom was infected with a mongoose-dog rabies virus variant in Puerto Rico (55, 57, 89).

modified because these and recent epidemiological data suggest that transmission of rabies may occur from minor or seemingly insignificant or unrecognized bites from bats (40, 48, 95, 108). The small degree of injury inflicted by a bat bite (in contrast to lesions caused by terrestrial carnivores) might cause it to remain undetected and unreported, thereby limiting the ability of health care providers to determine the rabies risk resulting from an encounter with a bat (2, 3, 40, 48).

The number of rabies cases in other wild animals is relatively small, although the number of such animals reported as rabid has increased markedly since 1990 because of the continuing spread of the raccoon rabies epizootic (Table 1). The majority of the 508 foxes (29 states), 52 rodents and lagomorphs (11 states), and 118 other wild animals (16 states) reported as rabid in 2002 attest to the ability of rabies virus in terrestrial reservoir species to infect other species via spillover. What appears to have been a relatively small focus of red fox (*V. vulpes*) rabies in northern New York, Vermont, and New Hampshire was in fact a remnant of the southern border of a large epizootic in Ontario, Canada, that was once continuous with the epizootic in Alaska. Unrelated foci of fox rabies associated with yet another variant of the rabies virus are found in gray foxes (*U. cinereoargenteus*) in western Texas and southeastern Arizona (105).

In 2002, 49 cases of rabies among groundhogs (*Marmota monax*) and 2 cases among beavers (*Castor canadensis*), the largest species of rodents in the United States, accounted for 98.1% of the reported rabies cases in rodents and lagomorphs. Smaller rodents (such as squirrels, hamsters, guinea pigs, gerbils, chipmunks, rats, and mice) and lagomorphs (rabbits and hares) are almost never found to be infected with rabies, probably because they rarely survive the bite of the larger wild animals that would expose them to rabies virus (61). Another important wildlife species is the mongoose *Herpestes javanicus*, which is a reservoir of rabies in Puerto Rico and other Caribbean islands (72).

Domestic Animals

Only two cases of human rabies acquired in the United States since 1980 have been attributable to domestic animals; the exact circumstances of disease transmission were not elucidated (33, 39). Although most rabies cases occur in wild

---

[b]Data for exposure history are reported only when the biting animal was available and tested positive for rabies, when plausible information was reported directly by the patient (if lucid or credible), or when a reliable account of an incident consistent with rabies exposure (e.g., dog bite) was reported by an independent witness (usually a family member). In some instances where the exposure history is unknown, there may have been known or inferred interaction which, especially for bats, could have involved an unrecognized bite.

[c]Variants of the rabies virus associated with terrestrial animals in the United States are identified with the name of the animal reservoir, whereas variants of the rabies virus acquired outside the United States are identified with the names of the reservoir animal (dog, in all cases shown), followed by the name of the most definitive geographic entity (usually the country) from which the variant has been identified. Variants of the rabies virus associated with bats are identified with the names of the species of bat(s) in which they have been found to be circulating. In some instances the known or presumed geographic locations of human beings when they were infected may rule out one of the species indicated in the name for the variant known as the silver-haired/pipistrella variant (Ln/Ps). Because information regarding the location of the exposure and the identity of the exposing animal is almost always gathered retrospectively and much information is frequently unavailable, the location of the exposure and the identity of the animal responsible for the infection are often limited to deduction. Ln/Ps, *L. noctivagans* or *P. subflavus*, the silver-haired bat or the eastern pipistrelle; Msp, *Myotis*, species unknown; Tb, *Tadarida brasiliensis*, the Brazilian (Mexican) free-tailed bat; Ef, *Eptesicus fuscus*, the big brown bat.

animals, the vast majority of humans are treated as a result of exposure to domestic animals (81, 87, 98). This results in a tremendous cost toward rabies prevention in domestic animals in the United States. While wild animals are more likely than domestic ones to be rabid in the United States, the amount of human contact with domestic animals greatly exceeds that with wild animals. This is especially true for companion species, which are therefore vaccinated to prevent them from acquiring rabies from wild animals and thereby transmitting it to humans. Hundreds of domestic animals acquire rabies from wild animals every year in the United States (~500 to 1,100 cases reported annually since 1980), which would seemingly justify the recommendation for and cost of vaccinating all dogs and cats. The occurrence of only two indigenously acquired human rabies cases possibly attributable to pet domestic animals in the United States since 1979 attests to the success of current prevention measures.

Rabid domestic animals accounted for only 7.4% of all rabies cases in 2002. Approximately three times as many rabid cats as either rabid dogs or cattle were reported, and the majority of these cases were reported from states where the disease is enzootic or epizootic in raccoons or skunks. The 299 rabid cats reported in 2002 make them the domestic species most commonly reported as rabid. In fact, although the dog is probably thought to be the domestic animal most commonly reported to be rabid, reported cases of rabies in cats have outnumbered those in dogs during all but 2 of the past 23 years. During 2002, most of the reported rabid cats were from states affected by the raccoon rabies epizootic, and a total of 32 states and Puerto Rico reported at least one rabid cat. Cattle were the second most commonly reported rabid domestic animal (116 cases), having lost their prior dominance of the 1980s due largely to the decline of skunk rabies during the same period. Most cases were reported from the north- and south-central states in areas affected by skunk rabies and from the mid-Atlantic and New England states in areas affected by raccoon rabies. Dogs were the third most commonly reported rabid domestic animal. The 99 reported cases of rabies in dogs were distributed primarily in central states in regions affected by skunk rabies, in eastern states affected by raccoon rabies, and in Puerto Rico, with Texas, Puerto Rico, and North Carolina reporting the largest numbers of cases (15, 14, and 10, respectively). Although Texas historically has reported higher numbers of rabid dogs, apparently successful intervention in the dog-coyote epizootic in south Texas has resulted in dramatic declines in numbers of reported rabid dogs. In recent years, Texas only infrequently reported animals (dogs and coyotes) infected with the dog-coyote variant of the rabies virus. During earlier years, most cases of rabies in dogs were reported from south Texas and were the result of the epizootic of dog-coyote rabies that reemerged in the late 1970s and early 1980s. This had been the only area in the United States where possible dog-to-dog (enzootic) transmission of rabies was still reported. In 2002, cases of rabies in 78 other domestic animals, mainly horses, sheep, and goats, were reported (Table 1) (89). Monoclonal antibody and genetic analyses of rabies virus isolates from rabid domestic animals have demonstrated that these animals are almost always infected by the dominant terrestrial wildlife reservoir in the area (108).

RABIES OUTSIDE THE UNITED STATES

Dogs are the major reservoir of rabies in most developing countries of Asia, Africa, and Central and South America. In these countries, rabid dogs are responsible for tens of thousands of human rabies-related deaths each year (12, 117). Rates of postexposure prophylaxis in developing countries are about 10 times higher than those in the United States, and rates of human rabies are approximately 100 times higher (12). According to surveillance conducted by the World Health Organization, of the more than 30,000 human rabies cases worldwide in 1996, 95.0% were attributable to dogs. The remaining 5% of cases were attributable to cats (<1.0%), other domestic animals (<0.1%), bats (1.0%), foxes (<0.1%), and other wild animals (<3.0%) (117). Seventeen of the 49 cases of human rabies reported in the United States and in U.S. citizens or residents living overseas during the period from 1980 to 2002 were acquired in other countries (Table 2). Eight of the patients were citizens or residents of the United States who were exposed to rabies and acquired rabies while living abroad (seven of whom were known to have been exposed to a dog in a country where dog rabies is enzootic). The remaining nine persons had come to the United States from countries where dog rabies is enzootic: one had been exposed to a dog only a few months earlier, five had been bitten by dogs, and three had no history of exposure to rabies. Of those nine people, two had emigrated from Asia years before the onset of illness; four were citizens of Mexico, three of whom were temporarily working in the United States; and one was a citizen of Ghana (51, 97, 107). Genetic analysis of the virus strains from three of these patients showed that the virus strains originated in their native countries and established incubation periods as long as 1, 5, and 7 years (106).

Travelers to countries where canine rabies is enzootic are at increased risk of exposure to rabies and have occasionally developed the disease when they failed to receive advice before departure about the risk of exposure or failed to heed recommendations regarding preexposure immunization (10). A second opportunity to prevent rabies may be missed when postexposure treatment is either not administered or administered incorrectly (69).

In addition to dogs and the wild animal species discussed above, other important rabies hosts include vampire bats (*Desmodus rotundus*) (in much of South America and parts of Central America and Mexico) and mongooses (*H. javanicus*) (in Cuba, Puerto Rico, Grenada, and the Dominican Republic) (7, 72, 91). In Europe, red foxes (*V. vulpes*) are the major host. Black-backed jackals (*Canis mesomelas*) and yellow mongooses (*Cynictis penicillata*) are important hosts in some parts of southern Africa, and wolves (*Canis lupus*) are an important reservoir in Iran and Turkey. In some areas of the former Soviet Union and parts of Poland and Finland, the raccoon dog (*Nyctereutes procyonoides*) has been an increasingly important host (60).

PREVENTION OF HUMAN RABIES

The marked decrease in the number of human rabies cases in the United States since 1950 has been the direct result of the control of canine rabies. The introduction of potent, safe, and efficacious tissue culture-derived vaccines in the 1980s served to further supplement an already effective public health infrastructure.

Education and Pet Vaccinations

Although only 32 persons are known to have acquired rabies in the United States from 1980 through 2002, tens of thousands of people in the United States are exposed each year to animals capable of carrying the disease. The most effective way to prevent exposure to rabies is to educate the public to avoid contact with all wild animals and unfamiliar domestic animals. In addition, all pet dogs, cats, and ferrets should be vaccinated against rabies, and wild animals (many of which may be extremely susceptible to rabies) should not be kept as pets (96). Because of the high incidence of human rabies and of postexposure treatments among both residents and visitors in developing countries, travelers to these countries should be advised to avoid contact with dogs and other potential reservoirs of the disease. In addition, persons at risk of possible unavoidable contact with such animals in areas where rabies is enzootic should carefully evaluate possible benefits of preexposure prophylaxis (3).

Evaluation of Possible Exposures of Humans to Rabies

Each year in the United States, as many as ~40,000 persons receive rabies postexposure prophylaxis (87) and perhaps 10,000 more receive preexposure prophylaxis. Although canine rabies has been controlled in the United States, the close association and frequent contact between dogs and humans are still the primary reasons for most of these antirabies treatments (81). Because of the fatal nature of the disease, medical personnel, public health officials, and persons exposed are almost always unwilling to accept even a minute risk of rabies developing in a person who has been bitten by a dog that cannot be observed or tested for rabies. Appropriate management of persons who may have been exposed to rabies requires reasonably rapid interpretation of the risk of infection. Each possible exposure to rabies should be evaluated by a physician, and local or state public health officials should be consulted if questions remain. In the United States, factors to be considered include the identity of the exposing species, the type and circumstances of the exposure, the local epidemiology of rabies, and, when appropriate, the health and vaccination status of the exposing animal (3).

Rabies is transmitted only when the virus is introduced into open cuts or wounds in skin or mucous membranes. Thus, if the virus could not have been introduced or the material containing the virus was dry, postexposure treatment is not necessary. Contact such as petting a rabid animal or contact with the blood, urine, or feces (e.g., guano) of a rabid animal does not by itself constitute an exposure and is not an indication for prophylaxis.

Types of Exposure

It is useful to differentiate possible exposures into bite and nonbite types. Any penetration of the skin by teeth constitutes a bite exposure. Almost all rabies cases are the result of animal bites. Although bites carry the highest risk when the face is involved and a lower risk when the lower extremity is involved, all bites present a potential risk of rabies transmission, and the site of the bite should not influence the decision to administer treatment (3, 79). Once the decision to treat has been made, however, the site of the bite often influences the urgency of such treatment.

Contamination of scratches, abrasions, open wounds, or mucous membranes with saliva or other potentially infectious material (such as brain tissue) from a rabid animal constitutes nonbite exposure. Although occasional reports of transmission by nonbite exposure suggest that such exposures are sufficient reason to begin postexposure prophylaxis, nonbite exposures rarely cause rabies (4) and are frequently unique and thus defy categorization. The limited risk of nonbite exposures (such as scratches and licks) from rabid animals is demonstrated by the unusual nature of human rabies cases that resulted from nonbite exposures frequently enough to allow grouping. Two types of nonbite exposures have been implicated in the transmission of rabies in humans: those resulting from corneal transplantation and those resulting from unusual aerosol scenarios. Eight cases of rabies in corneal transplant recipients have been reported (two each in Thailand, India, and Iran and one each in the United States and France), and they represent the only multiple instances of human-to-human transmission of rabies (3, 84, 116). Retrospective investigations found that each of the cornea donors had died of an illness compatible with or proven to be rabies. Of the four cases of rabies attributable to aerosol exposures, two were due to infections acquired in rabies research laboratories (15) and two were attributed to infections believed to have been acquired in a cave that was home to tens of millions of bats (66). In addition, two possible cases (not laboratory confirmed) of human-to-human transmission of rabies (one via a bite and one via a kiss) in Ethiopia have been described (73).

Animals Involved in the Exposures

Information about the epidemiology of animal rabies in the geographic area where the exposure occurred is essential to the proper treatment of the patient and prevention of the disease. Exposures to specific domestic and wild animal species are extremely dangerous in some parts of the country and relatively free of risk in other parts. Carnivorous wild animals (especially skunks, raccoons, and foxes) and bats are the animals most often reported to be rabid and were the cause of most of the indigenously acquired cases in human rabies in the United States from 1960 through the 1970s (CDC records and reference 71). These animals constitute the most important potential source of infection for humans in the United States. All bites by wild carnivores and bats must be considered as possible exposures to rabies; in areas where the disease in these animals is endemic, up to 60% of those animals submitted for testing are positive for the virus (raccoons [New York State Department of Health, unpublished annual rabies summary, 1993]). The signs of rabies and the period of rabies virus shedding in carnivorous wild animals and bats cannot be interpreted reliably (85); therefore, any such animal that bites or scratches a person should be killed at once (without unnecessary damage to the head), and the brain should be submitted for rabies testing. If a person is bitten by such an animal, postexposure prophylaxis should be initiated as soon as possible unless the animal has already been tested and found not to be rabid. Treatment can be discontinued if the brain tests negative by immunofluorescence.

Many types of exotic pets and domestic animals that are crossbred with wild animals are highly susceptible to rabies and thus should be considered wild animals when the need for postexposure rabies treatment is evaluated. The period of virus shedding in wild animals and the offspring of wild animals crossed with domestic animals is unknown. Such animals should not be kept as pets. When the biting animal is a particularly rare or valuable specimen (e.g., a zoo animal), public health authorities may choose to recommend postexposure treatment of the bite victim in lieu of killing the animal for rabies testing (96). Since rodents rarely are found to be rabid, state or local health department officials should be consulted before a decision is made to initiate postexposure antirabies prophylaxis for a person bitten by a rodent.

The likelihood that a domestic animal is infected with rabies varies from region to region; hence, the need for postexposure prophylaxis also varies. In the continental United States, dog rabies was reported most frequently along the U.S.-Mexico border and only sporadically from other areas of the United States with enzootic wildlife rabies. As mentioned above, rabid cats have been more common than rabid dogs for all but 2 of the past 23 years. This is possibly a result of fewer vaccination and leash laws for cats, the roaming habits of cats, and the popularity of cats as pets. Most cases of rabies in cats have occurred in states affected by the mid-Atlantic raccoon rabies epizootic.

In areas where canine rabies is not enzootic (including virtually all of the United States and its territories), a healthy domestic dog or cat that bites a person should be confined and observed for 10 days. Any illness in the animal during confinement should be evaluated by a veterinarian and reported immediately to the local health department. If signs suggestive of rabies develop or if the animal is a stray or unwanted dog or cat, the animal should be killed immediately and the head should be removed and shipped, under refrigeration, to a laboratory for rabies examination (96). If the dog or cat is unavailable for observation, other epidemiological factors should be taken into account. An unprovoked attack by a domestic animal is more likely than a provoked attack to indicate that the animal was rabid; however, evaluation of provocation and application to treatment decisions seldom prove to be of any merit because an animal's territorial nature may result in nonthreatening as well as threatening activities being taken as provocation. Bites inflicted on a person attempting to feed or handle an apparently healthy animal should generally be regarded as provoked. A fully vaccinated dog or cat is very unlikely to become infected with rabies. In a nationwide study of dog and cat rabies in 1988, only one dog and two cats that were currently vaccinated developed rabies; all three of these animals had received only a single dose of vaccine (70). Rare vaccine failures also have occurred in dogs or cats that received only two vaccinations (29). Another nationwide study (conducted in 1999) disclosed a single vaccination failure in a fully vaccinated dog that did not receive a booster vaccination following exposure to a possibly rabid animal (93).

Exposures to dogs carry an extremely high risk of rabies in most developing countries (114, 117). For dog and cat (and ferret) exposures that occur in these areas, postexposure rabies treatment should be initiated immediately after exposure; prophylaxis can be discontinued if the dog, cat, or ferret remains healthy during the 10-day observation period (3). All eight of the U.S. residents who acquired rabies while traveling or living outside the country since 1980 had exposures that were improperly managed. In each case, the victim either did not recognize the risk of rabies or obtained incorrect advice regarding treatment (17, 19–21, 34, 38, 46, 86). Although dogs are the main reservoir of rabies throughout much of the world, the epizootiology of the disease in other animals differs sufficiently from one region or country to another to warrant the evaluation of all animal bites in these countries.

Rabies Postexposure Treatment

The two essential components of postexposure prophylaxis are local treatment of wounds and immunization, including the administration, in most instances, of both rabies immune globulin (RIG) and vaccine. Extensive laboratory evidence and field experience in many areas of the world indicate that the combination of local wound treatment, including the administration of passive immunization, and vaccination is uniformly effective when appropriately administered (6, 8). However, rabies occasionally has developed in humans when key elements of postexposure prophylaxis were omitted or incorrectly administered. Treatment should begin as soon as possible (preferably immediately) after bites by animals strongly suspected of being or proven to be rabid.

The importance of immediate and thorough washing of all bite wounds and scratches with soap and water cannot be overemphasized, since it may, by itself, be one of the most effective measures for preventing rabies; tetanus prophylaxis and measures to control bacterial infection are given as indicated. In experimental animals, simple local wound cleansing has been shown to markedly reduce the likelihood of rabies (68). The decision to suture large wounds should take into account the potential for inoculating rabies virus more deeply into the wound, the possibility of bacterial infections, and cosmetic factors.

Postexposure immunization, consisting of the local and systemic administration of human RIG (HRIG) and vaccine, is recommended for both bite and nonbite exposures regardless of the interval between exposure and initiation of treatment. There have been instances in which the decision to begin treatment was made many months after the exposure because of delay in recognizing that an exposure had occurred and awareness that incubation periods of more than 1 year have been reported (106).

The first postexposure regimen to include tissue culture vaccines was one recommended by the World Health Organization in 1977. The regimen, which was based on studies in Germany and Iran, combined passive immunization with a single dose of RIG and active immunization with six doses of human diploid cell vaccine (HDCV) administered over a 90-day period.

Vaccine administered in this manner was found to be safe and effective in protecting persons bitten by animals proven to be rabid, and it induced an excellent antibody response in all recipients (8). Studies conducted in the United States by the CDC have shown that a regimen of HRIG and five doses of HDCV over a period of 28 days also induced an excellent antibody response in all recipients (6).

Three rabies vaccines are currently available in the United States; each is administered in conjunction with HRIG at the beginning of postexposure therapy. Five 1-ml doses of HDCV, rabies vaccine adsorbed (RVA), or purified chick embryo cell (PCEC) vaccine should be given intramuscularly (i.m.). The first dose should be given as soon as possible after exposure; one additional dose should be given on days 3, 7, 14, and 28 after the first vaccination. For adults, the vaccine should always be administered in the deltoid area. For children, the outer aspect of the thigh is also acceptable. The gluteal area should never be used for vaccine injections because administration in this area results in lower neutralizing-antibody titers (13).

HRIG is the only form of RIG available in this country (equine RIG is not licensed for use in the United States). HRIG is administered only once, at the beginning of antirabies prophylaxis, to provide immediate antibodies until the patient responds to HDCV, RVA, or PCEC by active production of antibodies. If HRIG was not given when vaccination was begun, it can be given through the seventh day after administration of the first dose of vaccine. From the eighth day onward, HRIG is not indicated, since an antibody response to cell culture vaccine is presumed to have occurred. The recommended dose of HRIG is 20 IU/kg of body weight. This concentration is applicable for all age groups, including children. As much of the dose of RIG as is anatomically feasible should be thoroughly infiltrated in the area around the wound, and the remainder should be administered i.m. at a site distal to the site of present and future vaccine administration (historically, often the gluteal area). The gluteal area is no longer considered appropriate for HRIG administration. HRIG should never be administered in the same syringe or into the same anatomical site as vaccine. Because HRIG may partially suppress active production of antibody, no more than the recommended dose should be given (82).

Persons who have been previously vaccinated should receive two i.m. doses (1.0 ml each) of vaccine: one dose should be administered as soon as possible after exposure, and the remaining dose should be administered 3 days later. In such cases, "previously vaccinated" refers to persons who previously have received one of the recommended preexposure or postexposure regimens of HDCV, RVA, or PCEC or who received another regimen and had a documented rabies virus antibody titer. HRIG is unnecessary and should not be given in these cases because an anamnestic antibody response will follow the administration of a booster regardless of the prebooster antibody titer (74).

Rabies Postexposure Treatment Failures

There have been no postexposure vaccine failures in the United States during the 18 years since the first cell culture vaccine was licensed; however, seven persons outside the United States have developed rabies after receiving postexposure treatment with both HRIG and HDCV. Six other people have developed the disease after receiving active immunization with other cell culture vaccines and HRIG or antirabies serum of equine origin. In each of these cases, there was some deviation from the recommended postexposure treatment protocol (27, 103, 113; R. Fescharek, U. Quast, and G. Dechert, Letter, *Vaccine* 8:409, 1990). Specifically, patients who developed rabies after postexposure prophylaxis did not have their wounds cleansed with soap and water or other antiviral agents, received their rabies vaccine injections in the gluteal area instead of the deltoid area, or did not receive passive immunization with HRIG around the site of the wound.

Primary, or Preexposure, Prophylaxis

Preexposure vaccination should be offered to persons in high-risk groups, such as veterinarians, animal handlers, and certain laboratory workers. Other persons whose activities bring them into frequent contact with rabies virus or with potentially rabid carnivores or bats and persons visiting areas where canine rabies is enzootic should also be considered for preexposure prophylaxis (3). Persons whose hobbies or vocations regularly bring them into frequent contact with rabies virus or potentially rabid dogs, cats, skunks, raccoons, or bats or other species at risk of having rabies should also be considered for preexposure prophylaxis. However, preexposure prophylaxis is not recommended for hunters and other outdoor enthusiasts who may occasionally be exposed to the disease. These persons should be able to recognize exposures and report them to medical authorities, and such exposures are rare enough that the cost of administering preexposure prophylaxis to the entire group at risk almost always exceeds that of administering postexposure prophylaxis to those who are exposed (92). Administration of preexposure prophylaxis to persons traveling to areas where rabies is enzootic is not strictly cost beneficial (10) but may be considered because it may provide a measure of protection for persons whose postexposure therapy might be delayed, and although preexposure immunization *does not* eliminate the need for additional therapy after a rabies exposure, it simplifies therapy by eliminating the need for RIG and decreasing the number of doses of vaccine needed. Moreover, in many areas where rabies is enzootic, products for immunizing against rabies may not be available or the available products may carry a high risk of adverse reactions; thus, preexposure prophylaxis might be prudent when one travels to such areas.

The regimen for primary, or preexposure, i.m. vaccination consists of three 1.0-ml injections of HDCV, RVA, or PCEC given in the deltoid area; one vaccination each should be administered on days 0, 7, and 21 or 28. An intradermal (i.d.) preexposure prophylaxis regimen was approved only for HDCV and then only when administered with a special syringe developed for that purpose and specially packaged for that regimen; the 0.1-ml dose was administered in the deltoid area according to the same schedule as the i.m. regimen discussed above (1). Routine serologic testing was not necessary except for persons suspected of being immunosuppressed. The three-dose 0.1-ml i.d. regimen was recommended by the Advisory Committee on Immunization Practices as a less costly alternative to the 1.0-ml i.m. regimen for rabies preexposure prophylaxis with HDCV; neither RVA nor PCEC *was to be given by the i.d. route* (2, 3, 30, 49). The specially packaged HDCV i.d. product is no longer being manufactured; however, information about the product is included here in the interest of completeness.

Chloroquine phosphate (administered for malaria chemoprophylaxis) interferes with the antibody response to HDCV (99). Thus, persons receiving chloroquine in preparation for travel to countries where malaria is endemic were not to be administered HDCV by the i.d. route for preexposure rabies prophylaxis; the i.m. route of preexposure prophylaxis provides a sufficient margin of safety in this situation (11). For persons who were to receive both rabies preexposure prophylaxis and chloroquine in preparation for travel to an area where rabies is enzootic, the i.d. route (HDCV only) was to be initiated at least 1 month before travel to allow completion of the full three-dose vaccine series before antimalarial prophylaxis begins. If this was not possible, the i.m. route was to be used. Although interference with the immune response to HDCV and other rabies vaccines by other antimalarials structurally related to chloroquine (e.g., mefloquine) has not been evaluated, following similar precautions for persons receiving these antimalarials seems prudent.

Persons who work with live rabies virus in research laboratories or vaccine production facilities are at the highest risk of inapparent exposures and therefore should submit a serum sample for rabies antibody testing every 6 months. Booster doses of vaccine should be given as needed to maintain a serum titer corresponding to at least complete neutralization at a 1:5 serum dilution by the rapid fluorescent focus inhibition test (RFFIT). Other laboratory workers (such as those doing rabies diagnostic testing), spelunkers, veterinarians and staff, animal control and wildlife officers in areas where animal rabies is epizootic, and international travelers living in or visiting areas where canine rabies is a constant threat should have a serum sample tested for rabies antibody every 2 years. If the titer is <1:5 (complete neutralization) by the rapid fluorescent focus inhibition test, these persons may receive a booster dose of vaccine. Veterinarians, animal control workers, and wildlife officers working in areas of low rabies enzooticity do not require routine testing and booster doses of vaccine following completion of primary preexposure immunization (3).

SUMMARY

Although widespread epizootics of rabies in terrestrial wildlife in the United States have expanded and even peaked during recent years (9,498 reported cases of rabies in 1993), there have been few human infections involving variants of rabies virus associated with terrestrial wildlife in this country since 1980. One human rabies death was the result of infection with a rabies variant associated with skunks, and two human infections were the result of rabies variants circulating in coyotes and unvaccinated dogs in south Texas (18, 33, 39). The exposures that led to these infections remain unknown; however, because it is presumed that exposures from coyotes would hardly go unnoticed, dogs are the most likely source of the latter two infections. No one recreationally (or vocationally) exposed to rabies is known to have acquired the disease since 1977, when a laboratory worker developed rabies following an accident in a research facility (16). During the period from 1980 through 2002, insectivorous bats appear to have been responsible for 29 of the 32 human rabies cases acquired in the United States, but none of these individuals were in groups known to be at increased risk of exposure. Available information is sometimes conflicting because of missing details and subsequent variable interpretations, but these 29 bat-associated cases may be summarized roughly as follows: a bite was reported in 2 or 3 cases; contact but no recognized bite was apparent in 13 to 15 cases; and no history of exposure to bats was elicited in 11 to 14 cases, although an undetected or unreported bat bite remains the most plausible explanation for the last group (3). Most of these cases appear to have been entirely unpreventable. In hindsight, however, the cases involving a definite bat bite in Texas in 1990 and Minnesota in 2000 and several cases that involved certain, unique bat contact would probably have resulted in postexposure treatment (especially following the revision of Advisory Committee on Immunization Practices recommendations) (3) if the exposure scenarios had been brought to the attention of public health officials. Although not involved in most human rabies infections since 1980, the large number of wild animals reported as rabid each year serves as a reminder of the potential threat that rabies in these animals poses to the naive camper, hiker, or other outdoor enthusiast. Persons in the United States should be advised to avoid contact with wild animals, especially bats, and stray or ill-appearing domestic animals.

In developing countries, enzootic canine rabies is the most serious threat to Americans, although casual travelers appear to be at lower risk than persons residing in those countries. Travelers to such countries can substantially reduce the risk of rabies exposure by avoiding all dogs and wild animals. Americans planning to travel to or reside in countries where canine rabies is enzootic should be informed about rabies risks and should consider and evaluate the possible benefits of rabies preexposure vaccination.

REFERENCES

1. **Advisory Committee on Immunization Practices.** 1986. Rabies prevention: supplementary statement on the preexposure use of human diploid cell rabies vaccine by the intradermal route. *Morb. Mortal. Wkly. Rep.* **35:**767–768.
2. **Advisory Committee on Immunization Practices.** 1991. Rabies prevention—United States, 1991. Recommendations of the Immunizations Practices Advisory Committee (ACIP). *Morb. Mortal. Wkly. Rep.* **40**(RR-3)**:**1–19.
3. **Advisory Committee on Immunization Practices.** 1999. Human rabies prevention—United States, 1999: recommendations of the Advisory Committee on Immunization Practices (ACIP). *Morb. Mortal. Wkly. Rep.* **48**(RR-1)**:**1–21.
4. **Afshar, A.** 1979. A review of non-bite transmission of rabies virus infection. *Br. Vet. J.* **135:**142–148.
5. **Anderson, L. J., K. G. Nicholson, R. V. Tauxe, and W. G. Winkler.** 1984. Human rabies in the United States, 1960 to 1979: epidemiology, diagnosis, and prevention. *Ann. Intern. Med.* **100:**728–735.
6. **Anderson, L. J., R. K. Sikes, C. W. Langkop, J. M. Mann, J. S. Smith, W. G. Winkler, and M. W. Deitch.** 1980. Postexposure trial of a human diploid cell strain rabies vaccine. *J. Infect. Dis.* **142:**133–138.
7. **Baer, G. M.** 1991. Vampire bat and bovine paralytic rabies, p. 389–403. *In* G. M. Baer (ed.), *The Natural History of Rabies.* CRC Press, Boca Raton, Fla.
8. **Bahmanyar, M., A. Fayaz, S. Nour-Salehi, M. Mohammadi, and H. Koprowski.** 1976. Successful protection of humans exposed to rabies infection. Postexposure treatment with the new human diploid cell rabies vaccine and antirabies serum. *JAMA* **236:**2751–2754.
9. **Bell, G. R.** 1967. Death from rabies in a ten-year-old boy (one of two cases in United States in 1966). *S. D. J. Med.* **20:**28–29.
10. **Bernard, K. W., and D. B. Fishbein.** 1991. Pre-exposure rabies prophylaxis for travellers: are the benefits worth the cost? *Vaccine* **9:**833–836.

11. **Bernard, K. W., D. B. Fishbein, K. D. Miller, R. A. Parker, S. Waterman, J. W. Sumner, F. L. Reid, B. K. Johnson, A. J. Rollins, C. N. Oster, L. B. Schonberger, G. M. Baer, and W. G. Winkler.** 1985. Pre-exposure rabies immunization with human diploid cell vaccine: decreased antibody responses in persons immunized in developing countries. *Am. J. Trop. Med. Hyg.* **34:**633–647.

12. **Bogel, K., and E. Motschwiller.** 1986. Incidence of rabies and post-exposure treatment in developing countries. *Bull. W. H. O.* **64:**883–887.

13. **Brooks, R.** 1990. Survey of the dog population of Zimbabwe and its level of rabies vaccination. *Vet. Rec.* **127:**592–596.

14. **Brown, C. I., and J. G. Szakacs.** 1997. Rabies in New Hampshire and Vermont: an update. *Ann. Clin. Lab. Sci.* **27:**216–223.

15. **Center for Disease Control.** 1977. Rabies in a laboratory worker—New York. *Morb. Mortal. Wkly. Rep.* **26:**183–184.

16. **Center for Disease Control.** 1977. *Rabies Surveillance Annual Summary 1976.* Center for Disease Control, Atlanta, Ga.

17. **Centers for Disease Control.** 1981. Human rabies acquired outside the United States from a dog bite. *Morb. Mortal. Wkly. Rep.* **30:**537–540.

18. **Centers for Disease Control.** 1981. Human rabies—Oklahoma. *Morb. Mortal. Wkly. Rep.* **30:**343–344, 349.

19. **Centers for Disease Control.** 1982. Human rabies—Rwanda. *Morb. Mortal. Wkly. Rep.* **31:**135.

20. **Centers for Disease Control.** 1983. Human rabies—Kenya. *Morb. Mortal. Wkly. Rep.* **32:**494–495.

21. **Centers for Disease Control.** 1983. Imported human rabies. *Morb. Mortal. Wkly. Rep.* **32:**78–80, 85.

22. **Centers for Disease Control.** 1983. Rabies—Michigan. *Morb. Mortal. Wkly. Rep.* **32:**159–160.

23. **Centers for Disease Control.** 1984. Human rabies—Pennsylvania. *Morb. Mortal. Wkly. Rep.* **33:**633–635.

24. **Centers for Disease Control.** 1984. Human rabies—Texas. *Morb. Mortal. Wkly. Rep.* **33:**469–470.

25. **Centers for Disease Control.** 1985. Human rabies acquired outside the United States. *Morb. Mortal. Wkly. Rep.* **34:**235–236.

26. **Centers for Disease Control.** 1985. Human rabies diagnosed 2 months postmortem—Texas. *Morb. Mortal. Wkly. Rep.* **34:**700, 705–707.

27. **Centers for Disease Control.** 1987. Human rabies despite treatment with rabies immune globulin and human diploid cell rabies vaccine—Thailand. *Morb. Mortal. Wkly. Rep.* **36:**759–760, 765.

28. **Centers for Disease Control.** 1988. Human rabies—California, 1987. *Morb. Mortal. Wkly. Rep.* **37:**305–308.

29. **Centers for Disease Control.** 1988. Imported dog and cat rabies—New Hampshire, California. *Morb. Mortal. Wkly. Rep.* **37:**559–560.

30. **Centers for Disease Control.** 1988. Rabies vaccine, adsorbed: a new rabies vaccine for use in humans. *Morb. Mortal. Wkly. Rep.* **37:**217–218, 223.

31. **Centers for Disease Control.** 1989. Human rabies—Oregon, 1989. *Morb. Mortal. Wkly. Rep.* **38:**335–337.

32. **Centers for Disease Control.** 1991. Human rabies—Texas, 1990. *Morb. Mortal. Wkly. Rep.* **40:**132–133.

33. **Centers for Disease Control.** 1991. Human rabies—Texas, Arkansas, and Georgia, 1991. *Morb. Mortal. Wkly. Rep.* **40:**765–769.

34. **Centers for Disease Control.** 1992. Human rabies—California, 1992. *Morb. Mortal. Wkly. Rep.* **41:**461–463.

35. **Centers for Disease Control and Prevention.** 1993. Human rabies—New York, 1993. *Morb. Mortal. Wkly. Rep.* **42:**799–806.

36. **Centers for Disease Control and Prevention.** 1994. Human rabies—Texas and California, 1993. *Morb. Mortal. Wkly. Rep.* **43:**93–96.

37. **Centers for Disease Control and Prevention.** 1994. Human rabies—California, 1994. *Morb. Mortal. Wkly. Rep.* **43:**455–462.

38. **Centers for Disease Control and Prevention.** 1994. Human rabies—Miami, 1994. *Morb. Mortal. Wkly. Rep.* **43:**773–775.

39. **Centers for Disease Control and Prevention.** 1995. Human rabies—Alabama, Tennessee, and Texas, 1994. *Morb. Mortal. Wkly. Rep.* **44:**269–272.

40. **Centers for Disease Control and Prevention.** 1995. Human rabies—Washington, 1995. *Morb. Mortal. Wkly. Rep.* **44:**626–627.

41. **Centers for Disease Control and Prevention.** 1995. Human rabies—West Virginia, 1994. *Morb. Mortal. Wkly. Rep.* **44:**86–93.

42. **Centers for Disease Control and Prevention.** 1996. Human rabies—California, 1995. *Morb. Mortal. Wkly. Rep.* **45:**353–362.

43. **Centers for Disease Control and Prevention.** 1996. Human rabies—Florida, 1996. *Morb. Mortal. Wkly. Rep.* **45:**719–727.

44. **Centers for Disease Control and Prevention.** 1997. Human rabies—Kentucky and Montana, 1996. *Morb. Mortal. Wkly. Rep.* **46:**397–400.

45. **Centers for Disease Control and Prevention.** 1997. Human rabies—Montana and Washington, 1997. *Morb. Mortal. Wkly. Rep.* **46:**770–774.

46. **Centers for Disease Control and Prevention.** 1997. Human rabies—New Hampshire, 1996. *Morb. Mortal. Wkly. Rep.* **46:**267–270.

47. **Centers for Disease Control and Prevention.** 1997. Update: raccoon rabies epizootic—United States, 1996. *Morb. Mortal. Wkly. Rep.* **45:**1117–1120.

48. **Centers for Disease Control and Prevention.** 1998. Human rabies—Texas and New Jersey, 1997. *Morb. Mortal. Wkly. Rep.* **47:**1–5.

49. **Centers for Disease Control and Prevention.** 1998. Availability of new rabies vaccine for human use. *Morb. Mortal. Wkly. Rep.* **47:**12.

50. **Centers for Disease Control and Prevention.** 1999. Human rabies—Virginia, 1998. *Morb. Mortal. Wkly. Rep.* **48:**95–97.

51. **Centers for Disease Control and Prevention.** 2000. Human rabies—California, Georgia, Minnesota, New York, and Wisconsin, 2000. *Morb. Mortal. Wkly. Rep.* **49:**1111–1115.

52. **Centers for Disease Control and Prevention.** 2000. Update: raccoon rabies epizootic—United States and Canada, 1999. *Morb. Mortal. Wkly. Rep.* **49:**31–35.

53. **Centers for Disease Control and Prevention.** 2002. Human rabies—California, 2002. *Morb. Mortal. Wkly. Rep.* **51:**686–688.

54. **Centers for Disease Control and Prevention.** 2002. Human rabies—Tennessee, 2002. *Morb. Mortal. Wkly. Rep.* **51:**828–829.

55. **Centers for Disease Control and Prevention.** 2003. Human rabies—Iowa, 2002. *Morb. Mortal. Wkly. Rep.* **52:**47–48.

56. **Centers for Disease Control and Prevention.** 2003. First human death associated with raccoon rabies—Virginia, 2003. *Morb. Mortal. Wkly. Rep.* **52:**1102–1103.

57. **Centers for Disease Control and Prevention.** 2004. Human death associated with bat rabies—California, 2003. *Morb. Mortal. Wkly. Rep.* **53:**33–35.

58. **Chang, H. G., M. Eidson, C. Noonan-Toly, C. V. Trimarchi, R. Rudd, B. J. Wallace, P. F. Smith, and D. L. Morse.** 2002. Public health impact of reemergence of rabies, New York. *Emerg. Infect. Dis.* **8:**909–913.

59. **Charlton, K. M., W. A. Webster, G. A. Casey, and C. E. Rupprecht.** 1988. Skunk rabies. *Rev. Infect. Dis.* **10**(Suppl. 4):S626–S628.

60. **Cherkasskiy, B. L.** 1988. Roles of the wolf and the raccoon dog in the ecology and epidemiology of rabies in the USSR. *Rev. Infect. Dis.* **10**(Suppl. 4):S634–S636.

61. **Childs, J. E., L. Colby, J. W. Krebs, T. Strine, M. Feller, D. Noah, C. Drenzek, J. S. Smith, and C. E. Rupprecht.** 1997. Surveillance and spatiotemporal associations of rabies in rodents and lagomorphs in the United States, 1985–1994. *J. Wildl. Dis.* **33:**20–27.

62. **Childs, J. E., A. T. Curns, M. E. Dey, L. A. Real, L. Feinstein, O. N. Bjornstad, and J. W. Krebs.** 2000. Predicting the local dynamics of epizootic rabies among raccoons in the United States. *Proc. Natl. Acad. Sci. USA* **97:**13666–13671.

63. **Childs, J. E., A. T. Curns, M. E. Dey, L. A. Real, C. E. Rupprecht, and J. W. Krebs.** 2001. Rabies epizootics among raccoons vary along a North-South gradient in the eastern United States. *Vector Borne Zoonotic Dis.* **1:**253–267.

64. **Clark, K. A., S. U. Neill, J. S. Smith, P. J. Wilson, V. W. Whadford, and G. W. McKirahan.** 1994. Epizootic canine rabies transmitted by coyotes in south Texas. *J. Am. Vet. Med. Assoc.* **204:**536–540.

65. **Constantine, D. G.** 1962. Rabies transmission by nonbite route. *Public Health Rep.* **77:**287–289.

66. **Constantine, D. G.** 1967. *Rabies Transmission by Air in Bat Caves*, p. 1–51. Public Health Service publication no. 1617. U.S. Government Printing Office, Washington, D.C.

67. **Constantine, D. G.** 1979. An updated list of rabies-infected bats in North America. *J. Wildl. Dis.* **15:**347–349.

68. **Dean, D. J., and G. M. Baer.** 1963. Studies on the local treatment of rabies infected wounds. *Bull. W. H. O.* **28:**477–486.

69. **Devriendt, J., M. Staroukine, F. Costy, and J. J. Vanderhaeghen.** 1982. Fatal encephalitis apparently due to rabies. Occurrence after treatment with human diploid cell vaccine but not rabies immune globulin. *JAMA* **248:**2304–2306.

70. **Eng, T. R., D. B. Fishbein, and the National Study Group on Rabies.** 1990. Epidemiologic factors, clinical findings, and vaccination status of rabies in cats and dogs in the United States in 1988. *J. Am. Vet. Med. Assoc.* **197:**201–209.

71. **Eng, T. R., T. A. Hamaker, J. G. Dobbins, T. C. Tong, J. H. Bryson, and P. F. Pinsky.** 1989. Rabies surveillance, United States, 1988. *Morb. Mortal. Wkly. Rep.* **38**(SS):1–21.

72. **Everard, C. O., and J. D. Everard.** 1992. Mongoose rabies in the Caribbean. *Ann. N. Y. Acad. Sci.* **653:**356–366.

73. **Fekadu, M., T. Endeshaw, W. Alemu, Y. Bogale, T. Teshager, and J. G. Olson.** 1996. Possible human-to-human transmission of rabies in Ethiopia. *Ethiop. Med. J.* **34:**123–127.

74. **Fishbein, D. B., K. W. Bernard, K. D. Miller, T. Van der Vlugt, C. E. Gains, J. T. Bell, J. W. Sumner, F. L. Reid, R. A. Parker, J. T. Horman, et al.** 1986. The early kinetics of the neutralizing antibody response after booster immunizations with human diploid cell rabies vaccine. *Am. J. Trop. Med. Hyg.* **35:**663–670.

75. **Gomez, M. R., R. G. Siekert, and E. C. Herrmann.** 1965. A human case of skunk rabies. Case report with comment on virological studies and the prophylactic treatment. *JAMA* **194:**333–335.

76. **Hanlon, C. A., J. R. Buchanan, E. Nelson, H. S. Niu, D. Diehl, and C. E. Rupprecht.** 1993. A vaccinia-vectored rabies vaccine field trial: ante- and post-mortem biomarkers. *Rev. Sci. Technol.* **12:**99–107.

77. **Hanlon, C. A., M. Niezgoda, A. N. Hamir, C. Schumacher, H. Koprowski, and C. E. Rupprecht.** 1998. First North American field release of a vaccinia-rabies glycoprotein recombinant virus. *J. Wildl. Dis.* **34:**228–239.

78. **Hattwick, M. A., F. H. Hochberg, P. J. Landrigan, and M. B. Gregg.** 1972. Skunk-associated human rabies. *JAMA* **222:**44–47.

79. **Hattwick, M. A. W.** 1974. Human rabies. *Public Health Rev.* **3:**229–274.

80. **Held, J. R., E. S. Tierkel, and J. H. Steele.** 1967. Rabies in man and animals in the United States, 1946–65. *Public Health Rep.* **82:**1009–1018.

81. **Helmick, C. G.** 1983. The epidemiology of human rabies postexposure prophylaxis, 1980–1981. *JAMA* **250:**1990–1996.

82. **Helmick, C. G., C. Johnstone, J. Sumner, W. G. Winkler, and S. Fager.** 1982. A clinical study of Merieux human rabies immune globulin. *J. Biol. Stand.* **10:**357–367.

83. **Humphrey, G. L., G. E. Kemp, and E. G. Wood.** 1960. A fatal case of rabies in a woman bitten by an insectivorous bat. *Public Health Rep.* **75:**317–326.

84. **Javadi, M. A., A. Fayaz, S. A. Mirdehghan, and B. Ainollahi.** 1996. Transmission of rabies by corneal graft. *Cornea* **15:**431–433.

85. **Jenkins, S. R., and W. G. Winkler.** 1987. Descriptive epidemiology from an epizootic of raccoon rabies in the Middle Atlantic States, 1982–1983. *Am. J. Epidemiol.* **126:**429–437.

86. **Krebs, J. W., R. C. Holman, U. Hines, T. W. Strine, E. J. Mandel, and J. E. Childs.** 1992. Rabies surveillance in the United States during 1991. *J. Am. Vet. Med. Assoc.* **201:**1836–1848.

87. **Krebs, J. W., S. C. Long-Marin, and J. E. Childs.** 1998. Causes, costs, and estimates of rabies postexposure prophylaxis treatments in the United States. *J. Public Health Manag. Pract.* **4:**57–63.

88. **Krebs, J. W., J. S. Smith, C. E. Rupprecht, and J. E. Childs.** 1998. Rabies surveillance in the United States during 1997. *J. Am. Vet. Med. Assoc.* **213:**1713–1728.

89. **Krebs, J. W., J. T. Wheeling, and J. E. Childs.** 2003. Rabies surveillance in the United States during 2002. *J. Am. Vet. Med. Assoc.* **223:**1736–1748.

90. **Linhart, S. B., F. S. Blom, R. M. Engeman, H. L. Hill, T. Hon, D. I. Hall, and J. H. Shaddock.** 1994. A field evaluation of baits for delivering oral rabies vaccines to raccoons (Procyon lotor). *J. Wildl. Dis.* **30:**185–194.

91 Lopez, A., P. Miranda, E. Tejada, and D. B. Fishbein. 1992. Outbreak of human rabies in the Peruvian jungle. *Lancet* **339**:408–411.

92. Mann, J. M. 1984. Routine pre-exposure rabies prophylaxis: a reassessment. *Am. J. Public Health* **74**:720–722.

93. McQuiston, J. H., P. A. Yager, J. S. Smith, and C. E. Rupprecht. 2001. Epidemiologic characteristics of rabies virus variants in dogs and cats in the United States, 1999. *J. Am. Vet. Med. Assoc.* **218**:1939–1942.

94. Meltzer, M. I. 1996. Assessing the costs and benefits of an oral vaccine for raccoon rabies: a possible model. *Emerg. Infect. Dis.* **2**:343–349.

95. Moran, G. J. 1997. Human rabies—Kentucky and Montana, 1996. *Ann. Emerg. Med.* **30**:334–336.

96. National Association of State Public Health Veterinarians, Inc. 2001. Compendium of animal rabies prevention and control, 2001. *Morb. Mortal. Wkly. Rep.* **50**:1–9.

97. Noah, D. L., C. L. Drenzek, J. S. Smith, J. W. Krebs, L. Orciari, J. Shaddock, D. Sanderlin, S. Whitfield, M. Fekadu, J. G. Olson, C. E. Rupprecht, and J. E. Childs. 1998. Epidemiology of human rabies in the United States, 1980 to 1996. *Ann. Intern. Med.* **128**:922–930.

98. Noah, D. L., G. M. Smith, J. C. Gotthardt, J. W. Krebs, D. Green, and J. E. Childs. 1996. Mass human exposure to rabies in New Hampshire: assessment of exposures and adverse reactions. *Am. J. Public Health* **86**:1149–1151.

99. Pappaioanou, M., D. B. Fishbein, D. W. Dreesen, I. K. Schwartz, G. H. Campbell, J. W. Sumner, L. C. Patchen, and W. J. Brown. 1986. Antibody response to preexposure human diploid-cell rabies vaccine given concurrently with chloroquine. *N. Engl. J. Med.* **314**:280–284.

100. Rosatte, R., D. Donovan, M. Allan, L. A. Howes, A. Silver, K. Bennett, C. MacInnes, C. Davies, A. Wandeler, and B. Radford. 2001. Emergency response to raccoon rabies introduction into Ontario. *J. Wildl. Dis.* **37**:265–279.

101. Rupprecht, C. E., A. N. Hamir, D. H. Johnston, and H. Koprowski. 1988. Efficacy of a vaccinia-rabies glycoprotein recombinant virus vaccine in raccoons (Procyon lotor). *Rev. Infect. Dis.* **10**(Suppl. 4):S803–S809.

102. Rupprecht, C. E., C. A. Hanlon, M. Niezgoda, J. R. Buchanan, D. Diehl, and H. Koprowski. 1993. Recombinant rabies vaccine: efficacy assessment in free ranging animals. *Onderstepoort J. Vet. Res.* **60**:463–468.

103. Shill, M., R. D. Baynes, and S. D. Miller. 1987. Fatal rabies encephalitis despite appropriate post-exposure prophylaxis. A case report. *N. Engl. J. Med.* **316**:1257–1258.

104. Smith, J. S. 1988. Monoclonal antibody studies of rabies in insectivorous bats of the United States. *Rev. Infect. Dis.* **10**(Suppl. 4):S637–S643.

105. Smith, J. S. 1989. Rabies virus epitopic variation: use in ecologic studies. *Adv. Virus Res.* **36**:215–253.

106. Smith, J. S., D. B. Fishbein, C. E. Rupprecht, and K. Clark. 1991. Unexplained rabies in three immigrants in the United States. A virologic investigation. *N. Engl. J. Med.* **324**:205–211.

107. Smith, J. S., L. A. Orciari, and P. A. Yager. 1995. Molecular epidemiology of rabies in the United States. *Semin. Virol.* **6**:387–400.

108. Smith, J. S., L. A. Orciari, P. A. Yager, H. D. Seidel, and C. K. Warner. 1992. Epidemiologic and historical relationships among 87 rabies virus isolates as determined by limited sequence analysis. *J. Infect. Dis.* **166**:296–307.

109. Uhaa, I. J., V. M. Dato, F. E. Sorhage, J. W. Beckley, D. E. Roscoe, R. D. Gorsky, and D. B. Fishbein. 1992. Benefits and costs of using an orally absorbed vaccine to control rabies in raccoons. *J. Am. Vet. Med. Assoc.* **201**:1873–1882.

110. Uhaa, I. J., E. J. Mandel, R. Whiteway, and D. B. Fishbein. 1992. Rabies surveillance in the United States during 1990. *J. Am. Vet. Med. Assoc.* **200**:920–929.

111. Wandeler, A. I., S. Capt, H. Gerber, A. Kappeler, and R. Kipfer. 1988. Rabies epidemiology, natural barriers and fox vaccination. *Parasitologia* **30**:53–57.

112. Wandeler, A. I., S. Capt, A. Kappeler, and R. Hauser. 1988. Oral immunization of wildlife against rabies: concept and first field experiments. *Rev. Infect. Dis.* **10**(Suppl. 4):S649–S653.

113. Wilde, H., P. Choomkasien, T. Hemachudha, C. Supich, and S. Chutivongse. 1989. Failure of rabies postexposure treatment in Thailand. *Vaccine* **7**:49–52.

114. Wilde, H., S. Chutivongse, W. Tepsumethanon, P. Choomkasien, C. Polsuwan, and B. Lumbertdacha. 1991. Rabies in Thailand: 1990. *Rev. Infect. Dis.* **13**:644–652.

115. **Wilson, M. L., P. M. Bretsky, G. H. Cooper, Jr., S. H. Egbertson, H. J. Van Kruiningen, and M. L. Cartter.** 1997. Emergence of raccoon rabies in Connecticut, 1991–1994: spatial and temporal characteristics of animal infection and human contact. *Am. J. Trop. Med. Hyg.* **57:**457–463.
116. **World Health Organization.** 1994. Two rabies cases following corneal transplantation. *Wkly. Epidemiol. Rec.* **44:**330
117. **World Health Organization.** 1998. *World Survey of Rabies No. 32: for the Year 1996,* p. 1–29. World Health Organization, Geneva, Switzerland.

Infections of Leisure, Third Edition
Edited by David Schlossberg
© 2004 ASM Press, Washington, D.C.

Chapter 11

Exotic and Trendy Cuisine

Jeffrey K. Griffiths

Fashions in food have always carried the cachet of class and trendiness, and some-times the cost of fashion is illness. As travel has expanded the locales that the trav-eler may visit, it has also expanded the range of food-related illnesses that may be acquired by the individual on vacation or on a business trip. Moreover, one need not be traveling to suffer these maladies, as sometimes they are imported to one's home given the globalization of food production. As the consumption of novel foods and the pleasures of international travel spread from the trendiest groups to society at large, the pool of people at risk for these illnesses increases. Indeed, as our societies and diets become more diverse, the opportunities for exotic, weird, and otherwise fascinating diseases multiply.

Many foods, such as seafood or dairy products, are preferentially eaten raw or unpasteurized in their most fresh and tasty form. This maximizes their potential to act as vectors for bacteria, viruses, and parasites. Some of these pathogens are well known to clinicians; others cause rare zoonoses that do not normally infect humans and may escape early recognition, and some may in fact cause newly emerging diseases. In recognition of this potential, the food industry has made some changes in how it processes foods. For example, fish destined to be eaten raw for sushi is now often frozen before consumption to kill *Anisakis* parasites. Alas, even cooked food can transmit prions, leading to diseases such as kuru, but since the ingestion of human brains is now rare, in this chapter I focus on more likely or exotic diseases.

With the current trends towards freshness and purity, there has also been a trend towards home or artisanal production of foods. Some of these, such as yo-gurt and mayonnaise, are wonderful culture media for specific bacteria such as *Staphylococcus aureus* and *Salmonella* species. For toxin-mediated diseases, cooking or heating the food (culture media) may kill the bacterium but leave the bacterial toxin to do its damage. Patterns of food storage can also predispose to disease. In

Jeffrey K. Griffiths • Graduate Programs in Public Health, Department of Community Medicine and Family Health, and Department of Medicine, Tufts University School of Medicine, 136 Harrison Ave., Boston, MA 02111.

some parts of the world, such as Africa and Asia, uneaten rice is stored overnight and eaten for breakfast. Unfortunately, *Vibrio cholerae*, the etiologic agent of cholera, has been shown (131) to be capable of increasing in number in cooked rice from 10^2/g to over 10^{10}/g during storage. The adventurous yet fastidious traveler who partakes of leftover rice for breakfast may be greatly surprised, to say the least, when this leads to cholera!

The capture or slaughter of some foods can also be risky. The recent pandemic of severe acute respiratory syndrome (SARS) caused by a coronavirus is illustrative. Molecular analysis of the SARS coronavirus has shown that it resembles a coronavirus found in civets, animals most closely related to the mongoose (38a). Civets are a delicacy in Chinese cuisine, and they are commonly kept alive at restaurants in anticipation of a gourmet's meal. SARS may have been introduced into a human population seeking the thrill of an exotic dinner. Outbreaks of Ebola virus in hunters have been linked to "bush meat" (monkeys or other primates) in Africa, and some have conjectured that human immunodeficiency virus (HIV) may have entered the human population through the same route (22a). This only goes to show that the simple pursuit of a delicious dinner can result in both personal illness and worldwide pandemics! Below I discuss the risks of *eating* but not *catching* these foods.

RAW FISH AND SEAFOOD: WORMS IN THE TIME OF CHOLERA

Perhaps no food has been trendier in the United States than sushi, in which the freshest of seafoods are matched with rice, pickled vegetables, and other condiments. Sushi is now a global mainstream food item. Originally from Japan and Korea, it has become commonly available throughout the world (I recently had excellent sushi in Nairobi, Kenya). In many cultures, raw seafoods, such as herring, anchovies, and oysters in Europe or sea urchins in the Mediterranean and Far East, have been popular. The Latin American and Caribbean dishes of raw seafood marinated in acidic fruit juices, such as ceviche, have also become widely favored. Through this spread of once regional cuisines, a number of pathogens have been brought to the naïve consumer.

Anisakiasis is a potentially catastrophic disease caused by the larval stages of marine nematodes of the family Anisakidae (82), sometimes called "herring worms." The adult forms of these parasites are typically found in the stomachs of large sea mammals, and humans are only infected by the larvae as dead-end hosts. *Pseudoterranova decipiens*, a common offender, is a pathogen of seals, sea lions, and walruses, while *Anisakis simplex* is a parasite of porpoises and whales. The larvae develop first in small crustaceans and then in fish and squid, which serve as transport hosts until the larvae are eaten by the definitive host. These transport larvae may be harbored in cod, sole, flounder, fluke, salmon, mackerel, herring, yellow corbina, sea eel, ling, yellowtail, octopus, and squid (55, 63); more than 200 species of fish have had anisakid larvae detected in them. Alas, many of these make delicate sushi and sashimi, and new aquatic hosts are described frequently. For example, American shad (*Alosa sapidissima*) from Oregon, a springtime delicacy for many, were recently shown to harbor *A. simplex* (124). Live larval forms are ingested when raw fish is eaten. Humans may be vulnerable to raw, lightly pickled, salted, insufficiently microwaved, or undercooked fish. The prevalence of this group of parasites is higher in the Pacific than in the Atlantic Ocean, perhaps reflecting the larger number of Pacific sea mammals. A recent survey from Okhotsk Sea basin fish in Russia showed that 58.8% of 9,223 examined fish had larvae of the Anisakidae (141).

The hallmark of acute anisakiasis, or anisakidosis, is sudden abdominal pain, either intermittent or constant, beginning 1 to 24 h after consumption of raw fish. Nausea, vomiting, fever, and epigastric pain are common. Not infrequently, the worm is regurgitated, ending the episode (70). Many people have gone to surgery after a presumptive diagnosis of a perforated viscus, appendicitis, or tumor. The most severe cases are apparently caused by *A. simplex*, with milder disease often caused by *P. decipiens*. If endoscopy is performed early, it is possible to retrieve the slender, 1- to 4-cm-long, larval worm in about half the cases, with immediate resolution of pain (53). A little more than half the time, the larvae will be found in the greater curvature, with severe mucosal edema (60). The parasite attempts to burrow into the stomach, expecting it to be the thick one of a sea mammal, and may perforate it. Eventually the parasite will perish in the inappropriate human host, leaving a granulomatous reaction in the stomach wall or wherever else it may have come to rest. A recent case series from Italy described the finding of anisakids in the gastric wall, the intestinal wall, the omentum, the spleen, the mesentery, and even the appendix (98). Freezing fish for 24 to 72 h at −20°C kills the larvae, and in fact most salmon served as sushi in the United States are now frozen after harvesting to decrease this risk.

With increased awareness, other syndromes associated with anisakiasis have emerged. First, there are a set of unusual syndromes, such as intestinal obstruction (134), esophageal disease in the setting of reflux esophagitis (139), tonsillar anisakiasis (9), continuous ambulatory peritoneal dialysis peritonitis (M. Ohta, K. Ikeda, H. Miyakoshi, K. Nishide, T. Horigami, T. Akao, S. Yamagishi, and S. Hirano, Letter, *Am. J. Gastroenterol.* **90:**1902–1903, 1995), and pulmonary disease (80). Respiratory anisakiasis can be accompanied by high fever and pleural effusions; curiously, in one case report, eosinophilia did not accompany the extraordinarily high anti-*Anisakis* immunoglobulin E (IgE) levels found during the disease. Small intestinal anisakiasis can be evaluated with ultrasonography, which typically reveals ascites, small bowel dilatation, and focal edema of Kerckring's folds. Giant gastric folds may be seen (94). The ascites is typically eosinophilic. In the clinical setting of an acute abdomen after the recent ingestion of seafood, eosinophilic ascites, and ultrasonographic findings as noted above, conservative management without laparotomy may be considered (52); in one study, symptoms resolved in 18 patients by the eighth day after onset when treated conservatively (125). Chronic infestation, marked by feelings of chronic ill health and abdominal pain, has been described (14). In such a case, serologic testing is often positive, and surgery is necessary for the resection of the eosinophilic lesion that (diagnostically) contains a larva with Y-shaped lateral cords. In contrast, the incidental detection of an *Anisakis* larva in continuous ambulatory peritoneal dialysis effluent (147) was recently reported, suggesting that not everyone with anisakiasis is clinically "ill."

Another emerging syndrome associated with anisakiasis is allergy and IgE-mediated anaphylaxis (28, 33, 40; A. Alonso, A. Daschner, and A. Moreno-Ancillo, Letter, *N. Engl. J. Med.* **337**:350–351, 1997; E. Buendia, Editorial, *Allergy* **52**:481–482, 1997). Anaphylaxis can occur in those who ingest cooked, killed *Anisakis* larvae— presumably after a preceding intimate exposure to the parasite, e.g., after an episode of anisakiasis (6). The overall prevalence of allergy to anisakid larvae is unknown. In one study from Spain, 14 (1.4%) of 1,008 sera showed high levels, and 47 (4.7%) showed intermediate levels, of antibody to *Anisakis* from individuals with no clinical suspicion of anisakiasis (43). It is thus not surprising that rheumatological complaints have now been identified following anisakiasis (23). Surveys of commercially important wild marine fish have frequently found that infection rates are high. One survey from Norway found that 99.6, 97.8, and 88.0% of saithe, cod, and redfish (respectively) contained *A. simplex* in the viscera or muscles (132). Another survey from the Bohai Sea, China, revealed that 5,992 third-stage larvae of *A. simplex* were found in 121 of 156 assorted fish (15 of 19 species) and from 15% of one species of squid (75). Thus, exposure to anisakid larvae must be common in those who consume these fishes. Commercial salmon farming has become common. Deardorff and Kent (29) found that all 50 wild sockeye salmon caught during their spawning migration were infected with *A. simplex* larvae, whereas none of 237 Atlantic, coho, and chinook salmon raised in commercial pens carried the parasite. Thus, for those who eat raw salmon, and especially for those with allergy to *Anisakis*, farmed fish may be safer than wild fish, no matter the potential compromise in taste that some claim only wild fish has.

Anisakiasis may be more prevalent than commonly recognized. Spanish workers have found that dyspeptic individuals undergoing upper digestive tract endoscopy have a higher seroprevalence of antibody to anisakid antigens, and this correlates well with the consumption of fish in vinegar, raw fish, or smoked fish (138). One series of 25 cases from Spain noted that all identified patients had eaten raw herring (107).

Another group of truly horrible parasites transmitted by raw freshwater fish and other creatures are the *Gnathostoma* species of worms. Adult worms live attached to the stomach walls of mammals such as felines, boars, weasels, and dogs. The eggs are passed in the feces of the definitive host, and water-living *Cyclops* species are the host for the first- and second-stage larvae. Fish, frogs, and snakes are the usual next hosts for the third-stage larvae. These animals, when eaten raw, are the usual vectors for transmission to humans, in whom the parasite cannot develop. Instead, larvae unable to complete development wander through the unfortunate person's tissues, sometimes for years, causing mayhem and pain as they search for the unobtainable (e.g., a dog's stomach) (3). It is hard to believe that the unfulfilled aspirations of a lost worm can cause such human misery.

Gnathostomiasis is a major problem in Thailand and Southeast Asia, where is it considered the most common symptomatic tissue helminth infection. It has also been described to occur in Japan, India, Latin America (including Mexico), the Middle East (25, 95), and, recently, Africa (48). Worms recovered from humans are 2 to 3 mm long and ~0.5 mm wide; adults in the definitive host are up to 5 cm in length. Soon after ingestion of the raw fish or other paratenic host, nausea, vomiting, diarrhea, and abdominal cramps are followed by malaise, chest discomfort, cough, myalgias, weakness, and migratory swellings. Most chronic clinical manifestations are related to the restless, relentless, and clinically cruel migration of the parasite through the host, and cutaneous migrations are accompanied by intensely pruritic swelling and eruptions. Concurrent marked eosinophilia, high IgE levels, and parasite-specific antibody are usually found. Most worrisome are invasions of the central nervous system (CNS) and ocular system, which may be fatal. Gnathostomiasis can cause an eosinophilic meningitis in association with painful radiculopathy, subarachnoid hemorrhage, and the cutaneous symptoms and signs already mentioned. The latter help to differentiate it from eosinophilic meningitis caused by *Angiostrongylus cantonensis*, the rat lungworm, in which the associated symptoms of *Gnathostoma* infection are not found (104, 122). *Angiostrongylus* eosinophilic meningitis is usually manifested by headache, paresthesias, generalized weakness, and, occasionally, visual difficulties and extraocular muscle palsies (64).

Concerning this disease, regions of interest to travelers, or their health care providers, include Mexico (93), Japan (56, 87), and most of Southeast Asia. The first recorded case of North American gnathostomiasis was in Mexico in 1970, and reporting of this disease is on the increase (45, 93). Most Thai cases of the disease are believed to be caused by *Gnathostoma spinigerum*. Both *Gnathostoma doloresi* and *Gnathostoma nipponicum* are well established in Japan, where wild boars and pigs can act as the final host, and fish, frogs, and snakes can act as the intermediate hosts of the former. Interestingly, recent work has suggested that small rodents and insectivores can also serve as paratenic intermediate hosts for *G. nipponicum* (97). Throughout Asia, raw carp, kokanee, ice fish, and loach are savored meals and excellent vectors for *Gnathostoma* parasites (136), and loach imported into Korea from China have been found to be infected with *Gnathostoma hispidum* (128). Thus, the indiscriminate individual who consumes the odd raw snake, frog, fish, mouse, or rat in east or Southeast Asia risks infection with the apparently equally indiscriminate and cosmopolitan *Gnathostoma*.

In 1988, 8 of 12 diplomats attending a dinner in Dhaka, Bangladesh (M. L. Bennish, C. Sullivan, and S. Michelson, *Program Abstr. 28th Intersci. Conf. Antimicrob. Agents Chemother.*, abstr. 1098, 1988), who ate a previously frozen, and subsequently marinated (pH 5.0), fish pâté developed *G. spinigerum* infection. Six of the eight developed intermittent, migratory subcutaneous swellings, and two had systemic symptoms, including diarrhea, weight loss, and abdominal and thoracic pain. Serologic studies performed at Mahidol University in Bangkok, Thailand, documented anti-*Gnathostoma* antibody titers of >1:1,600 in the symptomatic, and <1:25 in the asymptomatic, diplomats. Despite multiple courses of thiabendazole and mebendazole, symptoms and migratory swellings persisted beyond 10 months in five of the six. In a recently reported *Gnathostoma* outbreak in Mexico, everyone who ate a ceviche made from freshwater perch developed acute throat pain, chest and joint pains, headache, and fever, with edematous migrating skin lesions (34). These outbreak reports prove the point that the attack rate can be very high when infected fish are consumed. It is clear that freezing of the fish and subsequent marination in a mildly acidic lime juice solution were not sufficient to kill the parasite, although it is not known whether a temperature of −20°C was reached and sustained. Recent studies (59, 65) have reported that albendazole has an efficacy rate of >90%, and similar efficacy has been reported for ivermectin (90), yet in a recent case series from London, England, 3 of 16 (19%) patients treated with these agents required second courses of treatment (84).

The prevalence of gnathostomiasis is not well understood. The outbreak in Mexico mentioned above led to a seroepidemiological investigation. In the affected agricultural and fishing community of Sinaloa, 36% of households reported the consumption of raw fish, 35% of individuals were seropositive for *Gnathostoma*, and 12 additional individuals who had a history of migrating skin lesions were identified. Five fish species and four fish-eating bird species were infected with *Gnathostoma binucleatum*, a species found in Mexico and Ecuador. Gnathostomiasis may be a true emerging disease with far more affected people than heretofore recognized.

One may expect that with time, other parasites will be added to the list of those causing sushi-related (raw fish) diseases. Several groups have reported cases of *Eustrongylides* infection presenting as appendicitis (86, 146). This nematode is a parasite of fish-eating birds, and people have been infected by eating raw freshwater fish. Larvae are also found in reptiles and amphibians, which may serve as paratenic (transport) hosts (71, 99). Presenting with severe right lower quadrant pain and peritoneal signs, thought to be acute appendicitis, the afflicted individuals have undergone surgery and had small (~4-cm) pink-red worms recovered from the peritoneum. Three patients who swallowed live minnows in Maryland had a similar disease; in one the disease resolved spontaneously, but the other two underwent laparotomy and *Eustrongylides* larvae were found to have perforated their ceca (20). Probably even sushi devotees can be persuaded not to eat live minnows; one wonders if in the era of eating live goldfish these infections were more common.

Diphyllobothrium latum is a tapeworm acquired by eating the raw or undercooked muscle of fish. It is a big problem, primarily in the sense that it grows to a length of 20 to 30 ft. The adult worm is found in humans, cats, dogs, foxes, bears, wolves, and pigs, animals that eat freshwater and marine fish. Eggs passed in human or animal feces embryonate in water and are ingested by freshwater crustaceans. When a crustacean is eaten by a fish, the parasite penetrates the intestinal wall, where it develops into a plerocercoid, which is infectious to carnivores that subsequently eat the infected fish. These plerocercoids are 1 to 5 cm long and visible to the naked eye. Of note is the potential for worms such as *Diphyllobothrium* to cause sparganosis, a disease in which the undifferentiated plerocercoid is found in humans, instead of the usual hosts. The usual route of acquisition of sparganosis is the ingestion of raw frogs or snakes (21), or the direct application of raw snake flesh to the skin (66). Recent reports have included descriptions of ocular (12) and testicular (116) sparganosis, attesting to the variety of places where people put raw foods.

Fish species that have been found to be infected include salmon, whitefish, rainbow trout, pike, perch, turbot, and ruff (142). Areas of endemicity include subarctic and temperate Asia and Europe, the lake regions of the European Alps, the

Danube River basin, and many parts of North and South America where human immigration has carried the parasite. About 10% of people in Scandinavia are infected with *Diphyllobothrium*. Salmon spend a portion of their lives in freshwater, and fresh salmon from Alaska were implicated in an outbreak of fish tapeworm disease along the west coast of the United States in 1979 and 1980 (19). It is presumed that young salmon are infected after hatching in spawning rivers contaminated by infected bears as they are fishing. In a fascinating discovery, the existence of neolithic yuppies has now been confirmed: the analysis of human coprolites (feces) from the neolithic site of Chalain, France, has revealed eggs of *Diphyllobothrium* species (as well as the more mundane helminths *Trichuris* spp. and *Fasciola hepatica*) (13). Thus, the human association is an ancient one.

Like other physicians trained in New York City, I was taught to suspect *D. latum* infection in any vitamin B-deficient Jewish immigrant from eastern Europe who prepares gefilte fish in the traditional way. This ethnic delicacy is made with chopped freshwater fish, and the proper balance of spices can only be made as the (still uncooked) fish dish is being made. Indeed, pernicious megaloblastic anemia is sometimes caused by the special ability of the tapeworm to absorb vitamin B_{12} in the proximal small intestine. For reasons that are unclear, this complication of infection is more common in Europe than in the United States, where the worm can be found in Great Lake fish (117). Other nonspecific symptoms include abdominal pain and weight loss. Diagnosis is made by examination of the stool for proglottids and the oval eggs, which have a characteristic operculum (121). Several agents, including the time-tested niclosamide and praziquantel, are curative with single-dose treatment.

Other *Diphyllobothrium* species may well be involved in human infection. Curtis and Bylund have discussed the other species thought to infect humans in the circumpolar Arctic region (24), including *Diphyllobothrium dendriticum*, *Diphyllobothrium ursi*, *Diphyllobothrium dalliae*, and *Diphyllobothrium klebanovskii*. Interestingly, there are no reports of anemia in individuals infected with one of the above-mentioned non-*D. latum* species. It is not possible to distinguish infections with different *Diphyllobothrium* species by stool exam, as the eggs are very similar and the proglottids of the non-*D. latum* species are easily confused with those of *D. latum*. There is some evidence that the fish reservoirs for the different *Diphyllobothrium* species are separable; for example, *D. dendriticum* is usually found in salmonid fish such as salmon, trout, whitefish, and Arctic char and has never been reported to occur in perch and pike. Perch and pike are the usual intermediate hosts for *D. latum*, and salmonids rarely harbor *D. latum*.

Of note is the intestinal fluke *Nanophyetus salmincola*, which has been reported to cause disease in people who have eaten raw salmon, Pacific steelhead trout, or steelhead roe that was undercooked or smoked (38, 41). Unlike with many other flatworm infections, the majority of reported cases (13 of 20) involved abdominal pain, diarrhea, bloating, nausea and vomiting, weight loss, and fatigue. One individual reported fever. Ten of eighteen individuals examined had eosinophilia of >500 eosinophils per μl. One individual has been reported to have acquired the infection after handling a naturally infected coho salmon (49), reminiscent of the direct invasion of the human host from the raw flesh of frogs and snakes that leads to sparganosis. Diagnosis is made by examining stools for the oval, operculated eggs using concentrated fecal specimens or trichrome-stained stools. Most cases have been reported from the Pacific Northwest region, and praziquantel appears to be an effective therapy. Nanophyetiasis may be the most commonly encountered naturally occurring trematode infection in North America. Other trematodes, such as *Fasciola buski*, *Heterophyes heterophyes*, *Metagonimus yokogawai*, and *Echinostoma ilocanum*—endemic to Southeast Asia and the Nile Delta—may be increasingly found in North America after the ingestion of imported raw snails, freshwater plants, or fish and are on the increase (35).

Many lovers of sushi are aware that the puffer fish (species of *Fugu*) is highly poisonous, with high concentrations of tetrodotoxin found in the liver, ovaries, intestines, and skin of the fish (54). The toxin causes respiratory failure, paralysis, paraesthesias, numbness, nausea, and ataxia. Paresthesia is the usual early-presenting complaint, consisting of either numbness or tingling of the lips, tongue, mouth, hands, and feet, rapidly followed by flaccid paralysis and respiratory failure. Most individuals requiring respirator support recover in 12 to 48 h without sequelae (61). Even the dried fillets of the puffer fish, perhaps contaminated during preparation, can contain high levels of toxin and cause neurotoxic food poisoning (51). Recently, *Vibrio* species have been found to produce tetrodotoxin, and a theory has arisen that tetrodotoxin-containing fish and animals (puffer fish, the California newt, gobies, *Atelopus* frogs, gastropod mollusks, the blue-ringed octopus, etc.) bioaccumulate the toxin made by these symbiotic bacteria (69).

Unpleasant fish toxins probably are more widely extant than previously suspected. Sohn et al. reported a case of *Stellantchasmus falcatus* infection in a 33-year-old man in Seoul, Republic of Korea, who had eaten raw brackish-water fish; after a single dose of praziquantel and a magnesium-salt purge, 17 adult worms were found (127). The patient had had vague abdominal pain and discomfort. This mild illness pales in comparison to the acute renal failure and hepatitis suffered by 13 Korean persons who ate raw carp bile (100). All of the individuals initially reported gut upset after ingestion of the raw carp, followed by oliguria in 7, jaundice in 8, and hematuria in 10. The severity of the symptoms was related to the amount of bile ingested; all recovered with supportive therapy, including dialysis. Biopsy samples of the kidney and liver revealed changes consistent with an acute tubular necrosis produced by nephrotoxins, and those of the liver revealed changes of acute toxic hepatitis. Clearly, even lovers of sushi may wish to reconsider the ingestion of raw bile!

As already noted, ceviche is the generic name for raw fish dishes prepared in Latin and Central America. Depending upon the locale, the fish may be steeped in lime or lemon juice (and other condiments) for 24 h before being eaten or may be briefly rinsed in acidic fruit juice on its way to the mouth of the impatient diner. This dish is extremely popular with indigenous populations, and increasingly so with the adventurous tourist or business traveler from abroad. Citrus juices are added to many foodstuffs around the world, and they clearly have a protective effect against bacterial pathogens. Lime juice was found to be a protective factor during the 1994 cholera epidemic in Guinea-Bissau, decreasing the risk of infection by about 80% (109). A follow-up study during the 1996 epidemic of cholera in the same locale similarly found that lime juice in the sauce eaten with rice was strongly protective against infection (decrease of 69%) (110). Cranberry, lemon, and lime juices demonstrate at least a 5-log-unit inactivation of *Salmonella, Listeria,* and *Escherichia coli* O157:H7 in laboratory studies (89). My advice is to drown your ceviche with lime, and add plenty of lemon or lime juice when eating risky food!

Cholera

Epidemic cholera emerged throughout South and Central America in the 1990s, and it is endemic along the U.S. Gulf Coast. The world has suffered from seven pandemics since the first pandemic began in India in 1817. Cholera has been epidemiologically associated with the ingestion of raw seafood (74). It is difficult to convey how important this disease is, and how many people can be affected or even killed by it. For example, the Pan American Health Organization estimated during the onset of the western hemisphere epidemic in 1991, 322,562 cases of cholera occurred in Peru in that year alone; indeed, nearly a million cases were reported and over 9,000 people died (47). In a well-publicized outbreak of interest to travelers, 75 cases of acute cholera in 1991 were linked to the ingestion of a cold seafood salad aboard an airliner that flew from Peru to California. Presumably the salad was contaminated with *V. cholerae,* either by a handler or from the start, perhaps because preparation was inadequate to kill the bacterium. Similarly, 11 cases of cholera were associated with eating crab smuggled from Colombia into New Jersey. Episodic cases are being reported for U.S. citizens and foreigners returning from South and Central America after eating raw seafood (108). Gulf Coast raw shellfish and crabs have historically been the reservoir for a few cases per year in the United States; the risk of cholera from eating raw seafood in the more southern Americas has now become far greater and deserving of a cautionary word to those departing to those areas. With the transport of raw seafood delicacies across continents to appease the appetites of trendy epicureans, cholera may appear anywhere.

In an illustrative report, Swaddiwudhipong et al. described several sporadic outbreaks of El Tor cholera in the northern Chiang Mai region of Thailand (133). Two of the three outbreaks were associated with infected food handlers (one a butcher and one a food packer); in the other, six young men ate raw fish from a canal contaminated with *V. cholerae.* Thus, both marine and freshwater fish may carry and transmit cholera.

Cholera is the prototypical dehydrating diarrheal disease. It can lead to death in as little as 6 h after the onset of diarrhea. The key to treatment (and survival) is rehydration with fluids that contain the salts lost in the diarrheal flux. In the majority of cases, *vigorous* oral rehydration prevents death and restores euvolemia. Antimicrobials play a secondary role in the treatment of cholera, shortening the duration of illness and stopping further contamination of the environment with viable vibrios (62, 114). It is an error of management and judgment to focus on drug therapy and not on the fluid replacement needs in this disease, which can be prodigious.

For better or for worse, the profile of the modern traveler has changed: he or she is more likely to be obese. With corpulence come gastrointestinal reflux and the use of agents to neutralize stomach acid; use of such agents has been shown to decrease the infectious dose of *V. cholerae* by ~10,000-fold in volunteer studies (17). Individuals taking such agents should be warned about these increased risks, and the use of alternative agents may be prudent. Cannabis or marijuana smokers are at increased risk of cholera as well (85), since heavy cannabis users have lower mean and histamine-induced concentrations of gastric acid than nonsmokers. Marijuana-smoking, overweight travelers with reflux and adventurous tastes may run special risks!

RAW BEEF, RAW PORK, AND DYSENTERY

Raw beef and pork are famous for transmission of the beef and pork tapeworms, *Taenia saginata* and *Taenia solium*, respectively. Those epicureans who favor dishes such as steak tartare are protected in some countries by strict public health measures, but in some regions, such as Africa and the Middle East, the estimated prevalence of bovine cysticercosis exceeds 10%. In some parts of Europe, eastern and Southeast Asia, and Latin America, the rates are 0.1 to 5%. *T. saginata* infections are usually asymptomatic, though mild epigastric discomfort, nausea, vomiting, weight loss, and diarrhea may be reported. The most common complaint is the passage per anus of motile, muscular proglottids, which seems rarely to occur at a discreet time or location, but rather during public speeches, dinner parties, or similarly inconvenient events. Rarely, acute appendicitis, pancreatitis, bowel obstruction, or cholangitis may occur with an obstructing bolus of worm. Tissue invasion with larval forms of *T. saginata* is rare, and cysticercosis with this parasite is reportable.

In contrast, the pork tapeworm, *T. solium*, has a far higher potential to cause invasive disease. Though infection in humans with the mature tapeworm form is clinically indistinguishable from infection with *T. saginata*, infection with the *larval* form (cysticercoid), or cysticercosis, can be extremely unpleasant. This infection has been controlled in many countries by the mandatory freezing of pork before sale is allowed and by rigidly excluding potentially infected foodstuffs from swine feed. The larval stages of the parasite can be hematogenously spread from the gut to the liver, brain, long muscles, subcutaneous tissues, and eye, among other tissues. The cysticerci become surrounded by a connective tissue membrane and can live for up to 10 years after the acute infection. When the cysticerci die, antigens may leak into the surroundings and cause inflammation. In Mexico, cerebral cysticerci are found in 10 to 30% of patients undergoing craniotomies and in about 3% of individuals autopsied. In one series from Mexico City, neurocysticercosis was the main identified cause of adult-onset epilepsy (83). Fully half the 100 patients studied had evidence of cysticercal disease as documented by computed tomography, electroencephalography, cerebrospinal fluid (CSF) analysis, serologic testing, and (in some cases) angiography and surgical extirpation. Thirty-six of the 50 individuals had seizures, 41 had parenchymal calcifications, and 15 had two or more lesions.

Seizures, motor deficits, and visual impairment are common in this disease. About 5% of CNS cysticercosis cases involve the spinal cord. Peripheral eosinophilia is usually absent or low grade, and the CSF may be normal or show non-specific increases in protein concentration or cell counts, including of eosinophils and plasma cells. Computed tomography often shows parenchymal, subarach-noid, or intraventricular cysts, hydrocephalus, and punctate calcifications. En-hancement of the lesions with contrast agents is variable. Serologic studies are positive for only about 80% of individuals.

The therapy of cerebral cysticercosis has been filled with controversy; prazi-quantel and albendazole have been the two most frequently used agents recently (144). Steroids may be required to decrease the inflammatory sequelae after killing the parasites with antiparasitic agents, and seizures often warrant the use of anti-convulsants. Shunting procedures may be indicated when ventricular obstruction is present (31, 37, 129, 135). Vasquez and Sotelo reviewed the course of seizures af-ter treatment for cerebral cysticercosis (140) and found that treatment was usually associated with a remission or marked improvement in the associated seizure dis-order, correlating with a marked decrease in the number of cysts. While a propor-tion of cysts are destroyed by the host's immune response, scarring at the focus can lead to persistent seizures; in this study, drug therapy was least likely to lead to persistent seizures. In contrast, others have found that treatment may not alter the course of neurocysticercosis and have been more cautious as to the benefits of therapy (143). A recent consensus guideline recognized that clinical manifesta-tions of this disease are highly variable and depend on the number, stage, and size of the lesions, as well as the host response. Principles of therapy include individ-ual therapeutic decisions based on the number, location, and viability of the para-sites; the need to manage growing cysticerci with either drug therapy or surgical excision; prioritizing the management of intracerebral hypertension before any other form of therapy; and the management of seizures (42). Criteria for the diag-nosis of cysticercosis have also been published (30).

While there does not appear to be an increased incidence of cerebral cysticerco-sis in people with HIV, the lack of cellular immunity may change the expression of the disease. Giant cysts and racemose forms of the infection may be more frequent in HIV-infected persons. Delobel et al. have recently reported a case of epidural spinal racemose cysticercosis causing a cauda-equina syndrome (32).

A patient's abstinence from pork should not prevent the clever physician from considering *T. solium* infection in the proper clinical setting. Schantz and col-leagues investigated an outbreak of neurocysticercosis in an Orthodox Jewish community in New York City (118). Seven of 17 immediate family members were seropositive for the parasite, and two children had cystic CNS lesions. Of note, the afflicted families had employed housekeepers who were seropositive for the para-site or for whom stool exams were positive for *Taenia* eggs. The housekeepers were recent immigrants from Latin America and were the presumed sources of infec-tion for the Orthodox Jewish families. Even the vegetarian gourmet is at risk of neurocysticercosis!

Eating raw pork is well associated with infection by *Trichinella spiralis,* the cause of trichinosis. This disease is found everywhere in the world except for Australia and Puerto Rico. When undercooked meat is eaten, the larvae are released from cysts in the muscle tissue. The larvae move to the intestine, where they mature.

Following copulation, the adult female worms burrow into the gut, and the released larvae enter the systemic circulation and are distributed among the tissues, primarily skeletal muscle. Female worms are thought to be capable of producing about 1,500 larvae during their lifetime. Larvae enter single cells and encyst within them, remaining viable for months to years. The symptoms of trichinosis relate to both the intestinal stage and the dissemination of the new larvae into the tissues. When only a few larvae infect the host, symptoms may be absent. With heavy infections, diarrhea, cramps, and sometimes constipation result from the original infection of the small bowel. Secondary larval spread causes severe myositis, neurological, pulmonary, and cardiovascular manifestations, including inflammatory myocarditis, that can lead to death (101). In addition to the pig, larvae are found in bears, wild boars, walruses, and other carnivorous mammals. Recent data suggest that a number of *Trichinella* species can infect humans (10). Interestingly, species or genotypes from the Arctic survive the freezing of their rat hosts better than tropical isolates, suggesting a degree of adaptation to the environment (78). This means that even meat that has been frozen through the wintertime may still be infectious.

Many of the hosts for *Trichinella* are game animals, a particular delight of gourmets, especially when only lightly cooked. The Centers for Disease Control and Prevention recently reviewed its experience with trichinosis reported in the United States from 1997 to 2001. Wild game meat is now the most common source of infection, with transmission from bears, cougars, and boars well documented (113). Only 12 cases, 4 of them traced to a foreign source, could be traced to commercial pork products. For example, a recent epidemic of trichinosis in Ohio was linked to inadequately cooked meat from a bear shot in Ontario, Canada. The index patient "had eaten two bear burgers that were cooked rare in a microwave oven" (88). In another epidemic in Canada, patients with confirmed cases were more likely to have eaten dried bear meat than boiled meat (120). Dried prosciutto and other dried pork products from Europe (only recently allowed into the United States by the Department of Agriculture) are also salted. Satisfyingly, Smith and coworkers in Canada have shown that the appropriate salt curing process of these raw meat delicacies destroys *T. spiralis,* as demonstrated by rat bioassay and pepsin digestion methods (126). Recent outbreaks associated with eating wild boar meat and pig have been reported in Spain (111). In Italy, wild boar meat has been implicated in 9.4% of the 584 cases diagnosed since 1961, but it is not believed to play a major role in the sylvatic cycle of *Trichinella* in Piedmont and Liguria; none of 1,518 samples of wild boar muscle were found to be infected during the period from 1987 to 1990, whereas 14 of 608 wild foxes were infected (112).

In some countries, the incidence of trichinellosis remains high, with substantial mortality related to the migration of the parasites through the tissues. These cases represent the tip of the iceberg. For example, in Thailand, many thousands of people are estimated to have been infected with *Trichinella* in the last 30 years, and 85 of them have died. Pigs raised by hill tribes are thought to be the main source of human infections (102). The number of infected humans surely exceeds this figure by several orders of magnitude. To give some historical perspective to this study, epidemics in Germany during the 1800s were associated with mortality rates as high as 30% (46). In contrast, with the implementation of public health measures, the increasing use of frozen pork, and a trend away from home preparation of fresh pork sausage, the incidence has fallen dramatically in some countries. The number of reported cases in the United States fell from around 400 per year in the late 1940s, with 10 to 15 deaths yearly, to 57 per year, with 3 deaths, in the five years from 1982 to 1986 (7). One to two percent of human autopsy examinations of the diaphragm muscle are still positive for larvae, however. Pork products are responsible for about two-thirds of U.S. cases, with the rest associated with ground beef and wild animal meat. Cattle are not naturally infected with the parasite, and it is believed that ground beef products are accidentally contaminated with infected pork products. The number of cases attributable to commercial pork sources continues to fall, whereas the number of cases attributed to wild game (bear, wild boar, etc.) has remained relatively constant. There are marked variations in the incidence of infected porcine populations in the United States: no infected animals were found in the 3,245 sampled in 1983 to 1985 from the Midwest, whereas 0.73% of 5,315 hogs slaughtered in New England were infected. In contrast, colleagues in China have reported that the rate of pig trichinellosis is as high as 4% in some Chinese provinces (72). Many eastern European countries have had major increases in trichinellosis related to their difficult political and economic circumstances, and the breakdown of veterinary services, since 1990 (44). Alas, our gourmet friends in France were recently the victims of *Trichinella*-infected horsemeat imported from the United States, reinforcing the point that trendy foods that gourmets must fear need not originate in the developing world (68).

Special mention should be made of trichinosis in the Arctic regions, where among Inuit populations the ingestion of raw walrus and polar bear meat is common. Trichinosis in the Arctic is caused by a nematode biologically and genetically distinct from the temperate and tropical *Trichinella*, and it has been proposed that the northern variant is a distinct species, *Trichinella nativa* (15). In a variety of surveys, the prevalence of *Trichinella* in polar bears was 45%, that in wolves was 22.3%, that in Arctic foxes was 4%, and that in walruses was 2.6% (77), demonstrating the ubiquitous nature of the parasite in Arctic carnivores. Many cases have been linked to the ingestion of walrus meat, which is preferentially eaten raw among the Inuit, in contrast to polar bear meat, which is most often eaten cooked. A new syndrome has been described in the Arctic, marked by prolonged diarrhea, that is distinct from the classic myopathic form. The group that has described this new entity has presented evidence that it represents a secondary infection in previously sensitized individuals (76). Diarrhea is prominent, with >10 stools a day at the onset, and persistent diarrhea with two to five loose motions and prominent abdominal pain are common, accompanied by high-level eosinophilia.

The classic myopathic disease may begin with abdominal pain and diarrhea, thought to reflect the invasion of the gut by the adult nematode females. This intestinal stage usually begins within 7 days of ingestion of the cysts, and nausea, vomiting, diarrhea, constipation, malaise, epigastric or right lower abdominal pain, and low-grade fever are common. It is followed by a visceral stage which is manifested by fever, edema, muscle weakness, and myalgias; the last is the cardinal symptom that has been used in survey work. Chills, cough, diaphoresis, diarrhea or constipation, and pruritus may also be seen. Skin rashes, petechiae, and conjunctivitis may also be noted. Muscle pain and swelling are striking features, with the most commonly affected muscles being the diaphragm, extraocular, masseter, tongue, laryngeal, intercostal, neck, back, and deltoid muscles. Symptoms are related to the specific muscle groups affected; dyspnea is associated with the diaphragmatic and intercostal muscles, dysphagia is associated with the pharyngeal and tongue muscles, etc. CNS involvement results in generalized seizures, focal motor deficits, deafness, and encephalopathy. These neurological symptoms are seen in 10 to 24% of hospitalized patients. Cardiac involvement can lead to myocarditis, arrhythmias, congestive heart failure, and death. Eosinophilia is prominent, and elevated levels of muscle enzymes (creatine phosphokinase and serum glutamic oxalacetic transaminase) in serum are found, sometimes being extraordinarily high in severe cases. Other findings include decreased serum proteins, hypokalemia, leukocytosis, and mild elevations of hepatocellular enzymes. Muscle biopsy is diagnostic, as it shows the larvae within muscle cells. These are observed live and instantaneously by crushing the sample on a slide and viewing under low-power light microscopy. However, given the life cycle, muscle biopsy may not be positive until the third or fourth week of illness. The deltoid and gastrocnemius muscles are preferred tissue sites to sample. Stool examination is usually not helpful, as eggs are not produced by this viviparous worm, and larval or adult worms are rarely seen. Albendazole has been shown to be superior to thiabendazole for treatment, and the administration of steroids may be prudent in severe cases (119). Mebendazole appears to be ineffective (103). The convalescent stage is marked by the resolution of fever and myalgias, usually during the third or fourth week of illness. Treatment for this parasite, as well as the others, is summarized in Table 1.

Table 1. Worms in gourmet delights

Parasite	Therapy[a]
Anisakidae	Removal
D. latum	Niclosamide[b] or praziquantel[c]
Eustrongylides	Removal
Gnathostoma species	Albendazole[a,d]
N. salmincola	Praziquantel[d]
S. falcatus	Praziquantel[d]
T. saginata	Niclosamide or praziquantel
T. solium	Niclosamide or praziquantel for gut forms
Cysticerci	Praziquantel[e] or albendazole[f] for CNS disease, often with steroids and/or antiseizure medications as indicated. Surgery may be required.
T. spiralis	Albendazole[g] or thiabendazole[h]; steroids if symptoms are severe

[a]For some infections, only scanty data are available.
[b]2 g orally once in adults; body weight of 11 to 34 kg, 1 g orally once; >34 kg, 1.5 g once.
[c]10 to 20 mg/kg orally once.
[d]Unclear which regimen to use.
[e]Total of 50 mg/kg/day in three divided doses for 2 weeks.
[f]Total of 15 mg/kg/day for 1 month; some investigators believe that a 3-day course is sufficient.
[g]400 mg orally twice per day for 14 days; for some persons with AIDS, repeat treatment may be required.
[h]Total of 25 mg/kg twice daily (maximum, 3 g/day) for 5 days; for some people with AIDS, repeat treatment may be required.

An underappreciated consequence of eating poorly cooked beef may be exposure to bacterial pathogens that cause diarrhea and other intestinal complaints. *E. coli* O157:H7 is an enteric pathogen that causes hemorrhagic colitis and is strongly linked with hemolytic-uremic syndrome (HUS) and thrombotic thrombocytopenic purpura. In a classic study published by the Mayo Clinic in Rochester, Minn., it was the fourth most common bacterial pathogen isolated during a 6-month period (79). This organism produces toxins structurally and functionally similar to the prototypical Shiga toxin of *Shigella dysenteriae* type 1 (91); however, it is not enteroinvasive and does not produce the heat-labile or heat-stable enterotoxins associated with enterotoxigenic *E. coli*. Wells and colleagues investigated several outbreaks of HUS associated with raw-milk consumption in the United States and found that enterohemorrhagic *E. coli* (EHEC) organisms such as O157:H7 could be isolated from local dairy cattle (heifers and calves), milk samples, and raw beef samples (142a). Similar results have been obtained in Canada (105), where 10.4% of 225 beef samples were culture positive and where 26.4% of the samples harbored bacteria producing the cytotoxin, based upon cytotoxicity assays. Thus, EHEC is present in the food chain (specifically in cattle and dairy products) in areas where HUS occurs.

The direct association between HUS and infection with *E. coli* O157:H7 has been illuminated by several studies. Chart and colleagues found serologic evidence for infection in 44 of 60 patients with HUS and in none of 16 controls (22). Tarr and coworkers have published clear-cut evidence that the timing of initial stool cultures in cases of postdysenteric HUS in the United States directly affects the likelihood of isolating *E. coli* O157:H7 from the stool, with the highest success rate in the first 6 days of diarrheal illness (137). Thus, the pathogen that is linked epidemiologically with HUS is present in dairy cattle and in raw or undercooked meat. The magnitude of the problem is not yet known, as it is now recognized that children with hemorrhagic colitis routinely develop a spectrum of coagulation disorders related to the infection, and only a fraction develop overt HUS (92). HUS due to *E. coli* O157:H7 remains the most common cause of acute renal failure in children in the United States. The bloody hamburger enjoyed by many is, unhappily, ubiquitously at risk of containing *E. coli* O157:H7 (2).

Treatment of *E. coli* O157:H7 infections with antibiotics is controversial. Experimental evidence suggests that antibiotic treatment *increases* the release of the miscreant toxin from *E. coli* O157:H7 and leads to death in mice (148). No studies have shown that antibiotic treatment alters the course of the disease. A meta-analysis suggesting that treatment may not cause adverse events has been the subject of no little controversy (115). I do not treat *E. coli* O157:H7 infections with antibiotics.

Salmonella, ubiquitously present in animals of commercial food importance such as fowl and cattle, and in some household pets such as turtles, is discussed in chapters 7 and 8.

STEAK TARTARE AND TOXOPLASMOSIS

While McDonald's, Burger King, and Wendy's hamburgers have unintentionally been vehicles for EHEC, *Salmonella*, and other organisms and are the essence of Americana, they are not the trendiest of foodstuffs. Hence, I turn to steak tartare, a flavorful concoction of raw chopped beef, raw egg, onion, capers, and a vinaigrette. Unfortunately, other things get into steak tartare, including *Toxoplasma gondii*, the etiologic agent of toxoplasmosis. *T. gondii* is an obligate intracellular parasite found throughout the world. Infection with the parasite is followed by dissemination into the tissues, most often including the brain, heart, and skeletal muscle. Encysted *Toxoplasma* is usually asymptomatic, and chronic silent infection is the rule. The acute symptomatic infection is less common, accounting for 10 to 20% of infections in adults. Though symptomatic infection is usually benign and self-limiting, and often resembles an infectious mononucleosis-like syndrome, the severe end of the spectrum of clinical manifestations includes myocarditis, pneumonitis, and meningoencephalitis.

The definitive hosts for *Toxoplasma* are felines, in which both an enteroepithelial cycle and an extraintestinal cycle occur; in contrast, only the extraintestinal cycle occurs in other mammalian, avian, and saurian hosts. Tachyzoites are the form found in tissues during acute infection and invade all mammalian cells except red cells. Tissue cysts developing within host muscle cells are the infectious form eaten by epicureans ingesting raw meat. The intestinal digestive juices (peptic and tryptic) disrupt the cyst wall, liberating the tachyzoites, which invade gut enterocytes. From this focus the parasites disseminate systemically using lymphatic or hematogenous routes, usually setting up new foci in the brain, heart, and skeletal muscle, although all tissues can be affected. Once new tissue cysts develop in the newly infected host, these persistent forms may serve as a source of recrudescent disseminated disease, especially in the immunosuppressed. In felines (members of the family Felidae), parasites which infect gut cells go through both an asexual cycle (schizogony) and a sexual cycle (gametogony), leading to the development of oocysts, which are excreted in feces. The intestinal cycle in cats occurs primarily in young animals and for a limited period, with eventual resolution. Oocysts are hardy, environmentally resistant forms that can survive in warm, moist soil for months to a year. Ingestion of oocysts also causes infection in humans.

Infection is usually acquired by eating food with infectious tissue cysts, by ingesting infectious oocysts, or transplacentally. Rare cases have been reported of infection via contaminated water, transfusion, and transplantation and through laboratory accidents. The prevalence of cysts in raw beef is not well studied; according to Remington and McLeod (106), approximately 10% of lamb and 25% of pork is infected. In a recent study, viable *T. gondii* was isolated from 51 of 55 Massachusetts pigs destined for human consumption; 2 of the infected pigs were seronegative by the Sabin-Feldman dye test, the modified agglutination test, and Western blotting (36)! In the United States and Europe, the highest rates of seropositivity in humans are in young adults, which is thought to be secondary to eating undercooked pork, lamb, or beef. In contrast, in countries such as Burundi, Panama, and Somalia, undercooked meat is rarely eaten (especially pork), and there is widespread environmental contamination with oocysts. Infection is often acquired in early childhood, and children have the highest seropositivity rates (5, 39, 130).

Toxoplasmosis has always been of major public health importance because of the congenital disease that can occur (see below). This concern has increased considerably in the AIDS era. In countries such as Finland and Slovenia, where the prevalence of *Toxoplasma* antibody in adults is relatively low, the incidence of infection during pregnancy is around 3 per 1,000 pregnancies (67, 73), comparable to the range of 2.5 to 5.5 cases per 1,000 pregnancies in studies conducted in the United Kingdom (4). In contrast, in countries where raw meat is favored—such as France (58), Germany, Pakistan (8), Turkey (18), and Sudan (1)—the *Toxoplasma* antibody seropositivity rate is high, as is the seroconversion rate during pregnancy, and it poses more of a public health problem. In screening studies in Paris conducted between October 1981 and September 1983, the standardized prevalence rate in pregnant French women was 71% ± 4%, compared to 51% ± 5% in immigrant women, and the incidence of seroconversion in nonimmune pregnant women was estimated to be 1.6% (123)!

The rate of congenital toxoplasmosis infection is ~1 in 12,000 live births, based on 14 years of newborn screening data in Massachusetts. Interestingly, the odds ratios for infection are increased if the mother's educational level is that of a college graduate or higher (57). Since education is linked to income, this may be an indication that people who ingest trendy cuisines really are at elevated risk of this disease!

The usual infection in a child or adult results in a mononucleosis-like syndrome, with the most frequent manifestation being lymphadenopathy. Any and all lymph nodes can be involved; with involvement of the abdominal group, abdominal pain and fever can be dominant. The lymph nodes become enlarged and firm but do not suppurate. Other manifestations include hepatitis and hepatosplenomegaly, myalgias and arthralgias, urticaria and a maculopapular rash that spares the palms and soles, confusion, headache, and meningismus. These symptoms and signs usually resolve without specific therapy—and indeed are rarely recognized as being toxoplasmosis—in the healthy host. Unhappily, in some individuals more severe disease may be seen: hepatitis, pneumonitis, meningoencephalitis or encephalitis, pericarditis or myocarditis, and polymyositis.

Special mention of ocular and CNS disease should be made. Acute chorioretinitis can produce epiphora, photophobia, scotomata, pain, and blurred vision; if the macula is involved, central vision may be lost. In congenital disease, strabismus, nystagmus, anisometropia, cataracts, small cornea, and microophthalmia may result. In infants, the only site of clinically overt infection may be the eyes, and examination by an ophthalmologist is important; chronic infection and inflammation can cause scarring, vision loss, and optic nerve atrophy. In contrast, in AIDS patients significant inflammatory changes are less common, and necrotic eye disease is caused by the direct effects of the parasite.

CNS disease mainly occurs in two groups: the congenitally infected and those with HIV infection. Women who become infected while pregnant have an increased risk of transmitting the parasite to the fetus the nearer they are to term; however, the disease is most severe in the first trimester, less so in the second trimester, and rarely problematic in the third trimester. The parasites cause irremediable CNS and ocular disease in the still-developing early fetus, whereas damage to other organs and tissues can often be compensated for. Congenital infection can cause protean manifestations in newborns, affecting all organ systems.

In those with signs of active infection at birth, deafness, mental retardation, epilepsy, spasticity, palsies, and blindness may occur. Chorioretinitis occurs in about half of congenitally infected children, including the asymptomatic, and less commonly mental or physical retardation, epilepsy, blindness, and strabismus may result. In a study of 23,000 pregnancies (123), children born to highly seropositive (antibody titer of 256 to 512) mothers had a 60% increase in microcephaly, a 30% increase in low intelligence quotient (<70), and a doubling in the rate of deafness. In a subgroup of women with high indirect-hemagglutination antibody levels or seroconversions with IgM, there were 15 pregnancies: two children had congenital toxoplasmosis, and three were stillborn.

In individuals with AIDS, the most common manifestation of toxoplasmosis is recrudescent disease of the brain from old, formerly silent cysts. Acute infection does occur in regions of high prevalence and can result in a protean disseminated disease. The latter is often fulminant and rapidly fatal, but it is less common than the typical CNS presentation. In these patients, symptoms and signs of CNS toxoplasmosis are related to the mass lesions, meningoencephalitis, and encephalopathy that occur; thus, seizures, fever, focal neurological deficits, and headache are common. The basal ganglia are most often affected, followed by the frontal, parietal, and occipital lobes; the cerebellum is not often involved. Magnetic resonance imaging is even more sensitive than contrast-enhanced computed tomography for the detection of lesions. The CSF is usually abnormal, although a lumbar puncture may be contraindicated if cerebral edema exists. CNS toxoplasmosis is the most common CNS opportunistic infection in AIDS patients in the developed world (81). It is uniformly fatal if not treated.

There is evidence that treatment of pregnant women with acute toxoplasmosis leads to reduced risk of disease in the fetus. Daffos and colleagues (26) in Paris reported their experience using pyrimethamine and sulfa drugs in 15 women, in a cohort of 746, who developed acute toxoplasmosis in pregnancy and carried their infants to term. Of the 15 infants, 2 had chorioretinitis and the others remained clinically well during follow-up. Members of this group have published another study in which 52 women with *Toxoplasma* infection acquired during pregnancy were treated with spiramycin and monitored to term; 54 live infants were born. Forty-three of the 52 women were also treated with pyrimethamine and sulfonamides. Only one infant had severe congenital toxoplasmosis, and this child was the result of one of the nine pregnancies not additionally treated with pyrimethamine and sulfa. The researchers recommended that spiramycin be started as soon as the diagnosis of maternal *Toxoplasma* infection during pregnancy was proven or strongly suspected (50). It is less clear whether postnatal treatment of the congenitally infected infant is as helpful. Wilson and Remington have published suggested treatment regimens for toxoplasmosis in pregnant women and congenitally infected infants which incorporate their own experience with that of Jacques Couvreur at the Institut de Puériculture in Paris (145). It is recommended that sulfa drugs be avoided in the first trimester of pregnancy and at term, the latter related to the risk of kernicterus. Prenatal diagnosis of congenital toxoplasmosis using PCR tests of amniotic fluid may prove helpful (106); European workers have now reported that PCR diagnosis using amniotic fluid is as reliable as amniocentesis and fetal blood sampling (F. Forestier, P. Hohlfeld, Y. Sole, and F. Daffos, Letter, *Prenatal Diagn.* **18:**407–409, 1998).

In individuals with AIDS, a number of treatment regimens have been recognized as efficacious. The standard of treatment is pyrimethamine plus either sulfadiazine or clindamycin. Trimethoprim-sulfamethoxazole and pyrimethamine plus either clarithromycin, azithromycin, atovaquone, or dapsone are also efficacious in human trials or in in vitro and in vivo experiments (27, 106). Regimens such as trimethoprim-sulfamethoxazole, pyrimethamine-dapsone, and sulfadoxine-pyrimethamine provide prophylaxis against the development of clinical disease in individuals seropositive for both *Toxoplasma* and HIV (76). Recent studies have also shown pyrimethamine plus azithromycin to be an acceptable alternative to pyrimethamine plus sulfadiazine for ocular disease (11). Treatment regimens are summarized in Table 2.

There is no evidence that treatment is appropriate for the healthy individual with asymptomatic or mildly symptomatic toxoplasmosis.

UNPASTEURIZED MILK PRODUCTS

Unpasteurized milk products have always enjoyed a reputation for having a slightly fresher taste and aroma than their pasteurized cousins. Although unpasteurized milk has previously been used chiefly by the poor, many of the famous local cheeses of Europe can only be made, in the opinion of the local artisans, with unpasteurized milk, and this belief has been accepted on the far side of the Atlantic. Indeed, I often enjoy a glass of wine with locally produced, no doubt disease-ridden cheese of artisanal production. Pathogens that can be acquired from eating unpasteurized food products include *Mycobacterium bovis, Mycobacterium tuberculosis, Listeria monocytogenes, Salmonella* species, *Campylobacter jejuni, Yersinia enterocolitica, Brucella abortus,* and *Streptococcus zooepidemicus;* the toxin-mediated diseases caused by *E. coli* and *S. aureus* can also be acquired this way (2).

TURISTA

Travel expands the mind, and loosens the bowels.

Anonymous

"Turista" is a term that can be used to describe an affliction of the traveler: diarrhea. It is instructive to reflect upon the fact that foreigners who visit developed countries such as the United States also suffer from diarrhea; in other words, one needs to adapt to the indigenous bacterial and viral flora and fauna wherever one might travel.

In some studies, up to 98% of travelers, many of whom indulge in eating delicious but unhealthfully raw foods, developed diarrhea during a lengthy trip abroad. In addition to the usual viral offenders, a number of bacteria can wreak havoc with the traveler's bowels: in most studies, enterotoxigenic *E. coli* is high on the list, followed by *Salmonella, Campylobacter,* and *Shigella* species. Avoidance of

Table 2. Therapy for toxoplasmosis

Host characteristics	Therapy
Pregnant women	
Acute disease, first 18 wk of pregnancy, or at any time if fetal infection is excluded[a]	Spiramycin, 1 g orally 3 times daily. If fetal infection is documented at 18–20 wk by amniocentesis and PCR, begin pyrimethamine, sulfadiazine, and folinic acid (leucovorin) as outlined below. If infection is excluded, spiramycin may be continued to term.
Fetal infection confirmed after 17th wk of gestation or maternal infection acquired late in pregnancy	Pyrimethamine[b] + sulfadiazine[c] + folinic acid[d]
Congenital infection	
Infants without AIDS	Pyrimethamine[e] + sulfadiazine[f] + folinic acid[g] for 1 yr; some treat with this combination for 6 mo and then alternate monthly with spiramycin. If active chorioretinitis is present or CSF protein level is ≥1 g/dl, use steroids.[h]
Infants with AIDS	As for infants without AIDS; duration of therapy is unknown
Chorioretinitis in healthy older children or adults	Pyrimethamine, sulfadiazine, and folinic acid as for pregnant women until 1–2 wk after resolution, + steroids[h]
Life-threatening organ damage in healthy children or adults	Pyrimethamine, sulfadiazine, and folinic acid as for pregnant women, with duration of 4–6 wk or until 1–2 wk after symptoms and signs of infection are resolved. No indication for steroids unless chorioretinitis or CSF inflammation is present.
Immunocompromised children or adults (e.g., transplantation patients)	Pyrimethamine, sulfadiazine, and folinic acid as for chorioretinitis in healthy older children or adults, with a duration of 4–6 wk beyond resolution of symptoms and signs of infection; no steroids
AIDS patients (active treatment)	Pyrimethamine, sulfadiazine, and folinic acid as for chorioretinitis in healthy children and adults, to be continued indefinitely. Clindamycin[i] may replace sulfadiazine for adults (unclear for children). Other agents that may be useful and replace sulfadiazine in this regimen include azithromycin, atovaquone, dapsone, and clarithromycin. Steroids should be used only if there is evidence of cerebral edema. Another alternative regimen is trimethoprim-sulfamethoxazole.[j]

[a] Avoid sulfa drugs in first trimester; avoid them just before birth of infant, unless in combination with pyrimethamine and folinic acid for treatment of congenital infection.
[b] 50 mg twice daily for 2 days and then once daily thereafter; for adult patients with AIDS, 50 to 75 mg/day.
[c] 100 mg/kg/day in two to four divided doses (maximum, 4 g/day).

raw salads, food that is cold or has cooled, and ice cubes when in a hot and tropical clime is indeed difficult but is important nonetheless in avoiding the trots. Cholera has been thankfully rare among healthy, well-nourished travelers. However, as the world pandemic spreads and involves regions frequented by pleasure seekers, more malignant and profuse turista can be expected to occur.

Many of the foodstuffs discussed in this chapter can act as vectors of a diarrheal disease; I only wish to make a few personal suggestions. First, I do not recommend prophylactic drug treatment in the absence of diarrhea but do suggest the avoidance of risky foods, the use of only boiled or bottled beverages (preferably fine wines, of course, but carbonated water will do in a pinch), and, when appropriate, the use of prophylactic bismuth subsalicylate. When diarrhea is persistent, bloody, or associated with fever, I currently utilize empirical therapy with ciprofloxacin or azithromycin. I suggest these drugs because many of the pathogens around the world are resistant to drugs such as trimethoprim-sulfamethoxazole, ampicillin, and tetracycline, and untreated or mistreated shigellosis is not a mild disease.

The importance of turista should not be underestimated; through the ages, nasty tourists have died from turista—the Visigoths at the gates of Rome and the Imperial French army in Haiti after the slave revolt immediately come to mind. Great literature, such as *Love in the Time of Cholera* and *The Horseman on the Roof* (also about a cholera epidemic), may have been conceived by fertile writers after particularly bad cases of turista.

SUMMARY

You can get an unbelievable number of gross and unpleasant diseases by eating raw or contaminated foods, most of which are delicious and delightful. Enjoy!

REFERENCES

1. **Abdel-Hameed, A. A.** 1991. Sero-epidemiology of toxoplasmosis in Gezira. *Sudan J. Trop. Med. Hyg.* **94:**329–332.
2. **Acheson, D. W. K., and R. K. Levinson.** 1998. *Safe Eating: Protect Yourself against E. coli, Salmonella, and Other Deadly Food-Borne Pathogens.* Dell Publishing Co., New York, N.Y.
3. **Adame, J., and P. R. Cohen.** 1996. Eosinophilic panniculitis: diagnostic considerations and evaluation. *J. Am. Acad. Dermatol.* **34**(2 Pt. 1):229–234.
4. **Ades, A. E.** 1992. Methods for estimating the incidence of primary infection in pregnancy: a reappraisal of toxoplasmosis and cytomegalovirus data. *Epidemiol. Infect.* **108:**367–375.

---

[d]5 to 20 mg/day, adjusted for anemia, thrombocytopenia, or granulocytopenia; blood counts must be monitored.
[e]2 mg/kg/day for 2 days and then 1 mg/kg/day.
[f]100 mg/kg/day in two to four divided doses daily.
[g]5 to 10 mg/day, adjusted for anemia, thrombocytopenia, or granulocytopenia; blood counts must be monitored.
[h]1 mg of prednisone per kg per day, or equivalent. Steroids should be used until high CSF protein level or chorioretinitis has subsided and should then be tapered and discontinued; use only with pyrimethamine-sulfadiazine-folinic acid regimens.
[i]600 to 1,200 mg every 6 h, orally or intravenously.
[j]5-mg/kg trimethoprim portion every 6 h, orally or intravenously.

5. **Ahmed, H. J., H. H. Mohammed, M. W. Yusus, S. F. Ahmed, and G. Huldt.** 1988. Human toxoplasmosis in Somalia. Prevalence of *Toxoplasma* antibodies in a village in the lower Scebelli region and in Mogadishu. *Trans. R. Soc. Trop. Med. Hyg.* **82:**330–332.

6. **Audicana, M. T., I. J. Ansotegui, L. F. de Corres, and M. W. Kennedy.** 2002. Anisakis simplex: dangerous—dead and alive? *Trends Parasitol.* **18:**20–25.

7. **Bailey, T. M., and P. M. Schantz.** 1990. Trends in the incidence and transmission patterns of trichinosis in humans in the United States: comparisons of the periods 1975–1981 and 1982–1986. *Rev. Infect. Dis.* **12:**5–11.

8. **Bari, A., and G. A. Khan.** 1990. Toxoplasmosis among pregnant women in northern parts of Pakistan. *J. Pakistani Med. Assoc.* **40:**288–289.

9. **Bhargava, D., R. Raman, M. Z. El Azzouni, K. Bhargava, and B. Bhusnurmath.** 1996. Anisakiasis of the tonsils. *J. Laryngol. Otol.* **110:**387–388.

10. **Bolas-Fernandez, F.** 2003. Biological variation in Trichinella species and genotypes. *J. Helminthol.* **77**(2):111–118.

11. **Bosch-Driessen, L. H., F. D. Verbraak, M. S. Suttorp-Schulten, R. L. van Ruyven, A. M. Klok, C. B. Hoyng, and A. Rothova.** 2002. A prospective, randomized trial of pyrimethamine and azithromycin vs. pyrimethamine and sulfadiazine for the treatment of ocular toxoplasmosis. *Am. J. Ophthalmol.* **134:**34–40.

12. **Botterel, F., and P. Bouree.** 2003. Ocular sparganosis: a case report. *J. Travel Med.* **10:**245–246.

13. **Bouchet, F., P. Petrequin, J. C. Paicheler, and S. Dommelier.** 1995. First paleoparasitologic approach of the neolithic site in Chalain (Jura, France). *Bull. Soc. Pathol. Exot.* **88:**265–268. (In French.)

14. **Bouree, P., A. Paugam, and J. C. Petithory.** 1995. Anisakidosis: report of 25 cases and review of the literature. *Comp. Immunol. Microbiol. Infect. Dis.* **18:**75–84.

15. **Britov, V. A., and S. N. Boev.** 1972. Taxonomic rank of various strains of *Trichinella* and their circulation in nature. *Vestn. Akad. Med. Nauk SSSR* **28:**27–32.

16. **Carr, A., B. Tindall, B. J. Brew, D. J. Marriott, J. L. Harkness, R. Penny, and D. A. Cooper.** 1992. Low-dose trimethoprim-sulfamethoxazole prophylaxis for toxoplasmic encephalitis in patients with AIDS. *Ann. Intern. Med.* **117:**106–111.

17. **Cash, R. A., S. I. Music, J. P. Libonati, M. J. Snyder, R. P. Wenzel, and R. P. Hornick.** 1974. Response of man to infection with *Vibrio cholerae*. I. Clinical, serologic, and bacteriologic responses to a known inoculum. *J. Infect. Dis.* **129:**45–52.

18. **Cengir, S. D., F. Ortac, and F. Soylemez.** 1992. Treatment and results of chronic toxoplasmosis. Analysis of 33 cases. *Gynecol. Obstet. Investig.* **33:**105–108.

19. **Centers for Disease Control.** 1981. Diphyllobothriasis associated with salmon—United States. *Morb. Mortal. Wkly. Rep.* **30:**331–332, 337–338.

20. **Centers for Disease Control.** 1982. Intestinal perforation caused by larval *Eustrongylides*—Maryland. *Morb. Mortal. Wkly. Rep.* **31:**383–384, 389.

21. **Chang, K. H., J. G. Chi, S. Y. Cho, M. H. Han, D. H. Han, and M. C. Han.** 1992. Cerebral sparganosis: analysis of 34 cases with emphasis on CT features. *Neuroradiology* **34:**1–8.

22. **Chart, H., H. R. Smith, S. M. Scotland, B. Rowe, D. V. Milford, and C. M. Taylor.** 1991. Serological identification of *Escherichia coli* O157:H7 infection in haemolytic uraemic syndrome. *Lancet* **337:**138–140.

22a. **Courgnaud, V., S. Van Dooren, F. Liegeois, X. Pourrut, B. Abela, S. Loul, E. Mpoudi-Ngole, A. Vandamme, E. Delaporte, and M. Peeters.** 2004. Simian T-cell leukemia virus (STLV) infection in wild primate populations in Cameroon: evidence for dual STLV type 1 and type 3 infection in agile mangabeys (*Cercocebus agilis*). *J. Virol.* **78:**4700–4709.

23. **Cuende, E., M. T. Audicana, M. Garcia, M. Anda, L. Fernandez Corres, C. Jimenez, and J. C. Vesga.** 1998. Rheumatic manifestations in the course of anaphylaxis caused by Anisakis simplex. *Clin. Exp. Rheumatol.* **16:**303–304.

24. **Curtis, M., and G. Bylund.** 1991. Diphyllobothriasis: fish tapeworm disease in the circumpolar north. *Arct. Med. Res.* **50:**18–24.

25. **Daengsvang, S.** 1981. Gnathostomiasis in Southeast Asia. *Southeast Asian J. Trop. Med. Public Health* **12:**319–332.

26. Daffos, F., F. Forestier, M. Capella-Pavlovsky, P. Thulliez, C. Aufrant, D. Valenti, and W. L. Cox. 1988. Prenatal management of 746 pregnancies at risk for congenital toxoplasmosis. *N. Engl. J. Med.* **318:**271–275.

27. Dannemann, B., J. A. McCutchan, D. Israelski, D. Antoniskis, C. Leport, B. Luft, J. Nussbaum, N. Clumeck, P. Morlat, and J. Chiu. 1992. Treatment of toxoplasmic encephalitis in patients with AIDS. A randomized trial comparing pyrimethamine plus clindamycin to pyramethamine plus sulfadiazine. *Ann. Intern. Med.* **116:**33–43.

28. Daschner, A., C. Cuellar, S. Sanchez-Pastor, C. Y. Pascual, and M. Martin-Esteban. 2002. Gastro-allergic anisakiasis as a consequence of simultaneous primary and secondary immune response. *Parasite Immunol.* **24:**243–251.

29. Deardorff, T. L., and M. L. Kent. 1989. Prevalence of larval *Anisakis simplex* in pen-reared and wild-caught salmon (*Salmonidae*) from Puget Sound, Washington. *J. Wildl. Dis.* **25:**416–419.

30. Del Brutto, O. H., V. Rajshekhar, A. C. White, Jr., V. C. Tsang, T. E. Nash, O. M. Takayanagui, R. M. Schantz, C. A. Evans, A. Flisser, D. Correa, D. Botero, J. C. Allan, E. Sarti, A. E. Gonzalez, R. H. Gilman, and H. H. Garcia. 2001. Proposed diagnostic criteria for neurocysticercosis. *Neurology* **57:**177–183.

31. Del Brutto, O. H., and J. Sotelo. 1988. Neurocysticercosis: an update. *Rev. Infect. Dis.* **10:**1075–1087.

32. Delobel, P., A. Signate, M. El Guedj, P. Couppie, M. Gueye, D. Smadja, and R. Pradinaud. 2004. Unusual form of neurocysticercosis associated with HIV infection. *Eur. J. Neurol.* **11:**55–58.

33. del Pozo, M. D., I. Moneo, L. F. de Corres, M. T. Audicana, D. Munoz, E. Fernandez, J. A. Navarro, and M. Garcia. 1996. Laboratory determinations in Anisakis simplex allergy. *J. Allergy Clin. Immunol.* **97:**977–984.

34. Diaz Camacho, S. P., K. Willms, M. D. C. de la Cruz Otero, M. L. Zazueta Ramos, S. Bayliss Gaxiola, R. Castro Velazquez, I. Osuna Ramirez, A. Bojorquez Contreras, E. H. Torres Montoya, and S. Sanchez Gonzales. 2003. Acute outbreak of gnathostomiasis in a fishing community in Sinaloa, Mexico. *Parasitol. Int.* **52:**133–140.

35. Dixon, B. R., and R. B. Flohr. 1997. Fish- and shellfish-borne trematode infections in Canada. *Southeast Asian J. Trop. Med. Public Health* **28**(Suppl. 1):58–64.

36. Dubey, J. P., H. R. Gamble, D. Hill, C. Sreekumar, S. Romand, and P. Thuilliez. 2002. High prevalence of viable Toxoplasma gondii infection in market weight pigs from a farm in Massachusetts. *J. Parasitol.* **88:**1234–1238.

37. Earnest, M. P., L. B. Reller, C. M. Filley, and A. J. Grek. 1987. Neurocysticercosis in the United States; 35 cases and a review. *Rev. Infect. Dis.* **9:**961–979.

38. Easthurn, R. L., T. R. Fritsche, and C. A. Terhune, Jr. 1987. Human intestinal infection with *Nanophyetus salmincola* from salmonid fishes. *Am. J. Trop. Med. Hyg.* **36:**586–591.

38a. Enserink, M. 2004. Infectious disases: one year after outbreak, SARS virus reveals some secrets. *Science* **304:**1097.

39. Excler, J. L., E. Pretat, B. Pozzetto, B. Charpin, and J. P. Garin. 1988. Sero-epidemiological survey for toxoplasmosis in Burundi. *Trop. Med. Parasitol.* **39:**139–141.

40. Fernandez de Corres, L., M. Audicana, M. D. Del Pozo, D. Munoz, E. Fernandez, J. A. Navarro, M. Garcia, and J. Diez. 1996. Anisakis simplex induces not only anisakiasis: report on 28 cases of allergy caused by this nematode. *J. Investig. Allergol. Clin. Immunol.* **6:**315–319.

41. Fritsche, T. R., R. L. Easthurn, L. H. Wiggins, and C. A. Terhune, Jr. 1989. Praziquantel for treatment of human *Nanophyetus salmincola* (*Troglotrema salmincola*) infection. *J. Infect. Dis.* **160:**896–899.

42. Garcia, H. H., C. A. Evans, T. E. Nash, O. M. Takayanagui, A. C. White, Jr., D. Botero, V. Rajshekhar, V. C. Tsang, P. M. Schantz, J. C. Allan, A. Flisser, D. Correa, E. Sarti, J. S. Friedland, S. M. Martinez, A. E. Gonzalez, R. H. Gilman, and O. H. Del Brutto. 2002. Current consensus guidelines for treatment of neurocysticercosis. *Clin. Microbiol. Rev.* **15:**747–756.

43. Garcia-Palacios, L., M. L. Gonzalez, M. I. Esteban, E. Mirabent, M. J. Perteguer, and C. Cuellar. 1996. Enzyme-linked immunosorbent assay, immunoblot analysis and RAST fluoroimmunoassay analysis of serum responses against crude larval antigens of Anisakis simplex in a Spanish random population. *J. Helminthol.* **70:**281–289.

44. Geerts, S., J. de Borchgrave, P. Dorny, and J. Brandt. 2002. Trichinellosis: old facts and new developments. *Verh. K. Acad. Geneeskd. Belg.* **64**(4):233–248, discussion 249–250.

45. Gorgolas, M., F. Santos-O'Connor, A. L. Unzu, M. L. Fernandez-Guerrero, T. Garate, R. M. Troyas Guarch, and M. P. Grobusch. 2003. Cutaneous and medullar gnathostomiasis in travelers to Mexico and Thailand. *J. Travel Med.* **10**:358–361.

46. Gould, S. E. 1970. *Trichinosis in Man and Animals.* Charles C Thomas, Springfield, Ill.

47. Guthmann, J. P. 1995. Epidemic cholera in Latin America: spread and routes of transmission. *J. Trop. Med. Hyg.* **98**:419–427.

48. Hale, D. C., L. Blumberg, and J. Frean. 2003. Case report: gnathostomiasis in two travelers to Zambia. *Am. J. Trop. Med. Hyg.* **68**:707–709.

49. Harrell, L. W., and T. L. Deardorff. 1990. Human nanophyetiasis: transmission by handling naturally infected coho salmon (Oncorhynchus kisutch). *J. Infect. Dis.* **161**:146–148.

50. Hohlfeld P., F. Daffos, P. Thulliez, C. Aufrant, J. Couvreur, J. MacAleese, D. Descombey, and F. Forestier. 1989. Fetal toxoplasmosis: outcome of pregnancy and infant follow-up after in utero treatment. *J. Pediatr.* **115**:765–769.

51. Hwang, D. F., Y. W. Hsieh, Y. C. Shiu, S. K. Chen, and C. A. Cheng. 2002. Identification of tetrodotoxin and fish species in a dried dressed fish fillet implicated in food poisoning. *J. Food Prot.* **65**:389–392.

52. Ido, K., H. Yuasa, M. Ide, K. Kimura, K. Toshimitsu, and T. Suzuki. 1998. Sonographic diagnosis of small intestinal anisakiasis. *J. Clin. Ultrasound* **26**:125–130.

53. Ikeda, K., R. Kumashiro, and T. Kifune. 1989. Nine cases of acute gastric anisakiasis. *Gastrointest. Endosc.* **35**:304–308.

54. Isbister, G. K., J. Son, F. Wang, C. J. Maclean, C. S. Lin, J. Ujma, C. R. Balit, B. Smith, D. G. Milder, and M. C. Kiernan. 2002. Puffer fish poisoning: a potentially life-threatening condition. *Med. J. Aust.* **177**:650–653.

55. Ishikura, H., K. Kikuchi, K. Nagasawa, T. Ooiwa, H. Takamiya, N. Sato, and K. Sugane. 1993. Anisakidae and anisakidosis. *Prog. Clin. Parasitol.* **3**:43–102.

56. Ishiwata, K., S. P. Diaz Camacho, K. Amrozi, Y. Horii, N. Nawa, and Y. Nawa. 1998. Gnathostomiasis in wild boars from Japan. *J. Wildl. Dis.* **34**:155–157.

57. Jara, M., H. W. Hsu, R. B. Eaton, and A. Demaria, Jr. 2001. Epidemiology of congenital toxoplasmosis identified by population-based newborn screening in Massachusetts. *Pediatr. Infect. Dis. J.* **20**:1132–1135.

58. Jeannel, D., G. Niel, D. Costagliola, M. Danis, B. M. Traore, and M. Gentilini. 1988. Epidemiology of toxoplasmosis among pregnant women in the Paris area. *Int. J. Epidemiol.* **17**:595–602.

59. Jelinek, T., M. Ziegler, and T. Loscher. 1994. Gnathostomiasis nach Aufenthalt in Thailand. *Dtsch. Med. Wochenschr.* **119**:1618–1622.

60. Kakizoe, S., H. Kakizoe, K. Kakizoe, Y. Kakizoe, M. Maruta, T. Kakizoe, and S. Kakizoe. 1995. Endoscopic findings and clinical manifestation of gastric anisakiasis. *Am. J. Gastroenterol.* **90**:761–763.

61. Kanchanapongkul, J. 2001. Puffer fish poisoning: clinical features and management experience in 25 cases. *J. Med. Assoc. Thail.* **84**:385–389.

62. Keusch, G. T., and J. K. Griffiths. 1993. Cholera, p 634–636. *In* F. D. Burg (ed.), *Gellis and Kagan's Current Pediatric Therapy,* 14th ed. W. B. Saunders Company, Philadelphia, Pa.

63. Kliks, M. M. 1986. Human anisakiasis: an update. *JAMA* **255**:2605.

64. Koo, J., F. Pien, and M. M. Kliks. 1988. Angiostrongylus (Parastrongylus) eosinophilic meningitis. *Rev. Infect. Dis.* **10**:1155–1162.

65. Kraivichian, P., M. Kulkumthorn, P. Yingyourd, P. Akarbovorn, and C. C. Paireepai. 1992. Albendazole for the treatment of human gnathostomiasis. *Trans. R. Soc. Trop. Med. Hyg.* **86**:418–421.

66. Kron, M. A., R. Guderian, A. Guevara, and A. Hidalgo. 1991. Abdominal sparganosis in Ecuador: a case report. *Am. J. Trop. Med. Hyg.* **44**:146–150.

67. Lappalainen, M., P. Koskela, K. Hedman, K. Teramo, P. Ammala, V. Hiilesmaa, and M. Koskiniemi. 1992. Incidence of primary toxoplasma infections during pregnancy in southern Finland: a prospective cohort study. *Scand. J. Infect. Dis.* **24**:97–104.

68. Laurichesse, H., M. Cambon, D. Perre, T. Ancelle, M. Mora, B. Hubert, J. Beytout, and M. Rey. 1997. Outbreak of trichinosis in France associated with eating horse meat. *Commun. Dis. Rep. CDR Rev.* **7**:R69–R73.

69. **Lee, M.-J., D.-Y. Jeong, W.-S. Kim, H.-D. Kim, C.-H. Kim, W.-W. Park, Y.-H. Park, K.-S. Kim, H.-M. Kim, and D.-S. Kim.** 2000. A tetrodotoxin-producing *Vibrio* strain, LM-1, from the puffer fish *Fugu vermicularis radiatus*. *Appl. Environ. Microbiol.* **66:**1698–1701.

70. **Lichtenfels, J. R., and F. P. Brancato.** 1976. Anisakid larva from the throat of an Alaskan Eskimo. *Am. J. Trop. Med. Hyg.* **25:**691–693.

71. **Lichtenfels, J. R., and B. Lavies.** 1976. Mortality in red-sided garter snakes, *Thamnophis sirtalis parietalis*, due to larval nematode, *Eustrongylides* sp. *Lab. Anim. Sci.* **26:**465–467.

72. **Liu, M., and P. Boireau.** 2002. Trichinellosis in China: epidemiology and control. *Trends Parasitol.* **18**(12)**:**553–556.

73. **Logar, I., Z. Novak-Antolic, A. Zore, V. Cerar, and M. Likar.** 1992. Incidence of congenital toxoplasmosis in the Republic of Slovenia. *Scand. J. Infect. Dis.* **24:**105–108.

74. **Loury, P. W., A. T. Pavia, L. M. McFarland, B. H. Peltier, T. J. Barrett, H. B. Bradford, J. M. Quan, J. Lynch, J. B. Mathison, R. A. Gunn, and P. A. Blacke.** 1989. Cholera in Louisiana. Widening spectrum of seafood vehicles. *Arch. Intern. Med.* **149:**2079–2084.

75. **Ma, H. W., T. J. Jiang, F. S. Quan, X. G. Chen, H. D. Wang, Y. S. Zhang, M. S. Cui, W. Y. Zhi, and D. C. Jiang.** 1997. The infection status of anisakid larvae in marine fish and cephalopods from the Bohai Sea, China and their taxonomical consideration. *Korean J. Parasitol.* **35:**19–24.

76. **MacLean, J. D., L. Poirier, T. W. Gyorkos, J. F. Proulx, J. Bourgeault, A. Corriveau, S. Illisituk, and M. Staudt.** 1992. Epidemiologic and serologic definition of primary and secondary trichinosis in the Arctic. *J. Infect. Dis.* **165:**908–912.

77. **MacLean, J. D., I. Viallet, C. Law, and M. Staudt.** 1989. Trichinosis in the Canadian Arctic: report of five outbreaks and a new clinical syndrome. *J. Infect. Dis.* **160:**513–520.

78. **Malakauskas, A., and C. M. Kapel.** 2003. Tolerance to low temperatures of domestic and sylvatic Trichinella spp. in rat muscle tissue. *J. Parasitol.* **89:**744–748.

79. **Marshall, W. F., C. A. McLimans, P. K. W. Yu, F. J. Allerberger, R. E. Van Scoy, and J. P. Anhalt.** Results of a 6-month survey of stool cultures for *Escherichia coli* O157:H7. *Mayo Clin. Proc.* **65:**787–792.

80. **Matsuoka, H., T. Nakama, H. Kisanuki, H. Uno, N. Tachibana, H. Tsubouchi, Y. Horii, and Y. Nawa.** 1994. A case report of serologically diagnosed pulmonary anisakiasis with pleural effusion and multiple lesions. *Am. J. Trop. Med. Hyg.* **51:**819–822.

81. **McArthur, J. C.** 1998. Neurologic complications of human immunodeficiency virus infection, p. 956–973. *In* S. L. Gorbach, J. G. Bartlett, and N. R. Blacklow (ed.), *Infectious Diseases*. W. B. Saunders, Philadelphia, Pa.

82. **McKerrow, J., J. Sakanari, and T. L. Deardorff.** 1988. Revenge of the sushi parasite. *N. Engl. J. Med.* **319:**1228–1229.

83. **Medina, M. T., E. Rosas, F. Rubio-Donnadieu, and J. Sotelo.** 1990. Neurocysticercosis as the main cause of late-onset epilepsy in Mexico. *Arch. Intern. Med.* **150:**325–327.

84. **Moore, D. A., J. McCroddan, P. Dekumyoy, and P. L. Chiodini.** 2003. Gnathostomiasis: an emerging imported disease. *Emerg. Infect. Dis.* **9:**647–650.

85. **Nalin, D. R., M. M. Levine, J. Rhead, E. Bergquist, M. Rennls, T. Hughes, S. O'Donnell, and R. B. Hornick.** 1978. Cannabis, hypochlorhydria, and cholera. *Lancet* **ii:**859–862.

86. **Narr, L. L., J. G. O'Donnell, B. Lister, P. Alessi, and D. Abraham.** 1996. Eustrongylidiasis—a parasitic infection acquired by eating live minnows. *J. Am. Osteopath. Assoc.* **96:**400–402.

87. **Nawa, Y., H. Maruyama, and K. Ogata.** 1997. Current status of gnathostomiasis dorolesi [sic] in Miyazaki Prefecture, Japan. *Southeast Asian J. Trop. Med. Public Health* **28**(Suppl. 1)**:**11–13.

88. **Nelson, M., T. L. Wright, A. Pierce, and R. A. Krogwold.** 2003. A common-source outbreak of trichinosis from consumption of bear meat. *J. Environ. Health* **65**(9)**:**16–19, 24.

89. **Nogueira, M. C., O. A. Oyarzabal, and D. E. Gombas.** 2003. Inactivation of Escherichia coli O157:H7, Listeria monocytogenes, and Salmonella in cranberry, lemon, and lime juice concentrates. *J. Food Prot.* **66:**1637–1641.

90. **Nontasut, P., V. Bussaratid, S. Chullawichit, N. Charoensook, and K. Visetsuk.** 2000. Comparison of ivermectin and albendazole treatment for gnathostomiasis. *Southeast Asian J. Trop. Med. Public Health* **31:**374–377.

91. **O'Brien, A. D., G. D. LaVeck, M. R. Thompson, and S. B. Formal.** 1982. Production of *Shigella dysenteriae* type 1-like cytotoxin by *Escherichia coli*. *J. Infect. Dis.* **146:**763–769.

92. **Ochoa, T. J., and T. G. Cleary.** 2003. Epidemiology and spectrum of disease of Escherichia coli O157. *Curr. Opin. Infect. Dis.* **16**(3):259–263.

93. **Ogata, K., Y. Nawa, H. Akahane, S. P. Diaz Camacho, R. Lamothe-Argumedo, and A. Cruz-Reyes.** 1988. Short report: gnathostomiasis in Mexico. *Am. J. Trop. Med. Hyg.* **58**:316–318.

94. **Okanobu, H., J. Hata, K. Haruma, M. Hara, K. Nakamura, S. Tanaka, and K. Chayama.** 2003. Giant gastric folds: differential diagnosis at US. *Radiology* **226**:686–690. (Erratum, **228**:904.)

95. **Ollague, W., J. Ollague, A. Guevara de Veliz, and S. Penaherrera.** 1984. Human gnathostomiasis in Ecuador (nodular migratory eosinophilic panniculitis). First finding of the parasite in South America. *Int. J. Dermatol.* **23**:647–651.

96. **Reference deleted.**

97. **Oyamada, N. T., H. Kobayashi, T. Kindou, N. Kudo, H. Yoshikawa, and T. Yoshikawa.** 1996. Discovery of mammalian hosts to Gnasthostoma nipponicum larvae and prevalence of the larvae in rodents and insectivores. *J. Vet. Med. Sci.* **58**:839–843.

98. **Pampiglione, S., F. Rivasi, M. Criscuolo, A. De Benedittis, A. Gentile, S. Russo, M. Testini, and M. Villan.** 2002. Human anisakiasis in Italy: a report of eleven new cases. *Pathol. Res. Pract.* **198**:429–434.

99. **Panesar, T. S., and P. C. Beaver.** 1979. Morphology of the advanced-stage larva of *Eustongylides wenrichi* Canavan 1929, occurring encapsulated in the tissues of *Amphiuma* in Louisiana. *J. Parasitol.* **65**:96–104.

100. **Park, S. K., D. G. Kim, S. K. Kang, J. S. Han, S. G. Kim, J. S. Lee, and M. C. Kim.** 1990. Toxic acute renal failure and hepatitis after ingestion of raw carp bile. *Nephron* **56**:188–193.

101. **Pawlowski, Z. S.** 1983. Clinical aspects in man, p. 367–401. *In* W. C. Campbell (ed.), *Trichinella and Trichinosis.* Plenum Press, New York, N.Y.

102. **Pozio, E., and C. Khamboonruang.** 1989. Trichinellosis in Thailand: epidemiology and biochemical identification of the aetiological agent. *Trop. Med. Parasitol.* **40**:73–74.

103. **Pozio, E., D. Sacchini, L. Sacchi, A. Tamburrini, and F. Alberici.** 2001. Failure of mebendazole in the treatment of humans with Trichinella spiralis infection at the stage of encapsulating larvae. *Clin. Infect. Dis.* **32**:638–642.

104. **Punyagupta, S., T. Bunnag, and P. Juttijudata.** 1990. Eosinophilic meningitis in Thailand. Clinical and epidemiological characteristics of 162 pateints with myeloencephalitis probably caused by Gnathostoma spinigerum. *J. Neurol. Sci.* **96**:241–256.

105. **Read, S. C., C. L. Gyles, R. C. Clarke, H. Lior, and S. McEwen.** 1990. Prevalence of verocytotoxigenic *Escherichia coli* in ground beef, pork, and chicken in southwestern Ontario. *Epidemiol. Infect.* **105**:11–20.

106. **Remington, J. S., and R. McLeod.** 1998. Toxoplasmosis, p. 1620–1640. *In* S. L. Gorbach, J. G. Bartlett, N. R. Blacklow (ed.), *Infectious Diseases.* W. B. Saunders, Philadelphia, Pa.

107. **Repiso Ortega, A., M. Alcantara Torres, C. Gonzalez de Frutos, T. de Artaza Varasa, R. Rodriguez Merlo, J. Valle Munoz, and J. L. Martinez Potenciano.** 2003. Gastrointestinal anisakiasis. Study of a series of 25 patients. *Gastroenterol. Hepatol.* **26**:341–346. (In Spanish.)

108. **Ries, A. A.** 22 July 1992. Cholera epidemic in the Americas—update 92-13. Revised memorandum. Centers for Disease Control, Atlanta, Ga.

109. **Rodrigues, A., H. Brun, and A. Sandstrom.** 1997. Risk factors for cholera infection in the initial phase of an epidemic in Guinea-Bissau: protection by lime juice. *Am. J. Trop. Med. Hyg.* **57**:601–604.

110. **Rodrigues, A., A. Sandstrom, T. Ca, H. Steinsland, H. Jensen, and P. Aaby.** 2000. Protection from cholera by adding lime juice to food—results from community and laboratory studies in Guinea-Bissau, West Africa. *Trop. Med. Int. Health* **5**:418–422.

111. **Rodrigues-Osorio, M., V. Gomez-Garcia, J. Rodriguez-Perez, and M. A. Gomez Morales.** 1990. Seroepidemiological studies of five outbreaks of trichinellosis in southern Spain. *Ann. Trop. Med. Parasitol.* **84**:181–184.

112. **Rossi, L., and V. Dini.** 1990. Importance of the wild boar in the epidemiology of wild trichinellosis in Piedmont and Liguria. *Parassitologia* **32**:321–326. (In Italian.)

113. **Roy, S. L., A. S. Lopez, and P. M. Schantz.** 2003. Trichinellosis surveillance—United States, 1997–2001. *Morb. Mortal. Wkly. Rep.* **52**(SS-6):1–8.

114. **Sack, D. A.** 1998. Cholera and related illnesses caused by *Vibrio* species and *Aeromonas*, p. 738–748. *In* S. L. Gorbach, J. G. Bartlett, and N. R. Blacklow (ed.), *Infectious Diseases*. W. B. Saunders, Philadelphia, Pa.

115. **Safdar, N., A. Said, R. E. Gangnon, and D. G. Maki.** 2002. Risk of hemolytic uremic syndrome after antibiotic treatment of Escherichia coli O157:H7 enteritis: a meta-analysis. *JAMA* **288**:996–1001.

116. **Sakamoto, T., C. Gutierrez, A. Rodriguez, and S. Sauto.** 2003. Testicular sparganosis in a child from Uruguay. *Acta Trop.* **88**:83–86.

117. **Salokannel, J.** 1970. Intrinsic factor in tapeworm anaemia. *Acta Med. Scand. Suppl.* **517**:1–51.

118. **Schantz, P. M., A. C. Moore, J. L. Munoz, B. J. Hartman, J. A. Schaefer, A. M. Aron, D. Persaud, E. Sarti, M. Wilson, and A. Flisser.** 1992. Neurocysticercosis in an Orthodox Jewish community in New York City. *N. Engl. J. Med.* **327**:692–695.

119. **Schantz, P. M., and M. K. Michelson.** 1998. Trichinosis, p. 1616–1620. *In* S. L. Gorbach, J. G. Bartlett, and N. R. Blacklow (ed.), *Infectious Diseases*. W. B. Saunders, Philadelphia, Pa.

120. **Schellenberg, R. S., B. J. Tan, J. D. Irvine, R. Stockdale, A. A. Gajadhar, B. Serhir, J. Botha, C. A. Armstrong, S. A. Woods, J. M. Blondeau, and T. L. McNab.** 2003. An outbreak of trichinellosis due to consumption of bear meat infected with Trichinella nativa, in 2 northern Saskatchewan communities. *J. Infect. Dis.* **188**:835–843.

121. **Schmidt, G. D.** 1986. *Handbook of Tapeworm Identification. Key to the Genera Taeniidae*, p. 221–227. CRC Press, Boca Raton, Fla.

122. **Schmutzhard, E., P. Boongird, and A. Vejjajiva.** 1988. Eosinophilic meningitis and radiculomyelitis in Thailand, caused by CNS invasion of *Gnathostoma spinigerum* and *Angiostrongylus cantonensis*. *J. Neurol. Neurosurg. Psychiatry* **51**:80–87.

123. **Sever, J. L., J. H. Ellenberg, A. C. Ley, D. L. Madden, D. A. Fuccillo, N. R. Tzan, and D. M. Edmonds.** 1988. Toxoplasmosis. Maternal and pediatric findings in 23,000 pregnancies. *Pediatrics* **82**:181–192.

124. **Shields, B. A., P. Bird, W. J. Liss, K. L. Groves, R. Olson, and P. A. Rossignol.** 2002. The nematode Anisakis simplex in American shad (Alosa sapidissima) in two Oregon rivers. *J. Parasitol.* **88**:1033–1035.

125. **Shirahama, M., T. Koga, H. Ishibashi, S. Uchida, Y. Ohta, and Y. Shimoda.** 1992. Intestinal anisakiasis: US in diagnosis. *Radiology* **185**:789–793.

126. **Smith, H. J., S. Messier, and F. Tittinger.** 1989. Destruction of *Trichinella spiralis spiralis* during the preparation of the "dry cured" pork products proscuitto, proscuittini and Genoa salami. *Can. J. Vet. Res.* **53**:80–83.

127. **Sohn, W. M., J. Y. Chai, and S. H. Lee.** 1989. A human case of *Stellantchasmus falcatus* infection. *Kisaengch'ung Hak Chapchi* **27**:277–279.

128. **Sohn, W. M., and S. H. Lee.** 1996. Identification of larval Gnathostoma obtained from imported Chinese loaches. *Korean J. Parasitol.* **34**:161–167.

129. **Sotelo, J., F. Escobedo, J. Rodriguez-Carbajal, B. Torres, and F. Rubio-Donnadieu.** 1984. Therapy of parenchymal brain cysticercosis with praziquantel. *N. Engl. J. Med.* **310**:1001–1007.

130. **Sousa, O. E., R. E. Saenz, and J. K. Frenkel.** 1988. Toxoplasmosis in Panama: a 10-year study. *Am. J. Trop. Med. Hyg.* **38**:315–322.

131. **St. Louis, M. E., J. D. Porter, A. Helal, K. Drame, N. Hargrett-Bean, J. G. Wells, and R. V. Tauxe.** 1990. Epidemic cholera in West Africa: the role of food handling and high-risk foods. *Am. J. Epidemiol.* **131**:719–727.

132. **Stromnes, E., and K. Andersen.** 1998. Distribution of whaleworm (Anisakis simplex, Nematoda, Ascaridoidea) L3 larvae in three species of marine fish: saithe (Pollachius virens (L.)), cod (Gadus morhua L.) and redfish (Sebastes marinus (L.)) from Norwegian waters. *Parasitol. Res.* **84**:281–285.

133. **Swaddiwudhipong, W., P. Akarasewi, T. Chayaniyayodhin, P. Kunasol, and H. M. Foy.** 1989. Several sporadic outbreaks of El Tor cholera in Sunpathong, Chiang Mai, September-October, 1987. *J. Med. Assoc. Thail.* **72**:583–588.

134. **Takabe, K., S. Ohki, O. Kunihiro, T. Sakashita, I. Endo, Y. Ichikawa, H. Sekdo, T. Amano, Y. Nakatani, K. Suzuki, and H. Shimada.** 1998. Anisakidosis: a cause of intestinal obstruction from eating sushi. *Am. J. Gastroenterol.* **93**:1172–1173.

135. **Takayanagui, O. M., and E. Jardim.** 1992. Therapy for neurocysticercosis. Comparison between albendazole and praziquantel. *Arch. Neurol.* **49**:290–294.

136. Taniguchi, Y., K. Hashimoto, S. Ichikawa, M. Shimizu, K. Ando, and Y. Kotani. 1991. Human gnathostomiasis. *J. Cutan. Pathol.* **18:**112–115.
137. Tarr, P. I., M. A. Neill, C. R. Clausen, S. L. Watkins, D. L. Christie, and R. O. Hickman. 1990. *Escherichia coli* O157:H7 and the hemolytic uremic syndrome: importance of early cultures in establishing the etiology. *J. Infect. Dis.* **162:**553–556.
138. Toro, C., M. L. Caballero, M. Baquero, J. García-Samaniego, I. Casado, M. Rubio, and I. Moneo. 2004. High prevalence of seropositivity to a major allergen of *Anisakis simplex,* Ani s 1, in dyspeptic patients. *Clin. Diagn. Lab. Immunol.* **11:**115–118.
139. Urita, Y., M. Nishino, H. Koyama, E. Kondo, Y. Naruki, and S. Otsuka. 1997. Esophageal anisakiasis accompanied by reflux esophagitis. *Intern. Med.* **36:**890–893.
140. Vazquez, V., and J. Sotelo. 1992. The course of seizures after treatment for cerebral cysticercosis. *N. Engl. J. Med.* **327:**696–701.
141. Vitomskova, E. A., and A. S. Dovgalev. 2001. Rates of infection of fishes from Okhotsk sea with human Anisakidae. *Med. Parazitol. Parazit. Bolezni* **2001**(2):31–34. (In Russian.)
142. von Bonsdorff, B., and G. Bylund. 1982. The ecology of *Diphyllobothrium latum. Ecol. Dis.* **1:**21–26.
142a. Wells, J. G., L. D. Shipman, K. D. Greene, E. G. Sowers, J. H. Green, D. N. Cameron, F. P. Downes, M. L. Martin, S. M. Ostroff, M. E. Potter, R. V. Tauxe, and I. K. Wachsmuth. 1991. Isolation of *Escherichia coli* serotype O157:H7 and other Shiga-like-toxin-producing *E. coli* from dairy cattle. *J. Clin. Microbiol.* **29:**985–989.
143. White, A. C. 1997. Neurocysticercosis. *Clin. Infect. Dis.* **24:**101–115.
144. White, A. C., Jr. 2000. Neurocysticercosis: updates on epidemiology, pathogenesis, diagnosis, and management. *Annu. Rev. Med.* **51:**187–206.
145. Wilson, C. B., and J. S. Remington. 1992. Toxoplasmosis, p. 2057–2069. *In* R. D. Feigin and J. D. Cherry (ed.), *Pediatric Infectious Diseases,* 3rd ed. W. B. Saunders, Philadelphia, Pa.
146. Wittner, M., J. W. Turner, G. Jacquette, L. R. Ash, M. P. Salgo, and H. B. Tanowitz. 1989. Eustrongylidiasis—a parasitic infection acquired by eating sushi. *N. Engl. J. Med.* **320:**1124–1126.
147. Yeum, C. H., S. K. Ma, S. W. Kim, N. H. Kim, J. Kim, and K. C. Choi. 2002. Incidental detection of an Anisakis larva in continuous ambulatory peritoneal dialysis effluent. *Nephrol. Dial. Transplant.* **17:**1522–1523.
148. Zhang, X., A. D. McDaniel, L. E. Wolf, G. T. Keusch, M. K. Waldor, and D. W. Acheson. 2000. Quinolone antibiotics induce Shiga toxin-encoding bacteriophages, toxin production, and death in mice. *J. Infect. Dis.* **181:**664–670.

Infections of Leisure, Third Edition
Edited by David Schlossberg
© 2004 ASM Press, Washington, D.C.

Chapter 12

Transmission of Infectious Diseases during Sporting Activities

Arezou Minooee and Leland S. Rickman

Recreational sporting events and organized athletic competitions are popular pastimes of our generation. With a high level of spectator interest in, even reverence towards, national and international games such as the Super Bowl or World Cup, sporting events have become the focus of many societies. Not only is participation in fitness activities enjoyable and sometimes challenging, but also any type of physical exercise is ultimately beneficial to one's health. Still, there are hazards. In addition to the risk of enduring physical injuries, one of the potential dangers faced by athletes is the possibility of contracting infectious diseases (2, 15, 16, 22, 47, 57, 58, 64, 74, 86, 92, 100, 108, 112, 144, 146, 147; M. Dorman, Letter, *JAMA* 272:436, 1994).

There are several mechanisms by which infectious agents may be spread during sports. The main routes of transmission include direct- and indirect-contact, droplet, common-source, and airborne transmission. Direct-contact transmission involves person-to-person contact in which infectious agents are physically transferred to a susceptible host from an infected player. Indirect-contact transmission may occur when a susceptible host comes into contact with contaminated objects or fomites, such as equipment, towels, or clothing. A type of indirect contact is droplet transmission, which may occur when droplets containing infectious agents are generated through coughing, sneezing, or talking and are deposited on the host's conjunctivae, nasal mucosa, or mouth after being propelled in the air a short distance. Common-source transmission may occur when infectious agents are transmitted by contaminated items, such as food, water, beverage containers, or other equipment which more than one person may have contact with. Airborne transmission may occur when evaporated droplets or dust particles containing infectious agents are suspended in the air for long periods and are subsequently inhaled by the susceptible host.

Arezou Minooee • University of Vermont College of Medicine, Box 298, 89 Beaumont Ave., Burlington, VT 05405. *Leland S. Rickman (deceased)* • Epidemiology Unit, Division of Infectious Diseases, University of California, San Diego, San Diego, CA 92103.

Infections that may pose a risk to athletes or persons who come into contact with them during sporting events are examined below. Preventive strategies and treatments are also briefly discussed. Table 1 summarizes potential sports-related infectious diseases according to mode of transmission, and Table 2 briefly discusses several reported infectious disease cases relevant to athletics.

Table 1. Classification of sports-related infections according to mode of transmission

---

Blood borne
   HIV infection, AIDS
   Hepatitis B

Direct- and indirect-contact transmission
   Viral infections
      HSV infection
      Molluscum contagiosum
      Verrucae (warts)
   Bacterial infections
      Erythrasma
      Pitted keratolysis
      Staphylococcal skin infections
         Folliculitis
         Furunculosis
   Hot tub folliculitis
   Streptococcal infections
      Impetigo
      Pyoderma
   Miscellaneous infections caused by viruses and bacteria
      Conjunctivitis
      IM
      Meningitis
      URTI
   Fungal infections
      Tinea corporis
      Tinea cruris
      Tinea pedis
      Tinea versicolor

Common-source transmission
   Enteroviral infections
      Aseptic meningitis
      Pleurodynia
   Hepatitis A

Airborne transmission
   Measles
   Chickenpox
   Influenza

Water sports-associated transmission[a]
   Leptospirosis
   Otitis externa

---

[a]Refer to Table 3 for a list of related infections.

Table 2. Reported infectious disease cases involving athletes

Infection or pathogen	Reference(s)	Comment
Aseptic meningitis	7	Outbreak among members of a high school football team (six students and one teacher) caused by coxsackievirus B2 infection as a result of unhygienic practices such as the sharing of water bottles
Aseptic meningitis	12	Outbreak among seven high school football players caused by echovirus 16 infection resulting from common-source transmission such as the sharing of cups
Aseptic meningitis	30	Outbreak among members of a high school football team and several band members in Ohio; occurred either by person-to-person transmission or by a continuing common-source exposure
Aseptic meningitis	116	Seven outbreaks in four states involving high school football players; caused by enterovirus infections, probably as a result of person-to-person transmission, with evidence to implicate common-source transmission at two schools (possibly the sharing of water bottles)
Hepatitis A	118, 119	Epidemic affecting 90 members of a college football team; occurred as a result of an unusual common-source outbreak such as through a contaminated water supply
Hepatitis B	61, 131, 132	Outbreak involving 568 Swedish orienteers during a 5-yr period (1957–1962) as a result of indirect contact; the epidemic was brought to an end when adequate clothing was made compulsory, but another outbreak involving 42 cases occurred shortly after the regulations had been abolished
Hepatitis B	88	Apparent percutaneous transmission among five members of a high school sumo wrestling club in Japan
Hepatitis B	163	Horizontal transmission among five members of an American-football team at a university in Japan due to contact with open wounds during training
HIV	164	Poorly documented case involving a bloody head-on collision during a soccer match
Hot tub folliculitis	38	Two cases due to *P. aeruginosa* infection after bathing in a hot tub shared by several people and not cleaned for 10 days
Hot tub folliculitis	65	Case report of localized folliculitis infection due to *P. aeruginosa* in a football player following whirlpool treatment for an ankle strain
HSV	17	Survey indicating herpes gladiatorum as a common skin infection among college and high school wrestlers due to increased skin contact

Table continues

Table 2. *Continued*

Infection or pathogen	Reference(s)	Comment
HSV	20	HSV type 1 infection diagnosed among 60 wrestlers in a high school wrestling camp as a result of direct skin contact
HSV	51	Outbreak among 17 members of a college wresting team and one contact (girlfriend of wrestler)
HSV	90	Case report of a 16-yr-old high school wrestler in Missouri who became infected due to direct contract during an epidemic involving at least 17 of his teammates
HSV	107	Four cases reported among rugby players
HSV	127	Outbreak among seven members of a college wrestling team due to direct-contact transmission
HSV	135	Case report regarding a 17-yr-old male high school wrestler as a result of direct contact
HSV	143	Outbreak among five members of an amateur wrestling group over a 10-mo period
HSV	148	Reported outbreak among members of a rugby team as a result of direct contact
HSV	149	Outbreak among nine rugby players; managed by vaccination
HSV	157	Outbreak among nine college wrestlers, with the implication that abrasive shirts may contribute to the spread of infection
HSV	Verbov and Lowe, letter	Case report of two rugby players as a result of direct contact
HSV	170	Outbreak among six members of a college wrestling team and likely spread to another team
HSV	172	Outbreak among four members of a rugby team with ocular infection (conjunctivitis)
Leptospirosis	10	Seven cases associated with swimming in a creek in Tennessee
Leptospirosis	34	Outbreak among 26 white-water rafters as a result of contaminated river water in Costa Rica
Leptospirosis	36, 37, 142	Outbreak among athletes exposed to water from the Segama River while participating in the Eco-Challenge Sabah 2000 multisport expedition race in Borneo, Malaysia
Leptospirosis	35	Outbreak among athletes participating in triathlons in Illinois and Wisconsin, possibly as a result of contact with a contaminated lake
Leptospirosis	66, 117	Outbreak among triathlon participants whose swimming event took place in a freshwater lake in Springfield, Ill.
Leptospirosis	79	Outbreak among five boys who had been swimming in a pond in Illinois

Table 2. *Continued*

Infection or pathogen	Reference(s)	Comment
Leptospirosis	80	Four cases associated with ingestion of contaminated creek water during a kayaking trip in Missouri
Leptospirosis	89	Common-source waterborne outbreak associated with swimming on the island of Kauai, Hawaii
Leptospirosis	124	Five cases diagnosed in the area of Rochefort, France, in persons who had swum in the Genouillé Canal
Leptospirosis	161	Infection acquired among at least 17 participants of a jungle race in Southeast Asia
Measles	31	Three cases among athletes competing at an international gymnastics competition in Indiana
Measles	43	Outbreak of 137 cases associated with high school basketball game attendance in Montana
Measles	53	25 cases following an international sporting event in a domed stadium in Minneapolis, Minn., as a result of airborne transmission (primary patient was a track-and-field athlete from Argentina)
Molluscum contagiosum	Commens, letter	Case report of 48-yr-old female infected during an orienteering competition in Australia as a result of indirect-contact transmission
Molluscum contagiosum	Mobacken and Nordin, letter	Survey indicating prevalence of infection among cross-country runners in Sweden
Molluscum contagiosum	122	Outbreak among 517 children using communal swimming pools near Tokyo, Japan
Pitted keratolysis	160	Report of two cases involving a volleyball player and field athlete from Japan with infection on non-weight-bearing areas
Pleurodynia	76	Outbreak among players of a high school football team; associated with coxsackievirus B1 infection as a result of common-source transmission such as through sharing the same water container
Pustular follicular dermatitis	5	Outbreak of folliculitis caused by gram-negative bacteria among college students in Seattle, Wash., as a result of common exposure and skin trauma endured while mud wrestling
Staphylococcal infection	14	Outbreak of furunculosis among 26 members of a high school football team in Illinois
Staphylococcal infection	44	Outbreak of minor skin infections among river-rafting guides in Tennessee, South Carolina, and North Carolina
Staphylococcal infection	101	Methicillin-resistant skin infections in a high school wrestling team and surrounding community in Vermont
Staphylococcal infection	152	Outbreak of furunculosis among 31 high school football and basketball players in Kentucky as a result of direct-contact transmission

Table continues

Table 2. *Continued*

Infection or pathogen	Reference(s)	Comment
Staphylococcal infection	155	Outbreak of methicillin-resistant *S. aureus* infection involving five members of a rugby football team
Streptococcal infection	G. Falck, Letter, *Lancet,* **347**:840–841, 1996	Group A streptoccoccal skin infection among football players
Streptococcal infection	62	Pyoderma caused by nephritogenic streptococci among college football players in North Carolina as a result of direct contact
Streptococcal infection	104	Pyoderma caused by nephritogenic streptococci among five rugby players and a girlfriend as a result of close physical contact
Tinea corporis	19	Outbreak of tinea corporis gladiatorum among 21 high school wrestlers in Alaska
Tinea corporis	54	Epidemic caused by *T. tonsurans* among 46 juvenile wrestlers (ages 7–17) in Germany
Tinea corporis	75	Epidemic due to *T. tonsurans* among wrestlers in Sweden as a result of direct contact
Tinea corporis	126	An outbreak of tinea gladiatorum reported among 45 wrestlers in Lanzarote, Canary Islands, Spain
Tinea corporis	156	Five cases due to *T. tonsurans* among college wrestlers as a result of direct contact
Tinea corporis	Werninghaus, letter	Four reported cases among college wrestlers
Tinea pedis	11	Report indicating 22% prevalence of occult athlete's foot among marathon runners
URTI	125	Study suggesting that fast marathon runners are subject to more symptoms than slower or moderate-speed runners as a result of increased stress
URTI	129	Three cases related to deep-sea diving and caused by penicillin-resistant *S. pneumoniae*

BLOOD-BORNE PATHOGENS

HIV

The human retrovirus known as human immunodeficiency virus (HIV) is the etiologic agent leading to the suppression of the immune system and to the development of AIDS. Modes of transmission include sexual contact, parenteral exposure to blood or blood components, contamination of open wounds or mucous membranes by infected blood, blood inoculation or needle sharing, and perinatal transmission from infected mother to fetus (82). The virus is distributed throughout a variety of bodily fluids but resides in highest concentrations within cellular elements and in blood (27).

Millions of people worldwide have been affected by HIV and AIDS. In the absence of a cure or vaccine, there is much concern regarding infection during athletic competitions where bleeding and skin abrasions are common, such as in boxing or football (23, 26, 28, 49, 56, 59, 68, 81, 109, 133, 138, 165; J. Karjalainen and G. Friman, Letter, *Ann. Intern. Med.* **123**:635–636, 1995; C. Loveday, Letter, *Lancet* **335**:1532, 1990). Although AIDS was initially described in 1981, there have been no definitive studies indicating transmission of the virus through bodily fluids such as sweat, tears, urine, sputum, vomitus, saliva, or respiratory droplets (174, 175).

American football is the one sport for which the potential risk of HIV transmission has been investigated. Based on the frequency of bleeding injuries and player contact observed in one study, the risk of infection was estimated to be less than 1 per 85 million game contacts (25). Athletes actually have a greater probability of becoming infected off the field through unsafe sexual practices and injection of drugs or anabolic steroids. For example, in one reported case a bodybuilder who had been administering intramuscular-injection steroids with a shared, unsterilized needle became infected with HIV (M. J. Scott and M. J. Scott, Jr., Letter, *JAMA* **262**:207–208, 1989). Other risk factors were ruled out for this individual.

There has been only one documented case of HIV transmission during sports contact. The report concerned an Italian soccer player who allegedly seroconverted after a bloody head-to-head collision with an HIV-positive individual during a recreational soccer match (164). After careful review of the case, however, health officials were unable to rule out other risk factors to verify the actual mode of transmission (63).

At least two instances of HIV transmission have been reported to be due to fist fighting episodes involving bloody injuries (G. Ippolito, P. Del Poggio, C. Arici, G. P. Gregis, G. Antonelli, E. Riva, and F. Dianzani, Letter, *JAMA* **272**:433–434, 1994; N. O'Farrell, S. J. Tovey, and P. Morgan-Capner, Letter, *Lancet* **339**:246, 1992). Such reports reinforce the theoretical risks athletes face and indicate the necessity to take precautions during events in which blood exposure may occur. The following preventive strategies and recommendations adopted from the American Medical Society for Sports Medicine (9), American Academy of Sports Medicine (9), American Academy of Pediatrics (8), National Football League (24), National Collegiate Athletic Association (111), and World Health Organization (174) should be considered regarding HIV in sports:

1. If a skin lesion is observed, it should be immediately cleansed with a suitable antiseptic and securely covered with an occlusive dressing that will withstand the demands of competition.
2. If a bleeding wound occurs, the individual's participation should be interrupted until the bleeding has been stopped and the wound has been both cleansed with antiseptics and securely covered or occluded. Any participant whose uniform is saturated with blood, regardless of the source, must have it changed before returning to competition.
3. Coaches and athletic trainers should receive training in first aid and emergency care; they should also be provided with the necessary supplies to treat open wounds, such as latex or vinyl gloves, disinfectant, bleach, antiseptic, designated receptacles for soiled equipment or uniforms, bandages or dressings, and

a container for appropriate disposal of needles, syringes, or scalpels.

4. Athletic equipment that is visibly contaminated with blood should be wiped clean and disinfected with a bleach solution before being reused.

5. Gloves should be worn by persons attending to injuries when direct contact with blood or body fluids is anticipated. The gloves should be changed after individual participants have been treated, and the hands should be washed after every glove removal. Emergency care, however, should never be delayed when protective equipment is not available.

6. Athletes should not be restricted from participating in sports merely on the basis of their HIV status unless substantial numbers of cases of transmission in sporting competitions occur.

7. The enforcement of mandatory HIV testing in athletic settings is unnecessary. Instead, voluntary testing and HIV education should be promoted to achieve public health benefits.

Viral Hepatitis

Hepatitis B virus (HBV) is transmitted via the same routes as HIV: through sexual contact, through parenteral blood exposure, and perinatally (57). HBV is more readily transmitted than HIV, however, since it is usually present at higher concentrations in the blood (73, 120, 174). A well-documented outbreak of HBV infection was reported among several members of a high school sumo wrestling club (88). It was suggested that HBV was transmitted percutaneously through the cuts and abrasions suffered while wrestling. In another report, horizontal transmission of HBV was documented among five players of an American-football team at a university in Japan due to contact with open wounds during training (163).

Other sports-related outbreaks of HBV have occurred among Swedish orienteers (61, 131, 132). Orienteering is a sport where runners are given the bearings of a number of checkpoints and, with the aid of a compass and map, choose the route they prefer to take to the finish line. It was suggested that inoculation of HBV might have occurred when the runners scratched themselves on the same bushes or after the competition when the participants bathed in stagnant waters or shared the same plastic bathtubs. Immediately after preventive measures were applied, the incidence of HBV infection among the orienteers decreased.

DIRECT- AND INDIRECT-CONTACT TRANSMISSION

Viral Infections

HSV (Herpes Gladiatorum, Venatorum, and Rugbeiorum and Scrumpox)

Herpes simplex virus (HSV) is the cause of a contagious viral infection of the skin and mucous membranes. Herpes labialis and herpes progenitalis are two forms of the disease, so named because of their anatomical localization. Since HSV infection is so prevalent among rugby players and wrestlers, it is also referred to as herpes gladiatorum (143), herpes venatorum (107), herpes rugbeiorum (J. Verbov and N. J. Lowe, Letter, *Lancet* **ii**:1523–1524, 1974), and scrumpox (148). The virus may be transmitted directly through skin-to-skin contact and indirectly through the sharing of towels, clothes, or other equipment. Athletes participating in contact sports may be at greater risk of infection. Several cases have been reported to occur among wrestlers and rugby players as a result of close person-to-person contact (Table 2) (17, 20, 51, 90, 107, 127, 135, 143, 148, 149, 157, 170, 172; Verbov and Lowe, letter). Symptomatic athletes should refrain from participating in contact sports to avoid spreading the virus. Wearing protective clothing may also help prevent infection by eliminating contact with the lesions, although it has been suggested that abrasive shirts may actually contribute to infection (157).

Even though cutaneous HSV infections are rarely life threatening, herpetic lesions are unsightly and tend to cause discomfort. Events such as trauma, exposure to sunlight, illness, surgery, stress, or menstruation may trigger recurrence of the lesions. For example, recurrent herpes labialis was reported among Alpine skiers exposed to increased UV irradiation at high altitudes (113). The prophylactic use of acyclovir has been shown to reduce the incidence of UV light-induced herpes labialis in skiers (128, 153).

Molluscum Contagiosum

Molluscum contagiosum is a benign viral skin infection caused by a poxvirus. Minor skin injuries are thought to be the sites at which the virus is introduced. Athletes participating in close-contact sports where skin trauma is common are at risk of infection. Wrestlers and boxers, for example, are commonly infected in areas such as the hands, face, and upper body. The virus may also be spread in connection with bathing and washing. In one study, the infection was recognized among young children who used communal swimming pools (122). Infections may also arise if athletes come into direct skin contact with each other in the sauna or shower or on benches and also if they share their soap, brushes, and towels (H. Mobacken and P. Nordin, Letter, *J. Am. Acad. Dermatol.* **17**:519–520, 1987).

Cutaneous transmission of molluscum contagiosum was reported to occur in a 48-year-old female during an orienteering competition (C.A. Commens, Letter, *Med. J. Aust.* **146**:117, 1987) as well as in other cross-country runners (Mobacken and Nordin, letter). The female orienteer had endured minor abrasions around her knees after running through a bush and developed lesions in the same area several weeks later. The incubation period for molluscum contagiosum ranges between 14 and 50 days, and because this individual had had no other opportunity for contact with the virus, it was thought to have been spread by other athletes who had passed along the same track and brushed vigorously against the same plants.

Untreated infections are ultimately self-resolving but either may last between 6 and 9 months or may persist for years (72; Commens, letter). Some methods of treatment include curettage, skin abrasion with granules or an abrasive pad after bathing, topical tretinoin (Retin-A) gel or cream, liquid nitrogen, and chemical treatments with retinoic acid, phenol, salicylic acid, lactic acid, or cantharidin as well as a variety of other destructive procedures (21, 57). Protective clothing and good hygienic conditions are recommended to help prevent infection.

Verrucae (Warts)

Warts are benign epithelial tumors caused by several human papillomaviruses (HPV), with an average incubation period of approximately 6 months. Common warts seen on the hands appear as raised areas that are irregular and rough. Plantar warts, seen on weight-bearing surfaces such as the feet, appear as flat lesions extending deep into the skin with hyperkeratotic surfaces. Athletes are predisposed to infection due to the effects of perspiration, since moist environments create conditions favoring the spread of verrucae. Although the infectivity rate is generally low, it is postulated that repetitive trauma to wet skin surfaces increases the risk of inoculation of HPV (134). Individuals competing in sports in which calluses are likely to develop, such as gymnastics, track, football, tennis, baseball, and wrestling, are more susceptible to acquiring warts.

In the athletic setting, it is likely that plantar warts are transmitted by contaminated floors, such as swimming pool decks or shower rooms, while hand warts are transmitted by contaminated gym equipment or weight apparatus (41). To prevent the transmission of HPV, warts should always be covered during contact sports. Athletes who are prone to warts should consider using drying powders on their feet and wearing rubber sandals in the locker room and shower (60).

Since warts may cause irritation in disadvantageous locations, such as the fingers or hands, an athlete's performance in sports such as golf or bowling may be limited. Effective treatment methods are available but may sometimes cause short-term disabilities. For example, athletic participation is likely to be interrupted when cryotherapy and liquid nitrogen are applied. Surgical removal and electrical desiccation techniques are also quite disabling. Less aggressive treatments include the application of salicylic acid plasters or topical tretinoin gel as well as other available methods.

Bacterial Infections

Erythrasma

Erythrasma is an infection caused by *Corynebacterium minutissimum* that may clinically mimic a fungal infection in appearance. The typical rash develops as a reddish-brown patch with desquamation in the axilla and groin. The lesions are erythematous, with a fine scale, and are well demarcated at their borders. The infection may be quite pruritic and can be diagnosed using Wood's light (black light), which reveals a coral red fluorescence. It is not a fungal disorder and must, therefore, be treated with topical cleansing agents, topical germicidal agents, or oral antibiotics. Using antibacterial soaps and wearing loose clothing may help prevent or eliminate infection (46, 95).

Pitted Keratolysis

Pitted keratolysis, also known as "stinky foot" or "toxic-sock syndrome," is an asymptomatic skin infection associated with the growth of *Corynebacterium*. Athletes participating in basketball, tennis, volleyball, and track often develop pitted keratolysis. Lesions are typically seen on weight-bearing areas of the body, such as the feet and toes (159). Two cases of pitted keratolysis in non-weight-bearing areas, however, involved a volleyball player and a field athlete (160). It was suggested that non-weight-bearing areas of the body are likely to be infected with the organism following infection of the weight-bearing regions. Infections are precipitated by occlusive footwear as well as hyperhydrated environments caused by excessive sweating. The lesions may clear rapidly with the elimination of local moisture, which may be achieved by wearing absorbent cotton socks and with the application of drying agents to areas of the foot that may become moist. More resistant infections may require treatment with oral erythromycin or mupirocin ointment (144, 166).

Staphylococcal Skin Infections (Folliculitis and Furunculosis)

Folliculitis is an infection of hair follicles usually caused by *Staphylococcus aureus,* but it may also be caused by gram-negative organisms. Lesions usually emerge on areas of the skin that have been traumatized by maceration, such as under shoulder pads or sweaty garments and on the legs, arms, and trunks of wrestlers. Deep folliculitis lesions may ultimately produce furuncles or boils. The infection does not spread as epidemics, but astringent lotions or drying agents that remove the tops of pustules should be used to control and prevent furuncles from developing. In one case, an outbreak of pustular follicular dermatitis among college students was the result of skin trauma endured while mud wrestling (5).

Furunculosis is an infection pertaining to hair follicles, sebaceous glands, or skin compromised by abrasions, wounds, or burns. It is usually caused by *S. aureus* but may also arise from existing areas of folliculitis. Outbreaks of staphylococcal skin infections reported among high school football teams and river-rafting guides have been attributed to direct person-to-person contact, with an increased risk of infection in the presence of skin injuries (Table 2) (14, 44, 101, 152, 155; D. Joyce, Letter, *Am. J. Sports Med.* **18:**219–220, 1990). Wearing uniforms that cover all parts of the body may reduce the frequency of ecchymoses and microabrasions on the skin. To prevent the spread of infection, infected athletes should refrain from participation until lesions have resolved. Also, ointments and powders should not be distributed by hand from common containers. Treatment consists of warm compresses and benzoyl peroxide along with oral antibiotics.

"Hot Tub" Folliculitis

Hot tub folliculitis differs from typical folliculitis in that it is caused by *Pseudomonas aeruginosa.* This type of infection has been recognized as being associated with the use of hot tubs, whirlpools, Jacuzzis, and swimming pools. In one report, hot tub-associated folliculitis was described to occur among individuals who had bathed in a tub that was shared by several people and had not been cleaned for 10 days (38). In another report, infection was described to occur in a college football player following whirlpool use for treatment of an ankle strain (65). To prevent infection, it is necessary to reduce the quantity of the bacterial organism in the water. This may be achieved by close monitoring of the temperature, pH, disinfectant level, and chlorine concentration. Hot tub folliculitis is a self-limiting condition lasting 7 to 10 days and therefore requires no specific treatment.

Streptococcal Skin Infections (Impetigo and Pyoderma)

Impetigo is a contagious bacterial skin infection caused by staphylococcal or streptococcal species and is most commonly seen among wrestlers, swimmers, gymnasts, football players, and soccer players. Lesions vary from small vesicles to large bullae on the face and body. When ruptured, the erosions become covered with a heavy honey-colored serosanguineous crust. The infection spreads quickly to multiple areas of the body and may lead to deeper invasive infections. A bacterial skin culture may confirm the clinical diagnosis. Treatment consists of local cleansing and debridement with hydrogen peroxide. Administration of oral or topical antibiotic treatments directed at the specific causative agent may also be helpful. As the infection is contagious, epidemics may occur if coaches and athletes pay little attention to the lesions. To prevent the spread of infection, athletic equipment and towels should not be shared and infected athletes should be discouraged from participating until healed.

Pyoderma, which is caused by *Streptococcus pyogenes*, is typically transmitted by close physical contact and may eventually cause acute glomerulonephritis. Epidemic pyoderma caused by nephritogenic streptococci has been documented to occur among members of college athletic teams (62, 104). Strategies such as keeping players with cutaneous streptococcal infections from participating on the field and applying skin antiseptics to traumatized skin after competition may help prevent the spread of infection.

Miscellaneous Infections Caused by Viruses and Bacteria

Conjunctivitis

Several etiologic agents of conjunctivitis may be spread by direct contact, through contaminated swimming pools, or by fomites. The most common bacterial organisms involved are *S. aureus*, *Staphylococcus epidermidis*, and *Haemophilus* species (150). Direct contact with lesions of HSV infections may also result in conjunctival infection. Athletes competing in contact sports such as rugby or wrestling therefore are usually at greater risk.

In one reported case, follicular conjunctivitis was among the complications observed when two players of a rugby team contracted HSV infections while in competition (172). In another study, conjunctival erythema was encountered among seven members of a college wrestling team who had developed extensive cutaneous herpes infections during a 2-week period in the wrestling season (127). The best preventive strategy is to carefully screen out symptomatic athletes before competition. Swimmers with conjunctivitis must also refrain from entering swimming pools to avoid spreading viral agents in the water.

IM

Epstein-Barr virus, which is classified as a herpesvirus, is one agent causing infectious mononucleosis (IM). Cytomegalovirus and *Toxoplasma gondii* are other causes of IM. Transmission may occur by direct contact but more commonly through droplet transmission (i.e., through infected oral secretions, such as saliva). It has been demonstrated that repeated and prolonged exposure to the virus does not necessarily contribute to infection. In one study, it was concluded that college roommates of infected patients had no increased risk of infection as a result of constant exposure (139). The incubation period for primary Epstein-Barr virus infection is generally 30 to 45 days. The illness may persist for 1 to several weeks, while the infectious state may last for up to a year in some cases. Even though life-threatening complications are remarkably infrequent, spontaneous rupture of the spleen and airway obstruction due to massive lymphoid hyperplasia during the acute phase of illness have accounted for a number of reported deaths (106, 137, 154).

Treatment consists of rest, fluids, and analgesics. Acetaminophen is recommended for fever, headache, and muscle pain, along with lozenges, saltwater gargles, or viscous lidocaine for sore throats. Athletes may, however, recover from IM more quickly than nonathletes, although they may not be able to perform to the best of their abilities in competitions for up to 3 months. It is important to restrict all kinds of strenuous activity for at least a month after the onset of clinical illness, since most splenic ruptures occur within the first 21 days of affliction (106, 154). Treatment for IM should be individualized, and athletes should return to activity only when they feel physically ready.

Meningitis

Meningitis may be caused by one of several microorganisms, including bacteria or viruses. *Neisseria meningitidis,* for example, is transmitted by direct contact, including droplets and discharges from the noses and throats of infected persons. The infection is normally spread in places where people are living closely together, such as in school dormitories or military camps. Although no reported cases of meningococcal meningitis are cited pertaining to the crowding conditions of sporting events, there have been episodes of infections occurring in overcrowded environments such as in dance clubs and bars (42, 52, 77, 158).

Viral meningitis is commonly associated with enteroviral infections, especially those of echoviruses and coxsackie B viruses. Several outbreaks of aseptic meningitis have been reported to occur among members of high school football teams (Table 2) (7, 12, 30, 116). Most of the reports indicate that infection was associated with the peak seasonal incidence of aseptic meningitis (summer and fall) and occurred through close physical contact among the athletes or by common-source transmission, such as the unhygienic sharing of water containers or the dipping of cups into a common water source.

URTI

Upper respiratory tract infections (URTI), which are caused by a number of viruses and bacteria, are of the most common illnesses encountered in sports. Symptoms vary according to the type of agent and the individual's immune response. The most common symptoms include runny nose, sneezing, congestion, sore throat, cough, myalgias, and a general feeling of weakness. There are over 200 viruses that may cause URTI, but the most common ones include rhinoviruses, coronaviruses, respiratory syncytial viruses, parainfluenza viruses, and adenoviruses (57). Although viruses account for over 60 to 90% of URTI, bacteria may also cause respiratory infections. In one study, three cases of respiratory infection relating to deep-sea diving involved a penicillin-resistant strain of *Streptococcus pneumoniae* (129).

Transmission may occur by contact with respiratory secretions, such as virus-containing droplets produced by a cough or sneeze, or by contact with contaminated secretions from mucous membranes on hands or shared athletic equipment (71, 140). Good personal hygiene and avoidance of close contact with infected individuals may help prevent infections. It has been suggested, however, that there is a relationship between acute stress and susceptibility to infection. In one study, it was observed that faster marathon runners developed more URTI symptoms than slower or more moderate runners (125). Since the frequency of symptoms is inversely proportional to the time taken to complete a race, it is postulated that a moderate level of physical exercise may be more beneficial in reducing the incidence of respiratory illnesses.

Fungal Infections

Tinea Corporis, Cruris, Pedis, and Versicolor

Tinea is the name applied to fungal infections in the keratin of the skin, hair, and nails. They are named according to the site of infection, such as tinea corporis (body), tinea cruris (groin), tinea manes (hands), tinea pedis (feet), tinea capitis (scalp), and tinea onychomycosis (nail) (21). A definitive diagnosis may be made by fungal cultures or KOH preparations of skin scrapings. It is important for these disorders to be recognized early to avert cancelled practices and competitions. Treatment may vary according to the type of fungal organism involved and the site of infection. The factors contributing to most cases in athletes are the presence of increased moisture from sweat, occlusive footwear, shared towels, skin injuries, and contaminated floors in the locker room, gymnasium, or showering facilities (29, 60, 130).

Tinea pedis, also known as athlete's foot, is most commonly seen among marathon runners, swimmers, and professional ice hockey players, as well as persons active in basketball, judo, tennis, water polo, and football (85, 98, 115). *Trichophyton rubrum*, which generally causes an erythematous and scaling eruption on the plantar surface of the foot, and *Trichophyton mentagrophytes*, which may present as painful, pruritic blisters, are the most common organisms involved (11). One study suggests that fungal infection of the toenail (onychomycosis) is three times more prevalent among swimmers and athletes already infected with tinea pedis than among the general population (67). Keeping the feet dry by wearing appropriate shoes and socks, using drying powders, and wearing sandals in the locker room or shower may help prevent infection. Topical treatments with antifungal agents are effective and should be applied several times a day.

Tinea corporis, also known as tinea corporis gladiatorum or ringworm (156; K. Werninghaus, Letter, *J. Am. Acad. Dermatol.* **28:**1022–1023, 1993), is a type of tinea infection occurring on portions of the skin where hair is not present, such as the face, trunk, and limbs. Athletes participating in close-contact sports such as football, rugby, and wrestling are at risk of becoming infected. Several outbreaks involving *Trichophyton tonsurans* have been reported among high school and college wrestlers (Table 2) (4, 19, 54, 75, 94, 126, 156; Werninghaus, letter). Athletes should either cover lesions or refrain from participating in sports to prevent the spread of infection. Other preventive strategies include inspecting the skin regularly and avoiding the use of shared equipment. Prophylactic treatment of tinea gladiatorum has been investigated and proven effective with intermittent doses of oral itraconazole (70) and 100 mg of fluconazole once weekly (93). Though topical antifungal agents are effective treatment options, the cost, the increased risk of microbial resistance, and the potential adverse effects of the medications may make general prophylaxis for all team members unattractive (3).

Tinea cruris, also known as "jock itch," is an infection involving the groin and upper thighs. The fungal organisms and treatment methods involved are similar to those of tinea pedis. The pruritic rash appears as red, scaly patches, usually with sharp margins, covering the moist areas. Symptoms include pain and pruritus with occasional production of a weeping discharge. Keeping the areas dry and maintaining good hygiene may help prevent infection.

Tinea versicolor, or "fungus of many colors," is caused by a yeast called *Pityrosporum orbiculare*. The diagnosis is confirmed by KOH staining of a skin scraping, which shows the active fungal form called *Malassezia furfur*, and a characteristic yellow-orange color appears under inspection with Wood's light. Hyperpigmented or hypopigmented irregularly shaped scaly patches that are asymptomatic typically appear on the back, trunk, neck, arms, and upper extremities. It is suggested that other than acne, tinea versicolor is the most common affliction observed in athletes participating in college football and basketball (W. E. McDaniel, Letter, *Arch. Dermatol.* **113**:519–520, 1997). Topical antifungal treatments and oral regimens are effective therapeutic measures.

COMMON-SOURCE TRANSMISSION

Common-source exposure to infectious diseases in athletic settings normally occurs in cases where water or food containers are either shared or contaminated. Such outbreaks may involve a myriad of different infectious agents. For example, an outbreak of hepatitis A occurred among players and coaching staff of a college football team as a result of a contaminated water supply (118). Enteroviral infections, such as aseptic meningitis and pleurodynia, have also been documented to occur by similar means in other studies involving members of athletic teams (Table 2) (7, 12, 30, 76, 116).

AIRBORNE TRANSMISSION

There is a potential risk of spreading infectious diseases by airborne transmission during indoor sporting events, where large groups of people are gathered in a confined environment. A packed, humid gym or stadium provides the classic conditions for the spread of illnesses such as measles, chickenpox (which is caused by varicella-zoster virus), and influenza (108). Although usually not life threatening, such illnesses may keep an athlete from competing, postpone sporting events, or deteriorate a team's competitive edge. Airborne infections, however, are not confined to the athletes competing on the field. Spectators watching sporting events from afar are at risk of infection as well. For example, several outbreaks of measles have been reported in association with mass spectator sporting events (Table 2) (31, 43, 53). Outdoor sports, such as track and field, baseball, and football, do not pose a high risk for airborne infections because the viruses become inactivated in sunlight (171). Immunizations are recommended and may help prevent the spread of infections.

WATER SPORTS-ASSOCIATED INFECTIONS

Water acts as a passive carrier for numerous infectious agents. Athletes participating in water sports may be at risk, depending on type of activity and water quality (39, 45, 69, 91, 97, 102, 121, 145, 162, 168). Water-based infections known to have been acquired by athletes either by prolonged contact with water or by ingestion during a sporting event are listed in Table 3 and reference 50. Leptospirosis and otitis externa, two of the prominent water-based diseases faced by athletes, are discussed below.

Table 3. Potential infectious diseases associated with water sports

Disseminated infections
  Leptospirosis

Enteric infections
  Amoebic dysentery
  Cryptosporidiosis (32)
  Escherichia coli infections (1, 33)
  Gastroenteritis
  Giardiasis
  Infectious hepatitis
  Norwalk virus infection (13, 96)
  Salmonellosis
  Shigellosis (136, 151)
  Typhoid fever

Eye infections
  Acanthamoebic keratitis

Skin and soft tissue infections
  Conjunctivitis
  Otitis externa
  Schistosome dermatitis (swimmer's itch) (99)
  Schistosomiasis

Respiratory infections
  Legionnaires' disease (e.g., Pontiac fever) (105)
  Pneumonia following near drowning

Wound infections
  Aeromonas primary wound infection (83)

Leptospirosis

Leptospirosis is transmitted via ingestion of urine-contaminated water, exposure to contaminated lakes or streams, or contact with infected animals or their excretions. Symptoms include chills, fever, headache, and a rash. If left untreated, the disease may result in liver or kidney damage and may also be fatal. Enthusiasts participating in water sports in environmental waters are at greater risk of infection. Several leptospiral outbreaks involving white-water rafters, swimmers, kayakers, and other recreational water users have been documented (Table 2) (10, 34, 79, 80, 89, 124). Outbreaks involving athletes participating in triathlons (races consisting of swimming, biking, and running competitions) who may have had exposure to contaminated waters have also been reported (35, 36, 37, 66, 117, 142, 161). Antimicrobial agents should be administered to treat the disease, and preventive measures, such as wearing protective clothing to minimize contact with potentially contaminated water, should be implemented (173).

Otitis Externa

Acute otitis externa, also known as swimmer's ear, is an inflammation of the external auditory canal. It is typically seen among athletes participating in water sports who commonly experience mechanical trauma to the external ear. Swimmers, divers, surfers, sailboarders, and kayakers who participate in their sports in polluted bodies of water are usually at risk of infection. The infection is most commonly caused by *P. aeruginosa* but may also be caused by the fungus *Aspergillus* and other organisms (6, 18). Prolonged exposure to water causes maceration of the epithelial tissue in the ear canal and removes the ear wax, which normally aids in repelling water and maintaining an acidic pH to prevent bacterial and fungal growth. Cleaning the external auditory canal and keeping it as dry as possible are important aspects of therapy, along with other available treatments, such as the application of antibacterial and antifungal creams.

CONCLUSION

The objective of this chapter has been to focus upon infectious diseases commonly transmitted in sporting environments. Several types of infectious pathogens have been identified which have affected individual athletes, team members, persons who came into contact with the participants, or spectators who were merely watching the events from afar. Most of the reviewed cases, however, could have been prevented with proper hygiene, appropriate immunizations, early recognition, and subsequent exclusion of infected participants during the game. Physicians caring for athletes must play an active role in educating them about effective preventive strategies and in providing advice on appropriate treatment methods based on consideration of their individual situations. Fortunately, being a healthy population in general, athletes tend to respond well to treatments provided.

Acknowledgments. A.M. thanks Gerry Silverstein of the Department of Microbiology at the University of Vermont College of Medicine for his advice and editorial assistance.

REFERENCES

1. Ackman, D., S. Marks, P. Mack, M. Caldwell, T. Root, and G. Birkhead. 1997. Swimming-associated haemorrhagic colitis due to *Escherichia coli* O157:H7 infection: evidence of prolonged contamination of a fresh water lake. *Epidemiol. Infect.* **119**:1–8.
2. Adams, B. B. 2002. Dermatologic disorders of the athlete. *Sports Med.* **32**:309–321.
3. Adams, B. B. 2002. Tinea corporis gladiatorum. *J. Am. Acad. Dermatol.* **47**:286–290.
4. Adams, B. B. 2000. Tinea corporis gladiatorum: a cross-sectional study. *J. Am. Acad. Dermatol.* **43**:1039–1041.
5. Adler, A. I., and J. Altman. 1993. An outbreak of mud-wrestling-induced pustular dermatitis in college students. Dermatitis palaestrae limosae. *JAMA* **269**:502–504.
6. Agius, A. M., J. M. Pickles, and K. L. Burch. 1992. A prospective study of otitis externa. *Clin. Otolaryngol.* **17**:150–154.
7. Alexander, J. P., Jr., L. E. Chapman, M. A. Pallansch, W. T. Stephenson, T. J. Török, and L. J. Anderson. 1993. Coxsackievirus B2 infection and aseptic meningitis: a focal outbreak among members of a high school football team. *J. Infect. Dis.* **167**:1201–1205.
8. American Academy of Pediatrics Committee on Sports Medicine and Fitness. 1991. American Academy of Pediatrics Committee on Sports Medicine and Fitness: human immunodeficiency virus [acquired immunodeficiency syndrome (AIDS) virus] in the athletic setting. *Pediatrics* **88**:640–641.
9. American Medical Society for Sports Medicine and American Academy of Sports Medicine. 1995. Human immunodeficiency virus (HIV) and other blood-borne pathogens in sports (joint position statement): the American Medical Society for Sports Medicine (AMSSM) and the American Academy of Sports Medicine (AASM). *Am. J. Sports Med.* **23**:510–514.
10. Anderson, D. C., D. S. Folland, M. D. Fox, C. M. Patton, and A. F. Kaufmann. 1978. Leptospirosis: a common-source outbreak due to leptospires of the grippotyphosa serogroup. *Am. J. Epidemiol.* **107**:538–544.
11. Auger, P., G. Marquis, J. Joly, and A. Attye. 1993. Epidemiology of tinea pedis in marathon runners: prevalence of occult athlete's foot. *Mycoses* **36**:35–41.
12. Baron, R. C., M. H. Hatch, K. Kleeman, and J. N. MacCormack. 1982. Aseptic meningitis among members of a high school football team: an outbreak associated with echovirus 16 infection. *JAMA* **248**:1724–1727.
13. Baron, R. C., F. D. Murphy, H. B. Greenberg, C. E. Davis, D. J. Bregman, G. W. Gary, J. M. Hughes, and L. B. Schonberger. 1982. Norwalk gastrointestinal illness: an outbreak associated with swimming in a recreational lake and secondary person-to-person transmission. *Am. J. Epidemiol.* **115**:163–172.
14. Bartlett, P. C., R. J. Martin, and B. R. Cahill. 1982. Furunculosis in a high school football team. *Am. J. Sports Med.* **10**:371–374.
15. Basler, R. S. W. 1983. Skin lesions related to sports activity. *Prim. Care* **10**:479–494.
16. Basler, R. S. W. 1989. Sports-related skin injuries. *Adv. Dermatol.* **4**:29–50.
17. Becker, T. M., R. Kodsi, P. Bailey, F. Lee, R. Levandowski, and A. J. Nahmias. 1988. Grappling with herpes: herpes gladiatorum. *Am. J. Sports Med.* **16**:665–669.
18. Bell, D. N. 1985. Otitis externa: a common, often self-inflicted condition. *Postgrad. Med.* **78**:101–104, 106.
19. Beller, M., and B. D. Gessner. 1994. An outbreak of tinea corporis gladiatorum on a high school wrestling team. *J. Am. Acad. Dermatol.* **31**:197–201.
20. Belongia, E. A., J. L. Goodman, E. J. Holland, C. W. Andres, S. R. Homann, R. L. Mahanti, M. W. Mizener, A. Erice, and M. T. Osterholm. 1991. An outbreak of herpes gladiatorum at a high-school wrestling camp. *N. Engl. J. Med.* **325**:906–910.
21. Bergfeld, W. F. 1984. Dermatologic problems in athletes. *Prim. Care* **11**:151–160.
22. Bergfeld, W. F., and J. S. Taylor. 1985. Trauma, sports, and the skin. *Am. J. Ind. Med.* **8**:403–413.
23. Bitting, L. A., C. A. Trowbridge, and L. E. Costello. 1996. A model for a policy on HIV-AIDS and athletics. *J. Athl. Train.* **31**:356–357.
24. Brown, L. S., Jr., D. P. Drotman, A. Chu, C. L. Brown, Jr., and D. Knowlan. 1995. Bleeding injuries in professional football: estimating the risk of HIV transmission. *Ann. Intern. Med.* **122**:271–274.

25. **Brown, L. S., Jr., R. Y. Phillips, C. L. Brown, Jr., D. Knowlan, L. Castle, and J. Moyer.** 1994. HIV-AIDS policies and sports: the National Football League. *Med. Sci. Sports Exerc.* **26:**403–407.

26. **Calabrese, L. H., H. A. Haupt, L. Hartman, and R. H. Strauss.** 1993. HIV and sports: what is the risk? *Physician Sportsmed.* **21:**173–180.

27. **Calabrese, L. H., and D. Kelley.** 1989. AIDS and athletes. *Physician Sportsmed.* **17:**126.

28. **Calabrese, L. H., and A. LaPerriere.** 1993. Human immunodeficiency virus infection, exercise and athletics. *Sports Med.* **15:**6–13.

29. **Caputo, R., K. De Boulle, J. Del Rosso, and R. Nowicki.** 2001. Prevalence of superficial fungal infections among sports-active individuals: results from the Achilles survey, a review of the literature. *J. Eur. Acad. Dermatol. Venereol.* **15:**312–316.

30. **Centers for Disease Control.** 1981. Aseptic meningitis in a high school football team—Ohio. *Morb. Mortal. Wkly. Rep.* **29:**631–637.

31. **Centers for Disease Control.** 1992. Measles at an international gymnastics competition—Indiana, 1991. *Morb. Mortal. Wkly Rep.* **41:**109–111.

32. **Centers for Disease Control and Prevention.** 1994. Cryptosporidium infections associated with swimming pools—Dane County, Wisconsin, 1993. *Morb. Mortal. Wkly. Rep.* **43:**561–563.

33. **Centers for Disease Control and Prevention.** 1996. Lake-associated outbreak of *Escherichia coli* O157:H7—Illinois, 1995. *Morb. Mortal. Wkly. Rep.* **45:**437–439.

34. **Centers for Disease Control and Prevention.** 1997. Outbreak of leptospirosis among white-water rafters—Costa Rica, 1996. *JAMA* **278:**808.

35. **Centers for Disease Control and Prevention.** 1998. Update: leptospirosis and unexplained acute febrile illness among athletes participating in triathlons—Illinois and Wisconsin, 1998. *Morb. Mortal. Wkly. Rep.* **47:**673–676.

36. **Centers for Disease Control and Prevention.** 2001. Update on emerging infections: news from the Centers for Disease Control and Prevention. *Ann. Emerg. Med.* **38:**83–86.

37. **Centers for Disease Control and Prevention.** 2001. Update: outbreak of acute febrile illness among athletes participating in Eco-Challenge-Sabah 2000—Borneo, Malaysia, 2000. *Morb. Mortal. Wkly. Rep.* **50:**21–24.

38. **Chandrasekar, P. H., K. V. I. Rolston, D. W. Kannangara, J. L. Le Frock, and S. A. Binnick.** 1984. Hot tub-associated dermatitis due to *Pseudomonas aeruginosa. Arch. Dermatol.* **120:**1337–1340.

39. **Chang, W. J., and F. D. Pien.** 1986. Marine-acquired infections. Hazards of the ocean environment. *Postgrad. Med.* **80:**30–32, 37, 41.

40. Reference deleted.

41. **Conklin, R. J.** 1990. Common cutaneous disorders in athletes. *Sports Med.* **9:**100–119.

42. **Cookson, S. T.** 1998. Disco fever: epidemic meningococcal disease in northeastern Argentina associated with disco patronage. *J. Infect. Dis.* **178:**266–269.

43. **Davis, R. M., E. D. Whitman, W. A. Orenstein, S. R. Preblud, L. E. Markowitz, and A. R. Hinman.** 1987. A persistent outbreak of measles despite appropriate prevention and control measures. *Am. J. Epidemiol.* **126:**438–449.

44. **Decker, M. D., J. A. Lybarger, W. K. Vaughn, R. H. Hutcheson, Jr., and W. Schaffner.** 1986. An outbreak of staphylococcal skin infections among river rafting guides. *Am. J. Epidemiol.* **124:**969–976.

45. **Dewailly, E., C. Poirier, and F. M. Meyer.** 1986. Health hazards associated with windsurfing on polluted water. *Am. J. Public Health* **76:**690–691.

46. **Dodge, B. G., W. R. Knowles, M. E. McBride, W. C. Duncan, and J. M. Knox.** 1968. Treatment of erythrasma with an antibacterial soap. *Arch. Dermatol.* **97:**548–552.

47. **Dorman, J. M.** 2000. Contagious diseases in competitive sport: what are the risks? *J. Am. Coll. Health* **49:**105–109.

48. Reference deleted.

49. **Drotman, D. P.** 1996. Professional boxing, bleeding, and HIV testing. *JAMA* **276:**193.

50. **Dufour, A. P.** 1986. Diseases caused by water contact, p. 23–41. *In* G. F. Craun (ed.), *Waterborne Diseases in the United States.* CRC Press, Boca Raton, Fla.

51. **Dyke, L. M., U. R. Merikangas, O. C. Bruton, S. G. Trask, and F. M. Hetrick.** 1965. Skin infection in wrestlers due to herpes simplex virus. *JAMA* **194:**1001–1002.

52. **Edmond, M. B., R. J. Hollis, A. K. Houston, and R. P. Wenzel.** 1995. Molecular epidemiology of an outbreak of meningococcal disease in a university community. *J. Clin. Microbiol.* **33:**2209–2211.

53. **Ehresmann, K., C. Hedberg, and M. Grimm.** 1995. An outbreak of measles at an international sporting event with airborne transmission in a domed stadium. *J. Infect. Dis.* **171:**679–683.

54. **El-Fari, M., Y. Gräser, W. Presber, and H.-J. Tietz.** 2000. An epidemic of tinea corporis caused by *Trichophyton tonsurans* among children (wrestlers) in Germany. *Mycoses* **43:**191–196.

55. Reference deleted.

56. **Feller, A., and T. P. Flanigan.** 1997. HIV-infected competitive athletes. What are the risks? What precautions should be taken? *J. Gen. Intern. Med.* **12:**243–246.

57. **Fields, K. B., and P. A. Fricker (ed.).** 1997. *Medical Problems in Athletes.* Blackwell Science, Inc., Malden, Mass.

58. **Freeman, M. J., and W. F. Bergfeld.** 1977. Skin diseases of football and wrestling participants. *Cutis* **20:**333–341.

59. **Gauthier, M. M.** 1987. Sports health workers respond to AIDS. *Physician Sportsmed.* **15:**51–54.

60. **Gentles, J. C., E. G. V. Evans, and G. R. Jones.** 1974. Control of tinea pedis in a swimming bath. *Br. Med. J.* **1:**577–580.

61. **Gille, G., O. Ringertz, and B. Zetterberg.** 1967. Serum hepatitis among Swedish track-finders. II. A clinical study. *Acta Med. Scand.* **182:**129–135.

62. **Glezen, P. W., J. L. DeWalt, R. L. Lindsay, and H. C. Dillon.** 1972. Epidemic pyoderma caused by nephritogenic streptococci in college athletes. *Lancet* **i:**301–303.

63. **Goldsmith, M. F.** 1992. When sports and HIV share the bill, smart money goes on common sense. *JAMA* **267:**1311–1314.

64. **Goodman, R. A., S. B. Thacker, S. L. Solomon, M. T. Osterholm, and J. M. Hughes.** 1994. Infectious diseases in competitive sports. *JAMA* **271:**862–867.

65. **Green, J. J.** 2000. Localized whirlpool folliculitis in a football player. *Cutis* **65:**359–362.

66. **Guarner, J., W.-J. Shieh, J. Morgan, S. L. Bragg, M. D. Bajani, J. W. Tappero, and S. R. Zaki.** 2001. Leptospirosis mimicking acute cholecystitis among athletes participating in a triathlon. *Hum. Pathol.* **32:**750–752.

67. **Gudnadóttir, G., I. Hilmarsdóttir, and B. Sigurgeirsson.** 1999. Onychomycosis in Icelandic swimmers. *Acta Dermato-venereol.* **79:**376–377.

68. **Gunby, P.** 1988. Boxing: AIDS? *JAMA* **259:**1613–1614.

69. **Harris, J. R., M. L. Cohen, and E. C. Lippy.** 1983. Water-related disease outbreaks in the United States, 1981. *J. Infect. Dis.* **148:**759–762.

70. **Hazen, P. G., and M. L. Weil.** 1997. Itraconazole in the prevention and management of dermatophytosis in competitive wrestlers. *J. Am. Acad. Dermatol.* **36:**481–482.

71. **Heath, G. W., C. A. Macera, and D. C. Nieman.** 1992. Exercise and upper respiratory tract infections. Is there a relationship? *Sports Med.* **14:**353–365.

72. **Highet, A. S.** 1992. Molluscum contagiosum. *Arch. Dis. Child.* **67:**1248–1249.

73. **Ho, D. D., T. Moudgil, and M. Alam.** 1989. Quantitation of human immunodeficiency virus type 1 in the blood of infected persons. *N. Engl. J. Med.* **321:**1621–1625.

74. **Houston, S. D., and J. M. Knox.** 1977. Skin problems related to sports and recreational activities. *Cutis* **19:**487–491.

75. **Hradil, E., K. Hersle, P. Nordin, and J. Faergemann.** 1995. An epidemic of tinea corporis caused by *Trichophyton tonsurans* among wrestlers in Sweden. *Acta Dermato-venereol.* **75:**305–306.

76. **Ikeda, R. M., S. F. Kondracki, P. D. Drabkin, G. S. Birkhead, and D. L. Morse.** 1993. Pleurodynia among football players at a high school. An outbreak associated with coxsackievirus B1. *JAMA* **270:**2205–2206.

77. **Imrey, P. B., L. A. Jackson, P. H. Ludwinski, A. C. England III, G. A. Fella, B. C. Fox, L. B. Isdale, M. W. Reeves, and J. D. Wenger.** 1996. Outbreak of serogroup C meningococcal disease associated with campus bar patronage. *Am. J. Epidemiol.* **143:**624–630.

78. Reference deleted.

79. **Jackson, L. A., A. F. Kaufmann, W. G. Adams, M. B. Phelps, C. Andreasen, C. W. Langkop, B. J. Francis, and J. D. Wenger.** 1993. Outbreak of leptospirosis associated with swimming. *Pediatr. Infect. Dis. J.* **12:**48–54.

80. **Jevon, T. R., M. P. Knudson, P. A. Smith, P. S. Whitecar, and R. L. Blake, Jr.** 1986. A point-source epidemic of leptospirosis. Description of cases, cause, and prevention. *Postgrad. Med.* **80:**121–122, 127–129.

81. **Johnson, R. J.** 1992. HIV infection in athletes. What are the risks? Who can compete? *Postgrad. Med.* **92:**73–75, 79–80.

82. **Jones, W. K., and J. W. Curran.** 1994. Epidemiology of AIDS and HIV infection in industrialized countries, p. 91–108. *In* J. J. Pine (ed.), *Textbook of AIDS Medicine.* Williams & Wilkins, Baltimore, Md.

83. **Joseph, S. W., O. P. Daily, W. S. Hunt, R. J. Seidler, D. A. Allen, and R. R. Colwell.** 1979. *Aeromonas* primary wound infection of a diver in polluted waters. *J. Clin. Microbiol.* **10:**46–49.

84. Reference deleted.

85. **Kamihama, T., T. Kimura, J.-I. Hosokawa, M. Ueji, T. Takase, and K. Tagami.** 1997. Tinea pedis outbreak in swimming pools in Japan. *Public Health* **111:**249–253.

86. **Kantor, G. R., and W. F. Bergfeld.** 1988. Common and uncommon dermatologic diseases related to sports activities. *Exerc. Sport Sci. Rev.* **16:**215–253.

87. Reference deleted.

88. **Kashiwagi, S., J. Hayashi, H. Ikematsu, S. Nishigori, K. Ishihara, and M. Kaji.** 1982. An outbreak of hepatitis B in members of a high school sumo wrestling club. *JAMA* **248:**213–214.

89. **Katz, A. R., S. J. Manea, and D. M. Sasaki.** 1991. Leptospirosis on Kauai: investigation of a common source waterborne outbreak. *Am. J. Public Health* **81:**1310–1312.

90. **Keilhofner, M., and D. S. McKinsey.** 1988. Herpes gladiatorum in a high school wrestler. *Mo. Med.* **85:**723–725.

91. **Kincaid, C. K.** 1967. Lake pollution and human disease. *Wis. Med. J.* **66:**371–372.

92. **Klein, A. W., and D. C. Rish.** 1992. Sports related skin problems. *Compr. Ther.* **18:**2–4.

93. **Kohl, T. D., D. C. Martin, R. Nemeth, T. Hill, and D. Evans.** 2000. Fluconazole for the prevention and treatment of tinea gladiatorum. *Pediatr. Infect. Dis. J.* **19:**717–722.

94. **Kohl, T. D., D. P. Giesen, J. Moyer, and M. Lisney.** 2002. Tinea gladiatorum: Pennsylvania's experience. *Clin. J. Sport Med.* **12:**165–171.

95. **Kooistra, J. A.** 1965. Prophylaxis and control of erythrasma of the toe webs. *J. Investig. Dermatol.* **45:**399–400.

96. **Koopman, J. S., E. A. Eckert, H. B. Greenberg, B. C. Strohm, R. E. Isaacson, and A. S. Monto.** 1982. Norwalk virus enteric illness acquired by swimming exposure. *Am. J. Epidemiol.* **115:**173–177.

97. **Krishnaswami, S. K.** 1971. Health aspects of water quality. *Am. J. Public Health* **61:**2259–2268.

98. **Lacroix, C., M. Baspeyras, P. de-La-Salmonière, M. Benderdouche, B. Couprie, I. Accoceberry, F. Weill, and F. Derouin.** 2002. Tinea pedis in European marathon runners. *J. Eur. Acad. Dermatol. Venereol.* **16:**139–142.

99. **Lévesque, S., P. Giovenazzo, P. Guerrier, D. Laverdière, and H. Prud'Homme.** 2002. Investigation of an outbreak of cercarial dermatitis. *Epidemiol. Infect.* **129:**379–386.

100. **Levine, N.** 1980. Dermatologic aspects of sports medicine. *J. Am. Acad. Dermatol.* **3:**415–424.

101. **Lindenmayer, J. M., S. Schoenfeld, R. O'Grady, and J. K. Carney.** 1998. Methicillin-resistant *Staphylococcus aureus* in a high school wrestling team and the surrounding community. *Arch. Intern. Med.* **158:**895–899.

102. **Losonsky, G.** 1991. Infections associated with swimming and diving. *Undersea Biomed. Res.* **18:**181–185.

103. Reference deleted.

104. **Ludlam, H., and B. Cookson.** 1986. Scrum kidney: epidemic pyoderma caused by a nephritogenic *Streptococcus pyogenes* in a rugby team. *Lancet* **ii:**331–333.

105. **Lüttichau, H. R., C. Vinther, S. A. Uldum, J. Møller, M. Faber, and J. S. Jensen.** 1998. An outbreak of Pontiac fever among children following use of a whirlpool. *Clin. Infect. Dis.* **26:**1374–1378.

106. **Maki, D. G., and R. M. Reich.** 1982. Infectious mononucleosis in the athlete. Diagnosis, complications, and management. *Am. J. Sports Med.* **10:**162–173.

107. **Maré, J. B., C. M. J. Keyzer, and W. B. Becker.** 1978. Traumatic *Herpesvirus hominis* infection during rugby (herpes venatorum): a discussion of four cases. *S. Afr. Med. J.* **54:**752–754.

108. **Mast, E. E., and R. A. Goodman.** 1997. Prevention of infectious disease transmission in sports. *Sports Med.* **24:**1–7.

109. **Mast, E. E., R. A. Goodman, W. W. Bond, M. S. Favero, and D. P. Drotman.** 1995. Transmission of blood-borne pathogens during sports: risk and prevention. *Ann. Intern. Med.* **122:**283–285.

110. Reference deleted.

111. McGrew, C. A., R. W. Dick, K. Schniedwind, and P. Gikas. 1993. Survey of NCAA institutions concerning HIV/AIDS policies and universal precautions. *Med. Sci. Sports Exerc.* **25**:917–921.

112. Midtvedt, T., and K. Midtvedt. 1982. Sport and infection. *Scand. J. Soc. Med. Suppl.* **29**:241–244.

113. Mills, J., L. Hauer, A. Gottlieb, S. Dromgoole, and S. Spruance. 1987. Recurrent herpes labialis in skiers. Clinical observations and effect of sunscreen. *Am. J. Sports Med.* **15**:76–78.

114. Reference deleted.

115. Möhrenschlager, M., H. P. Seidl, C. Schnopp, J. Ring, and D. Abeck. 2001. Professional ice hockey players: a high-risk group for fungal infection of the foot? *Dermatology* **203**:271.

116. Moore, M., R. C. Baron, M. R. Filstein, J. P. Lofgren, D. L. Rowley, L. B. Schonberger, and M. H. Hatch. 1983. Aseptic meningitis and high school football players: 1978 and 1980. *JAMA* **249**:2039–2042.

117. Morgan, J., S. L. Bornstein, A. M. Karpati, M. Bruce, C. A. Bolin, C. C. Austin, C. W. Woods, J. Lingappa, C. Langkop, B. Davis, D. R. Graham, M. Proctor, D. A. Ashford, M. Bajani, S. L. Bragg, K. Shutt, B. A. Perkins, and J. W. Tappero. 2002. Outbreak of leptospirosis among triathlon participants and community residents in Springfield, Illinois, 1998. *Clin. Infect. Dis.* **34**:1593–1599.

118. Morse, L. J., J. A. Bryan, L. W. Chang, J. P. Hurley, J. F. Murphy, and T. F. O'Brien. 1970. Holy Cross football team hepatitis outbreak. *Antimicrob. Agents Chemother.* **10**:30–32.

119. Morse, L. J., J. A. Bryan, J. P. Hurley, J. F. Murphy, T. F. O'Brien, and W. E. C. Wacker. 1972. The Holy Cross college football team hepatitis outbreak. *JAMA* **219**:706–708.

120. Mullan, R. J., E. L. Baker, D. M. Bell, W. W. Bond, M. C. Chamberland, M. S. Favero, J. S. Garner, S. C. Hadler, J. M. Hughes, H. W. Jaffe, M. A. Kane, R. Marcus, W. J. Martone, M. J. Scally, and P. W. Strine. 1989. Guidelines for prevention of transmission of human immunodeficiency virus and hepatitis B virus to health-care and public safety workers. *Morb. Mortal. Wkly. Rep.* **38**:1–37.

121. Mumford, C. J. 1989. Leptospirosis and water sports. *Br. J. Hosp. Med.* **41**:519.

122. Niizeki, K., O. Kano, and Y. Kondo. 1984. An epidemic study of molluscum contagiosum: relationship to swimming. *Dermatologica* **169**:197–198.

123. Reference deleted.

124. Perra, A., V. Servas, G. Terrier, D. Postic, G. Baranton, G. André-Fontaine, V. Vaillant, and I. Capek. 2002. Clustered cases of leptospirosis in Rochefort, France, June 2001. *Eurosurveillance* **7**:131–136.

125. Peters, E. M., and E. D. Bateman. 1983. Ultramarathon running and upper respiratory tract infections: an epidemiological survey. *S. Afr. Med. J.* **64**:582–584.

126. Piqu, E., R. Copado, A. Cabrera, M. Olivares, M. C. Farina, P. Escalonilla, M. L. Soriano, and L. Requena. 1999. An outbreak of tinea gladiatorum in Lanzarote. *Clin. Exp. Dermatol.* **24**:7–9.

127. Porter, P. S., and R. D. Baughman. 1965. Epidemiology of herpes simplex among wrestlers. *JAMA* **194**:998–1000.

128. Raborn, G. W., A. Y. Martel, M. G. A. Grace, and W. T. McGaw. 1997. Herpes labialis in skiers: randomized clinical trial of acyclovir cream versus placebo. *Oral Surg. Oral Med. Oral Pathol. Oral Radiol. Endod.* **84**:641–645.

129. Raymond, L. W., D. T. Kingsbury, and J. F. Duncan. 1971. Penicillin resistance of *D. pneumoniae* in upper respiratory infections associated with diving. *Aerosp. Med.* **42**:196–198.

130. Resnik, S. S., L. A. Lewis, and B. H. Cohen. 1977. The athlete's foot. *Cutis* **20**:351–353, 355.

131. Ringertz, O. 1971. Some aspects of the epidemiology of hepatitis in Sweden. *Postgrad. Med. J.* **47**:465–472.

132. Ringertz, O., and B. Zetterberg. 1967. Serum hepatitis among Swedish track finders. An epidemiologic study. *N. Engl. J. Med.* **276**:540–546.

133. Risser, W. L. 1992. HIV makes caution necessary in sports settings. *Physician Sportsmed.* **20**:190.

134. Roach, M. C., and J. H. Chretien. 1995. Common hand warts in athletes: association with trauma to the hand. *J. Am. Coll. Health* **44**:125–126.

135. Rosenbaum, G. S., M. J. Strampfer, and B. A. Cunha. 1990. Herpes gladiatorum in a male wrestler. *Int. J. Dermatol.* **29**:141–142.

136. Rosenberg, M. L., K. K. Hazlet, J. Schaefer, J. G. Wells, and R. C. Pruneda. 1976. Shigellosis from swimming. *JAMA* **236**:1849–1852.

137. Rutkow, I. M. 1978. Rupture of the spleen in infectious mononucleosis. *Arch. Surg.* **113**:718–720.

138. Sadovsky, R. 1995. Transmission of blood-borne pathogens during sports contact. *Am. Fam. Physician* **51**:2011.

139. Sawyer, R. N., A. S. Evans, J. C. Niederman, and R. W. McCollum. 1971. Prospective studies of a group of Yale University freshmen. I. Occurrence of infectious mononucleosis. *J. Infect. Dis.* **123**:263–270.

140. Schouten, W. J., R. Verschuur, and H. C. G. Kemper. 1988. Physical activity and upper respiratory tract infections in a normal population of young men and women: the Amsterdam growth and health study. *Int. J. Sports Med.* **9**:451–455.

141. Reference deleted.

142. Sejvar, J., E. Bancroft, K. Winthrop, J. Bettinger, M. Bajani, S. Bragg, K. Shutt, R. Kaiser, N. Marano, T. Popovic, J. Tappero, D. Ashford, L. Mascola, D. Vugia, B. Perkins, N. Rosenstein, and the Eco-Challenge Investigation Team. 2003. Leptospirosis in "Eco-Challenge" athletes, Malaysian Borneo, 2000. *Emerg. Infect. Dis.* **9**:702–707.

143. Selling, B., and S. Kibrick. 1964. An outbreak of herpes simplex among wrestlers (herpes gladiatorum). *N. Engl. J. Med.* **270**:979–982.

144. Sevier, T. L. 1994. Infectious disease in athletes. *Med. Clin. N. Am.* **78**:389–412.

145. Seyfried, P. L., R. S. Tobin, N. E. Brown, and P. F. Ness. 1985. A prospective study of swimming-related illness. *Am. J. Public Health* **75**:1068–1070.

146. Sharp, J. C. 1994. ABC of sports medicine: infections in sport. *Br. Med. J.* **308**:1702–1706.

147. Sharp, J. C. 1989. Viruses and the athlete. *Br. J. Sports Med.* **23**:47–48.

148. Shute, P., D. J. Jeffries, and A. C. Maddocks. 1979. Scrum-pox caused by herpes simplex virus. *Br. Med. J.* **2**:1629.

149. Skinner, G. R. B., J. Davies, A. Ahmad, P. McLeish, and A. Buchan. 1996. An outbreak of herpes rugbiorum managed by vaccination of players and sociosexual contacts. *J. Infect.* **33**:163–167.

150. Snyder, R. W., and D. B. Glasser. 1994. Antibiotic therapy for ocular infection. *West. J. Med.* **161**:579–584.

151. Sorvillo, F. J., S. H. Waterman, J. K. Vogt, and B. England. 1988. Shigellosis associated with recreational water contact in Los Angeles county. *Am. J. Trop. Med. Hyg.* **38**:613–617.

152. Sosin, D. M., R. A. Gunn, W. L. Ford, and J. W. Skaggs. 1989. An outbreak of furunculosis among high school athletes. *Am. J. Sports Med.* **17**:828–832.

153. Spruance, S. L., M. L. Hamill, W. S. Hoge, L. G. Davis, and J. Mills. 1988. Acyclovir prevents reactivation of herpes simplex labialis in skiers. *JAMA* **260**:1597–1599.

154. Srivastava, K. P., E. C. Quinlan, and T. V. Casey. 1972. Spontaneous rupture of the spleen secondary to infectious mononucleosis. *Int. Surg.* **57**:171–173.

155. Stacey, A. R., K. E. Endersby, P. C. Chan, and R. R. Marples. 1998. An outbreak of methicillin resistant *Staphylococcus aureus* infection in a rugby football team. *Br. J. Sports Med.* **32**:153–154.

156. Stiller, M. J., W. P. Klein, R. I. Dorman, and S. Rosenthal. 1992. Tinea corporis gladiatorum: an epidemic of *Trichophyton tonsurans* in student wrestlers. *J. Am. Acad. Dermatol.* **27**:632–633.

157. Strauss, R. H., D. J. Leizman, R. R. Lanese, and M. F. Para. 1989. Abrasive shirts may contribute to herpes gladiatorum among wrestlers. *N. Engl. J. Med.* **320**:598–599.

158. Stuart, J. M., K. A. Cartwright, J. A. Dawson, J. Rickard, and N. D. Noah. 1988. Risk factors for meningococcal disease: a case control study in south west England. *Community Med.* **10**:139–146.

159. Takama, H., Y. Tamada, K. Yano, Y. Nitta, and T. Ikeya. 1997. Pitted keratolysis: clinical manifestations in 53 cases. *Br. J. Dermatol.* **137**:282–285.

160. Takama, H., Y. Tamada, K. Yokochi, and T. Ikeya. 1998. Pitted keratolysis: a discussion of two cases in non-weight-bearing areas. *Acta Dermato-venereol.* **78**:225–226.

161. Teichmann, D., K. Göbels, J. Simons, M. P. Grobusch, and N. Suttorp. 2001. A severe case of leptospirosis acquired during an iron man contest. *Eur. J. Clin. Microbiol. Infect. Dis.* **20**:137–138.

162. Tillett, H. E., J. de Louvois, and P. G. Wall. 1998. Surveillance of outbreaks of waterborne infectious disease: categorizing levels of evidence. *Epidemiol. Infect.* **120**:37–42.

163. Tobe, K., K. Matsuura, T. Ogura, Y. Tsuo, Y. Iwasaki, M. Mizuno, K. Yamamoto, T. Higashi, and T. Tsuji. 2000. Horizontal transmission of hepatitis B virus among players of an American football team. *Arch. Intern. Med.* **160**:2541–2545.

164. Torre, D., C. Sampietro, G. Ferraro, C. Zeroli, and F. Speranza. 1990. Transmission of HIV-1 infection via sports injury. *Lancet* **335**:1105.

165. **Tranquilli, C., O. Armignacco, and M. Ilardi.** 1994. Sport activity and HIV infection. *Med. Sport* (Turin) **47:**47–52.

166. **Vazquez-Lopez, F., and N. Perez-Oliva.** 1996. Mupirocin ointment for symptomatic pitted keratolysis. *Infection* **24:**55.

167. Reference deleted.

168. **Walker, A.** 1992. Swimming—the hazards of taking a dip. *Br. Med. J.* **304:**242–245.

169. Reference deleted.

170. **Wheeler, C. E., Jr., and W. H. Cabaniss, Jr.** 1965. Epidemic cutaneous herpes simplex in wrestlers (herpes gladiatorum). *JAMA* **194:**993–997.

171. **White, J.** 1991. Measles: a hazard of indoor sports. *Physician Sportsmed.* **19:**21.

172. **White, W. B., and J. M. Grant-Kels.** 1984. Transmission of herpes simplex virus type 1 infection in rugby players. *JAMA* **252:**533–535.

173. **World Health Organization.** 1982. Guidelines for the control of leptospirosis. *WHO Offset Publ.* **67:**1–171.

174. **World Health Organization.** 1992. World Health Organization consensus statement: consultation on AIDS and sports. *JAMA* **267:**1312.

175. **Wormser, G. P., S. Bittker, G. Forseter, I. K. Hewlett, I. Argani, B. Joshi, J. S. Epstein, and D. Bucher.** 1992. Absence of infectious human immunodeficiency virus type 1 in "natural" eccrine sweat. *J. Infect. Dis.* **165:**155–158.

Infections of Leisure, Third Edition
Edited by David Schlossberg
© 2004 ASM Press, Washington, D.C.

Chapter 13

Traveling Abroad

Martin S. Wolfe

Approximately 15 million Americans travel abroad each year, and about half of this number go to the developing world. Tourists usually visit these remoter parts of the world for a period of weeks, where they may be exposed to diseases that are not present, or are at most rare, in the United States. Other individuals may be longer-term travelers or residents in the developing world.

In response to the hazards posed to travelers, the medical specialty of travel medicine has evolved, and numerous travel clinics are in operation. Travel medicine involves both the prevention of travel-related diseases and the diagnosis and treatment of exotic, primarily tropical, diseases on the traveler's return (61).

The main areas involved in prevention include pretravel advice, preparation of an individualized medical kit, immunizations, malaria prophylactic measures, and prophylaxis and self-treatment of traveler's diarrhea.

PRETRAVEL ADVICE

A pretravel physical examination, best performed by a personal physician, is indicated for travelers with serious medical problems and for those planning a long or physically demanding trip. A medical summary, including recent chest X rays and electrocardiogram, should be carried. A serious medical condition can be summarized on a health card or an engraved bracelet. The names of recognized, preferably English-speaking, physicians or specialists in the countries to be visited should be known by the traveler.

In addition, adequate medical insurance should be obtained to cover conditions acquired abroad, and hospitalization and medical evacuation if required. Those with chronic illness should carry a supply of required drugs.

Individualized Medical Kit

Items to be included in an individualized medical kit depend on preexisting and other potential needs. General items could include a thermometer, bandages,

Martin S. Wolfe • Traveler's Medical Service, 2141 K St. NW, Suite 408, Washington, DC 20037.

gauze, tape, a germicidal soap solution, aspirin, antacids, anti-motion sickness medication, and a mild laxative. Particular antibiotic, antifungal, and anti-inflammatory ointments should be included. A sunscreen is indicated for tropical areas. Antibiotics can be carried by travelers to remote areas where medical assistance may not be readily available. Suggested specific items for a medical kit and information on their use can be found in a publication of the American Society of Tropical Medicine and Hygiene, *Health Hints for the Tropics* (67). Specific items are discussed below.

Immunizations

Vaccine requirements by country are published annually by the Centers for Disease Control and Prevention (*Health Information for International Travel* [15]) and by the World Health Organization (*International Travel and Health: Vaccination Requirements and Health Advice* [70]). A number of commercial computer programs are also available (see references 3, 20, 25, 33, and 34).

Yellow Fever

Yellow fever is presently the only disease for which vaccination is required for international travel. Yellow fever occurs in tropical Africa and South America, and vaccination can be required for entry into countries in these regions, or for travelers entering certain other countries if they have come from a country with regions where infections occur (15). Vaccination must be validated in an International Certificate of Vaccination. Yellow fever vaccine requires continuous cold storage and must be used within 60 min after reconstitution. Because of this, yellow fever vaccine is given only in approved state-licensed official vaccination centers. A single dose is valid for 10 years, and side effects are minimal. The vaccine is contraindicated in those with an altered immune status or known hypersensitivity to eggs, in children below age 9 months, and in pregnant women. These individuals must be advised not to enter any area with active yellow fever infection and should be given a letter of contraindication to satisfy any entrance requirement.

Cholera

At present, no countries officially require a cholera certificate and the vaccine is not recommended, even for travel to areas with epidemic cholera. Currently available vaccines offer only 50 to 70% protection for 6 months and can cause side effects (15). New and improved oral cholera vaccines are available abroad but not yet in the United States (44).

Smallpox

Smallpox is considered to be eradicated worldwide, and vaccine is no longer required or recommended for travelers.

Hepatitis A

Hepatitis A is the most common type of hepatitis contracted by unprotected travelers to areas of endemicity (66). Two hepatitis A vaccines are now available in the United States. Havrix (GlaxoSmithKline) was approved in 1995, and Vaqta

(Merck) became available in 1996. Adults receive an adult dose, and children and adolescents ages 2 to 17 years receive a reduced dose. An initial dose of either vaccine will induce protective immunity within 4 weeks (18). A booster dose given 6 to 12 months after the first dose is expected to lead to long-term protection (estimated at possibly >20 years) (51). A combined hepatitis A and B vaccine (Twinrix) is also available (4).

Hepatitis B

Vaccination against hepatitis B is recommended for travelers who anticipate direct contact with blood or sexual contact with residents of high-risk areas and for resident expatriates (15). Three doses are required, and the vaccine is expensive. At this time, there is no recommendation for booster doses, as the primary series leads to long-term protection.

Immunoglobulin

Immunoglobulin is an alternative method for short-term protection from hepatitis A. Persons undertaking travel for less than 3 months will be protected by a single intramuscular dose (0.02 ml/kg of body weight). Those traveling for longer periods, as well as expatriate residents, should receive an intramuscular dose of 0.006 ml/kg at 4-month to no more than 6-month intervals. Immunoglobulin offers no protection against hepatitis B, C, or E.

Influenza and Pneumococcal Vaccines

Travelers at high risk for contracting influenza and pneumococcal infections should receive the appropriate vaccines.

Japanese Encephalitis Vaccine

Japanese encephalitis is endemic in much of the Far East, Southeast Asia, and south Asia. Occasional cases have occurred in expatriates, usually those in long-term residence. Persons who plan to live in rural-agricultural locations of infected areas should consider receiving vaccine (17).

Meningococcal Meningitis

Epidemic meningococcal meningitis occurs annually in sub-Saharan Africa during the dry winter months (December through June). Immunization with meningitis type A/C/Y/W 135 vaccine is recommended for travelers to this area during the epidemic season. A single dose offers protection for 3 years. Pilgrims and some visa applicants to Saudi Arabia are required to have evidence of this vaccination for entry (39).

Plague

Plague occurs sporadically, usually in remote locations. Vaccine is particularly indicated in field workers who could have direct contact with potentially plague-infected wild rodents in rural areas where plague is endemic. A case of plague imported into the United States by an American rodent collector infected in rural Bolivia emphasizes the importance of vaccine for such workers (59). A primary series requires three doses, and periodic boosters are required when exposure risk continues.

Polio

Because of polio eradication efforts, the number of countries in which polio is endemic has decreased to approximately seven. The western hemisphere, the western Pacific region (including China), and the European region are now considered free of polio. Most of the remaining cases of poliovirus transmission occur in Afghanistan, India, Pakistan, Nigeria, and Niger. Most travelers have had a basic polio immunization series during childhood, but not all have had a necessary subsequent booster. A single inactivated polio vaccine booster dose is recommended for travelers to countries where polio is still endemic (15).

Rabies

Rabies is endemic in practically all of the developing world. The usual traveler is at minimal risk, and the expensive three-dose human diploid cell or purified chicken embryo cell vaccine preexposure series is rarely indicated in this group. This series can be recommended for higher-risk groups such as young children, joggers, animal handlers, and field workers (56). The preexposure series offers added protection but does not eliminate the need for additional therapy following rabies exposure. All travelers going to areas where rabies is endemic should not approach stray dogs or cats, primates, or other wild animals.

Tuberculosis (*Mycobacterium tuberculosis BCG*)

Although tuberculosis is a potential hazard to visitors to the developing world, the use of BCG vaccine is not usually recommended by American travel medicine specialists because of troublesome side effects and questionable efficacy of available vaccines. Pre- and posttravel tuberculin skin test screening is considered preferable.

Typhoid

Typhoid and paratyphoid fevers are endemic in much of the developing world. There are no available vaccines for paratyphoid, but there are oral and injectable typhoid vaccines. The oral live-attenuated Ty21a strain vaccine is administered in capsule form, with one capsule taken every other day for four doses. A booster dose is required every 5 years (10). A single-dose parenteral vaccine will offer similar (approximately 70%) protection for 2 years (65).

Typhus

No American traveler has contracted epidemic typhus in the last 40 years. Typhus vaccine is no longer recommended and is not available in the United States.

Routine and Childhood Vaccinations

All Americans should be up-to-date on the routine immunizations regardless of travel plans, and indicated boosters must be given before travel. Boosters of adult tetanus and diphtheria are necessary every 10 years. *Haemophilus influenzae* type b vaccine should be given to all children older than 2 months. Measles-mumps-rubella vaccine is usually given as a single dose at age 15 months. However, the age of vaccination should be lowered for children traveling to areas where they are at increased risk of endemic or epidemic measles (15). Adult travelers may also be at increased risk of measles infection. Persons born in or after 1957 should be vaccinated with a single-dose measles vaccine if they have not previously received two doses of measles vaccine or have no history of measles (D. R. Hill and

R. D. Pearson, Editorial, *Ann. Intern. Med.* **111**:699–701, 1989). Varicella vaccine should be considered for travelers who do not have immunity to varicella-zoster virus, especially if close personal contact with local populations is expected (72).

Malaria Prophylaxis

Malaria infection is a very serious risk for travelers to areas where malaria is endemic. The emergence and continued spread of chloroquine-resistant and other drug-resistant *Plasmodium falciparum* malaria, and the complexities involved with contraindications and toxic effects of available malaria prophylactic drugs, make it most difficult to offer appropriate advice to travelers. Expert opinion is required to determine the areas of drug resistance and to make decisions on the best drug and antimosquito measures for particular situations (19).

Chloroquine is the drug of choice for the relatively few malarious areas where *P. falciparum* parasites remain sensitive to it (Central America, Haiti, and parts of the Middle East). In all other malarious areas, chloroquine-resistant *P. falciparum* malaria occurs, and other drugs must be used. Drugs should be started before travel and should be taken while in and for at least 4 weeks after leaving the malarious area. Atovaquone-proquanil need be taken for only 7 days after leaving. Chloroquine tablets are available in the United States, and liquid preparations are available abroad. The dose is 500 mg of salt (300 mg of base) once weekly for adults and 5 mg/kg weekly for children. Chloroquine is considered safe for young children and pregnant women (58). Minor side effects are common, but marked intolerance is rare. Retinal toxicity is virtually nonexistent in the recommended malaria prophylaxis dose (7). In recent years, chloroquine-resistant *Plasmodium vivax* malaria has occurred in parts of Southeast Asia and South America (68).

In the United States there are presently three main drugs recommended for prophylaxis. Mefloquine (Lariam) has the advantage of being taken weekly. The adult dose is 250 mg, and the drug is administered in reduced doses by weight for children. There is a high degree of mefloquine resistance by *P. falciparum* along the Thai-Burmese and Thai-Cambodian borders and in western Cambodia; rare cases of confirmed resistance have been reported in tropical Africa. Reported side effects of mefloquine include insomnia, bad dreams, dizziness, headache, irritability, and gastrointestinal symptoms. More serious reactions, such as toxic psychosis, depression and suicidal thoughts, and hallucinations occur in approximately 1 in 10,000 users. Since many of these adverse reactions occur within the first 3 weeks of initial usage, first-time users should ideally begin taking mefloquine 3 weeks before travel to allow potential adverse events to occur prior to travel. Contraindications to mefloquine use include a history of epilepsy, serious psychiatric disorders, and cardiac conduction abnormalities. Mefloquine is considered safe for infants and young children, as well as for pregnant women when there is a significant risk of contracting malaria (19, 31).

Malarone, a fixed combination of atovaquone and proquanil, is an alternative to mefloquine. Dosage is on a daily basis, beginning 1 day before entering a malarious area, while in the area, and for 7 days after leaving the area. This drug is therefore particularly useful and cost-effective for trips of 14 days or less. The adult dose is one adult tablet daily. Pediatric dose tablets are available, and doses vary by weight. The available data on the safety and efficacy of atovaquone-proquanil for prevention of malaria in children weighing less than 11 kg and in pregnant women are insufficient; the drug is contraindicated for these groups. Severe renal impairment is another contraindication. Atovaquone-proquanil should not be used with tetracyclines, rifampin, or metoclopramide. The most common adverse effects with this drug are abdominal pain, nausea, vomiting, and headache (19, 31).

The third commonly recommended prophylactic drug is daily doxycycline. It is particularly indicated for travelers to mefloquine-resistant areas mentioned above. The daily dose for adults is 100 mg. This is begun 1 day before arrival in and continued for 4 weeks after leaving the malarious area. Doxycycline is contraindicated for pregnant women and children less than 8 years of age. Potential adverse effects include photosensitivity, gastrointestinal effects, and candidiasis (19, 31).

Particularly for short trips, primaquine in a daily dose of 30 mg can be taken the day before entering, while in, and for 7 days after leaving the malarious area (48). Primaquine is also used to prevent potential relapsing malaria due to persisting liver forms of *P. vivax* and *Plasmodium ovale* which are not eliminated by other antimalaria prophylactic drugs. This is particularly important for persons who have had intense or prolonged exposure in malarious areas. Primaquine is taken in a daily dose for 14 days, after completing the terminal suppressive doses of one of the above-mentioned drugs. The usual adult dose is 15 mg of base daily. However, in some malarious areas, including the southwest Pacific, Southeast Asia, and Central and South America, *P. vivax* parasites have acquired resistance to this standard dose of primaquine. Travelers returning from these areas for whom terminal primaquine is indicated should take a dose of 30 mg of base daily for 14 days (68). Primaquine may cause severe hemolysis in persons with glucose-6-phosphate dehydrogenase deficiency, and this condition must be ruled out before primaquine is used. Primaquine is contraindicated during pregnancy.

Some drugs are no longer recommended for prophylaxis by American experts because of potentially serious side effects; these include pyrimethamine-sulfadoxine (Fansidar), amodiaquine, and pyrimethamine-sulfone (Maloprim).

Travelers who are in very remote areas without access to medical care may take along a dose of antimalarial medication for emergency self-treatment. This should be promptly taken if fever, chills, or other influenza-like illness develops. This self-treatment is only a temporary measure, and prompt medical evaluation is imperative. The drug of choice for presumptive self-treatment is atovaquone-proguanil for those *not* taking this drug for prophylaxis. The adult dose is four tablets in a single dose daily for 3 days (15).

In addition to drug prophylaxis, mosquito avoidance measures should be practiced. Malaria transmission by mosquitoes occurs primarily between dusk and dawn. Measures to prevent mosquito bites during these hours include the following:

1. Remaining in well-screened areas
2. Use of permethrin-impregnated mosquito nets (Anonymous, Editorial, *Lancet* **337**:1515–1516, 1991)

3. Wearing clothes that cover most of the body
4. Application of permethrin repellent to clothing
5. Use of DEET-containing repellents on exposed parts of the body (24)
6. Use of pyrethrum-containing flying-insect spray in living areas

Traveler's Diarrhea

Up to 50% of travelers to the developing world are affected by traveler's diarrhea. This can be caused by bacteria (particularly toxigenic *Escherichia coli*), viruses, and, less commonly, parasites. Infection is usually contracted from contaminated water or food (60).

To prevent traveler's diarrhea, water should be boiled for 3 min or disinfected with iodine tablets or a portable iodine resin filter prior to ingestion (8). Foods should be well cooked, and hot salads and cold foods should be avoided. Raw or poorly cooked shellfish, unwashed vegetables and fruits, and suspect dairy products should not be eaten.

Prophylactic antibiotics are generally not recommended by experts because of the potential for side effects and widespread bacterial resistance (26). Bismuth subsalicylate (Pepto-Bismol), two tablets four times a day for up to 3 weeks, has proven to be a safe means of reducing the occurrence of traveler's diarrhea by about 65% (22).

Should diarrhea occur during travel, lost fluids should be replaced by drinking water, tea, broth, or carbonated beverages. Oral rehydration electrolyte mixtures are even better (23). Cramps or moderate diarrhea can be relieved by such anti-motility agents as loperamide (Imodium) (23). Pepto-Bismol liquid, 1 oz every half-hour for eight doses, is useful, particularly for diarrhea due to toxigenic *E. coli* (23). If these measures are not adequate, or if fever, chills, or blood or mucus in the stool occurs, a physician should be contacted for appropriate diagnosis and treatment. In an emergency, self-treatment, preferably with a quinolone antibiotic, can be administered (1).

POSTTRAVEL MANAGEMENT

The most common problems in returning travelers are diarrhea and other gastrointestinal difficulties, fever, unexplained eosinophilia, and skin rashes. Drugs for parasitic infections are summarized in reference 5.

Diarrhea and Other Gastrointestinal Difficulties

Diarrhea and gastrointestinal complaints are the most common problems for travelers, both during and after a trip. The most common cause of acute diarrhea during or just after return is toxigenic *E. coli*, but infection may also be due to a variety of viral, bacterial, fungal, and protozoal organisms or toxic marine organisms (i.e., fish or shellfish poisoning). Symptoms developing sometime following travel are most commonly due to pathogenic intestinal protozoa. Less likely causes are tropical sprue or enteropathy, postinfectious lactose intolerance, or intestinal helminths.

Viral Intestinal Infections

Rotavirus spread by the fecal-oral route is a cause of enteric disease worldwide (12). After an incubation period of less than 48 h, there is the onset of frequent watery diarrhea, nausea, and malaise. Symptoms usually last for 5 to 7 days. The viral etiology is usually suspected from the clinical picture and the absence of other organisms. Specific diagnosis can be made from a variety of assays which detect rotavirus in stool.

Norwalk virus also occurs worldwide, has an incubation period of 18 to 48 h, and causes a 24- to 48-h illness (12). There is currently no available diagnostic assay. Treatment of both of these viral infections is supportive, with particular emphasis on fluid replacement.

Bacterial Intestinal Infections

Toxigenic *E. coli* causes approximately 50% of traveler's diarrhea cases. Other relatively common bacterial etiologic agents include *Shigella* and *Salmonella* species, *Campylobacter jejuni*, and *Vibrio parahaemolyticus*. Less common etiologies include other *Vibrio* species (*Vibrio cholerae* is distinctly uncommon), *Clostridium* spp., *Staphylococcus aureus*, and *Yersinia enterocolitica* (60).

Most severe infections leading to dysentery with fever, chills, and blood and mucus in the stool are usually caused by large-bowel-invasive *C. jejuni*, *Shigella* species, and certain invasive *Salmonella* species. Other organisms, such as toxigenic *E. coli*, are noninvasive and usually cause symptoms by producing an enterotoxin, leading to watery diarrhea and a relatively short self-limiting illness. A wet mount of stool stained with methylene blue usually reveals sheets of polymorphonuclear leukocytes and red blood cells with the former more invasive organisms, while these cells are generally absent with noninvasive bacteria colonizing the smaller bowel (60).

Definitive diagnosis is made with stool culture using various media, including those for *Salmonella* and *Shigella* and special selective media for *C. jejuni* and *Vibrio* species. Symptoms caused by noninvasive *Vibrio* and *Salmonella* species are generally self-limiting and usually do not require treatment. The other invasive organisms are well treated with a quinolone antibiotic (1).

In a traveler who has recently taken antibiotics, diarrhea may be due to *Clostridium difficile* infection. This is diagnosed by detecting *C. difficile* toxin in the stool. If the toxin is present, treatment is carried out with metronidazole or vancomycin.

Fungal enteritis

Recent use of broad-spectrum antibiotics or metronidazole can eliminate normal intestinal bacteria and allow candidal overgrowth. In some cases, this can lead to diarrhea and other gastrointestinal symptoms. Intestinal candidiasis should be considered as the etiology when budding yeast and mycelial forms are found in large numbers on direct fecal examinations after antimicrobial treatment. Rapid improvement is seen with oral nystatin (36).

Fish and Shellfish Toxins

Fish and shellfish toxins may initially cause acute diarrhea, which can then be followed by prolonged neurological symptoms. Ciguatera poisoning from ingestion of large marine reef fish (including grouper, snapper, and barracuda) containing ciguatoxin is the most common form of fish poisoning (21).

Intestinal Parasites

Pathogenic intestinal protozoa commonly affecting travelers include *Giardia lamblia* (most frequently recognized), *Entamoeba histolytica*, and *Dientamoeba fragilis*. Less common are *Cryptosporidium parvum*, *Cyclospora cayetanensis*, and *Isospora belli*. As the incubation period of these organisms is generally considerably greater than that for viruses and bacteria, initial symptoms frequently do not develop until late in a trip or following return. Symptoms can also be more prolonged or recurrent.

G. lamblia is a worldwide threat to travelers. Infection is usually acquired from contaminated water, and the incubation period is approximately 9 to 15 days. Typical symptoms include recurrent or persistent soft, foul-smelling stools and flatus, intestinal bloating and gurgling, belching, indigestion, weight loss, and fatigue. Diagnosis is usually made from a series of stool specimens, best collected in a preservative. However, up to 30% of those infected can be "low excretors" of the parasite and can be difficult to diagnose by stool examination. An enzyme-linked immunosorbent assay to detect *Giardia* antigen in stool is available (2), but it remains to be proven that this test is consistently positive for stool-negative low excretors. Other methods which can be used to confirm infection include examination of upper intestinal fluid obtained with a nasogastric tube or with the Enterotest duodenal string test (9), examination of a biopsy impression smear, or histological examination of a small-bowel biopsy specimen. In some cases with typical travel and exposure history and typical *Giardia*-like symptoms, it is not possible to confirm infections. In this situation, empirical treatment is advocated. Available drugs in the United States include metronidazole (Flagyl) and furazolidone (Furoxone) (64). Quinacrine (Atabrine), a very effective treatment, is not presently commercially available but can be put into capsules by certain pharmaceutical compounders. A new Food and Drug Administration-approved drug, nitazoxanide (Alinia), is available as a liquid preparation for children 1 to 11 years old in a 3-day course. A tablet formulation of nitazoxanide for use in adults is under Food and Drug Administration review. This drug is generally well tolerated and effective (6). Tinidazole (Fasigyn), which can be administered in a single dose, is available outside of North America. Lactase deficiency is common with giardiasis and may persist after successful treatment, yielding symptoms mimicking persistent giardiasis (64).

E. histolytica is also contracted worldwide by travelers. Many of those infected with *Entamoeba* are asymptomatic cyst passers who harbor the nonpathogenic species *Entamoeba dispar*. *E. histolytica* and *E. dispar* are morphologically identical but can be differentiated with a rapid stool antigen detection kit (28). At the other clinical extreme, amoebic dysentery is uncommon. Intermediate nondysenteric symptoms include alternating constipation and diarrhea, lower abdominal cramps, bloating and flatus (not foul smelling), and fatigue. Diagnosis is made by finding typical cysts or trophozoites in the stool and confirming *E. histolytica* identification by stool antigen detection. In cases of dysentery, proctoscopic examination reveals typical ulcers; scrapings or biopsy of these ulcers can reveal E. histolytica trophozoites. Amoebic serology is usually positive with invasive amoebic bowel disease. In mild cases, a nonabsorbed luminal drug such as paromomycin (Humatin) or iodoquinol is usually curative. Moderate to severe (dysenteric) symptoms require initial metronidazole, followed by a luminal drug (57).

D. fragilis is an amoeba-like noninvasive flagellate of the large bowel found worldwide. This protozoan has no cyst form and occurs only in the very labile trophozoite form. To confirm infection with this parasite, stools must be collected in preservative and permanently stained slides must be examined. Not all those infected have symptoms, but diarrhea, abdominal bloating, flatulence, and fatigue may occur (27). Treatment is carried out with paromomycin, with iodoquinol as an alternative (57).

Cryptosporidium is usually associated with AIDS patients, but infection can occur in travelers with normal immune systems (46). The incubation period can be as little as 4 days, and symptoms can mimic those of giardiasis. Diagnosis may require special stool concentration tests and staining. Nitazoxanide is effective for treatment, although infection in nonimmunosuppressed persons is usually self-limiting within 7 to 30 days (6).

Cyclospora is present throughout the world and has been identified in travelers from various regions. The incubation period varies from 2 to 11 days. Symptoms include watery diarrhea, indigestion, cramps, weight loss, and marked fatigue. Left untreated, infection is self-limiting in immunocompetent persons, usually after 4 to 6 weeks. Diagnosis is based on finding oocysts on fecal examinations. Trimethoprim-sulfamethoxazole is effective for treatment (47).

I. belli is a rarely diagnosed parasite which can produce symptoms similar to those of giardiasis (45). Blastocystis hominis is a ubiquitous parasite whose pathogenicity is debated. It is frequently present in asymptomatic travelers. In one careful study of symptomatic individuals with only B. hominis parasites, most were later found to have another difficult-to-recognize pathogenic protozoan (38).

A number of nonpathogenic intestinal protozoa must be differentiated from pathogenic parasites. This requires fecal smears permanently stained with iron hematoxylin or trichrome. Intestinal helminths seldom cause chronic diarrhea; a major exception is Strongyloides stercoralis.

Travelers with chronic diarrhea who have had relatively prolonged residence in south Asia and Southeast Asia and parts of the Caribbean may have tropical sprue (35). This malabsorption syndrome is rare in short-term travelers. It should be considered in those with a history of geographic exposure who have persistent diarrhea, indigestion, flatulence, and weight loss, when no pathogenic organism can be found.

Fever in the Returned Traveler

Many febrile illnesses in the traveler have a cosmopolitan rather than an exotic etiology and are frequently self-limiting. The major exotic tropical fevers occurring in travelers include malaria, enteric fever, hepatitis, bacterial dysentery, and rickettsial and arboviral infections (29).

Malaria

A febrile traveler returning from an area where malaria is endemic must first and foremost be considered to have possible malaria. Most malaria infections occur in travelers who have had no, irregular, or inappropriate chemoprophylaxis. However, all febrile travelers from a malarious area must be examined for malaria, since no chemoprophylaxis regimen can be considered fully protective. Potentially lethal falciparum malaria usually occurs within 4 weeks after leaving a malarious area. *P. vivax* and *P. ovale* malaria may occur up to 3 years after exposure, if primaquine has not been taken to eliminate persistent latent parasites in the liver. *Plasmodium malariae* does not have a latent liver phase and is the least common species seen in travelers. Typical malaria symptoms are high fever, shaking chills, sweats, headache, and myalgias. Symptoms may be modified or masked depending on the malaria immune status (as in an immune native of an area of endemicity) or by the use of prophylactic antimalarial drugs. Severe *P. falciparum* infections can rapidly lead to such lethal complications as cerebral malaria, renal failure, severe hemolysis, and adult respiratory distress syndrome (69).

Diagnosis is made by appropriately prepared and carefully examined Giemsa-stained thin and thick malaria smears. A single negative set of smears cannot rule out malaria, and smears should be repeated at 6-h intervals for a 24- to 48-h period.

Falciparum malaria contracted in one of the relatively few areas with chloroquine-sensitive malaria can be treated with chloroquine alone. Initially, 1-g of chloroquine phosphate salt (600-mg base) is given orally. Six hours later, 500 mg of salt (300-mg base) is taken, and this dose is repeated 24 and 48 h later. For falciparum malaria contracted in chloroquine-resistant areas, with a low level of parasitemia (less than 1%) and no complications, oral treatment can be given. Atovaquone-proguanil (Malarone) can be taken in an adult course of four adult tablets as a single dose on three consecutive days. Mefloquine (Lariam) in a single adult 1,250-mg dose can be used for those without a contraindication to this drug. Vomiting and neuropsychiatric side effects can occur in a small percentage of those so treated. Alternatively, oral quinine, 650 mg of salt three times a day for 3 days, can be used, to be followed by oral tetracycline at 250 mg four times a day for 7 days (53). Patients with severe or complicated falciparum malaria must be hospitalized and managed with intensive care, immediate intravenous antimalarial drug treatment, and necessary supportive treatment (69). In the United States, intravenous quinine is not available, and treatment must be carried out with intravenous quinidine (43). A continuous infusion of quinidine gluconate is recommended. A loading dose of 10 mg of quinidine gluconate salt (equal to 6.2 mg of quinidine base) per kg of body weight is given over 1 to 2 h, followed by constant infusion of 0.02 mg of quinidine gluconate salt (0.0125-mg base) per kg per min. This regimen is highly effective and well tolerated in monitored patients. Quinidine is given for 3 days and is then followed by tetracycline, as described above. In patients with a malaria parasitemia level greater than 10%, or with marked clinical deterioration, exchange transfusion along with constant quinidine infusion can be lifesaving (40).

P. malariae, P. vivax, and *P. ovale* can be treated with chloroquine alone, like chloroquine-sensitive *P. falciparum*. Chloroquine-resistant *P. vivax* should be treated with atovaquone-proguanil or mefloquine. With *P. vivax* or *P. ovale,* this should be followed by primaquine, 15-mg base, daily for 14 days (30-mg base in areas where primaquine-resistant *P. vivax* is found), after normal glucose-6-phosphate dehydrogenase status is established.

Enteric Fever

Typhoid and paratyphoid fevers can be contracted from contaminated food or water in the developing world, where the prevalence of the causative bacteria is high. Currently available typhoid vaccines offer protection to no more than 70% of the recipients (10). Enteric fever should be suspected in travelers returning from an area of endemicity with fever, headache, abdominal pain, diarrhea, or cough. Symptoms may not develop until several weeks after return. Diagnosis is confirmed by positive blood, stool, or urine cultures. Febrile agglutinin (Widal) tests or salmonella antibodies may be useful. *Salmonella typhi* organisms worldwide have developed multiple antibiotic resistance, and a quinolone is the drug of choice. Paratyphoid organisms are generally sensitive to amoxicillin or trimethoprim-sulfamethoxazole.

Hepatitis

Travelers to the developing world who have not received immunoglobulin or hepatitis A vaccine run a significant risk of contracting hepatitis A from contaminated water or food. Rare cases of hepatitis E have been contracted in south Asia and elsewhere, and this type of hepatitis is not protected against by immunoglobulin (16). Hepatitis B is usually contracted through sexual contact and is uncommon in travelers. In the preicteric phase of acute hepatitis, fever, chills, myalgias, and fatigue may occur, and this syndrome can mimic malaria and other acute tropical fevers. Hepatitis serologic testing can confirm infection, but when these tests are negative for a patient with apparent hepatitis, cytomegalovirus or Epstein-Barr virus (mononucleosis) infection should be considered.

Amoebic Liver Abscess

A period of acute diarrhea frequently precedes development of an amoebic liver abscess. A returned traveler with fever and right upper quadrant pain should be suspected of this disorder. Sonography or scan of the liver shows a filling defect, and an amoebic serology test confirms infection. Needle aspiration is seldom required for diagnosis or treatment. There is usually a very rapid clinical response to oral or intravenous metronidazole. Follow-up treatment should be given with paromomycin or iodoquinol (as for intestinal amoebiasis) to eliminate any bowel cysts and prevent relapse. Abscess cavities may take some months to fill in.

Rickettsial Infections

Tick typhus can be contracted in West, East, and southern Africa and in the Mediterranean littoral. Infection typically begins with a skin eschar at the tick bite site, fever, chills, and headache; in a few days, a diffuse papular rash may develop. Epidemic, scrub, and murine typhus are much less commonly contracted by travelers. The Weil-Felix agglutination battery can be used for initial screening, and confirmation can be obtained from indirect fluorescent-antibody tests for specific rickettsial organisms. Tetracycline is a highly effective and rapid treatment (42).

Viral Fevers

Dengue fever is endemic in most parts of the tropical world and is the most commonly imported arbovirus infection. Symptoms include fever, headache, body aches, and eye pain (49). Typically, a diffuse rash appears on the third to fifth day as other symptoms abate. Japanese B encephalitis is a rare infection of travelers to rural areas of the Far East (17). A number of other rarer acute viral illnesses have been imported from areas of endemicity, including lethal Lassa, Ebola, and Marburg fever viruses from west and central Africa (30). Diagnosis is usually confirmed serologically. Treatment is generally supportive; ribavirin has been found to be useful in Lassa fever cases.

Less Common Febrile Illnesses

African trypanosomiasis. African trypanosomiasis was contracted by 15 American travelers from 1967 through 1987 (13). Although the actual risk is low, even short-term travelers to game parks of east and central Africa should take precautions against tsetse fly bites. Travelers should inform their physicians of exposure history if symptoms such as trypanosomal chancre at a bite site, fever, evanescent rash, headache, and lethargy develop up to 4 weeks following return.

Tuberculosis. Tuberculosis remains a threat worldwide. Although infection in travelers is uncommon, any returnee with fever, cough, and chest radiographic evidence of pulmonary disease should be evaluated for tuberculosis. Pre- and posttravel tuberculin skin testing is recommended for longer-term travelers.

Brucellosis. Brucellosis is contracted from contaminated raw goat's or cow's milk or soft cheese. Those infected can present with fever, chills, sweats, body aches, headache, monarticular arthritis, weight loss, fatigue, or depression. Generalized lymphadenopathy and splenomegaly are common. Diagnosis is made by blood culture and specific agglutination tests (71).

Leptospirosis. Leptospirosis is common in the tropics but is rarely contracted by travelers. Infection is acquired through direct or indirect contact with infected animals. Most infections are anicteric and mild. Initial symptoms can include high remittent fever, chills, headache, myalgias, nausea, and vomiting. No more than 10% of those infected develop jaundice. Diagnosis is usually made with serologic techniques. Early therapy with penicillin or doxycycline is usually beneficial (50).

Anthrax. Anthrax is very rarely contracted from contact with contaminated animal by-products such as hides and wool. Most infections occur on the face or arms after a minor abrasion, presenting as an initial painless papule which vesiculates and becomes hemorrhagic, necrotic, and covered with an eschar. Treatment is carried out with penicillin or tetracycline.

Melioidosis. Melioidosis is an uncommon infection in travelers to Southeast Asia. Presentation resembles acute pulmonary tuberculosis. Less commonly, chronic infection may develop (54).

Histoplasmosis. Histoplasmosis is a cosmopolitan disease and has rarely infected travelers to Latin America. Visitors to caves contaminated with bat droppings are at particular risk (52). Consideration should be given to possible histoplasmosis in a returned traveler with pulmonary or, less likely, disseminated disease.

Visceral leishmaniasis. Visceral leishmaniasis (kala-azar) is extremely rare in American tourists, though European travelers have been infected around the Mediterranean littoral. Symptoms include fever, hepatosplenomegaly, and wasting. Diagnosis is confirmed by demonstrating leishmanial organisms in a biopsy specimen of liver, spleen, or bone marrow (11).

American trypanosomiasis. American trypanosomiasis (Chagas' disease) is very common in Latin America, and travelers engaged there in hiking, camping, and archaeological projects can be exposed. However, naturally acquired, documented infection is extremely rare in travelers.

Lyme disease. Lyme disease occurs in Europe and may also be present in other parts of the world. Hikers in particular should take precaution against tick bites in any recognized area of endemicity.

HIV. Human immunodeficiency virus (HIV) infection is a particular hazard of sexual contact, blood transfusion, or contact with contaminated needles or syringes in areas of high-level endemicity in the tropics. A number of disposable syringes and needles can be carried by travelers who might need injections while traveling in areas where only nondisposable products are used. HIV serology screening should be done on any traveler with the above-mentioned exposure (14).

Eosinophilia in the Returned Traveler

A returned traveler with an eosinophilia greater than 5% who has been in the developing world should be considered to have possible helminthic infection. With some exceptions, protozoal infections do not cause eosinophilia. Allergic problems usually cause an eosinophilia of less than 15%, but some drug reactions can cause a much higher eosinophilia (62).

Helminth Infections

High eosinophilia, up to 80%, can occur during the acute stage of certain helminth infections, particularly those with a tissue larval migration.

Adult intestinal helminths can cause mild to moderate (6 to 30%) eosinophilia. Patients are usually asymptomatic with *Ascaris lumbricoides,* hookworms, *Trichuris trichiura, Enterobius vermicularis* (pinworms), and various tapeworms. Diagnosis is made by finding typical eggs or tapeworm segments in the stool. Pinworm eggs are best diagnosed by applying sticky paddles or cellophane tape to the perianal area. Treatment of all these infections is carried out with mebendazole (Vermox) or albendazole (Albenza) (5). *Ascaris* and hookworms have an early larval migration through the lungs which can yield pulmonary symptoms and infiltrates and quite high eosinophilia.

S. stercoralis and the much less commonly acquired *Trichostrongylus* species infect through the skin. *S. stercoralis* can complete its life cycle without leaving the host, and infections persisting for over 40 years have been recognized. Eosinophilia is particularly high during the early years of infection, but in long-established infections eosinophil counts can be normal. Many infections are asymptomatic, but some individuals may have epigastric pain, diarrhea, cough, and urticarial rashes occurring on the buttocks and thighs (related to larval migration from the anus). Unsuspected asymptomatic infections can become disseminated throughout the body in the presence of immunosuppression, with steroid treatment, or with cancer therapy. Definitive diagnosis is made by finding larvae in the stool, but larvae will not be present in all cases. Special stool concentration tests or examination of duodenal fluid may be required to find larvae. An enzyme-linked immunosorbent serologic test (available at the Centers for Disease Control and Prevention) is very useful in making a presumptive diagnosis. Treatment is carried out with ivermectin (Stromectol).

Schistosomiasis is acquired through contact with freshwater snails which are intermediate hosts. *Schistosoma mansoni* occurs in northeastern South America, certain Caribbean islands, Africa, and the Middle East. *Schistosoma hematobium* occurs in Africa and the Middle East. *Schistosoma japonicum* and *Schistosoma mekongi* are present in the Far East. *Schistosoma intercalatum* is an uncommon cause of intestinal infection in West and Central Africa. Acute schistosomiasis (Katayama syndrome) is more often associated with *S. mansoni* and *S. japonicum* infections, and symptoms occur 4 to 8 weeks after exposure, when adult worms begin producing eggs. Symptoms include hypereosinophilia, fever, chills, pulmonary complaints, headache, abdominal pain, and urticaria. The majority of established schistosome infections are asymptomatic, and eosinophilia seldom exceeds 3,000 eosinophils/mm^3. Intestinal infection with *S. mansoni*, *S. japonicium*, *S. mekongi*, and *S. intercalatum* can cause abdominal pain, diarrhea, and fatigue. *S. hematobium* can produce hematuria and other urinary tract symptoms. Diagnosis is made by finding eggs in the stool or urine, depending on the geographic area of exposure, symptoms, and species. Infection in travelers is often light, and eggs can be missed on routine stool and urine examinations. Special concentration tests of stool and urine and rectal or bladder biopsy may be required to confirm infection. Serologic tests may be used to screen travelers with an exposure history. Treatment is carried out with praziquantel (Biltricide) (55).

Liver flukes in their early acute phase can cause hypereosinophilia, painful liver, and fever. *Fasciola hepatica* occurs almost worldwide, and infection is contracted from eating watercress containing infective-stage metacercariae. *Clonorchis sinensis* and *Opisthorchis viverrini* occur in Southeast and East Asia and are contracted from eating raw fish containing metacercariae. In early *F. hepatica* infections, eggs may not occur in the stool and diagnosis is made by suggested filling defects in the liver and hypereosinophilia; diagnosis of *F. hepatica* infection is made on the basis of a positive serologic test. Ultrasonography or cholangiography can demonstrate *C. sinensis* or *O. viverrini* flukes in the bile ducts and gallbladder. In chronic infections, which are frequently asymptomatic, eggs may be found in the stool, and mild eosinophilia may be present. *F. hepatica* is best treated with bithionol, and *Clonorchis* and *Opisthorchis* are best treated with praziquantel (5).

Trichinosis and echinococcosis are extremely rare in travelers. A number of filariae infect humans and can cause quite high eosinophilia. *Wuchereria bancrofti* and *Brugia malayi* are rare in travelers; long-term residence in an area of high-level endemicity seems necessary for infection. *Mansonella perstans* is a common parasite in tropical Africa and is the most commonly diagnosed cause of filarial infection in the United Kingdom. *Loa loa* and *Onchocerca volvulus* are the two most commonly diagnosed causes of filarial infections in the United States, usually in longer-term residents from tropical Africa. The incubation period can be from 6 months to 1 year, and symptoms may develop some time after return from an area of endemicity. Classic presentation of *L. loa* is the migration of the adult worm across the eye and/or subcutaneous evanescent swellings (Calabar swellings) on the arms or legs, associated with hypereosinophilia. Onchocerciasis usually presents with a very pruritic maculopapular eruption on the hips, back, buttocks, and thighs in the presence of hypereosinophilia. Filariasis should be suspected in travelers from areas of endemicity with hypereosinophilia and suggestive signs and symptoms. Microfilariae should be searched for in the blood, or in the case of onchocerciasis, in skin snips or biopsy samples. Filariasis serology can be useful. If infection is confirmed or strongly suspected, diethylcarbamazine is the treatment of choice for all species except *Onchocerca* and *M. perstans*. Onchocerciasis is treated with ivermectin, and *M. perstans* infection is treated with mebendazole or albendazole (41).

Intestinal Protozoa

Eosinophilia is distinctly uncommon in pure infections with *E. histolytica* and *G. lamblia*. Eosinophilia has been associated with other pathogenic intestinal protozoa, i.e., *D. fragilis* and *I. belli.*

Skin Disorders in the Returned Traveler

The most common skin disorders acquired by travelers are cutaneous mycoses. Tinea versicolor is frequently contracted in the tropics, and depigmentation of the lesions may persist for some months after effective treatment. Tinea pedis ("athlete's foot") is particularly common in moist climates, as is Tinea cruris ("jock itch"). The former can be prevented by regular use of foot powder and dry socks, while the latter can be prevented by use of a drying powder and frequent change of clothing. Superficial mycoses are diagnosed from skin scrapings in potassium hydroxide or by culture. Treatment is carried out with a broad-spectrum antimycotic preparation.

Cutaneous myiasis is contracted by travelers to Latin America (*Dermatobia hominis*) and by travelers to Africa (*Cordylobia anthropophaga*, the tumbu fly). Infection with *C. anthropophaga* results from eggs deposited on clothes which are air dried and unironed. Larvae hatch in a few days and penetrate the skin, causing persistent, pruritic, and sometimes painful furuncular lesions with central necrosis. These lesions can often be confused with bacterial infections. A larva, which can be extracted, is seen in the center of the lesion, and healing is generally rapid after removal.

The sand flea, *Tunga penetrans*, invades the skin (often around the toes) when a person is walking barefoot. Sand fleas are easily removed with fine forceps.

Scabies and louse infestations are cosmopolitan conditions and are contracted when hygiene is poor. There is usually severe pruritus. Infection is confirmed by observing moving lice or, in the case of scabies, by examination of scrapings of scabietic burrows or papules. Scabies are treated with topical 5% permethrin or

10% crotamiton. Lice can be similarly treated. Oral ivermectin can also be used for both of these conditions.

Dog and cat hookworms deposited in sandy soil can penetrate exposed skin and lead to cutaneous larva migrans (creeping eruptions). This leaves migrating pruritic serpiginous tunnels in the epidermis. *S. stercoralis* can cause a particular form of hive-like cutaneous lesions, usually on the buttocks or thighs. These lesions can be treated with locally applied thiabendazole or with oral ivermectin (32).

A number of cutaneous ulcers are contracted in the tropics. Most common is cutaneous leishmaniasis transmitted by sand flies in the Middle East, in the Mediterranean littoral, and in parts of Asia, Africa, and Latin America. The incubation period can be 1 to 3 months, rarely longer. Typically, a papule develops which gradually enlarges and ulcerates into a painless sore with rolled edges. The causal Leishman-Donovan parasites can be identified in Giemsa-stained preparations, in cultures of aspirate, or in biopsy specimens from the edge of the ulcer. Treatment is carried out with pentavalent antimonial compounds (11). Similar, but rare, ulcers may occur in hot, dry tropical areas, caused by *Corynebacterium diphtheriae*.

A generalized macupapular eruption can be seen with various typhus infections. Most common is tick typhus contracted in Africa, which often presents with an eschar at a tick bite site associated with rash, fever, chills, and headache. This is very responsive to tetracycline.

ROUTINE POSTTRAVEL SCREENING

Posttravel evaluation is usually not necessary for the short-term traveler who remains well while traveling and after return. However, ill travelers and their physicians must be aware of the long latent period of some infections. Prior travel must then be considered in the presence of symptoms beginning some months or even a few years after travel or residence in the developing world. Longer-term travelers or residents from the tropics should have certain routine screening tests following return. These can include complete blood count, urinalysis, liver function tests, hepatitis B and HIV testing, tuberculin skin test, stool examinations for ova and parasites, and serologic testing for schistosomiasis if possible exposure has occurred (37, 63).

REFERENCES

1. **Adachi, J. A., L. Ostrosky-Zeichner, H. L. Du Pont, and C. D. Ericsson.** 2000. Empirical antimicrobial therapy for traveler's diarrhea. *Clin. Infect. Dis.* **31:**1079–1083.
2. **Aldeen, W. E. K., K. Carroll, A. Robison, M. Morrison, and D. Hale,** 1998. Comparison of nine commercially available enzyme-linked assays for detection of *Giardia lamblia* in fecal specimens. *J. Clin. Microbiol.* **36:**1338–1340.
3. **Angus, B. J.** 2001. Malaria on the World Wide Web. *Clin. Infect. Dis.* **33:**651–661.
4. **Anonymous.** 2001. Twinrix: a combination hepatitis A and B vaccine. *Med. Lett. Drugs Ther.* **43:** 67–68.
5. **Anonymous.** 2002. Drugs for parasitic infections. *Med. Lett. Drugs Ther.* April. [Online.] http://www.medletter.com.
6. **Anonymous.** 2003. Nitazoxanide (Alinia)—a new antiprotozoal agent. *Med. Lett. Drugs Ther.* **45:** 29–31.

7. **Appleton, B., M. S. Wolfe, and G. I. Mishtowt.** 1973. Chloroquine as a malarial suppressive: absence of visual effects. *Mil. Med.* **138:**225–226.

8. **Backer, H.** 2002. Water disinfection for international and wilderness travelers. *Clin. Infect. Dis.* **34:**355–364.

9. **Beal, C. B., P. Viens, R. G. L. Grant, and J. M. Hughes.** 1970. A new technique for sampling duodenal contents—demonstration of upper small bowel pathogens. *Am. J. Trop. Med. Hyg.* **19:**349–352.

10. **Bennish, M. L.** 1995. Immunization against *Salmonella typhi. Infect. Dis. Clin. Pract.* **4:**114–122.

11. **Berman, J.** 1997. Human leishmaniasis: clinical, diagnostic, and chemotherapeutic developments in the last 10 years. *Clin. Infect. Dis.* **24:**684–703.

12. **Blacklow, N. R., and H. B. Greenberg.** 1991. Viral gastroenteritis. *N. Engl. J. Med.* **325:**252–264.

13. **Bryan, R. T., H. A. Waskin, F. O. Richards, T. M. Bailey, and D. D. Juranek.** 1988. African trypanosomiasis in American travelers: a 20 year review, *In* R. Steffen, H. O. Lobel, J. Haworth, and D. J. Bradley (ed.), *Travel Medicine.* Springer-Verlag, Berlin, Germany.

14. **Castelli, F., and A. Patroni.** 2000. The human immunodeficiency virus infected traveler. *Clin. Infect. Dis.* **31:**1403–1408.

15. **Centers for Disease Control and Prevention.** 2003–2004. *Health Information for International Travel.* U.S. Department of Health and Human Services, Public Health Service, Atlanta, Ga.

16. **Centers for Disease Control and Prevention.** 1993. Hepatitis E among US travelers, 1989–1992. *Morb. Mortal. Wkly. Rep.* **42:**1–4.

17. **Centers for Disease Control and Prevention.** 1993. Inactivated Japanese encephalitis vaccine. Recommendations of the Advisory Committee on Immunization Practices (ACIP). *Morb. Mortal. Wkly. Rep.* **42**(RR–1):1–15.

18. **Centers for Disease Control and Prevention.** 1996. Prevention of hepatitis A through active or passive immunization. Recommendations of the Advisory Committee on Immunization Practices (ACIP). *Morb. Mortal. Wkly. Rep.* **45**(RR–15):1–30.

19. **Connor, B.** 2001. Expert recommendations for antimalarial prophylaxis. *J. Travel Med.* **8**(Suppl. 3):557–564.

20. **Dardick, K.** 2000. Travel advisory software. *Med. Software Rev.* **August:**1–11.

21. **Dembert, M. L., K. F. Strosahl, and R. L. Baumgarner.** 1981. Diseases from fish and shellfish ingestion. *Am. Fam. Physician* **24:**103–108.

22. **DuPont, H. L., C. D. Ericsson, P. C. Johnson, J. M. Bitsura, M. W. DuPont, and F. J. de la Cabada.** 1987. Prevention of travelers' diarrhea by the tablet formulation of bismuth subsalicylate. *JAMA* **257:**1347–1350.

23. **Ericsson, C. D.** 1998. Travelers' diarrhea: epidemiology, prevention, and self-treatment. *Infect. Dis. Clin. N. Am.* **83:**285–304.

24. **Fradin, M. S.** 1998. Mosquitoes and mosquito repellents: a clinician's guide. *Ann. Intern. Med.* **128:**931–940.

25. **Freedman, D. O.** 1998. Keeping current: travel medicine resources available on the internet. *Infect. Dis. Clin. N. Am.* **12:**543–547.

26. **Gorbach, S. L., and R. Edelman (ed.).** 1986. Travelers' diarrhea: National Institutes of Health Consensus Development Conference. Bethesda, Maryland, January 28–30, 1985. *Rev. Infect. Dis.* **8**(Suppl. 2):S109–S233.

27. **Grendon, J. H., R. F. Di Giacomo, and F. J. Frost.** 1995. Descriptive features of *Dientamoeba fragilis* infections. *J. Trop. Med. Hyg.* **98:**309–315.

28. **Haque, R., L. M. Neville, P. Hahn, and W. A. Petrie.** 1995. Rapid diagnosis of *Entamoeba* infection by using *Entamoeba* and *Entamoeba histolytica* stool antigen detection kits. *J. Clin. Microbiol.* **33:**2558–2561.

29. **Humar, A., and J. Keystone.** 1996. Evaluating fever in travelers returning from tropical countries. *BMJ* **312:**953–956.

30. **Isaacson, M.** 2001. Viral hemorrhagic fever hazards for travelers in Africa. *Clin. Infect. Dis.* **33:**1707–1712.

31. **Jong, E. C., and H. D. Nothdurft.** 2001. Current drugs for antimalarial chemoprophylaxis: A review of safety and efficacy. *J. Travel Med.* **8**(Suppl. 3):548–556.

32. **Kain, K. C.** 1999. Skin lesions in the returned traveler. *Med. Clin. N. Am.* **83:**1077–1102.

33. **Keystone, J. S.** 1999. Gideon computer program for diagnosing and teaching geographic medicine. *J. Travel Med.* **6**:152–154.
34. **Keystone, J. S., P. E. Kozarsky, and D. O. Freedman.** 2001. Internet and computer-based resources for travel medicine practitioners. *Clin. Infect. Dis.* **32**:757–765.
35. **Klipstein, F. A.** 1981. Tropical sprue in travelers and expatriates living abroad. *Gastroenterology* **80**:590–600.
36. **Levine, J., R. K. Dykoski, and E. N. Janoff.** 1995. *Candida*-associated diarrhea: a syndrome in search of credibility. *Clin. Infect. Dis.* **21**:881–886.
37. **MacLean, J. D., and M. Libman.** 1998. Screening returning travelers. *Infect. Dis. Clin. N. Am.* **12**:431–443.
38. **Markell, L. K., and M. P. Udkow.** 1986. *Blastocystis hominis:* pathogen or fellow traveler? *Am. J. Trop. Med. Hyg.* **35**:1023–1026.
39. **Memish, Z.** 2002. Meningococcal disease and travel. *Clin. Infect. Dis.* **34**:84–90.
40. **Miller, K. D., A. E. Greenberg, and C. C. Campbell.** 1989. Treatment of severe malaria in the United States with a continuous infusion of quinidine gluconate and exchange transfusion. *N. Engl. J. Med.* **321**:65–70
41. **Ottesen, E.** 1993. Filarial infections. *Infect. Dis. Clin. N. Am.* **7**:619–633.
42. **Raeber, P. A., S. Winteler, and J. Paget.** 1994. Fever in the returned traveler: remember rickettsial diseases. *Lancet* **344**:331.
43. **Rosenthal, P. J., C. Peterson, F. R. Geertsma, and S. Kohl.** 1996. Availability of intravenous quinidine for falciparum malaria. *N. Engl. J. Med.* **348**:621.
44. **Ryan, E. T., and S. B. Calderwood.** 2000. Cholera vaccines. *Clin. Infect. Dis.* **31**:561–565.
45. **Shaffer, N., and L. Moore.** 1989. Chronic travelers' diarrhea in normal host due to *Isospora belli. J. Infect. Dis.* **159**:596–597.
46. **Soave, R., and P. Ma.** 1985. Cryptosporidiosis. Traveler's diarrhea in two families. *Arch. Intern. Med.* **145**:70–72.
47. **Soave, R.** 1996. *Cyclospora.* An overview. *Clin. Infect. Dis.* **23**:429–437
48. **Soto, J., J. Toledo, M. Rodriguez, J. Sanchez, R. Herrera, J. Padilla, and J. Berman.** 1998. Primaquine prophylaxis in nonimmune Colombian soldiers: efficacy and toxicity. *Ann. Intern. Med.* **129**:241–244.
49. **Sung, V., D. P. O'Brien, E. Matchett, G. V. Brown, and J. Torresi.** 2003. Dengue fever in travelers returning from Southeast Asia. *J. Travel Med.* **10**:208–213.
50. **Van Creval, R., P. Speelman, and C. Gravekamp.** 1994. Leptospirosis in travelers. *Clin. Infect. Dis.* **19**:132–134.
51. **Van Damme, P., J. Banatvala, O. Fay, O. Iwarson, B. McMahon, K. Van Herck, P. Shouval, P. Bonanni, B. Connor, G. Cooksley, G. Leroux-Roels, and F. Von Sonnenburg.** 2003. Hepatitis A booster vaccination: is there a need? *Lancet* **362**:1065–1071.
52. **Weinberg, M., J. Weeks, S. Lance-Parker, M. Traeger, S. Wiersma, Q. Phan, D. Dennison, P. MacDonald, M. Lindsley, J. Guarner, P. Connolly, M. Cetron, and R. Hajjeh.** 2003. Severe histoplasmosis in travelers to Nicaragua. *Emerg. Infect. Dis.* **9**:1322–1325.
53. **White, N.** 1996. The treatment of malaria. *N. Engl. J. Med.* **335**:800–806.
54. **White, N.** 2003. Melioidosis. *Lancet* **361**:1715–1722.
55. **Whitty, C. J. M., D. C. Mabey, M. Armstrong, S. G. Wright, and P. Chiodini.** 2000. Presentation and outcome of 1107 cases of schistosomiasis from Africa diagnosed in a non-endemic country. *Trans. R. Soc. Trop. Med. Hyg.* **94**:531–534.
56. **Wilde, H., D. J. Briggs, F.-X. Meslin, T. Hemachudha, and V. Sitprija.** 2003. Rabies update for travel medicine advisors. *Clin. Infect. Dis.* **37**:96–100.
57. **Wolfe, M. S.** 1982. The treatment of intestinal protozoa. *Med. Clin. N. Am.* **66**:707–720.
58. **Wolfe, M. S., J. F. Cordero.** 1985. Safety of chloroquine in chemosuppression of malaria. *Br. Med. J.* **290**:1466–1467.
59. **Wolfe, M. S., C. Tuazon, and R. Schultz.** 1990. Imported bubonic plague—District of Columbia. *Morb. Mortal. Wkly. Rep.* **39**:895–901.
60. **Wolfe, M. S.** 1990. Acute diarrhea associated with travel. *Am. J. Med.* **88**(Suppl. 6A):34S–37S.
61. **Wolfe, M. S.** 1991. Travel medicine and travel clinics. *Infect. Dis. Clin. N. Am.* **5**:377–391.
62. **Wolfe, M. S.** 1999. Eosinophilia in the returning traveler. *Med. Clin. N. Am.* **83**:1019–1032.

63. **Wolfe, M. S.** 1991. Medical evaluation of the returning traveler, p. 26.1–26.15. *In* E. C. Jong and J. S. Keystone (ed.), *Travel Medicine Advisor.* American Health Consultants, Atlanta, Ga.

64. **Wolfe, M. S.** 1992. Giardiasis. *Clin. Microbiol. Rev.* **5:**93–100.

65. **Wolfe, M. S.** 1995. Typhim Vi: a new typhoid vaccine. *Infect. Dis. Clin. Pract.* **4:**186–188.

66. **Wolfe, M. S.** 1995. Hepatitis A and the American traveler. *J Infect Dis.* **171**(Suppl. 1):S29–S32.

67. **Wolfe, M. S. (ed.).** 1998. *Health Hints for the Tropics,* 12th ed. American Society of Tropical Medicine and Hygiene, Northbrook, Ill.

68. **Wongsrichanalai, C., A. L. Pickard, W. H. Wernsdorfer, and S. R. Meshnick.** 2002. Epidemiology of drug-resistant malaria. *Lancet Infect. Dis.* **2:**209–218.

69. **World Health Organization.** 2000. Severe falciparum malaria. *Trans. R. Soc. Trop. Med. Hyg.* **94**(Suppl. 1):S1–S74.

70. **World Health Organization.** 2003. *International Travel and Health: Vaccination Requirements and Health Advice.* World Health Organization, Geneva, Switzerland.

71. **Young, E. J.** 1983. Human brucellosis. *Rev. Infect. Dis.* **5:**821–842.

72. **Zimmerman, R. K.** 1996. Varicella vaccine: rationale and indications for use. *Am. Fam. Physician* **53:**647–652.

Infections of Leisure, Third Edition
Edited by David Schlossberg
© 2004 ASM Press, Washington, D.C.

Chapter 14

From Boudoir to Bordello:
Sexually Transmitted Diseases and Travel

Jonathan M. Zenilman

Travel has been historically an important risk factor for acquisition of sexually transmitted diseases (STDs). Travel is often associated with a sense of adventure, periods of loneliness, and exploration away from one's home environment—which often form the milieu in which sexual activity can occur with new partners. Some travel occurs specifically for sexual purposes, such as the organized junkets to Southeast Asia, particularly Thailand, which were popular during the 1980s. Some travel situations, such as military deployments, occur in the context of large groups of individuals exposed to high levels of stress.

The types of diseases acquired during travel are dependent on the types of sexual activity, the types of sexual partners, and the reasons for or type of travel that occurred. For example, the diseases and social situation of a military base are different from those of a refugee camp, which in turn are much different from those encountered by casual travelers. Travel is an important factor in the spread of new types of infections, such as antimicrobial-resistant *Neisseria gonorrhoeae* infection and human immunodeficiency virus (HIV) infection. In areas where STD incidence is low, travelers are often implicated in the reestablishment of new epidemic foci (reintroductions). In this chapter, I review the clinical syndromes and epidemiology of the most commonly encountered STDs and review the clinical and behavioral aspects of travel and STD epidemiology.

STDs have a major public health impact. In the United States, over 18 million cases of STDs (173) (Table 1) occur annually, with the highest incidence in adolescents and young adults.

TRANSMISSION MODE: THE DEFINITION OF AN STD

STDs are transmitted through sexual intercourse. Sexual intercourse is clinically and epidemiologically defined as sexual contact including vaginal intercourse,

Jonathan M. Zenilman • Division of Infectious Diseases, Johns Hopkins University, Johns Hopkins Bayview Medical Center, 4940 Eastern Ave., Baltimore, MD 21224.

Table 1. Major STDs

Genital ulcer diseases
  Syphilis (*Treponema pallidum*)
  Granuloma inguinale (*Calymmatobacterium granulomatis*)
  Lymphogranuloma venereum (*Chlamydia trachomatis* LGV serovars)
  Chancroid (*Haemophilus ducreyi*)
  Genital herpes (HSV-1 and -2)
  HPV infection

Exudative diseases
  Gonorrhea (*Neisseria gonorrhoeae*)
  Chlamydia (*Chlamydia trachomatis*)
  Trichomoniasis (*Trichomonas vaginalis*)
  BV (vaginal flora ecological disturbance)

Systemic diseases
  HIV
  Hepatitis B virus infection
  Human T-lymphotropic virus type 1
  Cytomegalovirus
  Human herpesvirus 8 (Kaposi sarcoma virus)

Infestations
  Scabies
  Pediculosis

---

oral intercourse (either type of receptive oral intercourse, i.e., fellatio or cunnilingus), or rectal intercourse. STDs can be transmitted between heterosexual or homosexual partners. Different types of sexual activity may result in increased risks. Receptive rectal intercourse and vaginal intercourse carry the highest risks of STD transmission (144).

STDs are completely dependent on behavioral factors for transmission. Abstinent individuals will not contract an STD. Acquisition of STDs is also dependent on the probability that one will come into contact with an STD-infected partner, the susceptibility of the host, and the efficiency of transmission of the organism through sexual intercourse (16). These factors are critical for understanding an STD epidemiological model.

Not only is the absolute number of sexual partners important, but also the type of sexual partner contributes to potential infection risk. Individuals with partners who are more likely to be infected with STDs (for example, those involved in commercial sex work or drug use or those from an environment where diseases are highly prevalent) are much more likely to contract an STD than are individuals who do not have high-risk sexual partners. Similarly, persons with serial partners (but only one sexual partner at a time) are less likely to spread STDs than are persons who have multiple concurrent sex partners (59, 61). In parts of the world, such as western Europe, where STD rates are low, travelers to areas of high-level endemicity account for over half of the new bacterial STD infections (3, 4).

STD COVARIATES

Socioeconomic factors have been associated with increased incidence of STDs (19, 91, 95, 171). Areas with decreases in available health services, and especially preventive health services, have also been associated with increased incidence of STDs. In eastern Europe, there have been tremendous social and economic disruption, disintegration of the health care system, increased levels of intravenous drug use, and loosening of travel restrictions. These factors have coalesced to drive development of a very large STD and HIV epidemic (89, 159).

Urbanization in developing countries has been strongly associated with increased incidence of STDs (103, 122). In the United States, illicit drug use and its associated sexual behaviors are associated with STD incidence, especially of syphilis (48, 58, 63, 98, 118, 119, 135, 141–143, 158). This is in part related to direct pharmacological activities of the drugs themselves (cocaine may stimulate increased sexual activity), but is more often due to the behaviors associated with drug use and the marketing of drugs, including prostitution.

Alcohol and other drug use is particularly associated with high-risk sexual activity. The relationship between alcohol and sexual activity is thought to be driven primarily by the disinhibitory effect. For example, recent data from the United States suggest that 25% of adolescents were using alcohol at the time of their last sexual intercourse (90). Studies in university settings found that alcohol use, especially "binge" drinking, was associated with increased rates of unintended sexual intercourse and lower rates of condom and contraceptive use (172). Alcohol use is consistently associated with high-risk sexual encounters in military populations (22, 69). Similarly, studies of travelers find consistent relationships between alcohol use and, in some studies (where it was assessed), marijuana use and having sex with a new partner (70, 71). Alcohol use is a frequent accompaniment of travel, and commercial sex workers' (CSWs') establishments often are bars. Strategies for disease prevention in these settings should focus on identifying triggers or high-risk situations before they occur. If sexual activity is a possibility, then the individual should prepare beforehand (i.e., by having condoms available). Furthermore, individuals should take care not to overindulge in alcohol or drug use, because the technical capacity to use a condom correctly may become impaired with high levels of use of these agents.

EPIDEMIOLOGY OF TRAVEL AND STDs

Despite the popular beliefs on the subject, few systematic studies have been performed on sexual behavior among travelers. Most studies were performed in western Europe. Of 1,011 women queried in a Swedish family planning setting, 276 (27%) reported a history of casual sex while traveling, mostly to destinations in western Europe (31). Casual sex was associated with more frequent alcohol and marijuana use, history of STD, and, paradoxically, a higher education level (although this may be correlated with income and ability to travel). A nonsystematic survey of a vacation area in southern England found that local residents of this area also had sex with visiting travelers (estimated 13% of females and 40% of males, but the data were collected in a biased fashion) (44). In Britain, a survey conducted in 1991 to 1992 of 757 patients returning for posttravel follow-up at the Hospital for Tropical Diseases in London found that 18.6% of persons had a new sexual partner while abroad; of these 18.6%, 48% reported two or more new partners (51). The predictor variables for having a new overseas sex partner were male gender, being abroad for a prolonged period (>3 months), having paid for sex in the past 5 years, and having had an STD in the past 5 years. Six percent had a self-reported history of STD. A similar study was conducted over a 3-month period in the largest STD clinic in London (50). Within the clinic population, 18% had traveled abroad within the previous 6 months, mostly to western Europe. Of this subgroup, 25% reported having a new sex partner while abroad; of these 25%, 19% were from developing countries. Twenty-two percent of heterosexual men who had new sex partners while abroad paid for sexual services, and two-thirds did not practice consistent condom use. A 2002 study in Australia suggested that up to a quarter of new HIV infections may be acquired overseas, especially in Vietnam, where transmission through injection drug use and sexual transmission have increased rapidly (51).

Most of the literature on travel describes persons from developed countries visiting developing countries. This approach ignores the risks associated with indigenous travel. Two examples have been recently reported from sub-Saharan Africa. Short-term mobility was found to be a risk for HIV infection in rural west Africa (99), especially for HIV type 2 (HIV-2). Similar results were seen in Tanzania, where STD risk was associated with personal mobility, as well as geographic proximity to trading centers in rural areas (11).

Travel has affected HIV epidemiology in developed countries, especially in Europe, where ties to Africa and Asia are often close. In the United Kingdom, diagnoses of HIV acquired in Africa accounted for 64% of new heterosexually acquired HIV in 2000. In Londoners of sub-Saharan ancestry, 40% of men and 21% of women reported acquiring a new sex partner when traveling home (53).

MILITARY POPULATIONS

Military and merchant marine personnel are demographically similar to the highest-risk groups for STDs—adolescents and young adults. Studies from the 1960s and 1970s suggest that the annual incidence rates of STDs in merchant seamen were 17 to 23% per year (38), with annualized rates of 17,000 to 23,000/100,000, which are extraordinary!

Historically, the travel and disruption induced by military campaigns have been associated with very high rates of STD acquisition. For example, in the Boer War, the STD rate among British soldiers was >50% (1). An attack rate of 37% was observed among Dutch soldiers in the East Indies in 1913; corresponding rates of 16% in Dutch East Indies troops in the late 1940s, 27% in Australian troops in Vietnam (69), and 10% in U.S. naval personnel and marines deployed to Mediterranean staging areas, South America, and Africa from 1989 to 1991 (107) have been noted. Similar problems were observed in military personnel deployed for noncombat roles. For example, of 1,885 Dutch marines deployed to Cambodia in 1992 and 1993, all received intensive STD education prior to deployment and condoms were available. A total of 842 (45%) reported sexual contact during deployment; 301 (36%) had had one to three contacts, and 541 (64%) had had four or more contacts (79). Sexual activity was associated with age (being younger) and not having a steady sexual partner at home. Inconsistent condom use was higher in older men. The overall unadjusted attack rate (including non-sexually active soldiers in the denominator) was 3.5%, and no cases were reported for consistent condom users. In the United States, studies on military installations have shown high overall prevalence rates of STDs. For example, military inductees have chlamydia rates of 9% (60), and the distribution of these infections is localized in high-density barracks settings (181). Risk factors included having a new sex partner, inconsistent condom use, and a history of STDs. A study of U.S. Navy personnel based in the western Pacific found that the prevalence of asymptomatic urethritis ranged from 3.4 to 6.9% (15, 147). An epidemic of syphilis in soldiers stationed at Fort Bragg, N.C., mirrored the epidemic that was occurring concurrently within the local civilian population (115). In particular, incidence in black soldiers was 10 times that in white soldiers—again reflecting the local epidemiology and also probably reflecting patterns of sexual mixing and partner recruitment.

Since 1987, all U.S. military personnel have been periodically tested for HIV. Significant risk of HIV-1 seroconversion was associated with age of >30 years, male gender, unmarried status, and lower ranks (132). Assignment to an area of HIV endemicity has been consistently shown to be a risk factor for seroconversion, which is almost exclusively due to sexual contact (92). Few data are available on the current military deployment to the Middle East.

EXPATRIATES

Another group known to be at high risk for STDs and HIV infection is expatriates. Because of increasing numbers of HIV/AIDS cases in Belgian expatriates, a case control study of 33 expatriate HIV patients and 119 seronegative controls was performed from 1985 to 1987; the study found that HIV patients were more likely to have had higher numbers of local sex partners (odds ratio >34) and CSW contacts (odds ratio >10) (20). A retrospective survey of Peace Corps volunteers serving in Zaire from 1985 to 1990 found high rates of STD incidence, ranging from 131/1,000 person-years in 1985 to 6.8/1,000 person-years in 1989 (18). Even so, this represents extremely high exposure rates. By the end of 1993, 10 Peace Corps volunteers had acquired HIV infection, all from presumed heterosexual exposures. A cross-sectional questionnaire study ($n = 1,602$) found that 60% of respondents had had sex while overseas, and 29% of these persons had had sex with a local-country partner (120). Only 32% of volunteers reported consistent condom use; alcohol use and low perceived HIV risk were the most important predictors of condom nonuse. A study of 847 Dutch expatriates found that 22% of men and 19% of women had a local steady sexual partner, and 29% of men and 17% of women had local casual partners (43). Condom use rates were 17 to 21% for those with steady partners and 64 to 69% for those with casual partners. Of the men with casual partners, 19% had CSW exposure. A follow-up study of the same group, accompanied by more intensive qualitative research, established three different groups of expatriates stratified by sexual risk. (i) The first consisted of those who had not planned to have sex, but it happened and they were unprepared. This group responds best to prevention campaigns which emphasize condom availability. (ii) The second group consisted of persons who had chaotic personal lives at home, to which posting abroad was a response; these individuals had multiple partners, often associated with alcohol. This group posed the biggest challenge for prevention, since they were the least likely to use condoms either at home or abroad. (iii) The third group consisted of persons who had sexual intercourse with multiple partners before and after posting abroad, and the changes did not alter the sexual context (42).

CSWs

Sexual intercourse with CSWs is very common among travelers, expatriates, and military personnel and is one of the major risk factors for HIV and other STDs (41). In most parts of the world, CSWs are economically stratified. The lowest strata include brothel-based workers or CSWs who recruit customers on the street ("street-walkers"). The next level are workers who recruit customers in bars (often karaoke bars in Asia) and have intercourse in hourly hotels. At the highest stratum are workers who have preset appointments and have one partner per day. The prices for services vary accordingly. Since STD rates are intrinsically tied to partner turnover rates and socioeconomic class, the lowest strata have the highest STD rates.

Besides unprotected sexual intercourse, several practices of CSWs may increase STD risk even more. For example, in a study of Thai CSWs, 36% had used prophylactic medications within the past year, often provided by the brothel owner (93). This potentiates the possibility of subsymptomatic infection; in addition, increased incidence of antimicrobial resistance is a major issue. Thai CSWs were also found to use commercial vaginal products (such as polycresulin) as disinfectant remedies. However, these products also cause increased cervical abrasion, mucosal ulcer, and exfoliation, all of which have the potential to increase the shedding rate of HIV and STD pathogens (94). Finally, a study of African CSWs found that tuberculosis incidence was extraordinarily high. In 587 HIV-infected CSWs, an incidence rate (new cases, not recurrent tuberculosis) of 34/1,000 patient-years was observed (62).

Condom use with CSWs may vary by locale, which may be attributed to socioeconomic disparity (between CSW and client), social and local norms, and enforcement. A study of Hong Kong residents found that condom use was higher when they used CSWs in Hong Kong (91%) than when they used CSWs in mainland China (66%) and that self-reported STD rates were four times higher in those who had traveled to the mainland (104). Thirty-three percent of travelers to the mainland have used the services of CSWs, 11% on the most recent trip (105).

From a human rights standpoint, CSWs present important issues. Many are engaged in commercial sex work because of poverty or oppression, especially in developing countries. The work environments are oppressive, because the activity is illegal in most settings and therefore prone to corruption and organized criminal syndicates. Health care services, including sexual health care services and contraception, are often nonexistent. In the developed world, commercial sex work is associated with drug use and lack of effective income and drug treatment options. In addition to the objective disease risks, travelers should also consider the social context of commercial sex work and its associated issues.

IMPLICATIONS OF TRAVEL-ASSOCIATED STDs: IMPORTATION

In parts of western Europe, endemic transmission of syphilis and gonorrhea is extremely low. Travelers returning from areas of endemicity play a major role in inducing new outbreaks or "miniepidemics." For example, over 25% of the cases of gonorrhea in Switzerland from 1989 to 1991 were acquired abroad (50). Studies performed in Sweden in the late 1980s and early 1990s found that of 857 gonorrhea patients evaluated, 43% of cases were imported from outside the community, 90% of these being acquired abroad (145). Nineteen percent of all infections were imported from Asia, with the largest group represented by men who had visited Thailand. These cases resulted in secondary transmission. At least 22% of the men and 16% of the women infected abroad had transmitted their infection to partners in Stockholm. Similar trends have been observed in Finland, where in 1994 and 1995, 54% of gonorrhea cases seen in Helsinki were imported (74). As a variant on this theme, another group in Sweden evaluated women who reported intercourse with men of foreign nationality, but within Sweden. Of 996 patients seen in family planning and adolescent clinics, 12% reported having intercourse with a foreigner. Among this group, 12.5% had gonorrhea and 26% had chlamydia (compared to 3 and 15%, respectively, in the nonexposed group).

TRAVEL FOR HEALTH CARE PROFESSIONALS

Few data are available on travel-associated STD and HIV risk for health care professionals. For example, 60 to 70% of British medical students spend time in developing countries, leading to debates of whether students should take with them "starter packs" for postexposure prophylaxis—ostensibly for blood-borne occupational exposure. Eighteen of 23 medical schools surveyed provided starter packs for postexposure prophylaxis (all for blood-borne exposure) (160). A high proportion of fluid exposure and invasive procedures were reported by students, which reflects a combination of setting, health care system supply shortages, and local practices, although medical students still perceived road accidents to be a bigger problem (57).

CLINICAL ASPECTS OF COMMON STDs

Gonorrhea and Chlamydia

Gonorrhea is caused by *N. gonorrhoeae*, a fastidious gram-negative coccus (77). In men, urethritis is the most common syndrome (39, 149). Discharge or dysuria usually appears within 1 week of exposure, although as many as 5 to 10% of patients never have signs or symptoms. Asymptomatic disease can exist in men up to several weeks after infection (68, 148). In women, gonorrhea typically causes cervical disease (cervicitis). Women with untreated gonococcal cervicitis develop upper tract infection or pelvic inflammatory disease (PID) (28, 112). Symptomatic anorectal gonococcal disease occurs in men with a history of receptive rectal intercourse (106). Approximately 50% have symptoms, which include rectal pain, discharge, constipation, and tenesmus. Because rectal gonorrhea in men implies a history of unprotected rectal intercourse, surveillance of rectal gonorrhea has been useful as a surrogate marker for HIV risk in gay men (26, 30).

Gonococcal pharyngitis (81, 178) occurs in men or women after oral sexual exposure and is clinically indistinguishable from any other bacterial pharyngitis. Disseminated gonococcal infection (gonococcal septicemia) occurs in approximately 0.1 to 0.5% of total gonococcal cases (124, 134).

Chlamydia trachomatis infections are the most common STD in the United States (128), with approximately 2.5 million cases estimated annually. The syndromes for chlamydia are similar to those seen in gonorrhea; however, they tend to be less aggressive in the acute context. Still, they cause significant numbers of complications, especially PID and adverse perinatal outcomes (72, 73, 146). In men, chlamydia urethritis accounts for approximately 40% of all cases of nongonococcal urethritis (153, 154). Urethritis in men typically presents as a mucoid discharge, often associated with dysuria. Asymptomatic infection occurs in over 30% of cases seen in clinical settings but >90% of cases diagnosed in population-based prevalence studies (117, 161). The time from infection to development of symptoms is longer than that for gonorrhea, usually about 7 to 14 days.

In women, cervical infection is the most commonly reported syndrome. Over half of women with cervical infection are asymptomatic. When symptoms occur, they may manifest as vaginal discharge or poorly differentiated abdominal or lower abdominal pain (85, 113). At clinical examination, there are often no clinical signs present. When they are present, they include mucopurulent cervical discharge, cervical friability, and cervical edema. Left untreated, approximately 30% of women with chlamydial infection develop PID (21, 138, 139).

Rectal chlamydia (139) infection occurs predominantly in homosexual men who have had receptive rectal intercourse, although cases in heterosexual women with similar exposures are reported. Oropharyngeal chlamydial infection appears not to be a clinically important entity.

Diagnosis

Traditional approaches to diagnosis of gonorrhea and chlamydia used culture or antigen-based detection tests. Major advances in DNA and RNA amplification have facilitated the development of highly sensitive and specific nucleic acid amplification techniques, including PCR, ligase chain reaction, and strand displacement (10, 33, 86, 87, 96). Furthermore, the high sensitivities of these techniques have allowed them to be used with urine and self-administered vaginal swabs.

Antimicrobial Resistance

Antimicrobial resistance is not a clinical issue in chlamydia treatment. Antimicrobial-resistant gonorrhea has been an ongoing problem since the development of plasmid-mediated β-lactam resistance (penicillinase-producing *N. gonorrhoeae* in 1976 [84], first diagnosed in returning travelers from Southeast Asia). Since 1989, quinolones and cephalosporins have been the drugs of choice, since they were effective against the known β-lactam and tetracycline resistance determinants. However, since the mid-1990s, resistance has rapidly developed, initiating from foci in Southeast Asia and widely disseminated by travelers with sexual contact in that region. Outbreaks have been reported in the western United States (31), the United Kingdom (54), Israel (40) (associated with sex workers from the former Soviet Union), Denmark (155), and Australia, among others. In surveillance programs conducted in the Southeast Asia Pacific basin, the proportion of gonorrhea cases which are due to quinolone-resistant *N. gonorrhoeae* (QRNG) exceeds 50% in over a third of the countries surveyed (157). Most authorities believe that QRNG developed in this area because of widespread use of quinolones for prophylaxis, usually at subtherapeutic doses. The rapid spread of QRNG demonstrates the ability of sexually transmitted organisms to disseminate throughout the world via travelers.

Gonorrhea treatment (32) for mucosal gonorrhea infections is based on providing single-dose regimens, preferably oral, that are effective against most or all of the known resistance determinants. Current single-dose oral regimens include ciprofloxacin (500 mg), ofloxacin (400 mg), and cefixime (400 mg). Ceftriaxone at 125 mg intramuscularly is an alternative when oral regimens are not available. For patients traveling to the western United States or any part of Asia, quinolones are not recommended (9, 31). All patients treated for gonorrhea should also be treated for chlamydia. The base chlamydia regimens are either azithromycin at 1 g (single dose) or doxycycline at 100 mg twice daily for 1 week.

PID

PID encompasses soft tissue upper tract inflammation, including endometritis, oophoritis, and pelvic peritonitis (7, 112). PID usually follows an untreated lower genital tract infection, such as gonorrhea or chlamydia. Organisms that are isolated from the upper tract, for example, at laparoscopy or surgery, include *N. gonorrhoeae*; *C. trachomatis*; organisms associated with vaginal flora, such as *Streptococcus* spp. (group B), *Gardnerella* spp., *Escherichia coli*, and *Veillonella* spp.; and intraabdominal colonic organisms, such as *Bacteroides* spp. and other anaerobes. The pathophysiological progression (140, 169) of PID is hypothesized to be a sexually transmitted lower tract (cervical) infection causing breakdown of the normal defense mechanisms, followed by ascent of bacteria into the uterus, fallopian tubes, and periovarian areas, causing inflammation.

The inflammation caused by PID often results in tubal scarring, which is the cause of later tubal infertility and increased risk of ectopic pregnancy (20, 176, 177). Accurate clinical diagnosis is difficult (7), because up to a quarter of PID cases may manifest no symptoms, especially when the disease is associated with chlamydia. Therefore, many practitioners currently treat women with mild cervical motion tenderness with treatment regimens effective against PID under the assumption that the benefit of preventing PID or curing early PID outweighs the costs in terms of increased expense of treatment and potential side effects.

Treatment strategies for PID are based on the underlying microbiology, including antimicrobial coverage for *N. gonorrhoeae*, *C. trachomatis*, streptococci, gram-negative rods, and anaerobes. Treatment regimens are therefore complex (32) and beyond the scope of this chapter. Despite efforts to develop effective antimicrobial regimens, treatment efficacy has been difficult to assess because of the need to evaluate long-term impact.

Vaginal Infections

When individuals with vaginal infections or vaginal discharge (Fig. 1) are evaluated, it is imperative to differentiate primary vaginal infections from cervical infections presenting as vaginitis. Vaginitis has a number of causes, including trichomoniasis, bacterial vaginosis (BV), and candidiasis. Since candidiasis is not a sexually transmitted infection and has very few long-term health effects, it is not considered here for the sake of brevity. However, the clinician should recognize that patients often confuse any vaginal discharge disorder with a yeast infection and treat it with over-the-counter drugs before seeking medical attention.

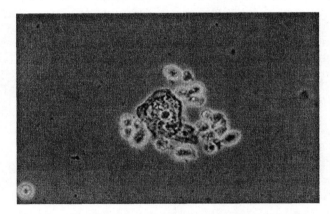

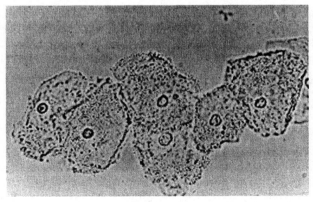

Figure 1. (Top) Vaginal discharge syndrome. *T. vaginalis* organisms on a wet mount are shown. (Bottom) BV. Clue cells with a ground-glass appearance are shown.

Trichomonas

Trichomonas infection occurs in approximately 3 million women annually and is caused by *Trichomonas vaginalis*, a flagellated protozoan (151, 152, 175). Signs and symptoms include a watery vaginal discharge, punctate hemorrhagic lesions on the cervix, and occasionally a frank cervicitis occurring in response to the vaginal infection. The prevalence of trichomoniasis in women is high; some studies report rate ranges of 5 to 40%. In men, *Trichomonas* infection can present as a nonchlamydial nongonococcal urethritis, and the prevalence in men in developing-country settings ranges from 6 to 12% (82).

Wet mount is the most inexpensive and widely used method for diagnosis. Treatment for trichomoniasis is metronidazole, 2 g as a single dose (32), which is considered safe during pregnancy (17). Metronidazole resistance is occasionally reported.

BV

BV is a disorder which occurs as a result of ecological disturbances in the vaginal flora (151). The normal vaginal flora overwhelmingly consists of lactobacilli. As a result, the vaginal host environment is acidic, with a pH of <4.5. In BV, alteration of the microflora occurs, with the population of lactobacilli replaced by gram-negative rods and anaerobes.

BV occurs most commonly as a secondary disorder due to cervical infection and inflammation (such as gonorrhea or chlamydia), alteration of vaginal microflora as a result of antibiotic use, or use of vaginal douches. Douching is particularly associated with development of BV (75). Therefore, clinical recommendations include specific recommendations not to douche. BV has been demonstrated to be a risk factor for premature rupture of membranes and premature delivery (114, 116, 121, 150). BV also is sexually transmitted in homosexual women (8, 109).

Diagnosis of BV is made on the basis of either evaluation of a vaginal smear Gram stain demonstrating the characteristic alteration of the vaginal flora or clinical criteria. The clinical criteria are three of the following: homogenous vaginal discharge, pH of >4.5, presence of an amine odor, and presence of "clue cells" (vaginal epithelial cells which have large amounts of adherent bacteria causing a ground-glass-type appearance) (27). Treatment of BV includes use of antimicrobials effective against anaerobes, such as metronidazole or clindamycin, which results in reestablishment of the normal vaginal microflora.

Genital Ulcer Diseases

Syphilis

Syphilis (78) is a multistage disease caused by *Treponema pallidum*. Syphilis is typically seen in situations where there are multiple opportunities for large numbers of anonymous sex partners such as homosexual bathhouses, drug "crack houses" (111), and situations where sex is exchanged for drugs.

Initial infection occurs through sexual contact at a mucosal membrane. The incubation period ranges between 10 and 30 days, and then a chancre develops (Fig. 2). The chancre is a painless lesion with an indurated border and has associated

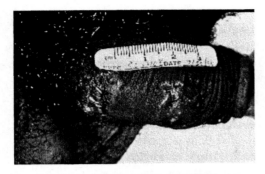

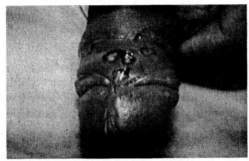

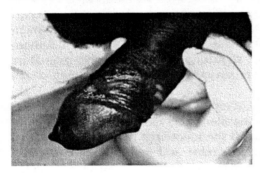

Figure 2. Classical and nonclassical examples of genital ulcers. These lesions could not be differentiated solely on the basis of physical examination. (Top) Primary syphilis chancre. Note that the edges are ragged and the lesion is hemorrhagic; in contrast to the classical description. (Middle) Chancroid. This multicentric ulcer was painful and had an undermined border. (Bottom) Primary herpes. These lesions were extremely painful and presented after the vesicle phase. There was large associated lymphadenopathy.

painless lymphadenopathy. Left untreated, the chancre heals spontaneously within 2 to 3 weeks. Four to 8 weeks later, the secondary syphilis syndrome develops. Secondary syphilis is a systemic vasculitis caused by high levels of *T. pallidum* in the blood and associated immunologic responses. The most characteristic findings are dermatologic, including the classic palmar plantar rash, but other manifestations include alopecia (hair loss), mucosal lesions, and visceral involvement which can include granulomatous hepatitis, nephrotic syndrome, optic neuritis, and, rarely, meningovascular syphilis. Left untreated, the secondary syphilis syndrome spontaneously resolves, usually within 1 to 2 months of onset.

The late complications of syphilis such as neurosyphilis, cardiovascular syphilis, and gummatous syphilis do not develop until 10 to 20 years after the resolution of early syphilis. For HIV patients, case reports have suggested that late complications may occur earlier and ulcers may be more severe (27, 100, 137).

Early latent syphilis is a serologic diagnosis made on the basis of a fourfold increase in titer (i.e., 2 dilutions; see below) within 1 year, with previous documentation of the earlier serology. Late latent syphilis is a serologic diagnosis of syphilis occurring more than 1 year after baseline diagnosis.

Diagnosis of primary syphilis. Dark-field examination of the ulcer exudate establishes the diagnosis. Realistically, dark-field microscopy is not available in most settings. False negatives may occur if patients apply bactericidal creams to the lesions. Therefore, diagnosis is most often clinically established by the presence of a lesion in association with serologic findings.

Serologic diagnosis. Serologic diagnosis of syphilis is a two-step procedure (102). Initially, a nontreponomal screening test is performed. The most widely used tests are the Venereal Disease Research Laboratory test and the rapid plasma reagin test. Results for these tests are reported as titers, i.e., the dilutions required to achieve a negative reaction using standard reagents. Patients with a positive nontreponemal test should have a confirmatory test such as the fluorescent treponemal antibody-absorbed (FTA-ABS) or microhemagglutination (microhemagglutination assay—*Treponema pallidum* [MHATP] or hemagglutination treponemal test for syphilis [HATTS]) test. Up to 20% of patients with positive nontrepenomal tests will have negative confirmatory tests. These are termed benign false positives. Most frequently, these are seen for patients with histories of intravenous drug abuse, pregnancy, systemic disorders such as lupus, and other infectious processes such as Lyme disease.

All stages of syphilis are seen more commonly in HIV-infected patients. Studies in STD clinics have demonstrated that HIV prevalence in patients with syphilis is up to three times higher than in nonsyphilis patients in these settings (2, 76, 80, 130).

Treatment. Treatment (5) of primary, secondary, and early latent syphilis with benzathine penicillin is recommended. For patients who are allergic to penicillin, doxycycline may be used. Patients with late latent syphilis, late syphilis, or syphilis of unknown duration (serologic syphilis in which an initial benchmark cannot be defined) should be treated with benzathine penicillin at 2.4×10^6 U intramuscularly for 3 weeks. Although there has been substantial concern about treatment failures in HIV-infected persons, in randomized clinical trials these concerns have been unfounded (136).

Chancroid

Chancroid is a genital ulcer disease caused by the organism *Haemophilus ducreyi*. Chancroid is predominantly seen in developing countries and in subtropical areas of the developing world. Occasional outbreaks are seen in the United States, usually associated with prostitution and drug use (45, 47, 118, 158).

The incubation period of chancroid is between 4 and 7 days. The ulcer develops initially as a tender papule with erythema. The ulcer typically is undermined and in contrast to syphilis is often painful and is not indurated, and it has a purulent exudate. Painful large adenopathy is seen in up to 50% of patients. This can develop into large purulent nodes spontaneously in sinus tracts and rupture (buboes). Chancroid does not disseminate and has not been associated with major perinatal or neonatal complications.

The classic identifying features of chancroidal ulcers are short incubation period; painful, tender ulcerations with an undermined, beefy appearance; purulent exudate; and rapid resolution with appropriate antimicrobial treatment.

Diagnosis of chancroid is difficult because the organism grows only on special medium at 33°C. Newer diagnostic tests using amplification of DNA from ulcer exudates (125) have been developed but are not yet widely available.

Current treatment regimens include expanded-spectrum cephalosporins, the quinolones, and azithromycin (32). In the United States, chancroid should be considered the sentinel event causing an epidemiological investigation, including evaluation of travel patterns of potential partners.

Genital Herpes Infection

Herpes simplex virus (HSV) infections are characterized by lifelong infection, latency, and recurrences. Genital herpes is almost exclusively sexually transmitted (34, 36). Historically, 90% of genital herpes cases were caused by HSV type 2 (HSV-2), and 10% were caused by HSV-1; in the past decade this has changed, especially in developed countries and among homosexual men (156, 180).

Primary infection is often asymptomatic (166). Genital herpes can occur at any mucosal exposed site (genitalia, rectum, and mouth). In primary disease, the ulceration develops 5 to 10 days after exposure; there may also be associated systemic signs (35), such as fever, myalgias, headache, and occasionally meningeal irritation. Recurrent herpes can develop at any time after the primary infection. In many settings, patients report a prodrome, which may consist of low-grade fever, pruritus, and tingling at the site of recurrence. Patients often report that they are able to feel the recurrence developing with nonspecific signs and symptoms, which is most likely related to irritation of the peripheral nerve roots.

Since many patients have asymptomatic primary infection, differentiation of a clinical first episode into primary disease or recurrence (in patients who have had an asymptomatic primary episode) is often not possible (101). In the research setting, primary infections are defined as an initial clinical episode with no serologic evidence of prior infection. Most patients, however, presenting with their initial episode actually have serologic evidence of prior infection. This is termed the first clinical episode of recurrent disease. This is often a very confusing point to clinicians but can be resolved using accurate serologic tests.

Recurrences are less symptomatic and heal faster than the primary episode. Recurrences often occur most frequently within the first year after primary infection, and frequency decreases thereafter.

Asymptomatic shedding plays a major role in transmission of HSV. Asymptomatic shedding occurs between clinical outbreaks, especially in the first few years after diagnosis. Initial culture studies of women with a recent diagnosis of primary herpes found that asymptomatic shedding occurred approximately 1% of the time (166, 167). The asymptomatic culture-diagnosed shedding definitely represents a potential infectious inoculum (about 10^4 viral particles). Further recent work with PCR demonstrated that shedding detectable by PCR occurred almost on a daily basis. From a transmission and public health standpoint, the implications of the PCR data are not yet fully understood. Serologic studies demonstrate that up to one in six members of the sexually active adult U.S. population is infected (37, 52, 55), and even higher proportions in developing countries are infected. Therefore, the data on asymptomatic shedding have profound implications for transmission, especially in unprotected sex with a new partner who has a high likelihood of infection.

Culture or other direct virus specific tests, such as a direct fluorescent antibody or DNA probe, are used to make the virological diagnosis of herpes. Directly obtained specimens are easily typed into HSV-1 and HSV-2 by using monoclonal antibody reagents. Treatment is effective in managing symptoms but is not curative. The nucleoside analogue drugs—acyclovir, famciclovir, and valacyclovir—all reduce symptom severity and shorten the time to healing of lesions. For individuals who have more than six recurrences per year, or who are profoundly immunosuppressed and have recurrent disease (such as those with advanced HIV disease, transplant recipients, and patients undergoing chemotherapy), suppressive therapy is indicated. Suppressive regimens are over 90% protective in preventing recurrences.

HPV Infection

Human papillomaviruses (HPVs) are small RNA viruses which have the unique capacity of causing chronic infection that can lead to malignant transformation resulting in vulvar, anal, cervical, and penile squamous cell carcinomas (97). HPVs cannot be cultured in vitro. There are over 80 subtypes of HPV; the HPV types that most commonly infect the genital tract are HPV types 6 (HPV-6), 11, 16, and 18. HPV-16 and -18 can cause malignant transformation and are frequently found in invasive cervical and other epithelial cancers and are thus classified as high-risk types (14).

The vast majority of HPV infections are asymptomatic. The incubation period is estimated to be 3 months (range of 3 weeks to 8 months). A small proportion of patients present with condylomata acuminata, or genital warts which are caused by proliferation of the keratinized epithelium. Lesions may occur anywhere on the external genitalia, the anus, and the rectum. In women, cervical warts are occasionally observed; in men, lesions may be present inside the urethra.

Treatment (32) for condylomata is based on surgical excision of the lesions, tissue-destructive therapy such as liquid nitrogen cryotherapy, chemical destruction with trichloroacetic acid or podophyllin, or local immunotherapy with imiquimod or interferons. An eradication of HPV-containing tissue is impossible because grossly and histologically normal-appearing tissues may be infected with HPV and cannot be identified unless specifically probed by DNA analysis. Therefore, the treatment of genital wart lesions due to HPV by traditional destructive methods such as liquid nitrogen or surgery leads to substantial recurrence rates because HPV infection is often present in the histologically normal surgical margins.

Estimates indicate that approximately 1% of the sexually active population in the United States have clinically apparent genital warts, and in STD clinic populations the percentage is much higher (6, 66, 67, 179). Estimates of infection range from 20% to above 90% depending on the specific populations studied, with college students, adolescents, and CSWs demonstrating the highest rates.

STD AND HIV RELATIONSHIPS

Sexually transmitted HIV is prevalent in many parts of the world, especially south Asia and Africa. As a sexually transmitted virus, HIV has a means of transmission that is facilitated by the same risk behaviors as are associated with the traditional STDs, e.g., multiple sexual partners, sex with CSWs, and drug-using sexual partners. Cross-sectional and prospective studies in the developed and developing world have firmly established that bacterial and viral STDs are biological cofactors in facilitating HIV transmission (56, 170). Since the late 1990s, there has been a resurgence of both HIV and traditional STDs, especially syphilis and gonorrhea, in gay men, often associated with high-risk sexual behavior at popular travel venues (129).

HIV prevalence studies demonstrate consistently three- to fivefold-increased odds for HIV positivity in a variety of patient populations with genital ulcer disease (46), including those with symptomatic and asymptomatic genital herpes (133, 163, 165). Most prospective studies of genital ulcers and increased risk for HIV infection have been performed with CSWs or STD clinic clients or defined populations such as military recruits (25). Prospectively, genital ulcer disease was associated with a sevenfold-increased seroconversion risk. Similarly, prospective studies in India and Zaire (12) conclusively demonstrated an association between exudative STD (gonorrhea and chlamydia) and HIV seroconversion. Careful large cohort studies in Africa have demonstrated that HIV transmission is increased stepwise by the presence of genital herpes (serologically defined), a genital ulcer, and incremental increases in HIV load facilitated by genital ulcers; this is important, especially in developing countries and in impoverished areas of developed countries (64, 131).

INTERVENTIONS TO REDUCE THE RISK OF SEXUAL EXPOSURE

Promoting condom use has been one of the central tenets of the HIV and STD risk reduction strategy both in the United States and abroad. Condoms are effective when used correctly and consistently. Studies of HIV-discordant heterosexual couples in California and Italy (29, 44, 126) have conclusively demonstrated that consistent use in controlled settings results in an approximately sevenfold decrease in HIV seroconversions. Condoms are also effective in reducing the risk of STDs, including herpes and HPV (22, 108, 164, 168, 174), which attains increasing importance as the relationships of STDs as cofactors continue to be elucidated.

Probably the most intensive and successful effort has been implemented in Thailand, where the "100% Condom" program (22, 24, 123) has been implemented since 1991. This program includes intensive advertising, an infrastructure to purchase and distribute condoms, and linkages in promoting condoms with stakeholders, including the army, provincial and municipal governments, and CSWs. Recent large-scale reductions in HIV seroincidence in Thailand have been in part attributed to this program. The Thai program provides a useful model for the development of an effective condom promotion and sexual risk reduction campaign.

The program includes open discussion of HIV prevention and condom promotion, mass media campaigns, and the active participation of a large variety of stakeholders, including the military, government, medical community, and even the brothels. In other words, this effective program's major accomplishment was to change the social norms across a broad spectrum of society to encourage condom use.

In developing countries, condom promotion and safer-sex education campaigns have often been innovative in responding to local situations. For example, a highly successful Kenyan campaign to increase condom use focused on truck drivers and their assistants and was conducted at truck and rest stops, which decreased STDs by >30% (83). In Nicaragua, the health ministry successfully implemented a condom promotion campaign in a CSW district by providing condoms on the beds of local motels (49). Both of these efforts utilize a harm reduction and nonjudgmental approach.

PREVENTION ISSUES SPECIFIC TO WOMEN

If a woman regularly takes hormonal contraceptives, she should continue her regimen if there is even a remote possibility of travel abroad. Under most circumstances, the risk of unintended pregnancy from unprotected intercourse is as high as or higher than that of STD. Hormonal contraceptives should be used *in addition* to condoms, i.e., the "dual method" approach.

There has been much interest in developing vaginal microbicides as a female-controlled method of STD prevention. The ideal vaginal microbicides should demonstrate physical and chemical stability in the vaginal environment, allowing insertion sometime before intercourse; should not interfere with sexual intercourse; and should also be inexpensive (110, 111, 127). The ideal compound would be bactericidal and viricidal while being nontoxic to the host epithelium. Besides the potential toxicity to host epithelium, another consideration is the potential effect on the commensal vaginal microflora, and the consequent BV and inflammation. To date, vaginal microbicides have been chemical detergents which are water soluble and can solubilize the lipid membranes of bacteria and spermatozoa. Nonoxynol-9 is the prototype. Nonoxynol-9 is effective against common bacterial STD pathogens. However, studies with African CSWs demonstrated that nonoxynol-9 increases the incidence of genital ulcer disease and is associated with increased risk of HIV seroconversion, most likely due to chemical irritation of the vaginal mucosa (162). There has therefore been increased interest in developing chemically stable, buffered, nonionic compounds that could be used as vaginal microbicides, and more than 20 are under development.

AN STD PREVENTION STRATEGY

The epidemiological data consistently show that travelers are sexually active. From the standpoint of primary prevention, abstinence would be an impractical approach—although this would clearly reduce the risk to zero! Preventing sexual infection in travelers therefore emphasizes reducing risk (Table 2). In developing

Table 2. STD prevention strategy

Reduce number of sex partners
Recognize trigger situations for intercourse with new partners, e.g., alcohol use, drug use
Eliminate or reduce contact with CSWs
100% condom use and hormonal contraceptives
Periodic screening for STDs and HIV at home and abroad
Postexposure
   Emergency contraception
   Syndromic treatment (postexposure prophylaxis)

---

countries, such as in Africa, Southeast Asia, and, more recently, the former Soviet Union, STD rates are extraordinarily high and heterosexual transmission of HIV is extremely common. Therefore, unprotected sexual contacts in these areas carry substantial risk. The context of sexual activity is clearly related to risk; for example, CSW contacts are more risky (in most situations) than expatriate contacts. However, the reader is cautioned that these conclusions are based on population-based statistics and that an individual's risk may vary substantially.

Those counseling travelers should emphasize that if there is even a remote possibility of sexual relations, the traveler should ensure that condoms are available and easily accessible. Counseling needs to be nonjudgmental and should also ascertain "triggers," or situations which put the traveler at risk. The best example above is the expatriate who does not anticipate being sexually active, but becomes so because of an unforeseen opportunity, often associated with alcohol use. Counseling in prior recognition of these settings is critical.

Persons who are sexually active with multiple partners should have periodic screening for STDs, especially gonorrhea, chlamydia, syphilis, and HIV, at least on an annual basis. Herpes serology, using new type-specific serologic tests, should also be considered to identify asymptomatic HSV infection.

MANAGEMENT STRATEGY AFTER EXPOSURE

Anyone who may have been exposed to an STD who develops either a vaginal or urethral discharge, an unexplained rash or genital lesion, or genital or pelvic pain should cease sexual activity and promptly seek competent medical care. However, STDs are often asymptomatic, especially in women; therefore, anyone who believes that he or she may have been exposed to an STD should consult his or her health care provider for possible screening for STD.

When available, diagnostic services should include a physical examination, including a pelvic examination for women, and diagnostic tests for *N. gonorrhoeae*, *C. trachomatis*, and syphilis. Women should have a vaginal wet mount to evaluate for *Trichomonas* infection and BV. Herpes simplex testing should be performed in the appropriate situation. All persons evaluated for a travel-related unprotected sexual exposure should also receive HIV counseling and testing. If the initial test is negative, the person should be tested a second time, >3 months after the last unprotected sexual exposure, to ensure that he or she is not in the "seroconversion window." Treatment for STDs should follow the current Centers for Disease

Control and Prevention guidelines. Persons should not have unprotected sex until the diagnostic and therapeutic process is completed and HIV testing is confirmed negative. If possible, partners should be notified as well of the potential exposure.

In many settings, however, diagnostic facilities and testing services are not available. In these situations, syndromic management strategies for STDs should be utilized, and HIV counseling and testing should still be offered.

ACUTE MANAGEMENT AFTER EXPOSURE

If there is an unprotected sexual exposure, women who are not contracepting should strongly consider emergency contraception protocols (65, 88). In most European, Asian, and African countries, emergency contraception can be purchased over the counter. There are no current guidelines for acute disease or disease prevention management after an unprotected sexual exposure. For STD prevention, if the contact was high risk (e.g., with a CSW), then preventive therapy should be considered. Under these circumstances a viable preventive therapy regimen would include an expanded-spectrum cephalosporin (such as cefixime [400 mg]) to cover gonorrhea and chancroid, azithromycin (1 g) to cover chlamydia as well as incubating syphilis, and metronidazole for *Trichomonas* exposure. HIV post-sexual exposure prophylaxis is another consideration (88); however, it is often impractical. Most authorities believe that for HIV postexposure prophylaxis to be effective, it needs to be instituted within 24 h of exposure, and the regimens need to be tailored to the community where the exposure took place, in order to account for resistant variants. These logistics are daunting to an individual traveler who is unfamiliar with local health care resources. Furthermore, the effectiveness of HIV postexposure prophylaxis is still controversial, and the regimens are associated with numerous side effects.

The Centers for Disease Control and Prevention Traveler's Health Service (http://www.cdc.gov/travel/diseases/stds.htm) states the following:

> International travelers are at risk of contracting STDs, including HIV, if they have sex with partners who have these diseases. . . . To avoid acquiring STDs, travelers should be advised not to have sexual contact with persons who might be infected. Persons most likely to be infected are those with numerous sex partners. In many places, persons who make themselves available for sex with travelers are likely to be persons, such as commercial sex workers, who have had many partners. In addition, injecting drug users are at high risk of being infected with HIV, regardless of the number of their sex partners. Travelers who wish to absolutely protect themselves from acquiring an STD should be advised to refrain from sexual contact. If, however, they choose not to do this, travelers should be advised that they can reduce their risk of acquiring infection by consistently and correctly using a latex condom during sexual contact, whether vaginal, oral, or anal.

If lubricants are used during sex, only water-based lubricants (e.g., K-Y Jelly or glycerine) should be used with latex condoms, because oil-based lubricants (e.g., petroleum jelly, shortening, mineral oil, or massage oils) can weaken latex condoms. Those who are sensitive to latex should use condoms made of polyurethane or other synthetic materials.

Any traveler who might have been exposed to an STD and who develops either a vaginal or urethral discharge, an unexplained rash or genital lesion, or genital or pelvic pain should be advised to cease sexual activity and promptly seek competent medical care. Because STDs are often asymptomatic, especially in women, travelers who believe that they might have been exposed to an STD should be advised to consult a physician regarding the advisability of screening for STDs.

In summary, health care providers should consider travel as a potential risk factor for unprotected intercourse and STD exposure, in both the pretravel counseling setting and the posttravel evaluation.

REFERENCES

1. **Adler, M. W.** 1980. The terrible peril: a historical perspective on the venereal diseases. *Br. Med. J.* **281**:206–211.
2. **Ansell, D. A., T. C. Hu, M. Straus, M. Cohen, and R. Sherer.** 1994. HIV and syphilis seroprevalence among clients with sexually transmitted diseases attending a walk-in clinic at Cook County Hospital. *Sex. Transm. Dis.* **21**:93–96.
3. **Arvidson, M., D. Hellberg, and P. A. Mardh.** 1995. Sexually transmitted diseases in Swedish women with experience of casual sex with men of foreign nationalities within Sweden. *Acta Obstet. Gynecol. Scand.* **74**:794–798.
4. **Arvidson, M., I. Kallings, S. Nilsson, D. Hellberg, and P. A. Mardh.** 1997. Risky behavior in women with history of casual travel sex. *Sex. Transm. Dis.* **24**:418–421.
5. **Augenbraun, M. H.** 2002. Treatment of syphilis 2001: nonpregnant adults. *Clin. Infect. Dis.* **35**:S187–S190.
6. **Bauer, H. M., Y. Ting, C. E. Greer, J. C. Chambers, C. J. Tashiro, J. Chimera, A. Reingold, and M. M. Manos.** 1991. Genital human papillomavirus infection in female university students as determined by a PCR-based method. *JAMA* **265**:472–477.
7. **Beigi, R. H., and H. C. Wiesenfeld.** 2003. Pelvic inflammatory disease: new diagnostic criteria and treatment. *Obstet. Gynecol. Clin. N. Am.* **30**:777–793.
8. **Berger, B. J., S. Kolton, J. M. Zenilman, M. C. Cummings, J. Feldman, and W. M. McCormack.** 1995. Bacterial vaginosis in lesbians: a sexually transmitted disease. *Clin. Infect. Dis.* **21**:1402–1405.
9. **Berman, S. M., J. S. Moran, S. A. Wang, and K. A. Workowski.** 2003. Fluoroquinolones, gonorrhea, and the CDC STD treatment guidelines. *Sex. Transm. Dis.* **30**:528–529.
10. **Black, C. M.** 1997. Current methods of laboratory diagnosis of *Chlamydia trachomatis* infections. *Clin. Microbiol. Rev.* **10**:160–184.
11. **Boerma, J. T., M. Urassa, S. Nnko, J. Ng'weshemi, R. Isingo, B. Zaba, and G. Mwaluko.** 2002. Sociodemographic context of the AIDS epidemic in a rural area in Tanzania with a focus on people's mobility and marriage. *Sex. Transm. Infect.* **78**(Suppl. 1):i97–i105.
12. **Bollinger, R. C., R. S. Brookmeyer, S. M. Mehendale, R. S. Paranjape, M. E. Shepherd, D. A. Gadkari, and T. C. Quinn.** 1997. Risk factors and clinical presentation of acute primary HIV infection in India. *JAMA* **278**:2085–2089.

13. **Bonneux, L., P. Van der Stuyft, H. Taelman, P. Cornet, C. Goilav, G. van der Groen, and P. Piot.** 1988. Risk factors for infection with human immmunodeficiency virus among European expatriates in Africa. *BMJ* **297:**581–584.

14. **Bosch, F. X., A. Lorincz, N. Munoz, C. J. Meijer, and K. V. Shah.** 2002. The causal relation between human papillomavirus and cervical cancer. *J. Clin. Pathol.* **55:**244–265.

15. **Brodine, S. K., M. A. Shafer, R. A. Shaffer, C. B. Boyer, S. D. Putnam, F. S. Wignall, R. J. Thomas, B. Bales, and J. Schachter.** 1998. Asymptomatic sexually transmitted disease prevalence in four military populations: application of DNA amplification assays for Chlamydia and gonorrhea screening. *J. Infect. Dis.* **178:**1202–1204.

16. **Brunham, R. C., and F. A. Plummer.** 1990. A general model of sexually transmitted disease epidemiology and its implications for control. *Med. Clin. N. Am.* **74:**1339–1352.

17. **Burtin, P., A. Taddio, O. Ariburnu, T. R. Einarson, and G. Koren.** 1995. Safety of metronidazole in pregnancy: a meta-analysis. *Am. J. Obstet. Gynecol.* **172:**525–529.

18. **Cappello, M., K. W. Bernard, B. Jones, H. Francis, and T. van der Vlugt.** 1991. Human immunodeficiency virus infection among Peace Corps volunteers in Zaire. No evidence for unusual modes of transmission. *Arch. Intern. Med.* **151:**1328–1330.

19. **Catania, J. A., D. Binson, M. M. Dolcini, R. Stall, K. H. Choi, L. M. Pollack, E. S. Hudes, J. Canchola, K. Phillips, J. T. Moskowitz, et al.** 1995. Risk factors for HIV and other sexually transmitted diseases and prevention practices among US heterosexual adults: changes from 1990 to 1992. *Am. J. Public Health* **85:**1492–1499.

20. **Cates, W., Jr., R. T. Rolfs, Jr., and S. O. Aral.** 1990. Sexually transmitted diseases, pelvic inflammatory disease, and infertility: an epidemiologic update. *Epidemiol. Rev.* **12:**199–220.

21. **Cates, W., Jr., and J. N. Wasserheit.** 1991. Genital chlamydial infections: epidemiology and reproductive sequelae. *Am. J. Obstet. Gynecol.* **164:**1771–1781.

22. **Celentano, D. D., K. C. Bond, C. M. Lyles, S. Eiumtrakul, V. F. Go, C. Beyrer, C. C. Na, K. E. Nelson, C. Khamboonruang, and C. Vaddhanaphuti.** 2000. Preventive intervention to reduce sexually transmitted infections: a field trial in the Royal Thai Army. *Arch. Intern. Med.* **160:**535–540.

23. Reference deleted.

24. **Celentano, D. D., K. E. Nelson, C. M. Lyles, C. Beyrer, S. Eiumtrakul, V. F. Go, S. Kuntolbutra, and C. Khamboonruang.** 1998. Decreasing incidence of HIV and sexually transmitted diseases in young Thai men: evidence for success of the HIV/AIDS control and prevention program. *AIDS* **12:**F29–F36.

25. **Celentano, D. D., K. E. Nelson, S. Suprasert, S. Eiumtrakul, S. Tulvatana, S. Kuntolbutra, P. Akarasewi, A. Matanasarawoot, N. H. Wright, N. Sirisopana, et al.** 1996. Risk factors for HIV-1 seroconversion among young men in northern Thailand. *JAMA* **275:**122–127.

26. **Centers for Disease Control.** 1984. Declining rates of rectal and pharyngeal gonorrhea among males—New York City. *Morb. Mortal. Wkly. Rep.* **33:**295–297.

27. **Centers for Disease Control.** 1987. Tertiary syphilis deaths—South Florida. *Morb. Mortal. Wkly. Rep.* **36:**488–491.

28. **Centers for Disease Control.** 1991. Pelvic inflammatory disease: guidelines for prevention and management. *Morb. Mortal. Wkly. Rep.* **40:**1–25.

29. **Centers for Disease Control.** 1992. Changes in sexual behavior and condom use associated with a risk-reduction program—Denver, 1988–1991. *Morb. Mortal. Wkly. Rep.* **41:**412–415.

30. **Centers for Disease Control and Prevention.** 1999. Increases in unsafe sex and rectal gonorrhea among men who have sex with men—San Francisco, California, 1994–1997. *Morb. Mortal. Wkly. Rep.* **48:**45–48.

31. **Centers for Disease Control and Prevention.** 2002. Increases in fluoroquinolone-resistant Neisseria gonorrhoeae—Hawaii and California, 2001. *Morb. Mortal. Wkly. Rep.* **51:**1041–1044.

32. **Centers for Disease Control and Prevention.** 2002. Sexually transmitted diseases treatment guidelines 2002. *Morb. Mortal. Wkly. Rep.* **51**(RR-6):1–78.

33. **Ching, S., H. Lee, E. W. Hook III, M. R. Jacobs, and J. Zenilman.** 1995. Ligase chain reaction for detection of *Neisseria gonorrhoeae* in urogenital swabs. *J. Clin. Microbiol.* **33:**3111–3114.

34. **Corey, L., and H. H. Handsfield.** 2000. Genital herpes and public health: addressing a global problem. *JAMA* **283:**791–794.

35. **Corey, L., and K. K. Holmes.** 1983. Genital herpes simplex virus infections: current concepts in diagnosis, therapy, and prevention. *Ann. Intern. Med.* **98**:973–983.

36. **Corey, L., and P. G. Spear.** 1986. Infections with herpes simplex viruses (2). *N. Engl. J. Med.* **314**:749–757.

37. **Cowan, F. M., A. M. Johnson, R. Ashley, L. Corey, and A. Mindel.** 1994. Antibody to herpes simplex virus type 2 as serological marker of sexual lifestyle in populations. *BMJ* **309**:1325–1329.

38. **Cross, A. B., and J. R. Harris.** 1976. Reappraisal of the problem of British mariners and sexually transmitted infection. *Br. J. Vener. Dis.* **52**:71–77.

39. **Daker-White, G., and D. Barlow.** 1997. Heterosexual gonorrhoea at St. Thomas'—I: patient characteristics and implications for targeted STD and HIV prevention strategies. *Int. J. STD AIDS* **8**:32–35.

40. **Dan, M., F. Poch, and B. Sheinberg.** 2002. High prevalence of high-level ciprofloxacin resistance in *Neisseria gonorrhoeae* in Tel Aviv, Israel: correlation with response to therapy. *Antimicrob. Agents Chemother.* **46**:1671–1673.

41. **Day, S., and H. Ward.** 1997. Sex workers and the control of sexually transmitted disease. *Genitourin. Med.* **73**:161–168.

42. **de Graaf, R., G. van Zessen, and H. Houweling.** 1998. Underlying reasons for sexual conduct and condom use among expatriates posted in AIDS endemic areas. *AIDS Care* **10**:651–665.

43. **de Graaf, R., G. van Zessen, H. Houweling, R. J. Ligthelm, and R. van den Akker.** 1997. Sexual risk of HIV infection among expatriates posted in AIDS endemic areas. *AIDS* **11**:1173–1181.

44. **de Vincenzi, I., and the European Study Group on Heterosexual Transmission of HIV.** 1994. A longitudinal study of human immunodeficiency virus transmission by heterosexual partners. *N. Engl. J. Med.* **331**:341–346.

45. **DiCarlo, R. P., B. S. Armentor, and D. H. Martin.** 1995. Chancroid epidemiology in New Orleans men. *J. Infect. Dis.* **172**:446–452.

46. **Dickerson, M. C., J. Johnston, T. E. Delea, A. White, and E. Andrews.** 1996. The causal role for genital ulcer disease as a risk factor for transmission of human immunodeficiency virus. An application of the Bradford Hill criteria. *Sex. Transm. Dis.* **23**:429–440.

47. **Dillon, S. M., M. Cummings, S. Rajagopalan, and W. C. McCormack.** 1997. Prospective analysis of genital ulcer disease in Brooklyn, New York. *Clin. Infect. Dis.* **24**:945–950.

48. **Edlin, B. R., K. L. Irwin, S. Faruque, C. B. McCoy, C. Word, Y. Serrano, J. A. Inciardi, B. P. Bowser, R. F. Schilling, S. D. Holmberg, and the Multicenter Crack Cocaine and HIV Infection Study Team.** 1994. Intersecting epidemics—crack cocaine use and HIV infection among inner-city young adults. *N. Engl. J. Med.* **331**:1422–1427.

49. **Egger, M., J. Pauw, A. Lopatatzidis, D. Medrano, F. Paccaud, and G. D. Smith.** 2000. Promotion of condom use in a high-risk setting in Nicaragua: a randomised controlled trial. *Lancet* **355**:2101–2105.

50. **Eichmann, A.** 1993. Sexually transmissible diseases following travel in tropical countries. *Schweiz. Med. Wochenschr.* **123**:1250–1255. (In German.)

51. **Elliott, J. H., A. M. Mijch, A. C. Street, and N. Crofts.** 2003. HIV, ethnicity and travel: HIV infection in Vietnamese Australians associated with injecting drug use. *J. Clin. Virol.* **26**:133–142.

52. **Emonyi, I. W., R. H. Gray, J. Zenilman, K. Schmidt, M. J. Wawer, K. N. Sewankambo, D. Serwadda, N. Kiwanuka, and F. Nalugoda.** 2000. Sero-prevalence of herpes simplex virus type 2 (HSV-2) in Rakai district, Uganda. *East Afr. Med. J.* **77**:428–430.

53. **Fenton, K. A., M. Chinouya, O. Davidson, and A. Copas.** 2001. HIV transmission risk among sub-Saharan Africans in London travelling to their countries of origin. *AIDS* **15**:1442–1445.

54. **Fenton, K. A., C. Ison, A. P. Johnson, E. Rudd, M. Soltani, I. Martin, T. Nichols, and D. M. Livermore.** 2003. Ciprofloxacin resistance in Neisseria gonorrhoeae in England and Wales in 2002. *Lancet* **361**:1867–1869.

55. **Fleming, D. T., G. M. McQuillan, R. E. Johnson, A. J. Nahmias, S. O. Aral, F. K. Lee, and M. E. St. Louis.** 1997. Herpes simplex virus type 2 in the United States, 1976 to 1994. *N. Engl. J. Med.* **337**:1105–1111.

56. **Fleming, D. T., and J. N. Wasserheit.** 1999. From epidemiological synergy to public health policy and practice: the contribution of other sexually transmitted diseases to sexual transmission of HIV infection. *Sex. Transm. Infect.* **75**:3–17.

57. Franklin, G. F., K. Gray, and D. Nathwani. 2001. Provision of drugs for post-exposure prophy-laxis of HIV for medical students on overseas electives. *J. Infect.* **43:**191–194.
58. Friedman, S. R., P. L. Flom, B. J. Kottiri, J. Zenilman, R. Curtis, A. Neaigus, M. Sandoval, T. Quinn, and J. Des. 2003. Drug use patterns and infection with sexually transmissible agents among young adults in a high-risk neighbourhood in New York City. *Addiction* **98:**159–169.
59. Garnett, G. P., and A. M. Johnson. 1997. Coining a new term in epidemiology: concurrency and HIV. *AIDS* **11:**681–683.
60. Gaydos, C. A., M. R. Howell, B. Pare, K. L. Clark, D. A. Ellis, R. M. Hendrix, J. C. Gaydos, K. T. McKee, Jr., and T. C. Quinn. 1998. Chlamydia trachomatis infections in female military recruits. *N. Engl. J. Med.* **339:**739–744.
61. Ghani, A. C., J. Swinton, and G. P. Garnett. 1997. The role of sexual partnership networks in the epidemiology of gonorrhea. *Sex. Transm. Dis.* **24:**45–56.
62. Gilks, C. F., P. Godfrey-Faussett, B. I. Batchelor, J. C. Ojoo, S. J. Ojoo, R. J. Brindle, J. Paul, J. Kimari, M. C. Bruce, J. Bwayo, F. A. Plummer, and D. A. Warrell. 1997. Recent transmission of tuberculosis in a cohort of HIV-1-infected female sex workers in Nairobi, Kenya. *AIDS* **11:**911–918.
63. Gomez, M. P., A. M. Kimball, H. Orlander, R. M. Bain, L. D. Fisher, and K. K. Holmes. 2002. Epidemic crack cocaine use linked with epidemics of genital ulcer disease and heterosexual HIV infection in the Bahamas: evidence of impact of prevention and control measures. *Sex. Transm. Dis.* **29:**259–264.
64. Gray, R. H., M. J. Wawer, R. Brookmeyer, N. K. Sewankambo, D. Serwadda, F. Wabwire-Mangen, T. Lutalo, X. Li, T. vanCott, T. C. Quinn, and the Rakai Project Team. 2001. Probability of HIV-1 transmission per coital act in monogamous, heterosexual, HIV-1-discordant couples in Rakai, Uganda. *Lancet* **357:**1149–1153.
65. Grimes, D. A., and E. G. Raymond. 2002. Emergency contraception. *Ann. Intern. Med.* **137:**180–189.
66. Hagensee, M. E., N. Kiviat, C. W. Critchlow, S. E. Hawes, J. Kuypers, S. Holte, and D. A. Gal-loway. 1997. Seroprevalence of human papillomavirus types 6 and 16 capsid antibodies in homo-sexual men. *J. Infect. Dis.* **176:**625–631.
67. Hagensee, M. E., L. A. Koutsky, S. K. Lee, T. Grubert, J. Kuypers, N. B. Kiviat, and D. A. Gal-loway. 2000. Detection of cervical antibodies to human papillomavirus type 16 (HPV-16) capsid antigens in relation to detection of HPV-16 DNA and cervical lesions. *J. Infect. Dis.* **181:**1234–1239.
68. Handsfield, H. H., T. O. Lipman, J. P. Harnisch, E. Tronca, and K. K. Holmes. 1974. Asympto-matic gonorrhea in men. Diagnosis, natural course, prevalence and significance. *N. Engl. J. Med.* **290:**117–123.
69. Hart, G. 1974. Factors influencing venereal infection in a war environment. *Br. J. Vener. Dis.* **50:**68–72.
70. Hawkes, S., G. J. Hart, E. Bletsoe, C. Shergold, and A. M. Johnson. 1995. Risk behaviour and STD acquisition in genitourinary clinic attenders who have travelled. *Genitourin. Med.* **71:**351–354.
71. Hawkes, S., G. J. Hart, A. M. Johnson, C. Shergold, E. Ross, K. M. Herbert, P. Mortimer, J. V. Parry, and D. Mabey. 1994. Risk behaviour and HIV prevalence in international travellers. *AIDS* **8:**247–252.
72. Hillis, S. D., L. M. Owens, P. A. Marchbanks, L. F. Amsterdam, and W. R. Mac Kenzie. 1997. Re-current chlamydial infections increase the risks of hospitalization for ectopic pregnancy and pelvic inflammatory disease. *Am. J. Obstet. Gynecol.* **176:**103–107.
73. Hillis, S. D., and J. N. Wasserheit. 1996. Screening for chlamydia—a key to the prevention of pelvic inflammatory disease. *N. Engl. J. Med.* **334:**1399–1401.
74. Hiltunen-Back, E., T. Rostila, H. Kautiainen, J. Paavonen, and T. Reunala. 1998. Rapid decrease of endemic gonorrhea in Finland. *Sex. Transm. Dis.* **25:**181–186.
75. Holzman, C., J. M. Leventhal, H. Qiu, N. M. Jones, and J. Wang. 2001. Factors linked to bacterial vaginosis in nonpregnant women. *Am. J. Public Health* **91:**1664–1670.
76. Hook, E. W., III. 1989. Syphilis and HIV infection. *J. Infect. Dis.* **160:**530–534.
77. Hook, E. W., III, and K. K. Holmes. 1985. Gonococcal infections. *Ann. Intern. Med.* **102:**229–243.
78. Hook, E. W., III, and C. M. Marra. 1992. Acquired syphilis in adults. *N. Engl. J. Med.* **326:**1060–1069.

79. **Hopperus Buma, A. P., R. L. Veltink, E. J. van Ameijden, C. H. Tendeloo, and R. A. Coutinho.** 1995. Sexual behaviour and sexually transmitted diseases in Dutch marines and naval personnel on a United Nations mission in Cambodia. *Genitourin. Med.* **71:**172–175.

80. **Hutchinson, C. M., A. M. Rompalo, C. A. Reichart, and E. W. Hook III.** 1991. Characteristics of patients with syphilis attending Baltimore STD clinics. Multiple high-risk subgroups and interactions with human immunodeficiency virus infection. *Arch. Intern. Med.* **151:**511–516.

81. **Hutt, D. M., and F. N. Judson.** 1986. Epidemiology and treatment of oropharyngeal gonorrhea. *Ann. Intern. Med.* **104:**655–658.

82. **Jackson, D. J., J. P. Rakwar, B. Chohan, K. Mandaliya, J. J. Bwayo, J. O. Ndinya-Achola, N. J. Nagelkerke, J. K. Kreiss, and S. Moses.** 1997. Urethral infection in a workplace population of East African men: evaluation of strategies for screening and management. *J. Infect. Dis.* **175:**833–838.

83. **Jackson, D. J., J. P. Rakwar, B. A. Richardson, K. Mandaliya, B. H. Chohan, J. J. Bwayo, J. O. Ndinya-Achola, H. L. Martin, Jr., S. Moses, and J. K. Kreiss.** 1997. Decreased incidence of sexually transmitted diseases among trucking company workers in Kenya: results of a behavioural risk-reduction programme. *AIDS* **11:**903–909.

84. **Jaffe, H. W., J. W. Biddle, S. R. Johnson, and P. J. Wiesner.** 1981. Infections due to penicillinase-producing Neisseria gonorrhoeae in the United States: 1976–1980. *J. Infect. Dis.* **144:**191–197.

85. **Johnson, B. A., R. M. Poses, C. A. Fortner, F. A. Meier, and H. P. Dalton.** 1990. Derivation and validation of a clinical diagnostic model for chlamydial cervical infection in university women. *JAMA* **264:**3161–3165.

86. **Johnson, R. E., W. J. Newhall, J. R. Papp, J. S. Knapp, C. M. Black, T. L. Gift, R. Steece, L. E. Markowitz, O. J. Devine, C. M. Walsh, S. Wang, D. C. Gunter, K. L. Irwin, S. DeLisle, and S. M. Berman.** 2002. Screening tests to detect Chlamydia trachomatis and Neisseria gonorrhoeae infections—2002. *Morb. Mortal. Wkly. Rep.* **51**(RR-15):1–38.

87. **Johnson, R. E., T. A. Green, J. Schachter, R. B. Jones, E. W. Hook III, C. M. Black, D. H. Martin, M. E. St. Louis, and W. E. Stamm.** 2000. Evaluation of nucleic acid amplification tests as reference tests for *Chlamydia trachomatis* infections in asymptomatic men. *J. Clin. Microbiol.* **38:**4382–4386.

88. **Kahn, J. O., J. N. Martin, M. E. Roland, J. D. Bamberger, M. Chesney, D. Chambers, K. Franses, T. J. Coates, and M. H. Katz.** 2001. Feasibility of postexposure prophylaxis (PEP) against human immunodeficiency virus infection after sexual or injection drug use exposure: the San Francisco PEP Study. *J. Infect. Dis.* **183:**707–714.

89. **Kalichman, S. C., J. A. Kelly, K. J. Sikkema, A. P. Koslov, A. Shaboltas, and J. Granskaya.** 2000. The emerging AIDS crisis in Russia: review of enabling factors and prevention needs. *Int. J. STD AIDS* **11:**71–75.

90. **Kann, L., S. A. Kinchen, B. I. Williams, J. G. Ross, R. Lowry, C. V. Hill, J. A. Grunbaum, P. S. Blumson, J. L. Collins, and L. J. Kolbe.** 1998. Youth risk behavior surveillance—United States, 1997. *MMWR CDC Surveill. Summ.* **47:**1–89.

91. **Karpati, A., S. Galea, T. Awerbuch, and R. Levins.** 2002. Variability and vulnerability at the ecological level: implications for understanding the social determinants of health. *Am. J. Public Health* **92:**1768–1772.

92. **Kelley, P. W., R. N. Miller, R. Pomerantz, F. Wann, J. F. Brundage, and D. S. Burke.** 1990. Human immunodeficiency virus seropositivity among members of the active duty US Army 1985–89. *Am. J. Public Health* **80:**405–410.

93. **Kilmarx, P. H., K. Limpakarnjanarat, M. E. St. Louis, S. Supawitkul, S. Korattana, and T. D. Mastro.** 1997. Medication use by female sex workers for treatment and prevention of sexually transmitted diseases, Chiang Rai, Thailand. *Sex. Transm. Dis.* **24:**593–598.

94. **Kilmarx, P. H., K. Limpakarnjanarat, S. Supawitkul, S. Korattana, N. L. Young, B. S. Parekh, R. A. Respess, T. D. Mastro, and M. E. St. Louis.** 1998. Mucosal disruption due to use of a widely-distributed commercial vaginal product: potential to facilitate HIV transmission. *AIDS* **12:**767–773.

95. **Kilmarx, P. H., A. A. Zaidi, J. C. Thomas, A. K. Nakashima, M. E. St. Louis, M. L. Flock, and T. A. Peterman.** 1997. Sociodemographic factors and the variation in syphilis rates among US counties, 1984 through 1993: an ecological analysis. *Am. J. Public Health* **87:**1937–1943.

96. **Koumans, E. H., C. M. Black, L. E. Markowitz, E. Unger, A. Pierce, M. K. Sawyer, and J. R. Papp.** 2003. Comparison of methods for detection of Chlamydia trachomatis and Neisseria gonorrhoeae

using commercially available nucleic acid amplification tests and a liquid Pap smear medium. *J. Clin. Microbiol.* **41:**1507–1511.

97. Koutsky, L. 1997. Epidemiology of genital human papillomavirus infection. *Am. J. Med.* **102:**3–8.

98. Kral, A. H., R. N. Bluthenthal, J. Lorvick, L. Gee, P. Bacchetti, and B. R. Edlin. 2001. Sexual transmission of HIV-1 among injection drug users in San Francisco, USA: risk-factor analysis. *Lancet* **357:**1397–1401.

99. Lagarde, E., M. Schim van der Loeff, C. Enel, B. Holmgren, R. Dray-Spira, G. Pison, J. P. Piau, V. Delaunay, S. M'Boup, I. Ndoye, M. Coeuret-Pellicer, H. Whittle, P. Aaby, and the MECORA Group. 2003. Mobility and the spread of human immunodeficiency virus into rural areas of West Africa. *Int. J. Epidemiol.* **32:**744–752.

100. LaGuardia, K. D., M. H. White, P. E. Saigo, S. Hoda, K. McGuinness, and W. J. Ledger. 1995. Genital ulcer disease in women infected with human immunodeficiency virus. *Am. J. Obstet. Gynecol.* **172:**553–562.

101. Langenberg, A., J. Benedetti, J. Jenkins, R. Ashley, C. Winter, and L. Corey. 1989. Development of clinically recognizable genital lesions among women previously identified as having "asymptomatic" herpes simplex virus type 2 infection. *Ann. Intern. Med.* **110:**882–887.

102. Larsen, S. A., B. M. Steiner, and A. H. Rudolph. 1995. Laboratory diagnosis and interpretation of tests for syphilis. *Clin. Microbiol. Rev.* **8:**1–21.

103. Larson, A. 1989. Social context of human immunodeficiency virus transmission in Africa: historical and cultural bases of east and central African sexual relations. *Rev. Infect. Dis.* **11:**716–731.

104. Lau, J. T., A. S. Tang, and H. Y. Tsui. 2003. The relationship between condom use, sexually transmitted diseases, and location of commercial sex transaction among male Hong Kong clients. *AIDS* **17:**105–112.

105. Lau, J. T., and J. Thomas. 2001. Risk behaviours of Hong Kong male residents travelling to mainland China: a potential bridge population for HIV infection. *AIDS Care* **13:**71–81.

106. Lebedeff, D. A., and E. B. Hochman. 1980. Rectal gonorrhea in men: diagnosis and treatment. *Ann. Intern. Med.* **92:**463–466.

107. Malone, J. D., K. C. Hyams, R. E. Hawkins, T. W. Sharp, and F. D. Daniell. 1993. Risk factors for sexually-transmitted diseases among deployed U.S. military personnel. *Sex. Transm. Dis.* **20:**294–298.

108. Manhart, L. E., and L. A. Koutsky. 2002. Do condoms prevent genital HPV infection, external genital warts, or cervical neoplasia? A meta-analysis. *Sex. Transm. Dis.* **29:**725–735.

109. Marrazzo, J. M., L. A. Koutsky, D. A. Eschenbach, K. Agnew, K. Stine, and S. L. Hillier. 2002. Characterization of vaginal flora and bacterial vaginosis in women who have sex with women. *J. Infect. Dis.* **185:**1307–1313.

110. Mauck, C., Z. Rosenberg, and L. Van Damme. 2001. Recommendations for the clinical development of topical microbicides: an update. *AIDS* **15:**857–868.

111. McCormack, S. 2002. Vaginal microbicides. *Curr. Opin. Infect. Dis.* **15:**57–62.

112. McCormack, W. M. 1994. Pelvic inflammatory disease. *N. Engl. J. Med.* **330:**115–119.

113. McCormack, W. M., B. Rosner, D. E. McComb, J. R. Evrard, and S. H. Zinner. 1985. Infection with Chlamydia trachomatis in female college students. *Am. J. Epidemiol.* **121:**107–115.

114. McGregor, J. A., and J. I. French. 2000. Bacterial vaginosis in pregnancy. *Obstet. Gynecol. Surv.* **55:**S1–S19.

115. McKee, K. T., Jr., W. E. Burns, L. K. Russell, P. R. Jenkins, A. E. Johnson, T. L. Wong, and K. B. McLawhorn. 1998. Early syphilis in an active duty military population and the surrounding civilian community, 1985–1993. *Mil. Med.* **163:**368–376.

116. Meis, P. J., R. L. Goldenberg, B. Mercer, A. Moawad, A. Das, D. McNellis, F. Johnson, J. D. Iams, E. Thom, W. W. Andrews, and the National Institute of Child Health and Human Development Maternal-Fetal Medicine Units Network. 1995. The preterm prediction study: significance of vaginal infections. *Am. J. Obstet. Gynecol.* **173:**1231–1235.

117. Mertz, K. J., G. M. McQuillan, W. C. Levine, D. H. Candal, J. C. Bullard, R. E. Johnson, M. E. St. Louis, and C. M. Black. 1998. A pilot study of the prevalence of chlamydial infection in a national household survey. *Sex. Transm. Dis.* **25:**225–228.

118. Mertz, K. J., J. B. Weiss, R. M. Webb, W. C. Levine, J. S. Lewis, K. A. Orle, P. A. Totten, J. Overbaugh, S. A. Morse, M. M. Currier, M. Fishbein, and M. E. St. Louis. 1998. An investigation of

genital ulcers in Jackson, Mississippi, with use of a multiplex polymerase chain reaction assay: high prevalence of chancroid and human immunodeficiency virus infection. *J. Infect. Dis.* **178:** 1060–1066.

119. Minkoff, H. L., S. McCalla, I. Delke, R. Stevens, M. Salwen, and J. Feldman. 1990. The relationship of cocaine use to syphilis and human immunodeficiency virus infections among inner city parturient women. *Am. J. Obstet. Gynecol.* **163:**521–526.

120. Moore, J., C. Beeker, J. S. Harrison, T. R. Eng, and L. S. Doll. 1995. HIV risk behavior among Peace Corps volunteers. *AIDS* **9:**795–799.

121. Morris, M., A. Nicoll, I. Simms, J. Wilson, and M. Catchpole. 2001. Bacterial vaginosis: a public health review. *Br. J. Obstet. Gynaecol.* **108:**439–450.

122. Moses, S., E. Muia, J. E. Bradley, N. J. Nagelkerke, E. N. Ngugi, E. K. Njeru, G. Eldridge, J. Olenja, K. Wotton, F. A. Plummer, et al. 1994. Sexual behaviour in Kenya: implications for sexually transmitted disease transmission and control. *Soc. Sci. Med.* **39:**1649–1656.

123. Nelson, K. E., D. D. Celentano, S. Eiumtrakol, D. R. Hoover, C. Beyrer, S. Suprasert, S. Kuntolbutra, and C. Khamboonruang. 1996. Changes in sexual behavior and a decline in HIV infection among young men in Thailand. *N. Engl. J. Med.* **335:**297–303.

124. O'Brien, J. P., D. L. Goldenberg, and P. A. Rice. 1983. Disseminated gonococcal infection: a prospective analysis of 49 patients and a review of pathophysiology and immune mechanisms. *Medicine* (Baltimore) **62:**395–406.

125. Orle, K. A., C. A. Gates, D. H. Martin, B. A. Body, and J. B. Weiss. 1996. Simultaneous PCR detection of *Haemophilus ducreyi, Treponema pallidum,* and herpes simplex virus types 1 and 2 from genital ulcers. *J. Clin. Microbiol.* **34:**49–54.

126. Padian, N. S., T. R. O'Brien, Y. Chang, S. Glass, and D. P. Francis. 1993. Prevention of heterosexual transmission of human immunodeficiency virus through couple counseling. *J. Acquir. Immune. Defic. Syndr.* **6:**1043–1048.

127. Pauwels, R., and E. De Clercq. 1996. Development of vaginal microbicides for the prevention of heterosexual transmission of HIV. *J. Acquir. Immune. Defic. Syndr. Hum. Retrovirol.* **11:**211–221.

128. Peipert, J. F. 2003. Clinical practice. Genital chlamydial infections. *N. Engl. J. Med.* **349:**2424–2430.

129. Poulton, M., G. L. Dean, D. I. Williams, P. Carter, A. Iversen, and M. Fisher. 2001. Surfing with spirochaetes: an ongoing syphilis outbreak in Brighton. *Sex. Transm. Infect.* **77:**319–321.

130. Quinn, T. C., D. Glasser, R. O. Cannon, D. L. Matuszak, R. W. Dunning, R. L. Kline, C. H. Campbell, E. Israel, A. S. Fauci, and E. W. Hook III. 1988. Human immunodeficiency virus infection among patients attending clinics for sexually transmitted diseases. *N. Engl. J. Med.* **318:** 197–203.

131. Quinn, T. C., M. J. Wawer, N. Sewankambo, D. Serwadda, C. Li, F. Wabwire-Mangen, M. O. Meehan, T. Lutalo, R. H. Gray, and the Rakai Project Study Group. 2000. Viral load and heterosexual transmission of human immunodeficiency virus type 1. *N. Engl. J. Med.* **342:**921–929.

132. Renzullo, P. O., W. B. Sateren, R. P. Garner, M. J. Milazzo, D. L. Birx, and J. G. McNeil. 2001. HIV-1 seroconversion in United States Army active duty personnel, 1985–1999. *AIDS* **15:**1569–1574.

133. Reynolds, S. J., A. R. Risbud, M. E. Shepherd, J. M. Zenilman, R. S. Brookmeyer, R. S. Paranjape, A. D. Divekar, R. R. Gangakhedkar, M. V. Ghate, R. C. Bollinger, and S. M. Mehendale. 2003. Recent herpes simplex virus type 2 infection and the risk of human immunodeficiency virus type 1 acquisition in India. *J. Infect. Dis.* **187:**1513–1521.

134. Rice, P. A., and D. L. Goldenberg. 1981. Clinical manifestations of disseminated infection caused by Neisseria gonorrhoeae are linked to differences in bactericidal reactivity of infecting strains. *Ann. Intern. Med.* **95:**175–178.

135. Rolfs, R. T., M. Goldberg, and R. G. Sharrar. 1990. Risk factors for syphilis: cocaine use and prostitution. *Am. J. Public Health* **80:**853–857.

136. Rolfs, R. T., M. R. Joesoef, E. F. Hendershot, A. M. Rompalo, M. H. Augenbraun, M. Chiu, G. Bolan, S. C. Johnson, P. French, E. Steen, J. D. Radolf, S. Larsen, and The Syphilis and HIV Study Group. 1997. A randomized trial of enhanced therapy for early syphilis in patients with and without human immunodeficiency virus infection. *N. Engl. J. Med.* **337:**307–314.

137. Rompalo, A. M., J. Lawlor, P. Seaman, T. C. Quinn, J. M. Zenilman, and E. W. Hook III. 2001. Modification of syphilitic genital ulcer manifestations by coexistent HIV infection. *Sex. Transm. Dis.* **28:**448–454.

138. **Rompalo, A. M., C. B. Price, P. L. Roberts, and W. E. Stamm.** 1986. Potential value of rectal-screening cultures for Chlamydia trachomatis in homosexual men. *J. Infect. Dis.* **153:**888–892.

139. **Rompalo, A. M., R. J. Suchland, C. B. Price, and W. E. Stamm.** 1987. Rapid diagnosis of Chlamydia trachomatis rectal infection by direct immunofluorescence staining. *J. Infect. Dis.* **155:**1075–1076.

140. **Ross, J.** 2003. Pelvic inflammatory disease. *Clin. Evid.* **2003:**1770–1775.

141. **Ross, M. W., L. Y. Hwang, L. Leonard, M. Teng, and L. Duncan.** 1999. Sexual behaviour, STDs and drug use in a crack house population. *Int. J. STD AIDS* **10:**224–230.

142. **Rothenberg, R. B., J. J. Potterat, D. E. Woodhouse, S. Q. Muth, W. W. Darrow, and A. S. Klovdahl.** 1998. Social network dynamics and HIV transmission. *AIDS* **12:**1529–1536.

143. **Rothenberg, R. B., C. Sterk, K. E. Toomey, J. J. Potterat, D. Johnson, M. Schrader, and S. Hatch.** 1998. Using social network and ethnographic tools to evaluate syphilis transmission. *Sex. Transm. Dis.* **25:**154–160.

144. **Royce, R. A., A. Sena, W. Cates, Jr., and M. S. Cohen.** 1997. Sexual transmission of HIV. *N. Engl. J. Med.* **336:**1072–1078.

145. **Ruden, A. K., A. Jonsson, P. Lidbrink, P. Allebeck, and S. M. Bygdeman.** 1993. Endemic versus non-endemic gonorrhoea in Stockholm: results of contact tracing. *Int. J. STD AIDS* **4:**284–292.

146. **Scholes, D., A. Stergachis, F. E. Heidrich, H. Andrilla, K. K. Holmes, and W. E. Stamm.** 1996. Prevention of pelvic inflammatory disease by screening for cervical chlamydial infection. *N. Engl. J. Med.* **334:**1362–1366.

147. **Shafer, M. A., C. B. Boyer, R. A. Shaffer, J. Schachter, S. I. Ito, and S. K. Brodine.** 2002. Correlates of sexually transmitted diseases in a young male deployed military population. *Mil. Med.* **167:**496–500.

148. **Shafer, M. A., V. Prager, J. Shalwitz, E. Vaughan, B. Moscicki, R. Brown, C. Wibbelsman, and J. Schachter.** 1987. Prevalence of urethral Chlamydia trachomatis and Neisseria gonorrhoeae among asymptomatic, sexually active adolescent boys. *J. Infect. Dis.* **156:**223–224.

149. **Sherrard, J., and D. Barlow.** 1996. Gonorrhoea in men: clinical and diagnostic aspects. *Genitourin. Med.* **72:**422–426.

150. **Silver, H. M., R. S. Sperling, P. J. St. Clair, and R. S. Gibbs.** 1989. Evidence relating bacterial vaginosis to intraamniotic infection. *Am. J. Obstet. Gynecol.* **161:**808–812.

151. **Sobel, J. D.** 1997. Vaginitis. *N. Engl. J. Med.* **337:**1896–1903.

152. **Soper, D.** 2004. Trichomoniasis: under control or undercontrolled? *Am. J. Obstet. Gynecol.* **190:**281–290.

153. **Stamm, W. E., C. B. Hicks, D. H. Martin, P. Leone, E. W. Hook III, R. H. Cooper, M. S. Cohen, B. E. Batteiger, K. Workowski, and W. M. McCormack.** 1995. Azithromycin for empirical treatment of the nongonococcal urethritis syndrome in men. A randomized double-blind study. *JAMA* **274:**545–549.

154. **Stamm, W. E., L. A. Koutsky, J. K. Benedetti, J. L. Jourden, R. C. Brunham, and K. K. Holmes.** 1984. Chlamydia trachomatis urethral infections in men. Prevalence, risk factors, and clinical manifestations. *Ann. Intern. Med.* **100:**47–51.

155. **Su, X., and I. Lind.** 2001. Molecular basis of high-level ciprofloxacin resistance in *Neisseria gonorrhoeae* strains isolated in Denmark from 1995 to 1998. *Antimicrob. Agents Chemother.* **45:**117–123.

156. **Sucato, G., A. Wald, E. Wakabayashi, J. Vieira, and L. Corey.** 1998. Evidence of latency and reactivation of both herpes simplex virus (HSV)-1 and HSV-2 in the genital region. *J. Infect. Dis.* **177:**1069–1072.

157. **Tapsall, J. W.** 2000. Surveillance of antibiotic resistance in Neisseria gonorrhoeae in the WHO Western Pacific Region, 1998. The WHO Western Pacific Gonococcal Antimicrobial Surveillance Programme. *Commun. Dis. Intell.* **24:**1–4.

158. **Telzak, E. E., M. A. Chiasson, P. J. Bevier, R. L. Stoneburner, K. G. Castro, and H. W. Jaffe.** 1993. HIV-1 seroconversion in patients with and without genital ulcer disease. A prospective study. *Ann. Intern. Med.* **119:**1181–1186.

159. **Tichonova, L., K. Borisenko, H. Ward, A. Meheus, A. Gromyko, and A. Renton.** 1997. Epidemics of syphilis in the Russian Federation: trends, origins, and priorities for control. *Lancet* **350:**210–213.

160. **Tilzey, A. J., and J. E. Banatvala.** 2002. Protection from HIV on electives: questionnaire survey of UK medical schools. *BMJ* **325:**1010–1011.

161. Turner, C. F., S. M. Rogers, H. G. Miller, W. C. Miller, J. N. Gribble, J. R. Chromy, P. A. Leone, P. C. Cooley, T. C. Quinn, and J. M. Zenilman. 2002. Untreated gonococcal and chlamydial infection in a probability sample of adults. *JAMA* **287:**726–733.

162. Van Damme, L., G. Ramjee, M. Alary, B. Vuylsteke, V. Chandeying, H. Rees, P. Sirivongrangson, L. Mukenge-Tshibaka, V. Ettiegne-Traore, C. Uaheowitchai, S. S. Karim, B. Masse, J. Perriens, and M. Laga. 2002. Effectiveness of COL-1492, a nonoxynol-9 vaginal gel, on HIV-1 transmission in female sex workers: a randomised controlled trial. *Lancet* **360:**971–977.

163. Wald, A., and L. Corey. 2003. How does herpes simplex virus type 2 influence human immunodeficiency virus infection and pathogenesis? *J. Infect. Dis.* **187:**1509–1512.

164. Wald, A., A. G. Langenberg, K. Link, A. E. Izu, R. Ashley, T. Warren, S. Tyring, J. M. Douglas, Jr., and L. Corey. 2001. Effect of condoms on reducing the transmission of herpes simplex virus type 2 from men to women. *JAMA* **285:**3100–3106.

165. Wald, A., and K. Link. 2002. Risk of human immunodeficiency virus infection in herpes simplex virus type 2-seropositive persons: a meta-analysis. *J. Infect. Dis.* **185:**45–52.

166. Wald, A., J. Zeh, S. Selke, R. L. Ashley, and L. Corey. 1995. Virologic characteristics of subclinical and symptomatic genital herpes infections. *N. Engl. J. Med.* **333:**770–775.

167. Wald, A., J. Zeh, S. Selke, T. Warren, A. J. Ryncarz, R. Ashley, J. N. Krieger, and L. Corey. 2000. Reactivation of genital herpes simplex virus type 2 infection in asymptomatic seropositive persons. *N. Engl. J. Med.* **342:**844–850.

168. Warner, L., D. R. Newman, H. D. Austin, M. L. Kamb, J. M. Douglas, Jr., C. K. Malotte, J. M. Zenilman, J. Rogers, G. Bolan, M. Fishbein, D. G. Kleinbaum, M. Macaluso, and T. A. Peterman. 2004. Condom effectiveness for reducing transmission of gonorrhea and Chlamydia: the importance of assessing partner infection status. *Am. J. Epidemiol.* **159:**242–251.

169. Wasserheit, J. N. 1987. Pelvic inflammatory disease and infertility. *Md. Med. J.* **36:**58–63.

170. Wasserheit, J. N. 1992. Epidemiological synergy. Interrelationships between human immunodeficiency virus infection and other sexually transmitted diseases. *Sex. Transm. Dis.* **19:**61–77.

171. Wasserheit, J. N., and S. O. Aral. 1996. The dynamic topology of sexually transmitted disease epidemics: implications for prevention strategies. *J. Infect. Dis.* **174**(Suppl. 2):S201–S213.

172. Wechsler, H., A. Davenport, G. Dowdall, B. Moeykens, and S. Castillo. 1994. Health and behavioral consequences of binge drinking in college. A national survey of students at 140 campuses. *JAMA* **272:**1672–1677.

173. Weinstock, H., S. Berman, and W. Cates, Jr. 2004. Sexually transmitted diseases among American youth: incidence and prevalence estimates, 2000. *Perspect. Sex Reprod. Health* **36:**6–10.

174. Weller, S., and K. Davis. 2002. Condom effectiveness in reducing heterosexual HIV transmission. *Cochrane Database Syst. Rev.* CD003255. [Online.]

175. Wendel, K. A. 2003. Trichomoniasis: what's new? *Curr. Infect. Dis. Rep.* **5:**129–134.

176. Westrom, L. 1975. Effect of acute pelvic inflammatory disease on fertility. *Am. J. Obstet. Gynecol.* **121:**707–713.

177. Westrom, L., R. Joesoef, G. Reynolds, A. Hagdu, and S. E. Thompson. 1992. Pelvic inflammatory disease and fertility. A cohort study of 1,844 women with laparoscopically verified disease and 657 control women with normal laparoscopic results. *Sex. Transm. Dis.* **19:**185–192.

178. Wiesner, P. J., E. Tronca, P. Bonin, A. H. Pedersen, and K. K. Holmes. 1973. Clinical spectrum of pharyngeal gonococcal infection. *N. Engl. J. Med.* **288:**181–185.

179. Xi, L. F., J. J. Carter, D. A. Galloway, J. Kuypers, J. P. Hughes, S. K. Lee, D. E. Adam, N. B. Kiviat, and L. A. Koutsky. 2002. Acquisition and natural history of human papillomavirus type 16 variant infection among a cohort of female university students. *Cancer Epidemiol. Biomark. Prev.* **11:**343–351.

180. Xu, F., J. A. Schillinger, M. R. Sternberg, R. E. Johnson, F. K. Lee, A. J. Nahmias, and L. E. Markowitz. 2002. Seroprevalence and coinfection with herpes simplex virus type 1 and type 2 in the United States, 1988–1994. *J. Infect. Dis.* **185:**1019–1024.

181. Zenilman, J. M., G. Glass, T. Shields, P. R. Jenkins, J. C. Gaydos, and K. T. McKee, Jr. 2002. Geographic epidemiology of gonorrhoea and chlamydia on a large military installation: application of a GIS system. *Sex. Transm. Infect.* **78:**40–44.

Infections of Leisure, Third Edition
Edited by David Schlossberg
© 2004 ASM Press, Washington, D.C.

Chapter 15

Infections from Body Piercing and Tattoos

Mukesh Patel and C. Glenn Cobbs

It appears that there has been an increase in the prevalence of body piercing and tattooing in the Western world in recent years. Temporary tattoos and body jewelry (without actual piercing) are popular decorative items for children. The term "body modification" has been used to describe procedures that "enhance" appearance, whether permanent or temporary, and also includes scarification, branding, and surgical modifications. An effect of the increased interest in tattoos and body piercing has been the development of standardized protocols of infection control to protect the client and the person performing the tattooing or piercing. Unfortunately, a significant number of tattoos and body piercings are still performed by personnel who do not follow the appropriate precautions. The purpose of this chapter is to summarize reports of tattoo- and body piercing-associated infections. We reviewed the English-language medical literature and a limited number of available foreign-language articles published from 1966 to the present via MEDLINE for articles that described an infectious process related to tattooing or body piercing. Articles predating MEDLINE were identified from more recent literature. In addition, we searched the Internet for related sites as well as books published on the topics of body piercing and tattooing.

TATTOOING

History

Tattooing has been performed since antiquity by numerous indigenous cultures throughout the world. Individual expression, decoration, storytelling, identification within a specific social group, and rites of passage are common reasons people have sought tattoos. More recently, tattooing has become a technique for application of permanent forms of makeup. An apparent increase in the popularity of tattoos in western cultures has been described since the 18th century, with members of the military and prison inmates commonly decorated with tattoos (32).

Mukesh Patel and C. Glenn Cobbs • Division of Infectious Diseases, University of Alabama at Birmingham, THT 229, 1530 3rd Ave. S., Birmingham, AL 35294-0006.

However, tattoos were also fashionable among high-society circles; Lady Randolph Churchill, Winston Churchill's mother, started a trend for tattooing among her peers in the late 19th century (62). It is estimated that more than 20 million people have tattoos in the United States alone (6). Tattoos are especially popular among adolescents and college students, with estimates of prevalence ranging from 13 to 23% (10, 36). Though the arms, legs, and back are most commonly decorated, virtually any part of the body may be tattooed, including the palms and soles, eyelids, face, genitals, and tongue.

Techniques

The tools of tattooing have changed over time, though the basic application techniques remain very similar. Pigment is deposited to a depth of 1 to 2 mm into the dermis with various devices. Traditional techniques involve using a sharp instrument to cut the surface of the skin, with the pigment pressed into the wound. Burning the skin followed by rubbing pigment into the wound is a less commonly used technique. Traditional Samoan tattooing remains popular and is performed with a sharpened, serrated bone or shark's tooth attached to the end of a long stick. The cutting edge is covered in ink, and the stick is tapped to create a shallow incision in the skin into which the ink is deposited (38). Tattoo dye or ink may be made from any number of pigmented substances, including ashes, oils, or synthetic dyes. Modern techniques of tattooing accomplish the same goal but with the aid of a motorized tattoo machine which allows a less painful and more controlled application of ink. However, some people prefer "homemade" or "prison" techniques using any available needle and ink. Others create their own tattoo machines from small motors obtained from household appliances. As the skin is punctured, minor bleeding accompanies application of the tattoo, and generally the fresh tattoo should remain covered with a bandage until the bleeding resolves.

Infectious Complications

Infectious disorders occurring after tattooing may be classified by the source of the infectious agent. Those due to endogenous agents represent diseases caused by normal flora following disruption of the skin's normal barriers. Infections associated with endogenous microorganisms are not completely preventable, although the use of the appropriate sterile techniques during tattoo application and proper aftercare of the new tattoo may serve to minimize the risk. Infections due to exogenous agents are due to inoculation of a microbe at the time of tattoo application and should also be preventable if hygienic techniques are followed. Viral hepatitis, tuberculosis, syphilis, and human immunodeficiency virus (HIV) disease are examples of infections following inoculation from an exogenous source.

Infectious Disorders due to Endogenous Flora

Streptococci and staphylococci are the most common bacterial causes of local infection and may cause cellulitis, impetigo, erysipelas, or furunculosis (32). More invasive syndromes including bacteremic illness may follow these disorders. Prevention of local infection involves proper sterilization of the equipment as well as aftercare of the tattoo.

Disseminated endogenous infection following tattooing has occurred, caused by both bacteria and fungi. Bacteremia typically complicates cellulitis. Polymicrobial sepsis with *Pseudomonas aeruginosa* and *Streptococcus pyogenes* (31) and *Staphylococcus aureus* epidural abscess (15) have been reported following tattooing. *S. aureus* aortic valve endocarditis following repeated tattooing occurred in a patient with a bicuspid aortic valve (52). *Candida albicans* endophthalmitis has been described for an asplenic individual with a recent tattoo application that required surgical drainage of the infected eye and long-term antifungal therapy with amphotericin B and fluconazole (3). There was no apparent local wound disease. Finally, tetanus has followed tattooing in Maori individuals in New Zealand (56) as well as in persons in the United States (11, 12). Of course, the risk of tetanus is inversely proportional to the level of anti-tetanus toxin antibody associated with prior immunization.

Infectious Disorders due to Exogenous Infections

Viral Hepatitis

Among the exogenously acquired diseases associated with tattoos, viral hepatitis has probably been best documented. The earliest reported outbreaks of acute hepatitis following tattooing occurred in military personnel who had received their tattoos at the same parlor (in which hygienic techniques were not employed) (55). Both hepatitis B virus (HBV) and HCV can be transmitted by transfusion of contaminated blood products, intravenous drug use (IVDU), and occupational needlestick injuries. HBV and HCV may both be transmitted sexually as well, though that route much more efficiently transmits HBV than HCV. Intranasal cocaine use is a risk factor for HCV infection. The risk of HBV transmission following needlestick with a hollow-bore needle is estimated to be between 2 and 40%, and risk of HCV transmission is estimated to be between 3 and 10% (22).

During the last 50 years, numerous common-source outbreaks of acute hepatitis have been associated with recent tattooing (cited in reference 32). In some instances, the person applying the tattoo had an illness with jaundice in the months preceding the outbreaks. Patients developed acute hepatitis when contaminated needles were reused, inadequate techniques were employed to sterilize needles or dye, or an infected tattoo artist tested the needle on himself before using it on a client. Earlier cases of hepatitis were mostly likely due to HBV, though HCV could have been implicated in some.

Nishioka and Gyorkos (41) have summarized a number of studies that evaluated the association between tattooing and seropositivity for viral hepatitides. Despite accounting for confounding variables in these studies, there was no consensus on the association between receiving a tattoo and chronic HBV or HCV infection. A recent study in the United States did not find tattoos to be a statistically significant risk factor for chronic viral hepatitis (HBV and HCV) when comparing tattooed emergency room patients to matched controls (53). Other risk factors for acquisition of viral hepatitis were noted for almost all of the individuals who had chronic viral hepatitis (e.g., body piercing, multiple sexual partners, and IVDU).

HIV

Concern about tattoo-associated HIV transmission is occasioned by the known risks of transmitting HIV by needlestick injury. Though the risk of transmitting HIV is relatively low for a single needle puncture (approximately 0.1%) (22), repeated punctures as utilized during application of a tattoo may increase the risk. Epidemiological studies suggest that tattoo application is a risk factor for acquiring HIV in some prison populations (9, 20) and in military personnel who travel to high-prevalence countries (43). In contrast, a study of HIV infection of prisoners in Canada did not find tattooing to be a risk factor for HIV infection (18). Therefore, although a substantial number of well-documented cases of HIV transmission following tattooing are lacking, at least one report has been published. In that instance, possible HIV transmission was reported for two prisoners who denied other risk factors (IVDU, sex with other men, or prior blood transfusions) but who had extensive tattooing with a needle used to apply tattoos on other prisoners (D. C. Doll, Letter, *Lancet* **i:**66–67, 1988). Both were found to be positive for HIV during incarceration, presumably with prior documented negative HIV tests. Of course, the potential risk of HIV transmission via tattooing may be much higher in regions of the world where HIV prevalence is itself significantly greater. Genital tattooing is practiced by some cultural groups in central and west Africa and has been considered a possible mode of HIV transmission through reuse of tattoo needles (27). Clearly, a theoretical risk for transmitting HIV exists and should be considered by those who wish to have tattoos applied outside of a "professional" setting.

Tuberculosis

Tuberculous cellulitis following cutaneous inoculation of *Mycobacterium tuberculosis* has been well described for many years. Historically, morticians and physicians who performed postmortem examinations on patients who died with active tuberculosis were prone to "prosector's wart"—cutaneous tuberculosis at the site of a skin injury with instruments contaminated by *M. tuberculosis*. Similarly, inoculation tuberculosis following application of a tattoo has been documented since the late 19th century. In one instance, a child with pulmonary tuberculosis used ink mixed with his saliva and tattooed three friends who subsequently developed pustules, local adenopathy, and giant cells as determined by skin biopsy at the site of the tattoos (16). Another report describes the development of presumed tuberculosis in a fresh tattoo contaminated by cow's milk that may have come from an infected cow. The use of nonhygienic techniques by modern standards was apparently commonplace at the time of the reported infections of inoculation tuberculosis (26, 32).

Syphilis

Both primary syphilis and secondary syphilis have been reported for patients following tattoo application. Syphilis is most commonly a sexually transmitted infection caused by the spirochete *Treponema pallidum*. It is spread person to person by infected body fluids, including semen, vaginal secretions, saliva, and blood.

Less commonly, kissing or other close contact with an active syphilitic lesion or direct inoculation may transmit infection. Primary syphilis is the first stage of infection, with the development of a painless papule at the site of inoculation occurring approximately 3 weeks after exposure. This lesion erodes and becomes indurated, forming the classic chancre. Chancres are usually encountered on or near the genitals, but they can appear almost anywhere depending on the site of inoculation. The chancre contains spirochetes and is infectious. Two to eight weeks after appearance of a chancre, bacteremic dissemination of spirochetes may lead to secondary syphilis, a generalized illness with diffuse skin lesions and systemic symptoms and signs. The rash can be macular, papular, pustular, or a combination of lesions. Any organ system may be involved, leading to the protean manifestations of secondary syphilis. If untreated, the rash will resolve over days to weeks, with potential for relapses. Chronic inflammation in an affected organ can lead to symptoms of tertiary syphilis (cardiovascular, neurological, and gumma late disease).

Primary syphilis at the site of a recently applied tattoo was described in the medical literature as early as 1853 (28) and subsequently reported by others (cited in reference 32). In the described cases, the tattoo artist had oral mucous patches thought to be chancres and used saliva to rewet the needle or ink, or saliva was applied directly to the tattoo site. Chancres formed within the newly applied tattoo. The lesions of secondary syphilis may localize within recently applied tattoos and may be due to chronic inflammation and decreased immune responses within the tattoo (50). Interestingly, rashes of secondary syphilis have been noted to preferentially affect portions of some tattoos, with higher concentrations of skin lesions in areas with blue ink and absent in areas with red pigment. This preference for blue-pigmented tattoos is due to the use of red cinnabar, or mercuric sulfide, in older formulations of red inks. Mercury compounds have been recognized to possess antiluetic activity for centuries and appear to prevent localization of disseminated treponemal disease in the red-pigmented areas, while the blue-pigmented areas are susceptible to the appearance of the rash of secondary syphilis.

Other Infections

Transmission of papillomavirus from contaminated ink or needles has resulted in the growth of warts within recently applied tattoos (32). Vaccinia has also been reported to occur near a recently applied tattoo and may have represented inoculation of virus (65). Tattoo-related fungal infections have also been reported. Sporotrichosis, typically a lymphocutaneous infection caused by the fungus *Sporothrix schenckii*, has been described to cause infection starting at the site of a tattoo recently applied using traditional Samoan techniques (14). The infection was likely due to inoculation of the skin with *S. schenckii* at the time of tattooing, and cutaneous nodules persisted for 6 years until definitively treated with itraconazole. Invasive mold disease with members of the zygomycete family usually occurs in immunocompromised individuals but also can occur in others. A subcutaneous infection with *Saksenaea vasiformis* at the site of a tattoo applied 7 years previously has been described to occur in an immunocompetent individual (46), though it is unclear if the mold infection was inoculated at the time of tattoo application or more recently acquired.

BODY PIERCING

Body piercing has gained popularity recently in developed countries but has been performed in primitive cultures for thousands of years, often as a rite of passage or associated with religious ceremonies. Piercing of the male genitals was described in the 4th-century Indian text the *Kama Sutra:* "In southern countries, the penis is pierced during childhood, just as one pierces the ears" (63). "Purists" of body piercing often do not consider earlobe piercings as true "body piercings" and prefer to consider piercings of the face, navel, nipples, and genitals to be true body piercings. More recently, "surface piercings," where jewelry is embedded in almost any surface of the body (especially the chest, neck, or arms), and implanting of jewelry or prosthetic material into the subcutaneous tissue have become popular. However, we were unable to find reports of infectious complications from these procedures. Since medical complications may involve any body piercing, for purposes of this discussion we define body piercing as Samantha et al. (51) do: "the use of needles, rings, steel posts, or other adornments that penetrate the skin and other structures of the human body." We include earlobe piercings in this definition.

Body Piercing Techniques

Specific techniques of body piercing vary depending on the site of the piercing but are generally similar. Most piercings are accomplished using a sharp, hollow needle designed for this purpose. The site to be pierced is usually held in place by a surgical clamp (Pennington or Foerster clamp) through which the needle is pushed by hand into a cork or rubber stopper. The needle is typically 14 or 16 gauge (though larger sizes are available) and is made of stainless steel. An open end of the jewelry is introduced into the rear blunt end of the piercing needle and pulled through the opening made by the needle.

Modern body jewelry implanted during piercing is fabricated of stainless steel, titanium, gold, niobium, or acrylic. Nickel-containing alloys are not recommended due to the risk of hypersensitivity. Frequently a barbell shaped device with two threaded beads at the ends or an open loop closed with a bead is used as the initial choice of jewelry. However, many styles of jewelry exist, with unique shapes being used with increasing frequency. Traditional jewelry used by cultures in developing countries in which body piercing is common includes items made of bone, wood, metal, shells, or feather quills.

General Infectious Complications

The risk of infection itself and the precise types of infectious disorders that follow body piercing depend upon the site of the piercing, extent of hygienic techniques utilized during the procedure, experience of the person performing the piercing, and aftercare of the pierced site. Healing time, generally a function of blood supply and tissue integrity, varies greatly with body location and is an important factor in the risk of infection. As with tattooing, infections associated with body piercing may be generally classified as either endogenous or exogenous depending on the suspected source of infection. Local inflammatory reactions must be distinguished from early local infections and may be due to direct mechanical irritation, allergic reactions to the metal, or granulomatous foreign-body reactions. Local cellulitis at the site of new piercings is the most common infectious complication, with an overall estimated prevalence ranging from 10 to 30% (23, 57). The most common sites where local infections have been described to occur include the navel, ear, nose, and nipple. Less commonly, piercings of the tongue, genitals, and other sites appear to be complicated by infectious disorders. Cellulitis, characterized by redness, swelling, pain, and purulent drainage from the piercing site, is most commonly caused by *S. aureus*, group A streptococci, and aerobic gram-negative bacilli, particularly *Pseudomonas* species. Table 1 summarizes the infectious disorders associated with body piercing.

Endogenously Acquired Infectious Complications by Site of Piercing

Ears

The ear remains the most commonly pierced site; as many as 80 to 90% of women in North America have at least one ear piercing (8, 54). In addition, a growing number of men have had their ears pierced. In addition to the earlobe, the cartilaginous portions of the ear, including the tragus, antitragus, helix, and antihelix, may be pierced. Techniques of ear piercing include use of a piercing "gun," which uses pressure to push the earring post through the earlobe, and use of a needle in the earlobe or cartilage to create a hole through which jewelry is placed. Piercing guns are apparently difficult to thoroughly disinfect. Local infections of the earlobe are most commonly caused by *S. aureus* and group A streptococci (39). Cellulitis and erysipelas at ear piercing sites have been well recognized since the 19th century (58). Chondritis following piercing of the cartilaginous portions of the ear is most commonly due to *Pseudomonas* species (21, 39, 61). The decreased vascularity of cartilage compared to the earlobe increases the risk of bacterial infection at that location (39, 61).

Cellulitis may occasionally be complicated by bacteremia. Lovejoy and Smith described the occurrence of severe disseminated *S. aureus* infection in three

Table 1. Overview of infectious complications of body piercing[a]

Site	Infectious complication(s)	Associated pathogens
General	Local infections, cellulitis, hepatitis, HIV	Staphylococci, streptococci, HBV, HCV
Ear	Chondritis, bacteremia, hepatic abscess, meningitis, osteomyelitis, toxic shock syndrome, glomerulonephritis, IE, tetanus, tuberculosis	*S. aureus*, group A streptococci, *Pseudomonas* species
Tongue	Glossitis, abscess, Ludwig's angina, Lemierre's syndrome, cerebellar abscess, IE, tetanus, warts	Oral flora, *H. aphrophilus*, *N. mucosa*, *S. aureus*, papillomavirus
Nose	IE	*S. aureus*
Nipple	Mastitis, IE, infected prosthetic breast implants	Staphylococci, streptococci, *M. abscessus*
Navel	Cellulitis, IE, tetanus	*S. aureus*
Genital	Warts, sexually transmitted infections	Papillomavirus

[a]See text for references.

children with recent earlobe piercings (two patients) or subacutely infected earlobe piercing sites (one patient): one case of bacteremia was complicated by hepatic abscesses, another case of bacteremia was complicated by osteomyelitis, and a third case of bacteremia was complicated by meningitis (33). Toxin-associated disease following ear piercing was described by Ahmed-Jushuf et al. (1), who reported poststreptococcal glomerulonephritis occurring in a boy who had recently pierced his own ear and developed group A streptococcal infection of the earlobe, and by McCarthy and Peoples (37), who reported toxic shock syndrome following earlobe piercing. In addition, tetanus has been noted following ear piercing (34, cited in reference 58). Finally, an unusual *Streptococcus viridans* aortic valve endocarditis complicated by a Gerbode ventricular septal defect may have been associated with recent ear piercing in an otherwise healthy 15-year-old boy (7).

Oral Piercings

Infections following oral soft tissue piercings have a broad variety of microbiological etiologies possible due to the many commensal organisms in the oral cavity. Oral piercing sites include the tongue, lip, cheek, and, rarely, the uvula. Distant infectious complications have been most frequently described with tongue piercings.

Tongue. Tongue piercings may be horizontal or vertical through the tongue or through the frenulum beneath the tongue. Despite the rich microbiological environment of the mouth, infections of tongue piercings remain uncommon, probably due to the rich vascularity of the tongue and the relatively rapid healing time for tongue injuries. Local inflammation following piercing is expected, with significant swelling and tenderness of the tongue, but this usually resolves in a few days to several weeks. Most tongue infections can be prevented with appropriate aftercare, usually involving regular use of antiseptic mouthwash during the initial healing period. Persistent swelling, tenderness, and pain may indicate glossitis, a local soft tissue infection of the tongue. If severe, glossitis requires removal of the jewelry and systemic antibiotics.

Development of a lingual abscess requiring surgical drainage has been reported to occur in an adolescent who attempted to pierce his tongue (44). Ludwig's angina, a rapidly spreading cellulitis involving the submandibular and sublingual spaces, has also been reported to occur 4 days after placement of a tongue piercing (47). A single case of postanginal septicemia, or Lemierre's disease, following tongue piercing has also been described (http://www.bmezine.com/risks/index.html). Lemierre's disease is a severe oropharyngeal infection caused by *Fusobacterium necrophorum* which may lead to internal jugular vein thrombosis and metastatic spread of infection to the lung, liver, joints, and other sites.

Bacteremia following tongue piercing may result in metastatic disease. A cerebellar abscess in a previously healthy woman who had a tongue piercing 4 weeks earlier has been reported (35). After the piercing, the patient appears to have had a self-limiting infection at the site, with purulent discharge. The patient's illness was characterized by headache, nausea, vomiting, and vertigo, and it required surgical drainage and long-term antimicrobial therapy. Cultures of the abscess revealed a polymicrobial infection with *S. viridans, Peptostreptococcus micros, Actinomyces* species, and *Eikenella corrodens*. The bacteria cultured were consistent with an oral source of infection, and no other infectious sources or predispositions could be found in this patient.

Infective endocarditis (IE) associated with tongue piercing has been reported for three individuals: *S. aureus* mitral valve IE occurred in a previously healthy woman 3 days after she replaced her tongue jewelry with (apparently) contaminated jewelry (24), *Neisseria mucosa* mitral valve IE occurred in a woman who had a tongue piercing 2 weeks prior to the development of systemic symptoms (59), and *Haemophilus aphrophilus* aortic valve IE occurred in a 25-year-old man with corrected congenital aortic stenosis whose tongue piercing was done 2 months earlier (2).

A single case of cephalic tetanus associated with tongue piercing has been described, manifesting as jaw pain, trismus, dysarthria, and flu-like symptoms (19).

Other Facial Piercings

Eyebrow, "antieyebrow" (piercings lateral to the eye or on the upper cheek below the eye), bridge, and nasal piercings are also common. Nasal piercing sites include the nostril or septum. In one reported complication of nasal piercing, *S. aureus* mitral valve IE occurred in a 14-year-old girl without known prior cardiac abnormalities (49). Nasal carriage of *S. aureus* was confirmed by culture and was the possible source of infection.

Nipples

Cellulitis may extend more deeply and has been noted to cause mastitis in both men and women after nipple piercing. Mastitis cases following nipple piercing and due to coagulase-negative staphylococci, group B streptococci, and microaerophilic staphylococci have been described (29). Mastitis following nipple piercing has been associated with the development of *Staphylococcus epidermidis* aortic valve IE in a 24-year-old man with a bicuspid aortic valve and corrected aortic coarctation (42). Also, a case of *Mycobacterium abscessus* mastitis presented as a tender breast mass in a 17-year-old girl with a prior nipple piercing (60). An unusual complication of nipple piercing is breast implant infection following local infection at the piercing site. Implant infection has been reported for both a female patient with silicone breast implants (30) and a male patient with solid pectoral implants who developed group A beta-hemolytic streptococcus infection after nipple piercing (17).

Navel

The navel is probably the most common site of body piercing after the ear. It is also the most likely body piercing site to experience a prolonged healing time (several months) and to be associated with infectious complications (57). Navel piercings may be placed through the subcutaneous tissue on any side of the navel. It should never include the umbilical remnant, which is more obvious in people with extroverted navels, as complications at this site may lead to intra-abdominal infectious disease. Prolonged healing at the navel is usually due to the presence of tight clothing irritating the pierced tissue and the presence of a persistent moist environment. There are few reports describing the precise bacterial etiology of cellulitis complicating navel piercing, but one may assume that staphylococci and streptococci are frequently implicated. A serious complication of navel piercing occurred in a 13-year-old girl with corrected D-transposition of the great arteries who developed *S. aureus* IE after she pierced her own navel (64). The patient did not take prophylactic antibiotics before the piercing, and a self-limiting local infection reportedly developed 2 days after the piercing, followed in 1 month by symptoms of IE. Tetanus has been reported to occur in a 27-year-old woman with remote history of tetanus vaccination who performed a navel piercing on herself and developed facial pain and trismus 10 days later (45).

Genital Piercings

Anatomical sites for male and female genital piercings are extremely diverse, and no part of the genitalia has been spared (5). "Traditional" male genital piercings include the Prince Albert piercing (a ring passes through the urethra and ventral surface of the penis), dydoe (piercing the coronal ridge of the glans), ampallang (horizontal bar through the glans), apadravya (vertical piercing through the glans), hafada (lateral scrotal tissue), guiche (piercing the tissue between the scrotum and anus), frenulum piercing, and foreskin piercing.

"Traditional" female genital piercings include piercing the labia majora or minora, clitoris, and clitoral hood and fourchette (a female version of the guiche piercing). As with other piercings, the popularity of body piercings has spawned numerous other variations on the traditional piercings (see http://www.bmezine.com for a thorough review).

Infectious complications appear to usually reflect the local flora of the perineum or acquisition of disease through sexual activity. Aerobic gram-negative bacilli, such as *Escherichia coli,* and other enteric bacteria that are common causes of genitourinary infections are also likely causes of genital piercing infections in addition to skin flora bacteria.

Recurrent genital warts have been noted at the site of a new penile frenulum piercing (4). The recent piercing caused local tissue damage that may have predisposed the patient to the recurrent papillomavirus infection.

Exogenously Acquired Diseases Associated with Body Piercing

Many studies have attempted to define the relationship between ear piercing and viral hepatitis, with the general consensus that ear piercing (and body piercing) is a risk factor for the spread of hepatitis B and C if aseptic techniques are not followed (25), and if the equipment used is contaminated by blood from prior infected clients.

Infection of the piercing recipient by HIV has been postulated but not well documented. A single case is described of a male with multiple documented seronegative tests for HIV antibody who subsequently seroconverted (48). During the year prior to seroconversion, he had multiple body piercings performed in several different countries. He also had three male sexual partners but did not report high-risk sexual activity. Certainly, it is possible that the patient acquired HIV during a body piercing procedure, though it is difficult to prove. Regardless, the possibility of HIV transmission exists if contaminated needles are reused.

Inoculation of infectious agents at the time of piercing or during the healing period has also been reported to cause disease. Primary tuberculosis of the earlobe has been reported for an infant following ear piercing by her mother, who had active pulmonary tuberculosis and may have moistened the piercing needle with her saliva (40). Growth of warts due to human papillomavirus at the site of new tongue piercing has been described, particularly following unprotected oral sex with a partner with genital warts (http://www.bmezine.com/risks/index.html). Piercing-associated warts usually do not resolve spontaneously and may require excision.

Sexually transmitted diseases are of particular concern in individuals with genital piercings. Unprotected sex with an unhealed piercing poses increased risk of transmission of many sexually transmitted diseases, including HIV, herpes simplex, syphilis, and gonorrhea. Even after a piercing is healed, it may cause mechanical irritation to mucous membranes and decrease the local barriers to transmission of viruses or bacteria.

PREVENTION AND AFTERCARE OF TATTOOS AND PIERCINGS

Prevention of infectious complications following tattooing or body piercing begins with the person performing the procedure. In recent years, most states in the United States, as well as many Western countries, have developed specific legislation that requires tattoo and piercing parlors to follow strict hygiene and infection control policies. Usually local public health departments (county and state) are responsible for ensuring that safe and sanitary practices are followed. In addition, professional piercing and tattooing associations have had some self-regulated infection control practices within their own industry. Generally, state laws mandate use of single-use needles, sterilization of nondisposable equipment, needles, and jewelry prior to use, and appropriate environmental disinfection guidelines. Piercing guns are not recommended, nor are home piercing kits. Persons not experienced in the appropriate tattooing or body piercing techniques, or using equipment and jewelry that has not been properly sterilized, should not perform tattooing or body piercing. Professional establishments should provide appropriate aftercare instructions depending on the site of the piercing. For persons with genital piercings, sexual activity should be avoided during the healing period. The Association of Professional Piercers (http://www.safepiercing.org) provides general aftercare recommendations and precautions for different body piercings.

TREATMENT OF INFECTIONS ASSOCIATED WITH TATTOOING AND BODY PIERCING

Most cases of local infection following body piercing may be managed with local care (mild antiseptics or irrigation with saline solution). Removal of jewelry is not advocated if a local infection occurs, as it may result in a loculated infection in the pierced tract. Rather, the jewelry maintains a patent drainage site aiding in healing of the infection. If the infection progresses, however, removal of the jewelry may be necessary, especially if a loculated abscess is already present, which would require irrigation and debridement. Systemic antibiotics may be indicated for local infections that do not resolve or for complicated infections. Antibiotic choices should take into account the role of the local flora at a specific piercing site.

Infected oral piercings should be treated with antimicrobials with broad aerobic and anaerobic coverage. Genital piercings are predisposed to infections caused by aerobic gram-negative bacilli, especially the *Enterobacteriaceae*, as well as anaerobes, staphylococci, and streptococci. Antipseudomonal antimicrobials should be considered for treatment of auricular chondritis. All body piercing-associated infections should have adequate antimicrobial coverage for staphylococci and streptococci. For complicated infections (metastatic infection, bacteremia, and deep abscesses), blood cultures should be performed, and in the case of abscesses, operative cultures at the time of drainage should be performed to guide antimicrobial therapy.

An experienced tattoo artist should generally evaluate local infection of a recently applied tattoo. Topical antibiotic preparations are discouraged. If cellulitis or metastatic or systemic infection is suspected, evaluation by a physician and systemic antibiotics are warranted.

PRECAUTIONS FOR SPECIAL POPULATIONS

Certain medical conditions may increase the risk of infectious complications of body piercing, especially for those patients with congenital cardiac abnormalities, cardiac valvular disease, and immunologic disorders that predispose them to bacterial infections. The incidence of bacteremia following tattooing or body piercing is unknown but may place individuals with valvular or congenital heart disease at risk for IE. Of the eight cases of IE that have been associated with body piercing and tattooing, four occurred in persons with cardiac predispositions (Table 2). The current literature suggests that patients with predisposing cardiac abnormalities be made aware of the risk of serious infection, especially IE, and some recommend avoidance of tattoos and body piercing or the use of prophylactic antibiotics to minimize the risk of infection (13). Similarly, patients who are predisposed to infections due to immunosuppression or immunocompromising disorders or those with chronic skin disorders should be aware of the risk of serious infection and consider avoidance of these procedures.

Table 2. Endocarditis associated with tattooing and body piercing

Procedure	Reference	Organism	Valve affected	Predisposition
Ear piercing	7	Viridans group streptococci	Aortic	None
Tongue piercing	2	*H. aphrophilus*	Aortic	Bicuspid valve, repaired aortic stenosis (valvuloplasty)
Tongue piercing	59	*N. mucosa*	Mitral	None
Tongue piercing	24	*S. aureus*	Mitral	None
Nasal piercing	49	*S. aureus*	Mitral	None
Nipple piercing	42	*S. epidermidis*	Aortic	Bicuspid valve, repaired aortic coarctation
Navel piercing	64	*S. aureus*	Pulmonary	Corrected transposition of the great arteries
Tattooing	52	*S. aureus*	Aortic	Bicuspid valve

SUMMARY

Medical practitioners and the general public should be aware of the potential risks of infection associated with tattooing and body piercing. Early recognition of infections following tattooing or body piercing is important to prevent potential complications, but such infections can be difficult to appreciate because most health care professionals are unfamiliar with the infections associated with these procedures or treatment strategies. More recently, the popularity of these procedures has led to greater awareness and application of hygienic techniques and use of sterile equipment, greatly reducing the risk of transmitting blood-borne infections. In addition, public health departments have helped to regulate safe practices and procedures. Most infections seen today are due to endogenously acquired bacteria that can contaminate the healing tissue. Persons interested in getting a tattoo or body piercing should seek professional artists who follow the established hygienic techniques. The Association for Professional Piercers (http://www.safepiercing.org) and the American Tattooing Institute (http://www.tatsmart.com) are resources that provide information to find reputable tattooists and piercers. Certain populations, especially those with significant immunocompromise, skin disorders, or predisposing cardiac disease, should consider the infectious risks of tattooing and body piercing and take the appropriate precautions or avoid these procedures altogether.

REFERENCES

1. **Ahmed-Jushuf, I. H., P. L. Selby, and A. M. Brownjohn.** 1984. Acute post-streptococcal glomerulonephritis following ear piercing. *Postgrad. Med. J.* **60:**73–74.
2. **Akhondi, H., and A. R. Rahimi.** 2002. *Haemophilus aphrophilus* endocarditis after tongue piercing. *Emerg. Infect. Dis.* **8:**850–851. [Online.]
3. **Alexandridou, A.** 2002. *Candida* endophthalmitis after tattooing in an asplenic patient. *Arch. Ophthalmol.* **120:**518–519.
4. **Altman, J. S., and K. S. Manglani.** 1997. Recurrent condyloma acuminatum due to piercing of the penis. *Cutis* **60:**237–238.
5. **Anderson, W. R., D. J. Summerton, D. M. Sharma, and S. A. Holmes.** 2003. The urologist's guide to genital piercing. *BJU Int.* **91:**245–251.
6. **Armstrong, M. L.** 1994. Adolescents and tattoos: marks of identity or deviancy? *Dermatol. Nurs.* **6:**119–124.
7. **Battin, M., L. V. Fong., and J. L. Monro.** 1991. Gerbode ventricular septal defect following endocarditis. *Eur. J. Cardio-thorac. Surg.* **5:**613–614.
8. **Biggar, R. J., and G. E. Haughie.** 1975. Medical problems of ear piercing. *N. Y. State J. Med.* **75:**1460–1462.
9. **Buavirat, A., K. Page-Shafer, G. J. van Griensven, J. S. Mandel, J. Evans, J. Chuaratanaphong, S. Chiamwongpat, R. Sacks, and A. Moss.** 2003. Risk of prevalent HIV infection associated with incarceration among injecting drug users in Bangkok, Thailand: case-control study. *BMJ* **326:**308–312.
10. **Carroll, S. T., R.H. Riffenburgh, T. A. Roberts, and E. B. Myhre.** 2002. Tattoos and body piercings as indicators of adolescent risk-taking behaviors. *Pediatrics* **109:**1021–1027.
11. **Centers for Disease Control and Prevention.** 1998. Tetanus surveillance—United States, 1995–1997. *Morb. Mortal. Wkly. Rep.* **47**(SS–02):1–13.
12. **Centers for Disease Control and Prevention.** 2003. Tetanus surveillance—United States, 1998–2000. *Morb. Mortal. Wkly. Rep.* **52**(SS–03):1–8.
13. **Cetta, F., L. C. Graham, R. C. Lichtenberg, and C. A. Warnes.** 1999. Piercing and tattooing in patients with congenital heart disease: patient and physician perspectives. *J. Adolesc. Health* **24:**160–162.
14. **Choong, K. Y., and L. J. Roberts.** 1996. Ritual Samoan body tattooing and associated sporotrichosis. *Australas. J. Dermatol.* **37:**50–53.

15. Chowfin, A., A. Pott, A. Paul, and P. Carson. 1999. Spinal epidural abscess after tattooing. *Clin. Infect. Dis.* **29:**225–226.

16. Collings, D. W., and W. Murray. 1895. Three cases of inoculation of tuberculosis from tattooing. *Br. Med. J.* **1:**1200–1201.

17. de Kleer, N., M. Cohen, J. Semple, A. Simor, and O. Antonyshyn. 2001. Nipple piercing may be contraindicated in male patients with chest implants. *Ann. Plast. Surg.* **47:**188–190.

18. Dufour, A., M. Alary, C. Poulin, F. Allard, L. Noel, G. Trottier, D. Lepine, and C. Hankins. 1996. Prevalence and risk behaviours for HIV infection among inmates of a provincial prison in Quebec City. *AIDS* **10:**1009–1015.

19. Dyce, O., J. R. Bruno, D. Hong, K. Silverstein, M. J. Brown, and N. Mirza. 2000. Tongue piercing . . .the new "rusty nail"? *Head Neck* **22:**728–732.

20. Estebanez-Estebanez, P., C. Colomo-Gomez, M. V. Zunzunegui-Pastor, M. Rua Figueroa, M. Perez, C. Ortiz, P. Heras, and F. Babin. 1990. Jails and AIDS. Risk factors for HIV infection in the prisons of Madrid. *Gac. Sanit.* **4:**100–105. (In Spanish.)

21. George, J., and M. White. 1989. Infection as a consequence of ear piercing. *Practitioner* **23:**404–406.

22. Gerberding, J. L. 1995. Management of occupational exposures to blood-borne viruses. *N. Engl. J. Med.* **332:**444–451.

23. Guiard-Schmid, J. B., H. Picard, L. Slama, C. Maslo, C. Amiel, G. Pialoux, M. G. Lebrette, and W. Rozenbaum. 2000. Piercing and its infectious complications: a public health issue in France. *Presse Med.* **29:**1948–1956.

24. Harding, P. R., M. W. Yerkey, G. Deye, and D. Storey. 2002. Methicillin-resistant *Staphylococcus aureus* (MRSA) endocarditis secondary to tongue piercing. *J. Miss. State Med. Assoc.* **43:**109.

25. Hayes, M. O., and G. A. Harkness. 2001. Body piercing as a risk factor for viral hepatitis: an integrative research review. *Am. J. Infect. Control.* **29:**271–274.

26. Horney, D. A., J. M. Gaither, R. Lauer, A. L. Norins, and P. N. Mathur. 1985. Cutaneous inoculation tuberculosis secondary to "jailhouse tattooing." *Arch. Dermatol.* **121:**648–650.

27. Hrdy, D. B. 1987. Cultural practices contributing to the transmission of human immunodeficiency virus in Africa. *Rev. Infect. Dis.* **9:**1109–1119.

28. Hutin, J. M. F. 1853. *Recherches sur les tatouages.* JB Baillier, Paris, France.

29. Jacobs, V. R., K. Golombeck, W. Jonat, and M. Kiechle. 2002. Three case reports of breast abscess after nipple piercing: underestimated health problems of a fashion phenomenon. *Zentbl. Gynaekol.* **124:**378–385. (In German.)

30. Javaid, M., and M. Shibu. 1999. Breast implant infection following nipple piercing. *Br. J. Plast. Surg.* **52:**676–677.

31. Korman, T. M., M. L. Grayson, and J. D. Turnidge. 1997. Polymicrobial septicaemia with *Pseudomonas aeruginosa* and *Streptococcus pyogenes* following traditional tattooing. *J. Infect.* **35:**203.

32. Long, G. E., and L. S. Rickman. 1994. Infectious complications of tattoos. *Clin. Infect. Dis.* **18:**610–619.

33. Lovejoy, F. H., Jr., and D. H. Smith. 1970. Life-threatening staphylococcal disease following ear piercing. *Pediatrics* **46:**301–303.

34. Mamtani, R., P. Malhotra, P. S. Gupta, and B. K. Jain. 1978. A comparative study of urban and rural tetanus in adults. *Int. J. Epidemiol.* **7:**185–188.

35. Martinello, R. A., and E. L. Cooney. 2003. Cerebellar brain abscess associated with tongue piercing. *Clin. Infect. Dis.* **36:**e32–e34.

36. Mayers, L. B., D. A. Judelson, B. W. Moriarty, and K. W. Rundell. 2002. Prevalence of body art (body piercing and tattooing) in university undergraduates and incidence of medical complications. *Mayo. Clin. Proc.* **77:**29–34.

37. McCarthy, V. P., and W. M. Peoples. 1988. Toxic shock syndrome after ear piercing. *Pediatr. Infect. Dis. J.* **7:**741–742.

38. Moe, I. 1989. Samoan navel tattoo, p. 117–119. *In* V. Vale and A. Juno (ed.), *Modern Primitives.* Re-Search, San Francisco, Calif.

39. More, D. R., J. S. Seidel, and P. A. Bryan. 1999. Ear-piercing techniques as a cause of auricular chondritis. *Pediatr. Emerg. Care* **15:**189–192.

40. Morgan, L. G. 1952. Primary tuberculosis inoculation of an ear lobe: report of an unusual case and review of the literature. *J. Pediatr.* **40:**482–485.

41. **Nishioka, S. A., and T. W. Gyorkos.** 2001. Tattoos as risk factors for transfusion-transmitted diseases. *Int. J. Infect. Dis.* **5:**27–34.

42. **Ochsenfahrt, C., R. Friedl, A. Hannekum, and B. A. Schumacher.** 2001. Endocarditis after nipple piercing in a patient with a bicuspid aortic valve. *Ann. Thorac. Surg.* **71:**365–366.

43. **Ollero, M., E. Pujol, A. Gimeno, A. Gea, P. Marquez, and J. M. Iturriaga.** 1991. Risky practices associated with HIV infection in seamen who travel in sub-Saharan West Africa. *Rev. Clin. Espanola* **189:**416–421. (In Spanish.)

44. **Olsen, J. C.** 2001. Lingual abscess secondary to body piercing. *J. Emerg. Med.* **20:**409.

45. **O'Malley, C. D., N. Smith, R. Braun, and D. R. Prevots.** 1998. Tetanus associated with body piercing. *Clin. Infect. Dis.* **27:**1343–1344.

46. **Parker, C., G. Kaminski, and D. Hill.** 1986. Zygomycosis in a tattoo, caused by *Saksenaea vasiformis*. *Aust. J. Dermatol.* **27:**107–111.

47. **Perkins, C. S., J. Meisner, and J. M. Harrison.** 1997. A complication of tongue piercing. *Br. Dent. J.* **182:**147–148.

48. **Pugatch, D., M. Mileno, and J. D. Rich.** 1998. Possible transmission of human immunodeficiency virus type 1 from body piercing. *Clin. Infect. Dis.* **26:**767–768.

49. **Ramage, I. J., N. Wilson, and R. B. Thomson.** 1997. Fashion victim: infective endocarditis after nasal piercing. *Arch. Dis. Child.* **77:**187.

50. **Rukstinat, G. J.** 1941. Tattoos. A survey, with special reference to tattoos and scars as indicators of syphilis. *Arch. Pathol.* **31:**640–655.

51. **Samantha, S., M. Tweeten, and L. S. Rickman.** 1998. Infectious complications of body piercing. *Clin. Infect. Dis.* **26:**735–740.

52. **Satchitnananda, D. K., J. Walsh, and P. M. Schofield.** 2001. Bacterial endocarditis following repeated tattooing. *Heart* **85:**11–12.

53. **Silverman, A. L., J. S. Sekhon, S. J. Sagninaw, D. Wiedbrauk, M. Balasumbramaniam, and S. C. Gordon.** 2000. Tattoo application is not associated with an increased risk for chronic viral hepatitis. *Am. J. Gastroenterol.* **95:**1312–1315.

54. **Simplot, T. C., and H. T. Hoffman.** 1998. Comparison between cartilage and soft tissue ear piercing complications. *Am. J. Otolaryngol.* **4:**305–310.

55. **Smith, B. F.** 1950. Occurrence of hepatitis in recently tattooed service personnel. *JAMA* **144:**1074–1076.

56. **Sow, P. S., B. M. Diop, H. L. Barry, S. Badiane, and A. M. Coll-Seck.** 1993. Tetanus and traditional practices in Dakar (report of 141 cases). *Dakar Med.* **38:**55–59.

57. **Stirn, A.** 2003. Body piercing: medical consequences and psychological motivations. *Lancet* **361:**1205–1215.

58. **Thorner, M.** 1894. Pathological conditions following piercing of the lobules of the ear. *JAMA* **22:**110–112.

59. **Tronel, H., H. Chaudemanche, N. Pechier, L. Doutrelant, and B. Hoen.** 2001. Endocarditis due to *Neisseria mucosa* after tongue piercing. *Clin. Microbiol. Infect.* **7:**275–276.

60. **Trupiano, J. K., B. A. Sebek, J. Goldfarb, L. R. Levy, G. S. Hall, and G. W. Procop.** 2001. Mastitis due to *Mycobacterium abscessus* after body piercing. *Clin. Infect. Dis.* **33:**131–134.

61. **Turkeltaub, S. H., and M. B. Habal.** 1990. Acute *Pseudomonas* chondritis as a sequel to ear piercing. *Ann. Plast. Surg.* **24:**279–282.

62. **Vale, V., and A. Juno.** 1989. Lyle Tuttle, p. 114–117. *In* V. Vale and A. Juno (ed.), *Modern Primitives.* Re-Search, San Francisco, Calif.

63. **Vatsyanyana.** 1994. *The Complete Kama Sutra: the First Unabridged Modern Translation of the Classic Indian Text.* Translated by Alain Danielou. Park Street Press, Rochester, N.Y.

64. **Weinberg, J. B., and R. A. Blackwood.** 2003. Case report of *Staphylococcus aureus* endocarditis after navel piercing. *Pediatr. Infect. Dis. J.* **22:**94–95.

65. **Wilde, A. G.** 1929–1930. Vaccinia infected tattoo: case report. *New Orleans Med. Surg. J.* **82:**385–386.

Chapter 16

Infectious Diseases at High Altitude

Buddha Basnyat, Thomas A. Cumbo, and Robert Edelman

Travel to areas at high altitude (>2,500 m) is a popular activity enjoyed by many persons with various levels of experience and physical fitness. Activities range from relatively low-impact trekking at moderate altitude to extreme technical climbing. High mountain ranges are distributed in diverse ecosystems, cover approximately one-fifth of the earth's surface, are home to >300 million persons, and are visited annually by millions who normally reside at low elevations (42). Many of these mountains exist in the developing world and require the sojourner to visit lowland areas for days to weeks prior to ascent where they are exposed to infectious agents common in developing countries. Other mountains exist in more developed countries where infections are less common but high altitude still stresses the upper limits of human physiological reserve. Many host and environmental factors enhance susceptibility to infections and infectious disease, such as altered immune responses, hypoxia, physiological adaptation or lack of such adaptation, environmental stressors, increased UV radiation, cramped quarters, inability to maintain personal hygiene, and isolation from adequate medical care. The risk of contracting an infection varies depending on location, length of exposure, and nature of the high-altitude activity. There are few published data on this topic, and as a result, portions of this chapter are anecdotal and based on personal medical experience (B.B. and T.A.C.). The majority of our experience was gained in the Himalayas (Fig. 1). The Himalayas are among the world's tallest peaks and exist among some of the most impoverished areas of the globe. Therefore, this range provides an example of the complexities associated with high-altitude medicine and infectious diseases (Table 1).

Buddha Basnyat • Nepal International Clinic, Himalayan Rescue Association, and Patan Hospital, Lal Durbar, GPO Box 3596, Kathmandu, Nepal. *Thomas A. Cumbo* • Division of Infectious Diseases, SUNY Buffalo School of Medicine and Biomedical Sciences, Buffalo VAMC, 3495 Bailey Ave., Buffalo, NY 14215. *Robert Edelman* • Center for Vaccine Development, Division of Geographic Medicine, Department of Medicine, and Division of Infectious Diseases and Tropical Pediatrics, Department of Pediatrics, University of Maryland School of Medicine, 685 West Baltimore St., Room 480, Baltimore, MD 21201.

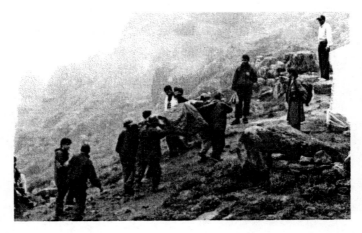

Figure 1. High-altitude evacuation of an ill Nepalese woman in the Himalayas during the Hindu festival of Janai Purnima in August 2000 near Lake Gosainkunda, Lang-Tang region, Nepal. Photo by Paul Joseph Cumbo.

Uniquely adapted flora and fauna exist in the low barometric pressure, hypoxic environment, and harsh conditions of the higher altitudes. This ecosystem is one of gradual transformation from a nurturing lowland to the inhospitable boundaries of space. Although the presence of microorganisms such as bacteria and fungi has been recorded in the outer stratosphere (40), there are no data linking such organisms with infections of trekkers. Moreover, the impact of high altitude on insect vectors and microbial biology is largely unknown.

More is known about the changes of mammalian adaptive physiological capacity and immunologic responses at high altitude. For example, in vitro studies using a hypobaric chamber reveal that T-lymphocyte function is compromised at high altitude, while B-cell function and mucosal immunity are not (28). T-cell-independent, B-cell antibody response to various antigens seems to be pre-

Table 1. Infectious risks at high altitude[a]

Type of infection	Infection(s)
Gastrointestinal	Enteropathogenic bacteria (*Escherichia coli*, *Salmonella*, *Shigella*, *Campylobacter*), viruses, protozoa (*Giardia*, *Cryptosporidium*, *Entamoeba*, *Cyclospora*), typhoid fever, hepatitis, abdominal tuberculosis in local persons
Neurological	Rabies, JE, bacterial meningitis
Respiratory	Sinusitis, upper respiratory tract infection, bronchitis, pneumonia, influenza, tuberculosis
Dermatologic	Pyoderma, furuncle, carbuncle, persistent wound infections, cellulitis, lymphangitis, herpes simplex, trauma and frostbite infections, scabies, lice, varicella
Urological and gynecological	STDs, genital candidiasis, urinary tract infections
Miscellaneous	Malaria, dengue, typhus, leptospirosis, dental caries, bone infections

[a]Adapted from reference 6 with permission from the publisher.

served (11). Some hypothesize that adrenocorticotropic hormone, cortisol, and endorphins may partially mediate the impaired T-lymphocyte function noted at low atmospheric pressures and hypoxic conditions (18). Murine studies have demonstrated an increased susceptibility to *Klebsiella pneumoniae, Salmonella enterica* serovar Typhimurium, *Escherichia coli, Chlamydia trachomatis,* and *Streptococcus* (29). Other work has shown an increased incidence of infectious symptoms such as coryza, cough, pharyngitis, and diarrhea, especially in those subjects also suffering from acute mountain sickness (30). Murine studies have shown a decreased susceptibility to influenza A virus in hypoxic conditions (29), although other studies have demonstrated increased pulmonary vascular edema and permeability in rats with a laboratory-induced viral upper respiratory infection later exposed to simulated high altitude (14). We know of at least two instances where well-acclimatized travelers (who had spent many days at 5,300 m) suffered from high-altitude pulmonary edema (HAPE) at 4,000 m after a bout of an upper respiratory tract infection. Respiratory infection may increase hypoxemia secondary to impaired diffusion capacity at high altitude. UV radiation exposure increases at high altitude because of the thin atmosphere. Although this energy results in the production of various immunomodulatory compounds (22), it is unclear if such compounds are clinically important. Other investigators have demonstrated increased amounts of systemic inflammatory markers such as interleukin-6, interleukin-1 receptor agonist, and C-reactive protein at high altitude (19). It is also postulated that free-radical-mediated change in the peripheral metabolism of amino acids such as glutamine, known to influence immune function, may enhance susceptibility to or delay recovery from opportunistic infections at high altitude (4).

The physician or other health care worker caring for patients at high altitude needs to recognize endogenous illness. Diagnosis in this environment is difficult because many diseases do not present in their typical fashion. For example, it can be difficult to differentiate bacterial pneumonia from HAPE or a pulmonary embolism.

The local population in the developing world is at greater risk for diseases such as tuberculosis or parasitic infections than travelers from developed countries. For this reason, hemoptysis at high altitude more likely represents tuberculosis in a local resident but HAPE in a trekker from North America, Europe, Australia, or other industrialized regions.

One must differentiate high-altitude travel in the developing world from such travel in more developed regions such as the Rocky Mountains or the Alps. The hypoxic and hypobaric stresses are essentially the same, but the surrounding lowlands of the nonindustrialized world contain a higher prevalence and variety of infectious agents which color the differential diagnosis. By contrast, medical problems at high altitude in the developed world are more often noninfectious by nature.

GASTROINTESTINAL INFECTIONS

Enteric infections are the leading cause of illness in travelers regardless of altitude (39). Ten percent of all helicopter evacuations in the Nepal Himalayas are related to severe diarrheal diseases (P. Pandey, D. R. Shlim, W. Cowe,

M. Springer, and H. Swinkels, *Seventh Conf. Int. Soc. Travel Med.*, abstr., 2001). One study performed in the Himalayas found that 14% of a cohort of foreign outdoor trekkers developed gastroenteritis (7). This is approximately one-half of the incidence found at lower altitudes in the same region. Nevertheless, risk factors for gastrointestinal illness do exist; they include cramped sleeping arrangements, poor hygiene, concurrent illness, and medications that increase gastric pH (23).

No systematic surveys have examined the prevalence and epidemiology of enteric pathogens encountered at high altitude. The enteropathogenic bacteria are presumably the most common cause of diarrhea (13, 34). Bacteria, *Giardia lamblia*, and amoebic dysentery are common causes in the Indian subcontinent (38), with *Cyclospora cayetanensis* occurring seasonally. *Campylobacter* spp, may cause a sizable number of diarrhea cases. Typhoid fever is one of the most common causes of fever within the Indian subcontinent (1). We have mistakenly diagnosed patients with high-altitude cerebral edema while they exhibited headache and fatigue found subsequently to be typhoid fever (unpublished data).

Local residents commonly develop large infestations with *Ascaris* worms, hookworms (21), or tapeworms. Travelers rarely develop symptomatic disease if they acquire low parasite inocula. If abdominal pain or unusual manifestations of diarrheal disease develop, however, stool screening examinations should be performed. Amoebic liver abscesses present with hepatomegaly and right upper quadrant abdominal pain. Abdominal tuberculosis manifests with ascites, wasting, and nonspecific signs and symptoms (24).

A fluoroquinolone effective against most aerobic bacterial pathogens and an antimotility drug are appropriate treatment for most cases of gastroenteritis in the tourist at high altitude (3). Fluid intake should be encouraged, and attention should be directed towards potential electrolyte loss.

HEPATITIS VIRUS INFECTIONS

Hepatitis A, B, and E virus infections occur commonly in developing countries. Before the introduction of the hepatitis A vaccine, many outdoor trekkers in the Himalayas acquired this infection. Hepatitis E is one of the most common causes of jaundice in the adult population of the Indian subcontinent (37). Appropriate immunization with hepatitis A, hepatitis B, and typhoid vaccines helps prevent liver and gastrointestinal disease. Women of childbearing age should be counseled about the high hepatitis E mortality rates that occur in pregnant women. Efficacy trials of hepatitis E vaccine are ongoing in Nepal (9).

NEUROLOGICAL INFECTIONS

Those going into high-altitude regions in Latin America, Africa, and Asia are at risk of rabies infection. It is very difficult to arrange expedient postexposure rabies prophylaxis so far from medical care. Preventive measures include preexposure rabies vaccination and counseling trekkers to descend for postexposure immunoglobulin in the event of a dog or monkey bite.

Japanese encephalitis (JE) exists in rural areas of Southeast Asia and parts of the Indian subcontinent. No tourists to high-altitude regions have been diagnosed with JE, probably due to the rarity of the *Culex* mosquito vector at high altitudes. In the Indian subcontinent, JE must be differentiated from tuberculosis meningitis, bacterial meningitis, and typhoid encephalopathy seen in the local population in areas of endemicity. Treatment of JE is symptomatic. Prevention involves mosquito avoidance and vaccination.

Tick-borne encephalitis is endemic to central and eastern Europe, the former Russian states, and sporadically throughout the eastern Mediterranean. Because areas of endemicity include deciduous forest below the altitude of 1,200 m, tick-borne encephalitis and perhaps its *Ixodes* tick vector may be uncommon in sojourners to the Alps and Ural Mountains unless the disease was acquired at lower altitude.

Bacterial meningitis, although endemic in many developing countries, is uncommon in the traveler to high-altitude regions. However, it is important to consider in cases of acute confusion or severe headache and as a potential danger to the outdoor trekker.

Cysticercosis of the brain is one of the most common causes of epilepsy in Nepal (20). Cysticercosis should be considered if a local inhabitant presents with neurological findings or an altered sensorium at high altitude.

RESPIRATORY INFECTIONS

Respiratory problems are common at high altitude (7, 10, 30). Pulmonary defense mechanisms are lessened by bronchospasm, congestion, and decreased mucociliary clearance (16). Symptoms are exacerbated by hypoxic conditions, crowding, and cold, dry air (41). Sinusitis, pharyngitis, bronchitis, and pneumonia are the result of such an environment. Presumably noninfectious sore throat and cough are common above 4,000 m. While not firmly established, respiratory infections may predispose to the development of acute mountain sickness (7, 10, 30).

The specific etiologic agents responsible for respiratory illness at high altitude remain unclear. Nonspecific prevention is important, which includes keeping the head warm, adequate hydration, use of nasal decongestants, and breathing through a silk scarf to keep the air humidified (17). The role of antibiotics is unclear, even with purulent sputum production (27). Respiratory infection can mimic HAPE. We maintain a low threshold for descent should respiratory infection or HAPE develop. Antibiotics may be used empirically. Influenza vaccine should be administered prior to departure. Pharyngitis accompanied by exudates and/or lymphandenopathy may represent a group A *Streptococcus* infection. Empirical antibiotics should be considered if medical care and a culture cannot be obtained in a timely manner.

It is important to consider active pulmonary tuberculosis in local inhabitants who present with cough. Recent work has demonstrated a lower incidence of *Mycobacterium tuberculosis* infection at higher altitudes, but an increased household clustering of tuberculosis occurs, hypothesized to be caused by crowded, poorly ventilated dwellings combined with increased UV light, hypoxia, and decreased humidity (32). An increased incidence of chronic obstructive pulmonary disease and cor pulmonale occurs in the mountain population of the Indian subcontinent. This is likely due to chronic smoke inhalation in poorly ventilated dwellings (33).

DERMATOLOGIC INFECTIONS

Pyoderma, carbuncles, furuncles, and wound infections are common problems encountered by those entering the mountains (8). Poor hygiene, prolonged exposure to moisture, local trauma from hiking boots, and frostbite are common in the mountain wilderness and can predispose to skin infections. Wounds heal slowly at high altitude despite therapy with antibiotics. Superficial infections are often accompanied by cellulitis and lymphangitis (35). Descent to lower altitude may be the only definitive treatment. Scabies and lice are common in shared living quarters. Cold and sun exposure increases the likelihood of a herpesvirus reactivation.

Local inhabitants commonly present with advanced cases of skin infections. Septicemia and osteomyelitis can develop as a result of such uncontrolled skin infections. Suppurative otitis media can predispose to facial infection, bone infection, hearing loss, and meningitis. Varicella is common in children. Visitors unsure of their varicella immune status should consider antibody testing if time permits or varicella vaccination prior to travel (6).

Prevention of skin conditions and infections at high altitude includes the use of sunscreen on skin and lips, adequate hydration, avoidance of even minor trauma (including insect bites), good hygiene, and antibiotic therapy when warranted. Provide booster doses of tetanus vaccine before travel to prevent tetanus in the event that *Clostridium tetani* contaminates traumatized skin.

INSECT-BORNE INFECTIONS

Arthropod-borne infections are extremely common in travel to developing countries, but arthropod vectors are less common at higher altitudes. Although malaria is an ever-present risk in most of the tropical world, *Plasmodium* species usually are not transmitted in higher-altitude locations (31); however, exceptions have been reported (15). Delayed febrile illness after initial plasmodial infection acquired at lower elevations may occur at higher elevations weeks or months later (12). Diagnosis is presumptive and must be followed by supervised evacuation to lower altitude. Mosquito avoidance and malaria chemoprophylaxis in lowland areas of endemicity before ascent to high altitude offer a high degree of protection.

Dengue fever is endemic to the tropics and subtropics (36). Like with malaria, travelers can become ill at high altitude with infection acquired in the lowlands. Diagnosis is presumptive, and descent is imperative.

Typhus may be an underdiagnosed cause of fever in mountain travelers, although the evidence of its prevalence is anecdotal. Typhus, as well as other rickettsial diseases, should be considered in patients coming from areas of endemicity, since a delay in diagnosis can be lethal. For example, an individual treated with ciprofloxacin for diarrhea while trekking did not improve and was subsequently diagnosed in Bangkok, Thailand, as having typhus; fortunately, treatment with doxycycline resulted in a rapid improvement (unpublished data).

Bartonella bacilliformis is transmitted by the *Phlebotomus* sand fly and occurs in the Andes Mountains between 600 and 2,500 m. Diagnosis is made by clinical presentation in the presence of anemia and by visualization of the pathogen in erythrocyte smears. Treatment options include tetracycline and chloramphenicol (26).

OTHER INFECTIONS

Leptospirosis is spread by direct contact of abraded skin or mucous membranes with contaminated water or soil. Floods and heavy rains common to the mountains can increase the concentration of spirochetes in water by washing hillside urinary waste contaminated with leptospires into lakes and streams. Treks and climbs usually pass through such areas. Treatment involves doxycycline or ampicillin depending on the severity of infection (25).

Sexually transmitted diseases (STDs), fungal vaginitis, and urinary tract infections usually present in typical fashion at high altitude. Increased frequency of sexual intercourse, new sexual partners, antibiotic use, and poor hygiene can predispose variably to gonorrhea, chlamydia, trichomoniasis, candidiasis, genital herpes, and acute human immunodeficiency virus infection. An increased index of suspicion is usually required to recognize STDs in this uncommon setting. Urinary tract infections can usually be diagnosed in the field with an adequate history and urine dipsticks to document the presence of white cells, leukocyte esterase, and nitrite in urine specimens. Treatment can often be instituted in the field if symptoms are mild and there is no indication of pyelonephritis.

SPECIAL CONSIDERATIONS

Immunocompromised travelers are at risk of contracting serious infections. Physicians counseling patients who travel with cancer, human immunodeficiency virus, chronic steroid or other immunosuppressive medication use, functional or anatomic asplenia, and renal insufficiency should familiarize themselves and their patients with the travel risks associated with these conditions. Elderly patients may be at increased risk for infectious disease because of comorbid conditions. Physicians and other health care professionals providing pretravel care should counsel such patients before they travel (2).

OTHER DISEASES AT HIGH ALTITUDE

The differential diagnosis of illness at high altitude includes other conditions that may be misdiagnosed as an infection. Documented examples include high-altitude cerebral edema and HAPE, subarachnoid hemorrhage, transient ischemic attack, seizures, cerebral neoplasm, migraine, syncope, Guillain-Barré syndrome, pulmonary embolism, chemical or plant toxin exposure, hypothermia, dehydration, carbon monoxide poisoning (from poorly ventilated indoor fires), acute psychiatric problems, asthma, and myocardial infarction (5).

Table 2. Preventive measures that may reduce morbidity at high altitude[a]

1. Descend to a lower altitude, especially if infections do not improve with antibiotics alone.
2. Wash hands with soap and/or liquid cleanser.
3. Use insect repellents with DEET to help avoid mosquito and tick bites. Cover exposed skin, especially when trekking.
4. Use pyrethrin-treated clothes and bed nets if necessary.
5. Sterilize water.
6. Avoid salads, ice, and other foods that can become easily contaminated.
7. Use a silk scarf to breathe through at high altitude to help humidify the cold air.
8. Use suncreen on all exposed skin, including lips and ears.
9. Maintain adequate hydration.
10. Get appropriate immunizations.
11. Review medical history, medication use, allergies, and pregnancy status prior to ascent.
12. Purchase evacuation insurance, register at the local embassy, and become familiar with evacuation procedures.

[a]Adapted from reference 6 with permission from the publisher.

Physicians who may treat infectious diseases at high altitude should carry appropriate chemotherapy and supportive equipment. Suggestions include a penicillin, ampicillin, dicloxacillin, trimethoprim-sulfamethoxazole, metronidazole, a macrolide, a fluoroquinolone, a tetracycline, hydrocortisone cream, a glucocorticoid, protective medical gloves, and water purification tablets or a reliable water filter. It is useful to carry both oral and intramuscular forms of the drugs if available. We also find it helpful to carry urine pregnancy test kits and urine dipsticks to help us modify therapy in the field. It should be emphasized that the ultimate treatment of many medical problems will require descent.

In essence, infections and infectious diseases at high altitude often parallel those in adjacent lowland environments. Hypoxemia, hypobaria, physiological adaptation, harsh environmental stressors, exposure to foreign agents, and reckless behavior can enhance susceptibility to pathogens. The ultimate treatment may require descent. Prevention is crucial; both counseling and immunization are essential (Table 2). Clearly, more research needs to be done on high-altitude infections to better understand their pathogenic mechanisms and epidemiology and to improve treatment and prevention.

REFERENCES

1. **Acharya, I. L., C. U. Lowe, R. Thapa, V. L. Gurubacharya, M. B. Shrestha, M. Cadoz, D. Schulz, J. Armand, D. A. Bryla, B. Trollfors, et al.** 1987. Prevention of typhoid in Nepal with the Vi capsular polysaccharide of *Salmonella typhi*: a preliminary report. *N. Engl. J. Med.* **317:**1101–1104.
2. **Albrecht, C., T. A. Cumbo, and S. Gambert.** 2003. Health issues, travel, and the elderly. *Clin. Geriatrics.* **11**(7):24–33.
3. **Ansdell, V. E., and C. D. Ericsson.** 1999. Prevention and empiric treatment of traveler's diarrhea. *Med. Clin. N. Am.* **83:**945–973.
4. **Bailey, D. M., B. Davies, L. M. Castell, D. J. Collier, J. S. Milledge, D. A. Hullin, P. S. Seddon, and I. S. Young.** 2003. Symptoms of infection and acute mountain sickness; associated metabolic sequelae and problems in differential diagnosis. *High Alt. Med. Biol.* **4:**319–331.
5. **Basnyat, B., T. A. Cumbo, and R. Edelman.** 2000. Acute medical problems in the Himalayas outside the setting of altitude illness. *High Alt. Med. Biol.* **1:**167–174.

6. **Basynat, B., T. A. Cumbo, and R. Edelman.** 2001. Infections at high altitude. *Clin. Infect. Dis.* **33:**1887–1991.

7. **Basnyat, B., J. Lemaster, and J. A. Litch.** 1999. Everest or bust: a cross sectional epidemiological study in the Himalayas at 4300 meters. *Aviat. Space Environ. Med.* **70:**867–873.

8. **Basnyat, B., and J. A. Litch.** 1997. Medical problems of porters and trekkers in the Nepal Himalaya. *Wilderness Environ. Med.* **8:**78–81.

9. **Basnyat, B., and R. M. Scott.** 2000. Update in hepatology. *Ann. Intern. Med.* **133:**747.

10. **Basnyat, B., D. Subedi, J. Sleggs, G. Bhasyal, B. Aryal, and N. Subedi.** 2000. Disoriented and ataxic pilgrims: an epidemiological study of acute mountain sickness and high-altitude cerebral edema at a sacred lake at 4300 meters in the Nepal Himalayas. *Wilderness Environ. Med.* **11:**89–93.

11. **Biselli, R., S. Le Moli, P. M. Matricardi, S. Farrace, A. Fattorossi, R. Nisini, and R. D'Amelio.** 1991. The effects of hypobaric hypoxia on specific B cell responses following immunization in mice and humans. *Aviat. Space Environ. Med.* **62**(9 Pt. 1):870–874.

12. **Bishop, R. A., and J. A. Litch.** 2000. Malaria at high altitude. *J. Travel Med.* **7:**157–158.

13. **Black, R. E.** 1990. Epidemiology of traveler's diarrhea and relative importance of certain pathogens. *Rev. Infect. Dis.* **12**(Suppl 1):S73–S79.

14. **Carpenter, R. C., J. T. Reeves, and A. G. Durmowicz.** 1998. Viral respiratory infection increases susceptibility of young rats to hypoxia-induced pulmonary edema. *J. Appl. Physiol.* **84:**1048–1054.

15. **Epstein, P. R., H. F. Diaz, S. Elias, G. Grabherr, N. E. Graham, W. J. M. Martens, E. Mosley-Thompson, and E. J. Susskind.** 1998. Biological and physical signs of climate change: focus on mosquito-borne disease. *Bull. Am. Meteorol. Soc.* **78:**409–417.

16. **Giesbrecht, G. G.** 1995. The respiratory system in a cold environment. *Aviat. Space Environ. Med.* **66:**890–902.

17. **Hackett, P. H., and R. C. Roach.** 2001. High-altitude medicine, p. 2–43. *In* P. S. Auerbach (ed.), *Wilderness Medicine.* C. V. Mosby, St. Louis, Mo.

18. **Harris, M. D., J. Terrio, W. F. Miser, and J. F. Yetter III.** 1998. High-altitude medicine. *Am. Fam. Physician.* **57:**1907–1914, 1924–1926.

19. **Hartmann, G., M. Tschop, R. Fischer, C. Bidlingmaier, R. Riepl, K. Tschop, H. Hautmann, S. Endres, and M. Toepfer.** 2000. High altitude increases circulating interleukin-6, interlukin-1 receptor antagonist and C-reactive protein. *Cytokine* **12:**246–252.

20. **Heap, B. J.** 1990. Cerebral cysticercosis as a common cause of epilepsy in Gurkhas in Hong Kong. *J. R. Army Med. Corps* **136:**146–149.

21. **Houston, R., and E. Schwartz.** 1990. Helmithic infections among Peace Corps volunteers in Nepal. *JAMA* **263:**373–374.

22. **Hug, D. H., J. K. Hunter, and D. D. Dunkerson.** 2001. Malnutrition, urocanic acid, and sun may interact to suppress immunity in sojourners to high altitude. *Aviat. Space Environ. Med.* **72:**136–145.

23. **Junkett, G.** 1999. Prevention and treatment of traveler's diarrhea. *Am. Fam. Physician* **60:**119–124, 135–136.

24. **Leader, R. A., and V. N. Low. 1995. Tuberculosis of the abdomen.** *Radiol. Clin. N. Am.* **33:**691.

25. **Magill, A. J.** 1998. Fever in the returned traveler. *Infect. Dis. Clin. N. Am.* **12:**445–469.

26. **Maquina, C., and E. Gotuzzo.** 2000. Bartonellosis: new and old. *Infect. Dis. Clin. N. Am.* **14:**1–22.

27. **McFadden, E. R.** 1987. The lower airway, p. 234–245. *In* J. R. Sutton, C. S. Houston, and G. Coates (ed.), *Hypoxia and Cold,* Prager, New York, N.Y.

28. **Meehan, R., U. Duncan, L. Neale, G. Taylor, H. Muchmore, N. Scott, K. Ramsey, E. Smith, P. Rock, R. Goldblum, and C. Houstan.** 1988. Operation Everest II: alterations in the immune system at high altitudes. *J. Clin. Immunol.* **8:**397–406.

29. **Meehan, R. T.** 1987. Immune suppression at high altitude. *Ann. Emerg. Med.* **16:**974–979.

30. **Murdock, D. R.** 1995. Symptoms of infection and altitude illness among hikers in the Mount Everest region of Nepal. *Aviat. Space Environ. Med.* **66:**148–151.

31. **Murphy, G. S., and E. C. Oldfield III.** 1996. Falciparum malaria. *Infect. Dis. Clin. N. Am.* **10:**747–775.

32. **Olender, S., S. Mayuko, J. Apgar, K. Gillenwater, C. T. Bautista, A. G. Lescano, P. Moro, L. Caviedes, E. J. Hsieh, and R. H. Gilman.** 2003. Low prevelance and increased household clustering of *Mycobacterium tuberculosis* infection in high altitude villages in Peru. *Am. J. Trop. Med. Hyg.* **68:**721–727.

33. **Pandey, M. R., B. Basnayt, and R. P. Neupane.** 1988. Chronic bronchitis and cor pulmonale in Nepal. *J. Inst. Med.* **10:**263–270.
34. **Petola, H., and S. L. Gorbach.** 1997. Travelers' diarrhea: epidemiology and clinical aspects, p. 78–86. *In* H. L. DuPont and R. Steffen (ed), *Textbook of Travel Medicine and Health.* BC Decker, Hamilton, Canada.
35. **Sarnquist, F. H.** 1983. Physicians on Mount Everest: a clinical account of the 1981 American medical research expedition to Everest. *West. J. Med.* **139(4):**480–485.
36. **Schwartz, E., E. Mendelson, and Y. Sidi.** 1996. Dengue fever among travelers. *Am. J. Med.* **101:**516–520.
37. **Shlim, D. R., and B. L. Innis.** 2000. Hepatitis E vaccine for travelers. *J. Travel Med.* **7:**167–169.
38. **Shlim, D. R.** 1999. Traveler's diarrhea. *Wilderness Environ. Med.* **10:**165–170.
39. **Steffen, R., F. van der Linde, K. Gyr, and M. Schar.** 1983. Epidemiology of diarrhea in travelers. *JAMA* **249:**1176–1180.
40. **Wainwright, M., N. C. Wickramasinghe, J. V. Narlikar, and P. Rajaratnam.** 2003. Microorganisms cultured from stratospheric air samples obtained at 41km. *FEMS Microbiol. Lett.* **218:**161–165.
41. **West, J. B.** 1998. *High Life: A History of High Altitude Physiology and Medicine,* p. 160. Oxford University Press, Oxford, United Kingdom.
42. **Zafren, K., and B. Honigman.** 1997. High-altitude medicine. *Emerg Med. Clin. N. Am.* **15:**191–222.

INDEX